Recent Breakthroughs in Neurodegenerative Disorders and Enzyme Therapy

Prashant Tiwari
https://orcid.org/0000-0003-4423-6819
Dayananda Sagar University, India

Sunil Kumar Kadiri
Dayananda Sagar University, India

Neha Minocha
https://orcid.org/0000-0002-0870-4972
K.R. Mangalam University, India

IGI Global
Scientific Publishing
Publishing Tomorrow's Research Today

Vice President of Editorial	Melissa Wagner
Director of Acquisitions	Mikaela Felty
Director of Book Development	Jocelynn Hessler
Production Manager	Mike Brehm
Cover Design	Jose Rosado

Published in the United States of America by
IGI Global Scientific Publishing
701 East Chocolate Avenue
Hershey, PA, 17033, USA
Tel: 717-533-8845 | Fax: 717-533-7115
Website: https://www.igi-global.com E-mail: cust@igi-global.com

Library of Congress Cataloging-in-Publication Data

LCCN: 2025941699 (CIP Data Pending)
ISBN13: 9798337346274
Isbn13Softcover: 9798337346281
EISBN13: 9798337346298
British Cataloguing in Publication Data
A Cataloguing in Publication record for this book is available from the British Library.

Table of Contents

Detailed Table of Contents

Neurotransmitters (NTs) are chemical messengers responsible for conveying signals across a synapse, through electrical and chemical pathways, by regulating excitatory and inhibitory mechanisms. Any disturbance in neurotransmission affects the synaptic plasticity and cognitive function. Antiepileptic drugs (AEDs) are designed to bind the receptors of neurotransmitters and activate, block, or modulate brain excitability to prevent or reduce seizures. They display multiple mechanisms of action, such as inhibiting voltage-gated Na+ and Ca+ channels, enhancing GABAergic inhibition, and modulating glutamate receptors in the brain, but also improperly affect neurotransmitter signals and activities. Adverse side effects include reduced dopamine and other neurotransmitters secretion which also leads to the development of several different types of neurodegenerative disorders (NDs) like Parkinson's disease and Alzheimer's disease. The authors aim to emphasize the need for careful monitoring of patients receiving long-term AED therapy and related cognitive decline due to neurotransmitter disruption.

One of the most complex organs in the body is the human brain, which is composed of numerous neuronal networks that maintain processes such as homeostasis,

cognition, and emotions. The purpose of this research is to detect brain cancer cells and leakage of CSF due to a breach of the BBB. We proposed two phases: the first is based on chemical testing to target the cancer cells in the brain using the UHPLC, which shows the presence of cancer and diagnoses the leakage symptoms of the CSF. The second phase is based on the hybrid k-mean cluster and Hidden Markov Model (HMM), namely kCHMM. In the first phase, we used UHPLC with immunotoxin antibodies. In the second phase, we used the hybrid k-mean cluster hidden Markov model (kCHMM) technique. The efficiency of the proposed datasets that we received after implementation of the kCHMM model is 0.9984.

Nanoparticles have emerged as pivotal components in medical applications, particularly in diagnostics, imaging and targeted therapy. Various types of nanoparticles facilitate precise therapeutic targeting while minimizing systemic side effects. Recent advancements in surface functionalization techniques have significantly improved nanoparticle stability and reduced immunogenicity, allowing for enhanced specificity in cellular targeting. Future directions in this field may include the exploration of smart nanoparticles capable of sequential drug delivery in response to real-time biomarkers and the development of biocompatible coatings that ensure prolonged stability.

Neurodegenerative diseases including Alzheimer's disease, Parkinson's disease, multiple sclerosis, amyotrophic lateral sclerosis, and Huntington's disease exerts a socio-economic burden and affecting a high percentage of population. Traditional medications of neurodegenerative disorders are asymptomatic and reliefs pain without halting progression of neuronal damage. Recently, nanotechnology is regarded as a very promising therapeutic approach for the prevention and treatment of several disorders, through enabling targeted and direct drug-delivery of active and therapeutic molecules to cross the Blood Brain Barrier in different neuropathological situations. The application of nanotechnology in neurology is a promising field and presenting a new horizon for treatment and diagnosis (Neurotheranostics) of neurodegenerative disorders. This review investigated the nano-based neurotherapeutics to manage CNS disorders. This review focuses on the recent application of iron oxide nanoparticles to act as drug carriers or as detection agents of brain disorders.

While radiation is often viewed solely as a damaging agent, emerging research suggests that certain doses and types of radiation may activate endogenous protective enzymes involved in cellular repair, redox balance, and inflammation modulation. This chapter explores the under-investigated concept of radiation-induced enzymatic activation in the central nervous system, positioning it as a potential gateway for neuroprotective drug development. We examine the paradoxical role of low-dose ionizing radiation and how it stimulates beneficial responses such as Nrf2 pathway activation, increased antioxidant enzyme expression, and DNA repair enzyme upregulation. The chapter

discusses the concept of radiation hormesis and how pre-conditioning the brain with controlled exposures may prime neuroprotective pathways.

Neurodegenerative disorders such as Alzheimer's disease, Parkinson's disease, Huntington's disease, and Amyotrophic Lateral Sclerosis present a growing global health burden due to their progressive nature, complex etiologies, and lack of effective disease-modifying therapies. Traditional drug discovery approaches that rely on single-target interventions have largely failed to yield successful treatments, primarily due to the multifaceted and overlapping pathological mechanisms involved, which range from protein misfolding and oxidative stress to neuroinflammation and synaptic dysfunction. This chapter explores the emerging paradigm of multi-target drug discovery, emphasizing the use of in silico techniques to identify ligands capable of modulating multiple disease-relevant targets such as β-secretase (BACE1), acetylcholinesterase (AChE), tau protein, NMDA receptors, MAO-B, and α-synuclein. The author has outline a comprehensive computational pipeline that integrates ligand-based and structure-based drug design approaches, including QSAR modeling, pharmacophore mapping, molecular docking.

Disorders of Consciousness (DoC), such as Unresponsive Wakefulness Syndrome (UWS) and the Minimally Conscious State (MCS), have an indelible effect on the patients and their families at very high stakes. Growing evidence shows that neuromodulation, especially deep brain stimulation, has the potential to restore consciousness in some DoC patients. There are efforts to propose an ai predictive model for the condition of coma-like patients undergoing treatment via neuromodulation. The research will center on the centromedian-parafascicular complex of the thalamus, especially when hypoxia or trauma affects one side of the brain more than the other. A longitudinal approach using EEG and neuroimaging methods for preprocessing and data segregation is combined with a GCSVM (Glasgow Coma Scale Support Vector Machine) model for continuous follow-up. AI model detects

Treatment based on the inhibition of tyrosine kinases can provide relief to patients with severe neurodegenerative phenomena, for example, Alzheimer's disease, multiple sclerosis, Parkinson's disease, and amyotrophic lateral sclerosis. All these conditions involve ongoing neuronal disruptions and neuro-degeneration, sharing several common traits: the build-up of abnormal protein aggregates, oxidative stress, mitochondrial dysfunction, DNA damage, neurotrophin irregularities, and persistent neuro-inflammation. Pathways participating in neurodegenerative diseases' progression and development, accompanied by the expression of biomarkers, are dependent on the activities of proteins called tyrosine kinases and phosphatases.

Neurodegenerative diseases like Alzheimer's, Parkinson's, ALS, and Huntington's are rising globally due to aging populations and longer life expectancy. Marked by progressive neuronal loss, these disorders share common features such as protein misfolding, mitochondrial dysfunction, oxidative stress, and chronic neuroinflammation. Current diagnostics often detect disease at late stages, and available treatments mainly alleviate symptoms without altering progression. However, advances in molecular biology, biotechnology, and imaging are enabling earlier detection and targeted interventions. Promising innovations include anti-amyloid antibodies, enzyme therapy, gene editing, and precision diagnostics. This chapter reviews key mechanisms, diagnostic challenges, and emerging therapies, highlighting the need for interdisciplinary research and policy support to translate scientific progress into effective clinical care.

Neurodegenerative diseases presents the pathways as promising therapeutic targets,such as protein aggregation, mitochondrial dysfunction, and lysosomal degradation. Enzymes like β-secretase in Alzheimer's disease and glucocerebrosidase in Parkinson's exemplify this therapeutic potential.Emerging therapeutic modalitiessuch as gene therapy and enzyme replacement therapypose additional regulatory scrutiny due to novel delivery mechanisms and long-term safety concerns. Ethical considerations, including informed consent in cognitively impaired patients and equitable trial access, further complicate the regulatory landscape. Ensuring compliance with GMP/GCP is critical but resource-intensive.enzyme pathways offer promising avenues for treating neurodegenerative diseases, overcoming regulatory, ethical, and clinical challenges will require coordinated efforts among researchers, regulators, clinicians, and industry stakeholders.

In today's world, neurological disorders, which encompass a variety of neurodegenerative, neuropsychiatric, and neurodevelopmental issues, are the leading causes of disability and mortality. One of the main causes of genesis of several brain disorders and the neuronal damage is oxidative stress, which is generated by an excess of reactive oxygen species (ROS). The aim of this study is to present an unbiased assessment of the evidence in favor of using phytomedicines to treat brain disorders. There is a captivating case for multidisciplinary teamwork among neuroscientists,

species, we highlight their potential to modulate enzymatic and oxidative pathways particularly through antioxidant, anti-inflammatory, and neuroprotective mechanisms. In addition, they are capable of interacting with targets such as acetylcholinesterase and neuroinflammatory mediators. By integrating traditional knowledge with pharmacological and biochemical analysis, we propose that phytomedicines from Mediterranean biodiversity can contribute to enzyme-based therapeutic strategies in neurodegeneration.

Vivek Pazhamalai, Department of Bioengineering, Vels Institute of Science, Technology, and Advanced Studies, India
M. Suriya, Department of Bioengineering, Vels Institute of Science, Technology, and Advanced Studies, India
V. Aarthi, Department of Bioengineering, Vels Institute of Science, Technology, and Advanced Studies, India
S. Ivo Romauld, Department of Bioengineering, Vels Institute of Science, Technology, and Advanced Studies, India
S. S. Meenambiga, Department of Bioengineering, Vels Institute of Science, Technology, and Advanced Studies, India
R. Chandrasekaran, Department of Biomedical Engineering, Vels Institute of Science, Technology, and Advanced Studies, India
N. M. Hariharan, Department of Biotechnology, Vel Tech Rangarajan Dr. Sagunthala R&D Institute of Science and Technology, India

This chapter explores the growing challenge posed by neurodegenerative and psychiatric disorders, which have underscored the limitations of conventional treatments. It focuses on the therapeutic potential of phytomedicines, particularly their antioxidant, anti-inflammatory, and neurotransmitter-modulating effects. Specifically, it examines the role of plant-derived compounds, such as terpenoids, alkaloids, and flavonoids, in mitigating symptoms of depression, anxiety, Parkinson's disease, and Alzheimer's disease. This chapter discusses the fusion of traditional wisdom with contemporary scientific methods, highlighting the need for rigorous standards and regulatory frameworks that prioritize ethical considerations. The integration of nanotechnology, AI, and personalized medicine is transforming phytomedicine, paving the way for innovative approaches to brain health and wellness.

As marketing moves into a time of hyper-personalization and algorithmic precision, the flaws in traditional self-report methods have become clearer. This study introduces the idea of "Neuromarketing 2.0," a new way of doing research that combines biometric feedback in real time with AI-driven emotion mapping to better understand how people act. The study uses primary data from a controlled experiment with EEG signals, eye-tracking metrics, and galvanic skin response (GSR) to train machine learning models to find cognitive engagement and emotional responses during digital ad exposure. The AI layer uses convolutional neural networks (CNNs) and recurrent neural networks (RNNs) to sort patterns of emotional valence and arousal, turning raw physiological data into useful marketing information.

Preface

INTRODUCTION

Neurodegenerative disorders continue to challenge the boundaries of medicine and science. These diseases—marked by relentless progression and complex pathophysiology—have long posed significant hurdles to effective diagnosis and treatment. Yet in recent years, we have witnessed extraordinary strides in understanding the molecular underpinnings of conditions such as Alzheimer's disease, Parkinson's disease, Huntington's disease, and amyotrophic lateral sclerosis (ALS). This book, *Recent Breakthroughs in Neurodegenerative Disorders and Enzyme Therapy*, was conceived as a response to these pivotal developments.

In assembling this volume, our objective was to capture the momentum of recent discoveries and highlight the therapeutic possibilities emerging from this rapidly evolving field. Particular attention is given to the role of enzyme therapy—an area that has shifted from experimental exploration to clinical relevance. The contributions within these pages reflect a growing body of work demonstrating that targeting protein misfolding, mitochondrial dysfunction, and neuroinflammation can not only deepen our understanding but also offer promising therapeutic avenues.

We have curated contributions from leading researchers and clinicians who provide insight into both foundational mechanisms and translational advances. Topics include lysosomal dysfunction, gene-editing techniques for enzyme delivery, and the development of enzyme-based therapeutics capable of modulating disease progression. By focusing on the interface between basic science and clinical application, this book serves as a bridge between the lab bench and bedside practice.

Equally important, this collection reflects a commitment to multidisciplinary collaboration. Progress in neurodegenerative disease research relies not only on neuroscientists and biochemists but also on the engagement of clinicians, healthcare policymakers, and emerging researchers across disciplines. It is our hope that this volume will inspire continued inquiry, inform clinical practice, and encourage the kind of cross-sector collaboration that leads to meaningful change for patients.

This book was developed with several guiding aims:

- To compile and present the latest research on neurodegenerative disorders and enzyme therapy advancements.

- To elucidate molecular mechanisms and therapeutic targets for conditions like Alzheimer's, Parkinson's, and ALS.
- To explore the role of enzyme-based therapies in modulating disease progression.
- To bridge basic science and clinical applications through multidisciplinary perspectives.
- To inspire further research and collaboration to improve patient outcomes in neurodegenerative disorders.

We believe this volume will serve as a valuable reference for neuroscientists, clinicians, medical researchers, and biochemists. It will also appeal to healthcare professionals, advanced students, and policymakers seeking informed perspectives on the future of neurodegenerative disease treatment and enzyme-based interventions.

We extend our sincere thanks to the contributors for their expertise, and to the readers for their commitment to advancing the science and care of neurodegenerative disorders.

ORGANIZATION OF THE BOOK

This volume opens with Chapter 1, which delves into the critical role of neurotransmitters in cognitive function and the adverse effects of long-term antiepileptic drug (AED) use. Disruption in neurotransmission—particularly involving dopamine and GABA pathways—has been increasingly linked to neurodegenerative disorders like Alzheimer's and Parkinson's disease. The chapter highlights the importance of monitoring AED therapy and emphasizes the broader implications of neurotransmitter dysregulation on cognitive decline.

In Chapter 2, the application of artificial intelligence in detecting cerebrospinal fluid (CSF) leakage and brain-blood barrier (BBB) compromise is explored. The chapter presents a two-phase approach combining ultra-high-performance liquid chromatography (UHPLC) with a novel hybrid k-means Hidden Markov Model (kCHMM), achieving high diagnostic precision. These findings underscore the potential of AI-assisted methods in early neurological diagnostics, especially in oncological and traumatic brain contexts.

Chapter 3 introduces medical nanoparticles as transformative agents in diagnostics and targeted therapies. With enhanced specificity, biocompatibility, and stability due to recent innovations in surface functionalization, nanoparticles are shaping the future of personalized medicine. The chapter anticipates a shift toward "smart" nanoparticles capable of responding to biomolecular signals for precision drug delivery.

Building upon this foundation, Chapter 4 focuses specifically on iron oxide nanoparticles and their application in neurotheranostics. By facilitating blood-brain barrier penetration and serving as both therapeutic and diagnostic agents, these nanoparticles represent a major advancement in treating CNS disorders such as multiple sclerosis and ALS. The chapter surveys their potential in modulating disease progression through targeted delivery.

In Chapter 5, a novel perspective on radiation is presented—not as a harmful force, but as a stimulator of protective enzyme systems. The concept of radiation hormesis is examined in the context of neuroprotection, showing how controlled exposure can activate endogenous antioxidant and DNA-repair pathways, offering a potential route to future neuroprotective drug discovery.

Chapter 6 shifts to in silico methods, exploring the design of multi-target ligands capable of modulating several disease-relevant proteins involved in neurodegeneration. Utilizing mo-

lecular docking, QSAR modeling, and pharmacophore-based design, the chapter demonstrates how computational approaches can accelerate the discovery of therapeutics targeting complex neurodegenerative mechanisms.

Chapter 7 examines the intersection of neuromodulation and AI in disorders of consciousness. Through deep brain stimulation and predictive modeling using EEG and imaging data, this chapter outlines how AI frameworks like the Glasgow Coma Scale Support Vector Machine (GCSVM) can detect subtle improvements in consciousness, offering hope for intervention in coma-like states.

The focus of Chapter 8 is enzyme-targeted therapy. By exploring the structural biology of key neurodegenerative enzymes through tools like AlphaFold and molecular docking, the chapter advocates for a shift from descriptive disease models to actionable therapeutic targets. Enzymes such as GSK3ß, MAO, and ASM emerge as central to this precision approach.

Chapter 9 continues this thread by reviewing enzymatic targets associated with protein misfolding and neuroinflammation in neurodegenerative disorders. Highlighting advances in biomarker development, early diagnostics, and enzyme-based interventions, the chapter emphasizes a translational approach that moves from molecular insights to clinical utility.

In Chapter 10, the spotlight turns to tyrosine kinases, whose dysregulation plays a critical role in several neurodegenerative conditions. The chapter outlines how targeting these kinases can modulate neuroinflammation, oxidative stress, and abnormal protein aggregation, offering new therapeutic strategies for conditions such as MS and ALS.

Chapter 11 reviews the rapidly evolving landscape of anti-amyloid monoclonal antibodies, presenting them as promising candidates for mitigating CNS disorders. It explores both the promise and the challenges of these biologics, from disease-modifying effects in Alzheimer's to the hurdles of early diagnosis and immune response regulation.

Chapter 12 addresses the regulatory complexities of enzyme-targeted and gene-based therapies. As emerging treatments grow more sophisticated, so too do the ethical, clinical, and procedural challenges—ranging from trial design and informed consent to GMP compliance. The chapter calls for integrated collaboration among regulators, scientists, and clinicians.

In Chapter 13, the book transitions to phytomedicine. This chapter presents an evidence-based analysis of plant-derived treatments for neurological disorders, particularly those addressing oxidative stress and inflammation. The potential of phytomedicines to complement conventional therapies is explored through interdisciplinary collaboration.

Chapter 14 expands upon this by highlighting the pharmacological mechanisms and clinical applications of bioactive plant compounds in neurological health. From polyphenols to alkaloids, the chapter emphasizes how phytochemicals can modulate neurotransmission, neuroinflammation, and cognitive function.

Chapter 15 further deepens the discussion, focusing on ethnobotanical resources widely used in traditional medicine. Plants such as Withania somnifera and Bacopa monnieri are examined for their neuroprotective and adaptogenic properties. The chapter supports the integration of these therapies as holistic alternatives to conventional drugs.

In Chapter 16, a case study from Talassemtane National Park in Morocco provides ethnobotanical evidence of traditional phytomedicine's value in modulating enzymatic pathways involved in neurodegeneration. The chapter bridges traditional knowledge with modern pharmacology, presenting a model for enzyme-targeted phytotherapy.

Chapter 17 concludes the phytomedicine triad by emphasizing cognitive restoration through plant-based therapies. It explores the future of personalized phytomedicine, leveraging tech-

nologies like AI and nanotechnology to tailor treatments that address depression, anxiety, and cognitive decline.

Finally, Chapter 18 steps outside traditional boundaries, examining how advances in neuroscience are being translated into neuromarketing. By integrating biometric feedback with AI-driven emotion mapping, this chapter illustrates how neurological insights are being applied in commercial contexts—revealing the expansive reach of neurotechnological innovation.

CONCLUSION

As we bring this volume to a close, it is evident that the field of neurodegenerative research stands at a critical juncture—where foundational discoveries in molecular biology, biotechnology, pharmacology, and data science are converging to redefine how we understand and treat disorders of the brain. Across the chapters presented in this book, we have highlighted not only the scientific advancements but also the collaborative, cross-disciplinary spirit that underpins them.

From the disruption of neurotransmitters and the promise of enzyme-targeted therapies to innovations in nanotechnology, artificial intelligence, and phytomedicine, the scope of inquiry reflected here is both vast and deeply focused. Each contribution illustrates how diverse approaches—whether computational, clinical, or ethnobotanical—can work in concert to address the urgent and complex challenges posed by neurodegenerative diseases.

Our aim with this edited volume has been to provide a comprehensive, accessible, and forward-looking resource for researchers, clinicians, policymakers, and students. By bridging the gap between basic science and real-world application, we hope to inspire further innovation and collaboration, ultimately accelerating the development of effective therapies that improve patient care and quality of life.

The path ahead will require continued interdisciplinary dialogue, regulatory flexibility, and ethical foresight. But with each breakthrough comes renewed hope—not only for slowing disease progression but for restoring cognitive and neurological function in ways once thought impossible.

We thank the contributors for their exceptional scholarship, and the readers for their dedication to advancing the field. It is our shared hope that this book will serve as both a catalyst and a compass for the next generation of breakthroughs in neurodegenerative research and enzyme therapy.

Chapter 1

Influence of Neurotransmitters Disruption on the Deterioration of Cognitive Function

Priyanka Gupta
https://orcid.org/0009-0002-7668-9169
CMP College, University of Allahabad, Prayagraj, India

Poornima Yadav
https://orcid.org/0009-0007-6942-8346
CMP College, University of Allahabad, Prayagraj, India

Sudhi Shrivastava
https://orcid.org/0009-0008-5474-0852
CMP College, University of Allahabad, Prayagraj, India

Ratnesh Kumar Soni
https://orcid.org/0000-0002-5774-8664
K.N. Government P.G. College, Gyanpur Bhadohi, India

ABSTRACT

Neurotransmitters (NTs) are chemical messengers responsible for conveying signals across a synapse, through electrical and chemical pathways, by regulating excitatory and inhibitory mechanisms. Any disturbance in neurotransmission affects the synaptic plasticity and cognitive function. Antiepileptic drugs (AEDs) are designed to bind the receptors of neurotransmitters and activate, block, or modulate brain excitability to prevent or reduce seizures. They display multiple mechanisms of action, such as inhibiting voltage-gated Na+ and Ca+ channels, enhancing GABAergic inhibition, and modulating glutamate receptors in the brain, but also improperly affect neurotransmitter signals and activities. Adverse side effects include reduced dopamine and other neurotransmitters secretion which also leads to the development of several different

DOI: 10.4018/979-8-3373-4627-4.ch001

types of neurodegenerative disorders (NDs) like Parkinson's disease and Alzheimer's disease. The authors aim to emphasize the need for careful monitoring of patients receiving long-term AED therapy and related cognitive decline due to neurotransmitter disruption.

INTRODUCTION

Neurotransmitters are endogenous chemical signals that convey signals between nerve cells and other target cells in the nervous system. They are fundamental to brain function, enabling the communication essential for behavior, thought, etc. There are approximately one hundred identified neurotransmitters, which are typically classified into major categories such as amino acid (Glutamate, GABA), monoamine (Dopamine, serotonin, Norepinephrine), peptides (endorphins), and others, like acetylcholine, Nitric oxide, etc. (Manca et al., 2025). Each neurotransmitter has distinct functions and is often localised to specific regions. Neurotransmitters can be of two types: excitatory, inhibitory, and modulatory. Inhibitory neurotransmitters like dopamine or serotonin can have various effects depending on the receptor type and area in the brain. On the other hand, Excitatory neurotransmitters like glutamate promote the firing of nerve cells. Balanced neurotransmitter activity is mandatory for normal brain function. Dysfunction or Dysregulation can result in neurodegenerative disorders such as Alzheimer's and Parkinson's disease, (Chen & Zhang 2025).

Both of these diseases are neurodegenerative disorders. Parkinson's disease primarily results from the loss of dopamine-producing nerve cells in a specific area of the brain called the Substantia Nigra. On the other hand, Alzheimer's disease affects memory, behaviour, thinking, and the ability to perform everyday tasks, (Miranda & Bermúdez-Rattoni, 2007). They are involved in the progressive degeneration and death of brain cells because of an imbalance of Neurotransmitters., This chapter aims to summarize and discuss the structure, secretion, and role of neurotransmitters, and the effects of AED therapy on neurotransmission, including its physical activity, which is mandatory for a better understanding of some of the most severe neurological diseases, (Teleanu et al., 2022)

Figure 1. Neurotransmitter diversity and function

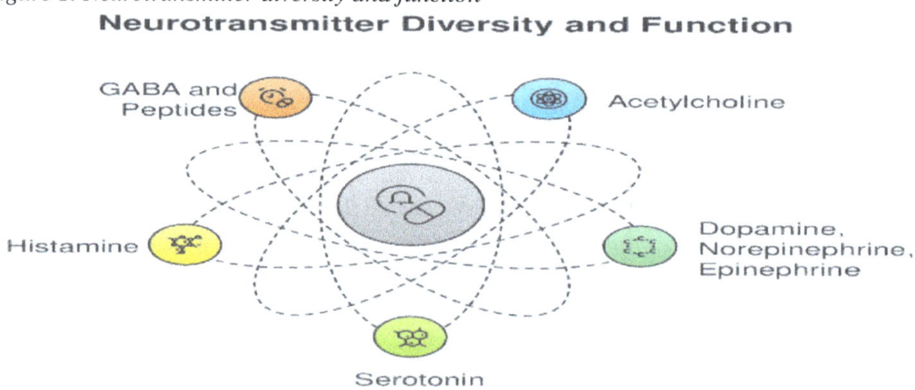

Epilepsy is a chronic neurological condition marked by abnormal electrical activity in the brain, causing recurring and unpredictable disruptions in brain function (Fisher etal.,2005). It is one of the most prevalent brain disorders worldwide, affecting a significant number of people, with estimated annual incidence rates between 50.4 and 817 cases per 100,000 individuals (Feigin etal.,2019). The development and progression of epilepsy involve intricate processes, including neuronal dysfunction, neurotransmitter imbalance, and genetic susceptibility, further influenced by inflammatory and oxidative stress response (Brodie & Sills, 2011). Over 30 antiepileptic drugs are available for clinical use targeting various mechanisms, such as modulating ion channels, enhancing GABAergic activity, and inhibiting glutamate receptors. Cognitive dysfunction frequently accompanies epilepsy, and factors such as the underlying cause, treatment success, and seizure control impact the extent and progression of impairment (Halmstaedter, 2001).

Antiepileptic drugs (AEDs), also known as anticonvulsants, comprise a diverse group of medications that help manage and reduce the frequency and severity of seizures associated with various neurological conditions. AEDs affect neurotransmitters such as GABA (Gamma–Aminobutyric Acid), which is an inhibitory neurotransmitter in the central nervous system, playing a crucial role in regulating neuronal activity in the context of epilepsy. AEDs reduce glutamate-mediated excitatory neurotransmission by targeting α-amino-3-hydroxy-5-methyl-4-isoxazolepropionic acid (AMPA) and N-methyl-D-aspartate receptors (NMDA). Perampanel, an AMPA receptor antagonist, is used to treat epilepsy but may cause dizziness, irritability, and psychiatric side effects (Paul et al.,2023; Cheli et al.,2021). Ketamine, an NMDA receptor antagonist, is used for anaesthesia and treatment-resistant depression, but carries risks of abuse, dissociative effects, and cognitive impairment (Manganotti et al, 2021; Alqahtani et al., 2020). Voltage-gated ion channels, such as sodium, potassium, and calcium channels, are modulated by certain AEDs (Main et al., 2000). These include phenytoin, carbamazepine, oxcarbazepine, and lacosamide, which are used to treat epilepsy, (Vezzani et al., 2022).

The research confirmed that antiepileptic drugs can affect cognitive abilities. The selection of antiepileptic medications requires careful consideration to balance effective seizure control with minimizing cognitive side effects, as some antiepileptics have more pronounced cognitive impacts than others. Regular cognitive monitoring is vital in epilepsy management, allowing for early detection of cognitive changes and guiding treatment modifications to optimize patient outcomes. Dysregulated synaptic pruning activity can result in an imbalance between excitatory and inhibitory neurotransmission, (Andoh et al., 2019). Reactive astrocytes, through synaptic remodeling and disruption of GABAergic networks, may significantly contribute to neural circuit reorganization in epilepsy, (Weissberg et al., 2015).

The brain neuronal network, comprising over 100 billion neurons, functions with remarkable precision. Specific signaling molecules can trigger abnormal neuronal changes, such as axonal sprouting and synaptic reorganization, (Tang et al., 2017). Inflammation-induced dysconnectivity in brain networks can result in impaired cognitive and motor functions. The adverse effects of these medications are often dose-dependent and can be mitigated through gradual dose titration. In contrast, levetiracetam may cause side effects in older adults, including difficulty concentrating, drowsiness, depression, and behavioral changes, without negatively impacting cognitive function. Medications like eslicarbazepine and oxcarbazepine can lead to hyponatremia and related symptoms, whereas gabapentin, lamotrigine, lacosamide, and pregabalin do not appear to cause significant cognitive side effects, (Goldsmith et al., 2023; Kitzbichler et al., 2021).

STRUCTURE OF NEUROTRANSMITTERS (NTS)

The earliest Neurotransmitter to be found was a mini molecule known as acetylcholine. Nearly all neurotransmitters are made of a tiny Amino acid backbone, an amine molecule, aromatic ring, ester of choline, short amino acid chain, Nucleotides, and simple diatomic molecules. These vary in chemical structure depending on their type and function. (Thomas suudhof;2008). Their structural diversity enables a wide range of physiological effects in the nervous system. Their chemical nature also influences how they are synthesized, stored, released, and degraded in the nervous system. Dopamine, Norepinephrine, and epinephrine have a catechol ring and an ethylamine side chain. Serotonin consists an indole ring and a hydroxyl with its side chain. Histamine contains an imidazole ring and is derived from histidine. GABA and peptides determine their mode of action, duration of effects, and role in neural communication and brain health, (Sheffler et al., 2025).

Figure 2. Elucidates the structure of different types of neurotransmitters

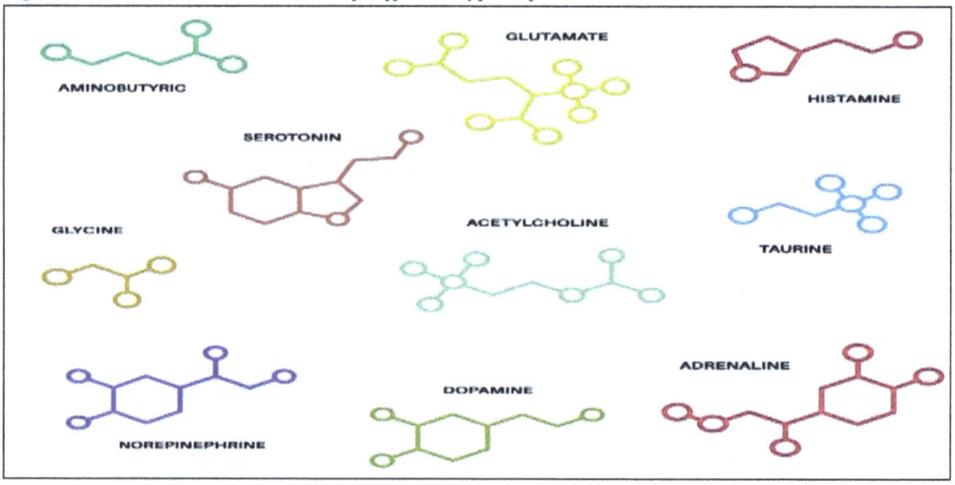

Neurotransmitters Can Be Classified Based on their Chemical Composition

Glutamate

It is also known as L-glutamic acid, is made of the 20 amino acids and most abundant excitatory neurotransmitter. Its chemical formula is C5H9NO4 and it has a molecular weight of 147.13 g/mol. The chemical composition consists of an amino acid group (-NH2), a carboxylic acid (-COOH), a side chain and hydrogen atom. This chemical composition allows glutamate to function both as an amino acid in protein synthesis and as a neurotransmitter in the brain. (Kazemi and hoop;1991). Glutamate is synthesized from glutamine via the enzyme glutaminase, primarily in presynaptic neurons. It is stored in vesicles and released into the synaptic cleft in

response to action potentials. The glutamate receptor are Ionotropic receptors and Metabotropic receptors which modulate synaptic transmission and neuronal excitability. In the normal brain, glutamate do a central role in learning, memory formation, synaptic plasticity, and overall cognition. (Iovino etal.,2020). It is a key modulator of long -term potentiation (LTP)- a process vital for strengthening synaptic connections during memory formation. Targeting the glutamatergic system has become a focus of research to prevent or slow cognitive decline. (Meldrum, 2000).

Norepinephrine

Norepinephrine is also called noradrenaline, is both a neurotransmitter and a hormone that plays a neurotransmitter and a hormone that plays essential roles in the brain and body. Its chemical formula is C8H11NO3 and molecular weight 169.18g/mol. The chemical composition consists a benzene ring with two hydroxyl groups, an ethylamine side chain, with an additional hydroxyl group. (Paul ;2021). Norepinephrine is produced in the brain primarily by neurons in the locus coerules (LC), a small nucleus in the pons. These neurons project throughout the cerebral cortex areas vital for attention, arousal, learning, memory and executive function. There are two receptor inhibitory (alpha1, alpha2) and stimulatory (beta1, beta2) modulates cognitive processes. The LC is one of the earliest brain region affected in Alzheimer's and Parkinson's disease, and loss neuron leads to a decline in norepinephrine production. (Silverberg etal;1978). Norepinephrine depletion contributes to non-motor symptoms like cognitive slowing, depression, and sleep disturbances. However, with aging and neurodegeneration, norepinephrine signaling is diminished- leading to executive dysfunction, memory deficits, and neuroinflammation. (Marks etal;2009).

Serotonin

Serotonin plays a critical role in regulating mood, emotion, sleep, appetite and cognition. It is also called 5- hydroxytryptamie, and its chemical formula is C10H12N2O. The chemical composition consists an indole ring, a hydroxyl group and an ethylamine side chain and its molecular weight is 176.22 g/mol, (Seyedabadi et al., 2014). Serotonin is synthesized in serotonergic neurons located primarily in the raphe nuclei of the brainstem and is stored in synaptic vesicles before being released into the synaptic cleft during neurotransmission. It exerts its effects via multiple serotonin receptors, excepts 5-HT, which is a ligand -gated ion channel. As people age or develop neurodegenerative disease, serotonergic dysfunction has been increasingly linked to cognitive decline, through both direct neuronal mechanism and indirect modulation of other systems. Serotonin regulates long- term potentiation (LTP) and long- term depression (LTD) in the hippocampus, both essential for memory formation. Loss of 5-HT reduce synaptic plasticity, impairs spatial learning and recall etc. serotonin exerts anti-inflammatory effects in the brain microglial cells. (Paredes-Rodriguez et al., 2020). Restoring or preserving serotonin levels through pharmacological, nutritional, 0r neuroprotective strategies represents a compelling direction for managing cognitive decline and more effective treatments for Parkinson's and Alzheimer's diseases, (Kanova & Kohout, 2021).

Acetylcholine

Acetylcholine is a kind of neurotransmitter in both the central and peripheral nervous systems. The acetylcholine chemical formula is C7H16NO2+ and its molecular weight 146.21g/mol. The chemical composition consists of an acetyl group (CH3CO-) and a choline moiety. (Picciotto etal;2012). It is a small water dissolves molecule that does not cross the blood brain barrier, so it must be synthesized in the brain. Acetylcholine binds to two main types of receptors that is Nicotinic acetylcholine receptors (nAChRs) and Muscarinic acetylcholic receptors (mAChRs). The basal forebrain cholinergic system, particularly the nucleus basalis of meynert, projects extensively to the hippocampus, amygdala, and neocortex, making it central to cognitive processing. (Brown, 2006). Studies show a marked decrease in ChAT activity in the brains of individuals with AD and PD. Understanding acetylcholine's role in brain health has led to some of the most widely used treatments for dementia today. Protecting or restoring path for slowing or mitigating cognitive decline, especially in the early stages of Alzheimer's disease. (R M Nitsch 1996).

Histamine

The chemical composition of an imidazole ring and ethylamine side chain with 111.15g/mol molecular weight. It is a biogenic amine taking part in various physiological processes, including immune responses, gastric secretion, neurotransmission in the brain. (yuan and Silberstein;2018). It is a hydrophilic, positively charged molecule under physiological conditions, which limits its ability to cross the blood brain barrier thus histamine used in the brain synthesised in situ. Although histamine is more widely known for its role in allergic reaction and gastric acid secretion, in the central nervous system (CNS), it acts as a modulatory neurotransmitter. (J C Schwartz;1975). They have H1, H2, H3 and H4 receptors acts through G-protein coupled receptors. Changes in central histaminergic neurotransmission have been increasingly associated with age- related cognitive decline and neurodegenerative such as PD, AD, HD, etc. In Parkinson's and Alzheimer's, H1 and H2 receptor expression is reduced, impairing histamine signaling. Animal studies show that blocking histamine receptors, especially H1 and H2, impairs memory, while stimulating histaminergic signaling enhance learning and recall. (Schwartz etal;1979). Targeting histamine pathways, particularly through H3 receptor anatagonists, presents a promising therapeutic direction for mitigating cognitive impairment in conditions like Alzheimmer's, Parkinson's, age related memory loss, (Wada et al., 1988).

Glycine

Glycine is the building block of protein and neurotransmitter in the central nervous system (CNS) and the chemical formula is C2H5NO2. It is a non- amino acid in human body and the molecular weight if glycine is 75.07g/mol. The chemical composition consists of amino group(-NH2), Carboxyl group (-COOH), and a hydrogen atom. (Gundersen etal;2004). Glycine also functions as a co-agonist with glutamate at the NMDA (N-methyl-D-aspartate receptor) in the brain. Essential for NMDA receptor activation, which is involved in learning, memory, and synaptic plasticity. Changes in glycine levels or receptor function are implicated in several neurodegeneration and cognitive disoders. Understanding and targeting glycine related pathways

could offer novel therapeutic strategies for cognitive impairment and dementia. (Hernandes & Troncone, 2009).

Taurine

The chemical name of taurine is 2-Aminoethanesulfonic acid, that is not used in protein synthesis but is abundantly present in various tissues, especially in the brain, heart, retina and skeletal muscle. The chemical formula of taurine is $C2H7NO3S$ and molecular weight 125.15g/mol. (oja and saransaari;2013). In the CNS, taurine behaves similarly to GABA and glycine acting as an inhibitory neuromodulator. Taurine has been implicated in the prevention of age related cognitive impairment and neurodegeneration. Its reactive oxygen species (ROS) and inhibits lipid peroxidation. (ocha-de la paz etal;2019). Taurine has been show to reduce amyloid-beta aggregation and tau hyperphosphorylation in preclinical models of Alzheimer's disease. Animal studies show that taurine supplementation improves learning and memory in aging and Alzhemier's models. (kumari etal;2013).

Aminobutyric

The most important inhibitory neurotransmitter is aminobutyric acid and it is also called Y-aminobutyric acid (GABA). The chemical formula is $C4H9NO2$ and its molecular weight 103.12g/mol. It plays a vital role in reducing neuronal firing, maintaining excitatory-inhibitory balance, regulating anxiety, mood, cognition and sleep. (Leon and tadi; 2025). Disruption of the GABAergic system is strongly linked to cognitive dysfunction and neurodegenerative disease, especially Alzhemier's parkinson's, age related memory impairment. This cause a shift toward excitatory neurotransmission, resulting in neurotoxicity and synaptic damage and leads to deficits in long term potentiation (LTP) and memory encoding. (Hepsomali etal;2020). Post mortem studies of AD brains show reduced GABA levels and receptor expression, especially in the hippocampus and cortex. Animals models of AD and aging show that GABA enhancers (benzodiazepines, muscimol) improve cognitive performance, (Krnjević & Schwartz, 1967).

Dopamine

Dopamine has a catechol structure and an amine group, classifying it as both a catecholamine and a monoamine. Its chemical formula is $C8H11NO2$ and molecular weight is 153.18g/mol. Dopamine is a precursor to norepinephrine and epinephrine in the catecholamine pathway. (Speranza etal;2021). Cognitive decline, particularly in aging and neurodegenerative diseases like Alzheimer's and parkinson's is strongly associated with dopaminergic dysfunction. Beyond motor symptoms, PD patients exhibit cognitive Impairments, attributed to reduced dopamine in frontostriatal circuits. (Yingfang Tian;2024). Research into doamine-enhancing nutraceuticals, reuptake inhibitors, and receptor modulators is ongoing for potential cognitive benefits. Targeting dopamine pathways offers a promising strategy for preserving cognitive function and treating neurodegenerative disorders. (Shohamy and Adcock;2010).

Adrenaline

Adrenaline is also called epinephrine, is a catecholamine hormone and neurotransmitter. The chemical name of adrenaline is 4-{(1-hydroxy-2-(methylamino)ethyl}benezene-1,2-diol and molecular weight 183.20g/mol. The catechol ring, hydroxyl group and methylamino group is a chemical composition. (A M Andersen;1975). Adrenaline is released in response to stress (fight or flight response) and exerts effects by binding to adrenergic receptor (alpha and beta). Although adrenaline is mostly known for its peripheral actions, it plays a modulatory role in memory, attention, and stress response, all of which impact cognitive impairment and neuro-degenerative processes through several mechanism. (Ring etal;2013). Acute stress and short term adrenaline elevation enhance memory consolidation via the amygdala and hippocampus. Animals studies show that acute adrenaline can enhance emotional memory. Thus, maintaining a balanced adrenergic system is essential for healthy cognitive aging and prevention of cognitive decline. (Ibragimov etal;2021).

MECHANISM OF NEUROTRANSMITTERS

Neurotransmitters allow nerve cells to communicate with the brain signals and their activities. The mechanism of neurotransmitters' action involves several key pathways like the Cerebral dopaminergic system, cerebral cholinergic system, cerebral Noradrenergic system, cerebral GABAergic and glutamatergic system. (Alarcon etal;2023). Each pathway is precisely regulated to maintain proper neural function and is crucial for processes such as movement, emotions, cognition, and memory. (Moghaddam etal;2017). Disruption in these mechanisms is implicated in numerous neurological and psychiatric disorders like Parkinson's and Alzheimer's disease. Understanding these pathways not only deepens our knowledge of the nervous system but also guides the development of effective therapies for brain disorders. (Polo & Kruss, 2016).

Dopaminergic Pathways (Cerebral Dopaminergic System)

Dopaminergic pathways involve neurons that produce and secrete dopamine. These pathways include the nigrostriatal, mesolimbic, mesocortical, and tuberoinfundibular tracts. It controls movement with the help of the nigrostriatal pathway, which causes Parkinson's, and the meso-cortical pathway involved in cognitive function. (Luo and Huang;2016). Dopaminergic Neurons in the Substantia Nigra pars compacta gradually degenerate. This leads to dopamine deficiency in the striatum, disrupting motor control. (Singaram etal;1995).

Nigrostriatal

Originating in the substantia nigra pars compacta and projecting to the dorsal striatum (caudate and putamen), this pathway is critical for motor control. It is severely affected in parkinson's disease. (Faure etal;2005).

Mesolimbic

Arising from the ventral tegmental area (VAT) and hippocampus, it regulates rewards, emotion, and motivation. Dysfunction in this pathway is linked to mood disorders and contributes to non-motor symptoms in neurodegeneration. (Alcaro etal;2007).

Mesocortical

The ventral tegmental area (VTA) to the prefrontal cortex; part taken in cognition, memory, and executive function. Reduced dopamine transmission in the prefontal cortex leads to impaired executive function, decreased working memory etc., (Quessy et al., 2021).

Tuberoinfundibular

Hypothalamus to the pituitary gland regulates hormone secretion, especially prolactin. Tuberoinfundibular pathway is not classically associated with cognition, its neuroendocrine control, dopaminergic modulation etc., effects on brain regions essential for cognitive Performance, (Qi-Lytle et al., 2023).

Cholinergic Pathways (Cerebral Cholinergic System)

The cerebral cholinergic pathways mention to a network of Neurons in the brain that generate and utilize acetylcholine. Imbalance in this system causes Alzheimer's, Parkinson's disease. It is especially damaging to the cerebral cortex, the Hippocampus, and the thalamus area, which regulates higher cognitive functions, (Hampel et al., 2018). Neuroinflammation and impaired neurotrophic signalling affect cholinergic neuron survival. This reduce in cholinergic activity is related with the following symptoms: -

- Memory loss
- Decreased attention span
- Cognitive impairment
- Behavioural changes

The key cholinergic pathways derive from specific basal forebrain and brainstem nuclei and predict to different regions are Basal forebrain cholinergic system and brainstem cholinergic system which is involve in learning, memory, sleepwake etc., (Katsari et al., 2022). In AD marked loss of cholinergic neurons in the basal forebrain and decreased ChAT activity and reduced Ach levels. In PD degeneration of PPN and LDT cholinergic neurons contributes to postural instability, sleep disturbances, and cognitive deficits, (Nemy et al., 2023).

Noradrenergic Pathways (Cerebral Noradrenergic System)

It comprises neurons that produce and utilize Norepinephrine (NE). These Neurons primarily originate in the locus coeruleus (LC) of the brainstem, (Leslie et al., 1985). Loss of Norepinephrine leads to the Amyloid-beta plaque deposition and tau tangle formation by reducing

Neuroprotective and anti-inflammatory signalling. Locus coeruleus degeneration contributes to non-motor symptoms, including depression, anxiety, sleep disturbances, and cognitive decline. The resulting decline in Norepinephrine levels contributes to: -

- Impaired attention and working memory
- Disruption of the sleep-wake cycle
- Increased Neuroinflammation
- Control of stress response via the hypothalamic-pituitary-adrenal axis, (Berridge et al., 1993)

Noradrenergic exhibits neuroprotective properties through modulation of microglial activity, reduction of oxidative stress, and maintenance of blood brain barrier integrity. Reduced NE levels in AD diminished these Protectives mechanism, leading to increased inflammation, neuronal vulnerability, and cognitive decline, (Sara, 1985). Furthermore, the NEs modulates amyloid precursor protein processing thus, its dysregulation may accelerate amyloid deposition. NE dysfunction in PD exacerbates the dopaminergic deficit by impairing compensatory mechanism and accelerating neurodegeneration. NE deficiency leads to increased neuroinflammation and impaired alpha synuclein clearance, contributing to neuronal toxicity. (Downs & McElligott, 2020). Pharmacological strategies targeting noradrenergic reuptake inhibitors have showed promise in ameliorating attention deficient and executive dysfunction in PD. Additionally, restoring NE levels may alleviate autonomic dysfunction and orthostatic hypotension associated with PD, (Paredes-Rodriguez et al., 2020). Severa mechanism explain how noradrenergic pathways impairment contributes to neurodegenerative diseases is neuroinflammation, oxidative stress, amyloidogenesis and protein aggregation, synaptic plasticity etc. understanding the mechanism of noradrenergic dysfunction offers new insights into disease progression and opens up avenues for novel therapeutic interventions targeting this critical neurotransmitter system, (Szabadi, 2013). As research advance, preserving noradrenergic function may become a cornerstone in combating cognitive decline and enhancing the quality of life in patients with neurodegenerative disorders, (Szabadi., 2013).

Cerebral GABAergic System

Cerebral is an inhibitory or modulatory signalling network in the brain that utilize GABA as its primary neurotransmitter. GABA is integrate in presynaptic neurons form glutamate by the enzyme glutamic acid decarboxylase (GAD), which exists in two isoforms: GAD65 and GAD67. Once synthesized, GABA is stored in synaptic vesicles by the vesicular GABA transporter (VGAT) and released into the synaptic cleft in reaction to an action potential, (Wu & Sun, 2015). The GABAergic system plays a crucial role in regulating brain excitability and maintaining neural circuit stability. Dysfunction in the GABAergic system is implicated in various neurodegenerative diseases. Neuronal hyperexcitability, which worsens cognitive decline, impaired GABA receptor function reduced synaptic plasticity, (Alharbi et al., 2024). Studies have shown reduced expression of GABAA receptor subunits and decreased GAD67 levels in the hippocampus and cortex of AD patients. GABAergic interneurons are relatively spared in early AD, but their functional impairment contributes to network hyperexcitability and cognitive decline. Abnormal GABA levels have been detected in various brain region in PD patients, contributing to both motor and

non-motor symptoms. Moreover, neuroprotective strategies aiming to restore GABAergic tone may delay disease progression and improve quality of life.

Glutamatergic System

Glutamate is synthesized in the presynaptic terminal from glutamine by the enzyme glutaminase. It is stored in synaptic vesicles and released into synaptic cleft in response to an action potential. NMDA (N-methyl-D-aspartate) receptor allow ca2+, Na2+, and k+ influx, (Wang, et al., 2011). They are highly permeable to Ca2+ and involved in synaptic plasticity, learning, and memory. This excitatory signalling must be tightly regulated as prolonged or excessive activation of glutamate receptors- especially NMDA receptors-can leads to neuronal damage, (Crombie et al., 2022). The glutamatergic pathway can become harmful, a substance known as excitotoxicity, which is a key mechanism in the development and progression of many neurodegenerative diseases. Overactivation of receptors leads to excessive calcium influx, triggering oxidative metabolism, etc.

Mechanism of Neurotransmission Dysregulation involves: -

- Blockage of voltage-gated sodium.
- Development of GABAergic inhibition.
- Inhibition of the mTOR pathway.
- Block of T-type calcium channels.
- Choke calcium voltage-gated channel.
- Oxidative stress and metabolic dysfunction.
- Epigenetics modulation.
- Neuroinflammation suppression
- Mitochondrial dysfunction. (Yelamanchi et al., 2015).

Figure 3. Signalling pathways of neurotransmitter receptor with synaptic cleft

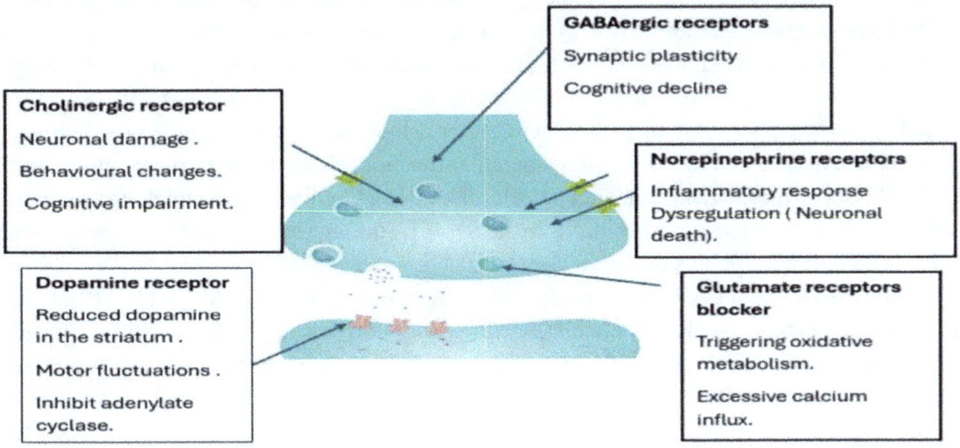

In AD, glutamatergic dysfunction contributes to cognitive decline and synaptic loss. It blocks excessive glutamate activity without interfering together normal synaptic transmission, offering symptomatic relief and neuroprotection, (Puranik & Song, 2024). PD is marked by dopaminergic neuron degeneration in the substantia nigra and disruption basal ganglia circuitry, where glutamate plays a central role. Excessive cortico-striatal glutamate release leads to NMDA receptor overactivation and striatal neuron death, (Johnson, Conn, & Niswender, 2009). Future research focused on modulating glutamate signalling while preserving its physiological roles will be key in developing effective treatments for neurodegenerative disorders., (Zhou & Danbolt, 2014).

NEUROTRANSMITTERS DISRUPTION AND COGNITIVE ALCHEMY

Neurotransmitters are chemical messengers in the brain and nervous system that transmit signals between nerve cells across synapses. Neurotransmitters present in the brain, such as Dopamine, serotonin, Norepinephrine, GABA, and Acetylcholine etc, play a vital role in regulating mood, memory, movement, and cognitive functions. Any dysfunction in the secretion, regulation, and functions of these neurotransmitters induces neurodegeneration and cognitive decline. (Nimgampalle et al., 2023).

In Neurodegenerative disease i.e. Parkinson's disease linked to Dopamine (DA) disruption. DA plays a crucial role in neural development, influencing processes like neuronal proliferation, migration, maturation, and connectivity. Disrupting dopamine signaling during developmental periods can alter embryonic development. Dopaminergic neurons are primarily found in three key areas: the substantia nigra (SN), ventral tegmental area (VTA), and a caudal extension of the SN containing dopamine-producing cells (Fallon & Moore,1978; Deutch et al., 1991). The substantia nigra (SN) and ventral tegmental area (VTA) play significant roles in cognition and are implicated in affective and behavioral disorders (Roeper, 2013), partly due to their overlap with the brain reward and limbic systems (Koob & Swerdlow, 1988). Dopamine in the SN and VTA regions is also involved in stimulus-conditioned responses (Bassareo & De Luca, 2002) and regulating locomotor activity. Mesocortical dopaminergic projections from the VTA and medial SN densely innervate multiple cortical areas, including prefrontal, cingulate, and entorhinal regions, as well as the hippocampus. The mesostriatal pathway originates from dopaminergic neurons in the SN ventral tier, projecting to the dorsal striatum (Fallon & Moore, 1978; Voorn et al., 1988), where dopamine modulates GABAergic and cholinergic neurons, influencing striatal output. Dopamine signaling in the dorsal striatum is integral to motor activity regulation, reward-based learning, and motor sequence control, supporting cognitive function and motor performance (Calabresi et al., 2000; Leisman, Braun-Benjamin, & Melillo, 2014). Cortical glutamatergic inputs to the striatum influence dopaminergic neurons in the SN-VTA through striatal feedback mechanisms. (Voorn et al., 1988; Robbins & Everitt, 1992; Calabresi et al., 2000).

Serotonin (5-HT) plays a critical role in mood regulation in the CNS. Altered 5-HT function is linked to various disorders, including, anxiety, and sleep disorders and cognitive slowing (Stockmeier, 2003; Albert et al., 2014). Additionally, 5-HT is implicated in the acquisition and retrieval of knowledge (Meneses et al. 1999; Faulkner & Deakin, 2014). Glutamate is a prevalent amino acid that acts as a crucial neurotransmitter in the brain, primarily stored in and released by glutamatergic neurons to facilitate neural signaling.

Dopamine (DA) disruption linked to Parkinson's disease, serotonin (5-HT) disruption contributes to depression, anxiety and cognitive slowing, Norepinephrine deficiency leads to attention deficits poor focus, GABA (gamma -aminobutyric acid) dysfunction may result in cognitive inhibition and Parkinson's disease, Acetylcholine (ACh) deficiency linked to Alzheimer's disease. Norepinephrine deficiency leads to attention deficits poor focus, GABA (gamma -aminobutyric acid) dysfunction may result in cognitive inhibition and Parkinson's disease, Acetylcholine (ACh) deficiency linked to Alzheimer's disease. (Babić Leko & Šimić, 2021). Neurotransmitter disruption is a central mechanism in various cognitive disorders. Targeting this disruption, pharmacological or behavioural interventions hold potential for improving cognitive function and quality of life. (Davis et al., 2023).

Antiepileptic drugs (AEDs) impact cognition by reducing neuronal excitability or enhancing inhibitory neurotransmission. While monotherapy typically results in modest cognitive side effects, these can still be clinically significant. Epilepsy patients treated with AEDs in a specialty clinic experienced significant declines in perceived quality of life due to subtle neurotoxic symptoms, despite several overt signs of toxicity on neurological examination. Increased risk of cognitive impairment is associated with polytherapy or high serum levels of AEDs. Common cognitive side effects of AED therapy include sedation, somnolence, distractibility, insomnia, and dizziness. Sedation is a frequent side effect of AEDs. Adults typically experience cognitive depression, whereas children may experience behavioural changes like aggression and hyperactivity. Multiple factors beyond AEDs can impact cognitive function in epilepsy patients, highlighting the complexity of managing the condition. Neurotransmitters are the brain's signaling molecules, bridging the gaps between nerve cells to enable transmission of neural messages. It is found in the brain, such as Dopamine, serotonin, Norepinephrine, GABA, and Acetylcholine, etc, play a critical role in regulating mood, memory, movement, and cognitive functions. Any dysfunction. In secretion, regulation, and functions of these neurotransmitters induce neurodegeneration and cognitive decline.

Glutamate production involves the conversion of glutamine by phosphate-activated glutaminase (PAG), followed by storage in synaptic vesicles via VGLUT1 and VGLUT2 transporters (Albrecht et al., 2007). Membrane depolarization triggers Ca^{2+} influx, prompting synaptic vesicle fusion and it is release into the synaptic cleft via exocytosis. Glutamate is cleared from the synaptic cleft through reuptake by excitatory amino acid transporters (EAATs) located on neurons and glial cells. Astrocytes convert glutamate to glutamine using glutamine synthase, and glutamine is subsequently transferred to neurons, potentially via system N and A transporters (Albrecht et al., 2007; Liguz-Lecznar & Skangiel-Kramska, 2007; Lee & Pow, 2010). After being released, glutamate binds to specific postsynaptic receptors, enabling excitatory transmission between neurons. Glutamate effects are mediated by two main receptor types: ionotropic and metabotropic receptors, which have distinct molecular, biochemical, and physiological properties (Kew, 2005; Kim et al., 2001). Presynaptic glutamate receptors also modulate glutamate release. Ionotropic glutamate receptors are categorized into three subgroups: AMPA, NMDA, and kainate receptors (Dingledine et al., 1999; Horning & Mayer, 2004). AMPA and kainate receptors primarily mediate fast excitatory transmission in the CNS. NMDA receptors are blocked by Mg^{2+} at resting potentials, but depolarization relieves this block, enabling Ca^{2+} and Na^{+} entry (Cull-Candy, Brickley, & Farrant, 2001). These receptors typically consist of GluN1 and GluN2 subunits (Prybylowski & Wenthold, 2004).

Physical Cognitive Impairment

Physical cognitive impairment in Parkinson's and Alzheimer's disease includes Resting tremor, muscle stiffness, postural instability, Bradykinesia, incontinence, risk of infections, shuffling gait, masked facial expression, speech and swallowing difficulties. These types of physical issues develop in later stages. (Zhao etal;2024). Physical cognitive impairment in Parkinson's and Alzheimer's disease includes Resting tremor, muscle stiffness, postural instability, Bradykinesia, incontinence, risk of infections, shuffling gait, masked facial expression, speech and swallowing difficulties. These types of physical issues develop in later stages.

Epilepsy, a prevalent neurological condition, involves recurring seizures and frequently co-occurs with neurocognitive impairments. Learning and memory deficits in epilepsy reflect hippocampal network disruptions that are similarly implicated in various neurodegenerative conditions (Knierim, 2015; Holmes, G.L.,2015). Aging is linked to declines in learning and working memory (Schneider-Garces, etal.,2010). Both mild cognitive impairment (MCI) and Alzheimer disease (AD) affect verbal information processing, with AD patients showing more pronounced deficits, (Guerreiro, et al., 2006; Mast & Allaire, 2006; Greenaway et al., 2006). Impaired verbal learning, despite repeated exposure, is a hallmark of AD and a predictor of functional decline (Mast, & Allaire, 2006; Greenaway, et al., 2006). The role of immature neurons in human cognition, particularly in specific functions, is still unknown. Deficits in hippocampal neurogenesis, seen in early MCI and AD could broadly impact verbal learning and memory in neurological disorders, (Tobin et al., 2019).

DIAGNOSTIC TOOLS AND BIOMARKERS FOR NDs

Neurodegeneration, characterized by progressive neuronal loss and dysfunction, underlies various neurological disorders, including Alzheimer; s disease (AD), Parkinson's disease (PD), amyotrophic lateral sclerosis (ALS), and multiple sclerosis (MS). The prevalence of these conditions is rising, largely due to the growing aging population. Detecting neurodegenerative diseases in their earliest stages presents the highest likelihood of successful medical intervention (Gómez-Río et al., 2016). Identifying NDs as early as possible can help slow or even stop disease progression, offering a critical window for intervention. The term & quot; biomarker & quot; covers various molecules, from small to large, including nucleic acids, proteins, and metabolites, identifiable using advanced technologies like genomics and Proteomics. MicroRNAs (miRNAs) in circulation show potential as biomarkers for detecting neurodegenerative diseases. (Laterza, et al.,2007).

To well sense the invisible and ongoing changes in the brain, the crossing of technology and medicine stands out as a precautionary strategy. Many different diagnostic tools and biomarkers detect Neurological disease depends on identifying neurotransmitter-related changes.

Table 1. Diagnostic tools and Biomarker for diagnosis neurodegenerative disorders

S.NO.	Diagnostic tools	Biomarkers	Disorders
1)	Positron emission tomography (PET)	Serotonergic biomarker (5-Hydroxyindoleacetic acid). Noradrenergic biomarker(3-Methyoxy-4-hydroxyphenylglycol). Cholinergic biomarkers (choline acetyltransferase). Dopaminergic biomarkers (Isoflurane).	Parkinson's and Alzheimer's disease.
2)	Magnetic Resonance spectroscopy (MRS)	GABAergic biomarker and Glutamatergic biomarker	Alzheimer's and Huntington's disease.

MicroRNAs are considered promising biomarkers due to their detectability in various bodily fluids, such as CSF and blood, with high specificity across different biological samples (Quinlan, et al.,2017). miRNAs are implicated in the modulation of synaptic plasticity, neuro-genesis, and neuronal differentiation, highlighting their importance in neural development and function (Grasso, et al.,2014). MicroRNAs are small, 21-22 nucleotide long RNA molecules that constitute about 1% of human genes code for proteins (O'Brien et al., 2018). It modulated post-transcriptional gene expression, impacting key cellular processes, including cell growth, development, and programmed cell death (apoptosis) (Saliminejad, etal.,2019). MiRNAs are considered promising biomarkers due to their detectability in various bodily fluids, such as CSF and blood, with high specificity across different biological samples (Quinlan, etal.,2017). Studies in animal models have demonstrated that disturbed miRNA binding causes defects in healthy brain development, highlighting the importance of miRNAs in neurodevelopment (Quinlan, S.; Kenny, A. et al.2017). Research by Burgos et al. identified specific miRNAs in blood and CSF of patients with neurodegenerative diseases, mirroring those found in brain samples (Burgos, et al.,2014). The dysregulation of miRNAs has been linked to various neurodegenerative disorders,

including AD, PD, ALS, and MS, characterized by neuronal death (Juźwik, C.A.; Drake, S.S. etal.,2019; Manna, I.; De Benedittis, S.et al.,2020). The main pathological hallmarks of Alzheimer disease (AD) include amyloid plaques composed of Aβ deposits and tau protein accumulation in neurofibrillary tangles (Crews, etal;2010). Additionally, neuroinflammation is a key feature of AD, associated with oxidative stress triggered by inflammatory processes in the brain (Calsolaro, et al; 2016). The diagnostic biomarkers for Alzheimer s disease in cerebrospinal fluid are Aβ, tTau, and pTau (Blennow, etal;2018). Amyloid-β is relesed into biological fluids like CSF during normal APP metabolism, even in the absence of disease (Haass, et al; 1992). Research confirms that AD patients often have decreased levels of circulating Aβ, contrasting with healthy controls (Galozzi, et al. 2015). Tau dysfunction leads to synaptic impairment, and phosphorylated tau protein is the primary component of neurofibrillary tangles (NFTs) (Blennow, et al; 2018). Elevated CSF levels of total tau (tTau) have been observed in AD patients, correlating with disease severity. miRNAs may regulate tau protein, particularly its phosphorylation. Aβ can induce reactive oxygen species (ROS), leading to oxidative stress (Cheignon, C.; Tomas, M. et al.,2018). Notably, miR-125b promotes APP and BACE1 expression, increasing Aβ production, as shown in an in vitro AD model (Jin.etal.,2018). Parkinson disease (PD) is the second most common neurodegenerative disorder globally (Elbaz, et al. 2016). Characterized by progressive motor symptoms, PD involves degeneration of the nigrostriatal dopaminergic pathway, affecting both motor and non-motor neurons. Parkinson disease motor symptoms comprise bradykinesia, resting tremor, limb rigidity, and postural instability, affecting balance and coordination (Ling, etal.,2012). Other proteins that frequently aggregate in ALS include wild-type superoxide dismutase 1 (SOD1) and ubiquilin 2 (Qin, et al.,2012; Bosco, et al.,2010). Neuroinflammation, featuring microgliosis and astrogliosis, is a component of ALS pathology, occurring with neurodegeneration (Brown, 2006; Philips & Rothstein, 2014). The C9orf72 mutation leads to increased toxicity, resulting in loss of function of neurons, including motor and non-motor neurons (Balendra & Isaacs, 2018). Over 50 mutations have been identified, primarily associated with cognitive impairment in ALS patients (Ishigaki & Sobue, 2018). Neurofilaments, abundant in neurons, have been implicated in this pathology (Vu & Bowser, 2017).

The progressive degeneration of upper and lower motor neurons in ALS results in symptoms like muscle stiffness, spasticity, and twitching. In ALS, disease progression leads to neuromuscular junction loss and muscular atrophy (Brown, 2006), with cognitive impairment observed in around 50% of patients (van etal.,2017). ALS like other neurodegenerative diseases, involves the accumulation of misfolded proteins, notably TDP-43, which undergoes pathological modifications like phosphorylation and mislocalization in motor neurons (Neumann, etal.,2006).

Neurofilaments, released into CSF and blood following axonal injury, show promise as ALS biomarkers. Specifically, phosphorylated neurofilament heavy chains (pNfH) are elevated in ALS patients compared to healthy controls (Vu & Bowser, 2017; Brettschneider et al., 2006). Multiple sclerosis (MS) is a chronic autoimmune disease characterized by demyelination, inflammation, and neurodegeneration in the central nervous system (Axisa & Hafler, 2016). Multiple sclerosis typically affects young to middle-aged adults (20-40 years), with a notable female predominance (Harbo, etal.,2013). In MS, activated T and B cells are thought to cross the blood-brain barrier, entering the CNS and triggering inflammatory responses that target the myelin sheath (Maglione, etal.,2021).

FUTURE DEVELOPMENT DIRECTIONS FOR RESEARCH

Neurodegeneration is a chronic neurological disorder characterized by recurrent seizures, is commonly managed with antiepileptic drugs (AEDs). Future research in NDs focus on understanding how dopaminergic, cholinergic and glutamatergic system interact across stage of diseases like Parkinson's and Alzheimer's and understand the future remedies for Neuroprotection, Enzyme pathway based drugs discovery, Stem cell therapy, regenerative medicine, Neuroimmune modulation, Biomarkers discovery (Muti- target and early -stage interventions), Neuroimaging advance, Combination therapies (reduce risks of NDS). (Hermans etal;2025). Future drugs will be targeted to specific neurotransmitter receptors or receptor subtypes, reducing side effects and increasing efficiency. Understanding these interactions offers a critical opportunity to design safer therapeutic with neuroprotective and cognition sparing profiles. The future of AED research lies in detailed mapping of neurotransmitter disruptions associated with each class of AED. Modern technologies like liquid chromatography-mass spectrometry (LC-MS), Magnetic resonance spectroscopy (MRS), and PET imaging can provide quantitative insight into neurotransmitter concentrations in specific brain regions. (Song etal;2025). Future research directions should integrate molecular studies (e.g., choline acetyltransferase, acetylcholinesterase), genetic markers (e.g., COMT, MAO-A/B POLYMORPHISM) and pharmacogenomic profiling. Future research should invest in advanced 3D human brain organoids, ipsc-derived neurons, and computational models to predict neurotransmitter disruption patterns of new AEDS, Simulate long term cognitive effects based on molecular signatures. (Barthel etal;2022). To better assess the cognitive impact of AEDs in clinical setting, there is a growing need for standardized cognitive biomarkers and digital cognitive assessments. Traditional neuropsychological test may lack sensitivity or consistency. The innovations may include EEG-based cognitive load markers, functional MRI and wearable technologies. (Amartumur etal;2024). However; the future of research holds immense promise through multi-dimensional strategies that integrate molecular, neurochemical, and behavioural neuroscience. Understanding these interactions offers a critical opportunity to design safer therapeutics with neuroprotective and cognition sparing profiles. (Gao etal;2025).

CONCLUSION

AEDs exert their antiepileptic effects by modulating the excitatory and inhibitory balance in the brain, primarily through interaction with major neurotransmitter system such as gamma- aminobutyric system such as gamma- aminobutyric (GABA), glutamate, acetylcholine, dopamine, serotonin and norepinephrine. While targeting these system is necessary to control hyperexcitability, the non-selective and chronic alteration of these neurotransmitters can disrupt synaptic homeostasis and neuroplasticity, both of which are essential for learning and memory. However; excessive GABAergic stimulation may impair long term potentiation (LTP), a cellular correlate of learning and memory, particularly in the hippocampus. Furthermore, chronic GABAergic enhancement can cause sedation, attentional deficits, and psychomotor slowing, which cumulatively contribute to cognitive decline. The cognitive burden associated with these AEDs often present as word finding difficulty, working memory impairment and reduced verbal fluency. Despite these challenges, it is important to note that cognitive outcomes are not uniform across all patients or AEDs. Factor such as drug type, dosages, duration of treatment, age of the patient, comorbidi-

ties, polypharmacy, genetic predisposition, and even the type of neurodegeneration all influence the degree of cognitive impairment. In summary, the intersection of antiepileptic drug therapy, neurotransmitter disruption, and cognitive decline is a complex yet critically important area of research. While AEDs remain essential for seizure control, their impact on brain chemistry and cognition must not be overlooked. Continued research into the mechanism of neurotransmitter disruption, coupled with technological innovations and patient centered care strategies, will be essential for advancing safe, effective, and neuroprotective treatment options for people with neurodegeneration. The future of neurodegeneration management should aim not only at seizure freedom but also at preserving and enhancing cognitive health recognizing that cognitive well beings is fundamental to overall quality of life.

REFERENCES

Alarcón, T. A., Presti-Silva, S. M., Simões, A. P. T., Ribeiro, F. M., & Pires, R. G. W. (2023). Molecular mechanisms underlying the neuroprotection of environmental enrichment in Parkinson's disease. *Neural Regeneration Research, 18*(5), 1050–1057. DOI: 10.4103/1673-5374.360264

Albert, P. R., Vahid-Ansari, F., & Luckhart, C. (2014). Serotonin-prefrontal cortical circuitry in anxiety and depression phenotypes: Pivotal role of pre- and post-synaptic 5-HT1A receptor expression. *Frontiers in Behavioral Neuroscience, 8*, 199. Advance online publication. DOI: 10.3389/fnbeh.2014.00199

Alharbi, B., Al-Kuraishy, H. M., Al-Gareeb, A. I., Elekhnawy, E., Alharbi, H., Alexiou, A., & Batiha, G. E. S. (2024). Role of GABA pathway in motor and non-motor symptoms in Parkinson's disease: A bidirectional circuit. *European Journal of Medical Research, 29*(1), 205. Advance online publication. DOI: 10.1186/s40001-024-01788-5

Alqahtani, F., Assiri, M. A., Mohany, M., Imran, I., Javaid, S., Rasool, M. F., & Alamri, F. F. (2020). Coadministration of ketamine and perampanel improves behavioral function and reduces inflammation in acute traumatic brain injury mouse model. *BioMed Research International, 2020*, 3193725. Advance online publication. DOI: 10.1155/2020/3193725

Amanollahi, M., Jameie, M., Heidari, A., & Rezaei, N. (2023). The dialogue between neuroinflammation and adult neurogenesis: Mechanisms involved and alterations in neurological diseases. *Molecular Neurobiology, 60*(3), 1613–1633. DOI: 10.1007/s12035-022-03102-z

Ammothumkandy, A., Corona, L., Ravina, K., Smith, J. A. D., & Bonaguidi, M. A. (2025). Human adult neurogenesis loss corresponds with cognitive decline during epilepsy progression. *Cell Stem Cell, 32*(2), 293–301. DOI: 10.1016/j.stem.2024.11.002

Ammothumkandy, A., Ravina, K., Wolseley, V., Tartt, A. N., Yu, P. N., & Corona, L. (2022). Altered adult neurogenesis and gliogenesis in patients with mesial temporal lobe epilepsy. *Nature Neuroscience, 25*(4), 493–503. DOI: 10.1038/s41593-022-01044-2

Andersen, A. M. (1975). Structural studies of metabolic products of dopamine. III. Crystal and molecular structure of (—)-adrenaline. *Acta Chemica Scandinavica, Series B, 29*(2), 239–244. DOI: 10.3891/acta.chem.scand.29b-0239

Andoh, M., Ikegaya, Y., & Koyama, R. (2019). Synaptic pruning by microglia in epilepsy. *Journal of Clinical Medicine, 8*(12), 2170. Advance online publication. DOI: 10.3390/jcm8122170

Ascherio, A. (2013). Environmental factors in multiple sclerosis. *Expert Review of Neurotherapeutics, 13*(12, Suppl.), 3–9. DOI: 10.1586/14737175.2013.865866

Axisa, P. P., & Hafler, D. A. (2016). Multiple sclerosis: Genetics, biomarkers, treatments. *Current Opinion in Neurology, 29*(3), 345–353. DOI: 10.1097/WCO.0000000000000319

Babić Leko, M., & Šimić, G. (2021). 5-HT interaction with other neurotransmitters: Experimental evidence and therapeutic relevance. In Progress in brain research. Elsevier. DOI: 10.1016/bs.pbr.2021.01.001

Balendra, R., & Isaacs, A. M. (2018). C9orf72-mediated ALS and FTD: Multiple disease pathways. *Nature Reviews. Neurology, 14*(7), 399–413. DOI: 10.1038/s41582-018-0047-2

Barthel, H., Villemagne, V. L., & Drzezga, A. (2022). Future directions in molecular imaging of neurodegenerative disorders. *Journal of Nuclear Medicine, 63*(Suppl. 1), 36S–41S. DOI: 10.2967/jnumed.121.263202

Bassareo, V., & De Luca, M. A. (2002). Differential expression of motivational stimulus properties by dopamine in nucleus accumbens shell versus core and prefrontal cortex. *The Journal of Neuroscience : The Official Journal of the Society for Neuroscience, 22*(11), 4709–4719. DOI: 10.1523/JNEUROSCI.22-11-04709.2002

Berridge, C. W., Arnsten, A. F. T., & Foote, S. L. (1993). Noradrenergic modulation of cognitive function: Clinical implications of anatomical, electrophysiological and behavioural studies in animal models. *Psychological Medicine, 23*(3), 557–564. DOI: 10.1017/S0033291700025332

Blennow, K., & Zetterberg, H. (2018). Biomarkers for Alzheimer's disease: Current status and prospects for the future. *Journal of Internal Medicine, 284*(6), 643–663. DOI: 10.1111/joim.12816

Bosco, D. A., Morfini, G., Karabacak, N. M., Song, Y., Gros-Louis, F., Pasinelli, P., Goolsby, H., Fontaine, B. A., Lemay, N., McKenna-Yasek, D., & Brown, R. H.Jr. (2010). Wild-type and mutant SOD1 share an aberrant conformation and a common pathogenic pathway in ALS. *Nature Neuroscience, 13*(11), 1396–1403. DOI: 10.1038/nn.2660

Brettschneider, J., Petzold, A., Süssmuth, S. D., Ludolph, A. C., & Tumani, H. (2006). Axonal damage markers in cerebrospinal fluid are increased in ALS. *Neurology, 66*(6), 852–856. DOI: 10.1212/01.wnl.0000203120.85850.54

Brodie, M. J., & Sills, G. J. (2011). Combining antiepileptic drugs—Rational polytherapy? *Seizure, 20*(5), 369–375. DOI: 10.1016/j.seizure.2011.01.004

Brown, D. A. (2006). Acetylcholine. *British Journal of Pharmacology, 147*(S1), S120–S129. DOI: 10.1038/sj.bjp.0706474

Burgos, K., Malenica, I., Metpally, R., Courtright, A., Rakela, B., Beach, T., Shill, H., Adler, C., Sabbagh, M., Villa, S., & Craig, D. W. (2014). Profiles of extracellular miRNA in cerebrospinal fluid and serum from patients with Alzheimer's and Parkinson's diseases correlate with disease status and features of pathology. *PLoS One, 9*(5), e94839. Advance online publication. DOI: 10.1371/journal.pone.0094839

Calabresi, P., Centonze, D., Gubellini, P., Marfia, G. A., Pisani, A., Sancesario, G., & Bernardi, G. (2000). Synaptic transmission in the striatum: From plasticity to neurodegeneration. *Progress in Neurobiology, 61*(3), 231–265. DOI: 10.1016/S0301-0082(99)00030-1

Calsolaro, V., & Edison, P. (2016). Neuroinflammation in Alzheimer's disease: Current evidence and future directions. *Alzheimer's & Dementia, 12*(6), 719–732. DOI: 10.1016/j.jalz.2016.02.010

Campos-Bedolla, P., Feria-Romero, I., & Orozco-Suárez, S. (2022). Factors not considered in the study of drug-resistant epilepsy: Drug-resistant epilepsy: Assessment of neuroinflammation. *Epilepsia Open, 7*(3), 404–409. DOI: 10.1002/epi4.12590

Chartier, S., & Duyckaerts, C. (2018). Is Lewy pathology in the human nervous system chiefly an indicator of neuronal protection or of toxicity? *Cell and Tissue Research*, *373*(1), 149–160. DOI: 10.1007/s00441-018-2854-6

Cheignon, C., Tomas, M., Bonnefont-Rousselot, D., Faller, P., Hureau, C., & Collin, F. (2018). Oxidative stress and the amyloid beta peptide in Alzheimer's disease. *Redox Biology*, *14*, 450–464. DOI: 10.1016/j.redox.2017.10.014

Cheli, M., Dinoto, A., Biaduzzini, F., Tomaselli, M., Mazzon, G., Roman-Pognuz, E., & Manganotti, P. (2021). Super refractory post-traumatic status epilepticus treated by combining perampanel and ketamine. *Journal of the Neurological Sciences*, *429*, 119103. Advance online publication. DOI: 10.1016/j.jns.2021.119103

Chen, X., & Zhang, Y. (2025). A review of the neurotransmitter system associated with cognitive function of the cerebellum in Parkinson's disease. *Neural Regeneration Research*, *20*(2), 379–384. DOI: 10.4103/1673-5374.379042

Chen, Z. P., Wang, S., Zhao, X., Fang, W., Wang, Z., Ye, H., & Zhang, J. (2023). Lipid-accumulated reactive astrocytes promote disease progression in epilepsy. *Nature Neuroscience*, *26*(4), 542–554. DOI: 10.1038/s41593-023-01288-6

Coan, A. C., & Cendes, F. (2013). Epilepsy as a progressive disorder: What is the evidence that can guide our clinical decisions, and how can neuroimaging help? *Epilepsy & Behavior*, *26*(3), 313–321. DOI: 10.1016/j.yebeh.2012.09.027

Crews, L., & Masliah, E. (2010). Molecular mechanisms of neurodegeneration in Alzheimer's disease. *Human Molecular Genetics*, *19*(R1), R12–R20. DOI: 10.1093/hmg/ddq160

Crombie, G. K., Palliser, H. K., Shaw, J. C., Hodgson, D. M., Walker, D. W., & Hirst, J. J. (2022). Evaluating changes in GABAergic and glutamatergic pathways in early life following prenatal stress and postnatal neurosteroid supplementation. *Trends in Neurosciences*, *16*(3), 187–198. DOI: 10.1016/j.tins.1993.03.005

Cull-Candy, S., Brickley, S., & Farrant, M. (2001). NMDA receptor subunits: Diversity, development and disease. *Current Opinion in Neurobiology*, *11*(3), 327–335. DOI: 10.1016/S0959-4388(00)00215-4

Davis, S. E., Cirincione, A. B., & Jimenez-Torres, A. C. (2023). The impact of neurotransmitters on the neurobiology of neurodegenerative diseases. *International Journal of Molecular Sciences*, *24*(20), 15340. Advance online publication. DOI: 10.3390/ijms242015340

Deng, X., Shao, Y., Xie, Y., Feng, Y., Wu, M., Wang, M., & Liao, W. (2019). MicroRNA-146a-5p downregulates the expression of P-glycoprotein in rats with lithium-pilocarpine-induced status epilepticus. *Biological & Pharmaceutical Bulletin*, *42*(5), 744–750. DOI: 10.1248/bpb.b18-00937

Deutch, A. Y., Lee, M. C., Gillham, M. H., Cameron, D. A., Goldstein, M., & Iadarola, M. J. (1991). Stress selectively increases fos protein in dopamine neurons innervating the prefrontal cortex. *Cerebral Cortex (New York, N.Y.)*, *1*(4), 273–292. DOI: 10.1093/cercor/1.4.273

Dingledine, R., Borges, K., Bowie, D., & Traynelis, S. F. (1999). The glutamate receptor ion channels. *Pharmacological Reviews*, *51*(1), 7–61. https://pubmed.ncbi.nlm.nih.gov/10049997/

Doroszkiewicz, J., Groblewska, M., & Mroczko, B. (2022). Molecular biomarkers and their implications for the early diagnosis of selected neurodegenerative diseases. *International Journal of Molecular Sciences*, *23*(9), 4610. Advance online publication. DOI: 10.3390/ijms23094610

Downs, A. M., & McElligott, Z. A. (2020). Noradrenergic circuits and signaling in substance use disorders. *Current Topics in Behavioral Neurosciences*, *49*, 249–270. DOI: 10.1007/7854_2020_178

Elbaz, A., Carcaillon, L., Kab, S., & Moisan, F. (2016). Epidemiology of Parkinson's disease. *Revue Neurologique*, *172*(1), 14–26. DOI: 10.1016/j.neurol.2015.09.012

Fallon, J. H., & Moore, R. Y. (1978). Catecholamine innervation of the basal forebrain. IV. Topography of the dopamine projection to the basal forebrain and neostriatum. *The Journal of Comparative Neurology*, *180*(3), 545–580. DOI: 10.1002/cne.901800310

Faulkner, P., & Deakin, J. F. (2014). The role of serotonin in reward, punishment, and behavioural inhibition in humans: Insights from studies with acute tryptophan depletion. *Neuroscience and Biobehavioral Reviews*, *46*(Pt. 3), 365–378. DOI: 10.1016/j.neubiorev.2014.07.024

Feigin, V. L., Nichols, E., Alam, T., Bannick, M. S., Beghi, E., Blake, N., Culpepper, W. J., Dorsey, E. R., Elbaz, A., Ellenbogen, R. G., & Murray, C. J. L. (2019). Global, regional, and national burden of epilepsy, 1990–2016: A systematic analysis for the Global Burden of Disease Study 2016. *Lancet Neurology*, *18*(4), 357–375. DOI: 10.1016/S1474-4422(18)30454-X

Feng, L., Murugan, M., Bosco, D. B., Liu, Y., Peng, J., Worrell, G. A., & Wu, L. J. (2019). Microglial proliferation and monocyte infiltration contribute to microgliosis following status epilepticus. *Glia*, *67*(8), 1540–1554. DOI: 10.1002/glia.23616

Fisher, R. S., van Emde Boas, W., Blume, W., Elger, C., Genton, P., Lee, P., & Engel, J.Jr. (2005). Epileptic seizures and epilepsy: Definitions proposed by the International League Against Epilepsy (ILAE) and the International Bureau for Epilepsy (IBE). *Epilepsia*, *46*(4), 470–472. DOI: 10.1111/j.0013-9580.2005.66104.x

Gallagher, D. A., Lees, A. J., & Schrag, A. (2010). What are the most important nonmotor symptoms in patients with Parkinson's disease, and are we missing them? *Movement Disorders*, *25*(15), 2493–2500. DOI: 10.1002/mds.23394

Galozzi, S., Marcus, K., & Barkovits, K. (2015). Amyloid-β as a biomarker for Alzheimer's disease: Quantification methods in body fluids. *Expert Review of Proteomics*, *12*(4), 343–354. DOI: 10.1586/14789450.2015.1065183

Garg, N., & Smith, T. W. (2015). An update on immunopathogenesis, diagnosis, and treatment of multiple sclerosis. *Brain and Behavior*, *5*(9), e00362. Advance online publication. DOI: 10.1002/brb3.362

Giraldez, A. J., Cinalli, R. M., Glasner, M. E., Enright, A. J., Thomson, J. M., Baskerville, S., Hammond, S. M., Bartel, D. P., & Schier, A. F. (2005). MicroRNAs regulate brain morphogenesis in zebrafish. *Science*, *308*(5723), 833–838. DOI: 10.1126/science.1109020

Goldsmith, D. R., Bekhbat, M., Mehta, N. D., & Felger, J. C. (2023). Inflammation-related functional and structural dysconnectivity as a pathway to psychopathology. *Biological Psychiatry*, *93*(5), 405–418. DOI: 10.1016/j.biopsych.2022.11.003

Gómez-Río, M., Moreno Caballero, M., Górriz Sáez, J. M., & Mínguez-Castellanos, A. (2016). Diagnosis of neurodegenerative diseases: The clinical approach. *Current Alzheimer Research*, *13*(5), 469–474. DOI: 10.2174/1567205013666151116141603

Grasso, M., Piscopo, P., Confaloni, A., & Denti, M. A. (2014). Circulating miRNAs as biomarkers for neurodegenerative disorders. *Molecules (Basel, Switzerland)*, *19*(5), 6891–6910. DOI: 10.3390/molecules19056891

Greenaway, M. C., Lacritz, L. H., & Binegar, D. (2006). Patterns of verbal memory performance in mild cognitive impairment, Alzheimer's disease, and normal aging. *Cognitive and Behavioral Neurology*, *19*(2), 79–84. DOI: 10.1097/01.wnn.0000208290.57370.a3

Guerreiro, M., Ribeiro, F., & de Mendonça, A. (2006). P3–039: Mild cognitive impairment: Neuropsychological performance. *Alzheimer's & Dementia*, *2*(3, Suppl.), S390. DOI: 10.1016/j.jalz.2006.05.1306

Gülçin, İ. (2009). Antioxidant activity of L-adrenaline: A structure-activity insight. *Chemico-Biological Interactions*, *179*(2–3), 71–80. DOI: 10.1016/j.cbi.2008.09.023

Gundersen, Y., Vaagenes, P., Dreiem, A., & Fonnum, F. (2004). Glycine. In *Encyclopedia of neuroscience* (pp. 1–10). Elsevier. DOI: 10.1016/B0-12-227210-2/00158-8

Haass, C., Schlossmacher, M. G., Hung, A. Y., Vigo-Pelfrey, C., Mellon, A., Ostaszewski, B. L., Lieberburg, I., Koo, E. H., Schenk, D., Teplow, D. B., & Selkoe, D. J. (1992). Amyloid beta-peptide is produced by cultured cells during normal metabolism. *Nature*, *359*(6393), 322–325. DOI: 10.1038/359322a0

Hampel, H., Mesulam, M. M., Cuello, A. C., Farlow, M. R., Giacobini, E., Grossberg, G. T., & Khachaturian, Z. S. (2018). The cholinergic system in the pathophysiology and treatment of Alzheimer's disease. *Brain*, *141*(7), 1917–1933. DOI: 10.1093/brain/awy132

Harbo, H. F., Gold, R., & Tintoré, M. (2013). Sex and gender issues in multiple sclerosis. *Therapeutic Advances in Neurological Disorders*, *6*(4), 237–248. DOI: 10.1177/1756285613488434

Helmstaedter, C. (2001). Behavioral aspects of frontal lobe epilepsy. *Epilepsy & Behavior*, *2*(5), 384–395. DOI: 10.1006/ebeh.2001.0253

Helmstaedter, C., Elger, C. E., & Witt, J. A. (2016). The effect of quantitative and qualitative antiepileptic drug changes on cognitive recovery after epilepsy surgery. *Seizure*, *36*, 63–69. DOI: 10.1016/j.seizure.2016.02.001

Helmstaedter, C., & Kurthen, M. (2001). Memory and epilepsy: Characteristics, course, and influence of drugs and surgery. *Current Opinion in Neurology*, *14*(2), 211–216. DOI: 10.1097/00019052-200104000-00013

Hermann, B., Seidenberg, M., & Lee, E.-J. (2007). Cognitive phenotypes in temporal lobe epilepsy. *Journal of the International Neuropsychological Society, 13*(1), 12–20. DOI: 10.1017/S135561770707004X

Hermans, A. M. M., Bakker, E., Starokozhko, V., den Otter, L., Elferink, A. J. A., Bradshaw, A., Guizzaro, L., Mol, P. G. M., & Pasmooij, A. M. G. (2025). Biomarkers for neurodegenerative diseases in regulatory decision-making by the European Medicines Agency. *Alzheimer's & Dementia: Translational Research & Clinical Interventions, 11*(1), e70072. Advance online publication. DOI: 10.1002/trc2.70072

Hernandes, M. S., & Troncone, L. R. P. (2009). Glycine as a neurotransmitter in the forebrain. *Journal of Neural Transmission (Vienna, Austria), 116*(11), 1473–1480. DOI: 10.1007/s00702-009-0326-6

Holmes, G. L. (2015). Cognitive impairment in epilepsy: The role of network abnormalities. *Epileptic Disorders, 17*(2), 101–116. DOI: 10.1684/epd.2015.0739

Horning, M. S., & Mayer, M. L. (2004). Regulation of AMPA receptor gating by ligand binding core dimers. *Neuron, 41*(3), 379–388. DOI: 10.1016/S0896-6273(04)00003-0

Ibragimov, S., Rustamova, D., Ganieva, A., & Zubaydilloeva, Z. (2021). Adrenaline, and what processes occur under its action in our body. *Grail of Science, 9*, 377–381. DOI: 10.36074/grail-of-science.22.10.2021.71

Iovino, L., Tremblay, M. E., & Civiero, L. (2020). Glutamate-induced excitotoxicity in Parkinson's disease: The role of glial cells. *Journal of Pharmacological Sciences, 144*(3), 151–164. DOI: 10.1016/j.jphs.2020.07.011

Ishigaki, S., & Sobue, G. (2018). Importance of functional loss of FUS in FTLD/ALS. *Frontiers in Molecular Biosciences, 5*, 44. Advance online publication. DOI: 10.3389/fmolb.2018.00044

Jin, Y., Tu, Q., & Liu, M. (2018). MicroRNA-125b regulates Alzheimer's disease through SphK1 regulation. *Molecular Medicine Reports, 18*(2), 2373–2380. DOI: 10.3892/mmr.2018.9156

Johnson, K. A., Conn, P. J., & Niswender, C. M. (2009). Glutamate receptors as therapeutic targets for Parkinson's disease. *CNS & Neurological Disorders - Drug Targets, 8*(6), 475–491. DOI: 10.2174/187152709789824606

Juźwik, C. A., Drake, S. S., Zhang, Y., Paradis-Isler, N., Sylvester, A., Amar-Zifkin, A., Douglas, C., Morquette, B., Moore, C. S., & Fournier, A. E. (2019). MicroRNA dysregulation in neurodegenerative diseases: A systematic review. *Progress in Neurobiology, 182*, 101664. Advance online publication. DOI: 10.1016/j.pneurobio.2019.101664

Kanova, M., & Kohout, P. (2021). Serotonin—Its synthesis and roles in the healthy and the critically ill. *International Journal of Molecular Sciences, 22*(9), 4837. Advance online publication. DOI: 10.3390/ijms22094837

Katsari, M., Angelopoulou, G., Laskaris, N., Potagas, C., & Kasselimis, D. (2022). Common neuroanatomical substrate of cholinergic pathways and language-related brain regions as an explanatory framework for evaluating the efficacy of cholinergic pharmacotherapy in post-stroke aphasia: A review. *Brain Sciences*, *12*(10), 1390. Advance online publication. DOI: 10.3390/brainsci12101390

Kazemi, H., & Hoop, B. (1991). Glutamic acid and gamma-aminobutyric acid neurotransmitters in central control of breathing. *Journal of Applied Physiology*, *70*(1), 1–7. DOI: 10.1152/jappl.1991.70.1.1

Kim, J. H., Anwyl, R., Suh, Y. H., Djamgoz, M. B., & Rowan, M. J. (2001). Use-dependent effects of amyloidogenic fragments of β-amyloid precursor protein on synaptic plasticity in rat hippocampus in vivo. *The Journal of Neuroscience : The Official Journal of the Society for Neuroscience*, *21*(4), 1327–1333. DOI: 10.1523/JNEUROSCI.21-04-01327.2001

Kitzbichler, M. G., Aruldass, A. R., Barker, G. J., Wood, T. C., Dowell, N. G., Hurley, S. A., & Bullmore, E. T. (2021). Peripheral inflammation is associated with micro-structural and functional connectivity changes in depression-related brain networks. *Molecular Psychiatry*, *26*(12), 7346–7354. DOI: 10.1038/s41380-021-01272-3

Klement, W., Garbelli, R., Zub, E., Rossini, L., Tassi, L., Girard, B., & Aronica, E. (2018). Seizure progression and inflammatory mediators promote pericytosis and pericyte-microglia clustering at the cerebrovasculature. *Neurobiology of Disease*, *115*, 70–81. DOI: 10.1016/j.nbd.2018.02.002

Knierim, J. J. (2015). The hippocampus. *Current Biology*, *25*(23), R1116–R1121. DOI: 10.1016/j.cub.2015.10.049

Koob, G. F., & Swerdlow, N. R. (1988). The functional output of the mesolimbic dopamine system. *Annals of the New York Academy of Sciences*, *537*(1), 216–227. DOI: 10.1111/j.1749-6632.1988.tb42108.x

Krnjević, K., & Schwartz, S. (1967). The action of γ-aminobutyric acid on cortical neurones. *Experimental Brain Research*, *3*(4), 320–336. DOI: 10.1007/BF00237558

Kumari, N., Prentice, H., & Wu, J.-Y. (2013). Taurine and its neuroprotective role. In *Advances in experimental medicine and biology* (Vol. 775, pp. 19–27). Springer. DOI: 10.1007/978-1-4614-6130-2_2

Laterza, O. F., Hendrickson, R. C., & Wagner, J. A. (2007). Molecular biomarkers. *Therapeutic Innovation & Regulatory Science*, *41*(5), 573–585. DOI: 10.1177/009286150704100504

Lee, A., & Pow, D. V. (2010). Astrocytes: Glutamate transport and alternative splicing of transporters. *The International Journal of Biochemistry & Cell Biology*, *42*(12), 1891–1896. DOI: 10.1016/j.biocel.2010.09.016

Leisman, G., Braun-Benjamin, O., & Melillo, R. (2014). Cognitive-motor interactions of the basal ganglia in development. *Frontiers in Systems Neuroscience*, *8*, 16. Advance online publication. DOI: 10.3389/fnsys.2014.00016

Leslie, F. M., Loughlin, S. E., Sternberg, D. B., McGaugh, J. L., Young, L. E., & Zornetzer, S. F. (1985). Noradrenergic changes and memory loss in aged mice. *Brain Research*, *359*(1–2), 292–299. DOI: 10.1016/0006-8993(85)91439-8

Librizzi, L., Noè, F., Vezzani, A., de Curtis, M., & Ravizza, T. (2012). Seizure-induced brain-borne inflammation sustains seizure recurrence and blood-brain barrier damage. *Annals of Neurology*, *72*(1), 82–90. DOI: 10.1002/ana.23567

Liguz-Lecznar, M., & Skangiel-Kramska, J. (2007). Vesicular glutamate transporters (VGLUTs): The three musketeers of the glutamatergic system. *Acta Neurobiologiae Experimentalis*, *67*(3), 207–218. https://pubmed.ncbi.nlm.nih.gov/17957903/

Ling, H., Massey, L. A., Lees, A. J., Brown, P., & Day, B. L. (2012). Hypokinesia without decrement distinguishes progressive supranuclear palsy from Parkinson's disease. *Brain*, *135*(4), 1141–1153. DOI: 10.1093/brain/aws038

Maes, O., Chertkow, H., Wang, E., & Schipper, H. (2009). MicroRNA: Implications for Alzheimer's disease and other human CNS disorders. *Current Genomics*, *10*(3), 154–168. DOI: 10.2174/138920209788185252

Maglione, A., Zuccalà, M., Tosi, M., Clerico, M., & Rolla, S. (2021). Host genetics and gut microbiome: Perspectives for multiple sclerosis. *Genes*, *12*(8), 1181. Advance online publication. DOI: 10.3390/genes12081181

Main, M. J., Cryan, J. E., Dupere, J. R., Cox, B., Clare, J. J., & Burbidge, S. A. (2000). Modulation of KCNQ2/3 potassium channels by the novel anticonvulsant retigabine. *Molecular Pharmacology*, *58*(2), 253–262. DOI: 10.1124/mol.58.2.253

Manca, R., De Marco, M., Soininen, H., Ruffini, L., & Venneri, A. (2025). Changes in neurotransmitter-related functional connectivity along the Alzheimer's disease continuum. *Brain Communications*, *7*(1), fcaf008. Advance online publication. DOI: 10.1093/braincomms/fcaf008

Manganotti, P., Cheli, M., Dinoto, A., Biaduzzini, F., Tomaselli, M., Mazzon, G., & Meletti, S. (2021). Combining perampanel and ketamine in super refractory post-traumatic status epilepticus: A case report. *Seizure*, *89*, 114–116. DOI: 10.1016/j.seizure.2021.04.026

Manna, I., De Benedittis, S., Quattrone, A., Maisano, D., Iaccino, E., & Quattrone, A. (2020). Exosomal miRNAs as potential diagnostic biomarkers in Alzheimer's disease. *Pharmaceuticals*, *13*(9), 243. Advance online publication. DOI: 10.3390/ph13090243

Marks, D. M., Shah, M. J., Patkar, A. A., Masand, P. S., Park, G.-Y., & Pae, C.-U. (2009). Serotonin-norepinephrine reuptake inhibitors for pain control: Premise and promise. *Current Neuropharmacology*, *7*(4), 331–336. DOI: 10.2174/157015909790031201

Mast, B. T., & Allaire, J. C. (2006). Verbal learning and everyday functioning in dementia: An application of latent variable growth curve modeling. *The Journals of Gerontology: Series B*, *61*(3), 167–P173. DOI: 10.1093/geronb/61.3.P167

Milo, R., & Kahana, E. (2010). Multiple sclerosis: Geoepidemiology, genetics and the environment. *Autoimmunity Reviews*, *9*(5), A387–A394. DOI: 10.1016/j.autrev.2009.11.010

Miranda, M. I., & Bermúdez-Rattoni, F. (2007). Cholinergic activity in the insular cortex is necessary for acquisition and consolidation of contextual memory. *Neurobiology of Learning and Memory*, *87*(3), 343–351. DOI: 10.1016/j.nlm.2006.09.009

Moreno-Jiménez, E. P., & Flor-García, M. (2019). Adult hippocampal neurogenesis is abundant in neurologically healthy subjects and drops sharply in patients with Alzheimer's disease. *Nature Medicine*, *25*(4), 554–560. DOI: 10.1038/s41591-019-0375-9

Nemy, M., Dyrba, M., Brosseron, F., Buerger, K., Dechent, P., Dobisch, L., Ewers, M., Fliessbach, K., Glanz, W., & Goerss, D. (2023). Cholinergic white matter pathways along the Alzheimer's disease continuum. *Brain*, *146*(5), 2075–2088. DOI: 10.1093/brain/awac385

Neumann, M., Sampathu, D. M., Kwong, L. K., Truax, A. C., Micsenyi, M. C., Chou, T. T., Bruce, J., Schuck, T., Grossman, M., Clark, C. M., & Lee, V. M.-Y. (2006). Ubiquitinated TDP-43 in frontotemporal lobar degeneration and amyotrophic lateral sclerosis. *Science*, *314*(5796), 130–133. DOI: 10.1126/science.1134108

Nimgampalle, M., Chakravarthy, H., Sharma, S., Shree, S., Bhat, A. R., Pradeepkiran, J. A., & Devanathan, V. (2023). Neurotransmitter systems in the etiology of major neurological disorders: Emerging insights and therapeutic implications. *Ageing Research Reviews*, *89*, 101994. Advance online publication. DOI: 10.1016/j.arr.2023.101994

Nitsch, R. M. (1996). From acetylcholine to amyloid: Neurotransmitters and the pathology of Alzheimer's disease. *Neurodegeneration*, *5*(4), 477–482. DOI: 10.1006/neur.1996.0066

O'Brien, J., Hayder, H., Zayed, Y., & Peng, C. (2018). Overview of microRNA biogenesis, mechanisms of action, and circulation. *Frontiers in Endocrinology*, *9*, 402. Advance online publication. DOI: 10.3389/fendo.2018.00402

Ochoa-de la Paz, L., Zenteno, E., Gulias-Cañizo, R., & Quiroz-Mercado, H. (2019). Taurine and GABA neurotransmitter receptors, a relationship with therapeutic potential? *Expert Review of Neurotherapeutics*, *19*(4), 289–291. DOI: 10.1080/14737175.2019.1593827

Oja, S. S., & Saransaari, P. (2013). Taurine and epilepsy. *Epilepsy Research*, *104*(3), 187–194. DOI: 10.1016/j.eplepsyres.2013.01.010

Ortinski, P., & Meador, K. J. (2004). Cognitive side effects of antiepileptic drugs. *Epilepsy & Behavior*, *5*(Suppl. 1), S60–S65. DOI: 10.1016/j.yebeh.2003.11.008

Pajares, M., Rojo, A. I., Manda, G., Boscá, L., & Cuadrado, A. (2020). Inflammation in Parkinson's disease: Mechanisms and therapeutic implications. *Cells*, *9*(7), 1687. Advance online publication. DOI: 10.3390/cells9071687

Paredes-Rodriguez, E., Vegas-Suarez, S., Morera-Herreras, T., De Deurwaerdère, P., & Miguelez, C. (2020). The noradrenergic system in Parkinson's disease. *Journal of Psychopharmacology (Oxford, England)*, *34*(8), 787–799. DOI: 10.1177/0269881113490326

Paul, G. Y., Yeh, P. G., Spruyt, K., DelRosso, L. M., & Walters, A. S. (2023). A narrative review of the lesser-known medications for treatment of restless legs syndrome and pathogenetic implications for their use. *Tremor and Other Hyperkinetic Movements (New York, N.Y.), 13*, 1. Advance online publication. DOI: 10.5334/tohm.739

Philips, T., & Rothstein, J. D. (2014). Glial cells in amyotrophic lateral sclerosis. *Experimental Neurology, 262*(Pt. B), 111–120. DOI: 10.1016/j.expneurol.2014.05.015

Picciotto, M. R., Higley, M. J., & Mineur, Y. S. (2012). Acetylcholine as a neuromodulator: Cholinergic signaling shapes nervous system function and behavior. *Neuron, 76*(1), 116–129. DOI: 10.1016/j.neuron.2012.08.036

Polo, E., & Kruss, S. (2016). Nanosensors for neurotransmitters. *Analytical and Bioanalytical Chemistry, 408*(11), 2727–2741. DOI: 10.1007/s00216-015-9160-x

Potschka, H. (2010). Targeting regulation of ABC efflux transporters in brain diseases: A novel therapeutic approach. *Pharmacology & Therapeutics, 125*(1), 118–127. DOI: 10.1016/j.pharmthera.2009.10.004

Prybylowski, K., & Wenthold, R. J. (2004). N-Methyl-D-aspartate receptors: Subunit assembly and trafficking to the synapse. *Annals of the New York Academy of Sciences, 1038*(1), 125–130. DOI: 10.1196/annals.1315.020

Puranik, N., & Song, M. (2024). Glutamate: Molecular mechanisms and signaling pathway in Alzheimer's disease, and potential therapeutic targets. *Molecules (Basel, Switzerland), 29*(23), 5744. Advance online publication. DOI: 10.3390/molecules29235744

Qi-Lytle, X., Sayers, S., & Wagner, E. J. (2023). Current review of the function and regulation of tuberoinfundibular dopamine neurons. *Frontiers in Endocrinology, 13*, 1068335. Advance online publication. DOI: 10.3389/fendo.2022.1068335

Qin, X., Peng, Q., Zeng, Z., Chen, Z., Lin, L., Deng, Y., Huang, X., Xu, J., Wu, H., Huang, S., & Xiao, Z. (2012). Interleukin-1A -889C/T polymorphism and risk of Alzheimer's disease: A meta-analysis based on 32 case-control studies. *Journal of Neurology, 259*(8), 1519–1529. DOI: 10.1007/s00415-011-6381-6

Quessy, F., Bittar, T., Blanchette, L. J., Lévesque, M., & Labonte, B. (2021). Stress-induced alterations of mesocortical and mesolimbic dopaminergic pathways. *Scientific Reports, 11*(1), 11000. Advance online publication. DOI: 10.1038/s41598-021-90166-8

Quinlan, S., Kenny, A., Medina, M., Engel, T., & Jimenez-Mateos, E. M. (2017). MicroRNAs in neurodegenerative diseases. *International Review of Cell and Molecular Biology, 334*, 309–343. DOI: 10.1016/bs.ircmb.2017.04.002

Robbins, T. W., & Everitt, B. J. (1992). Functions of dopamine in the dorsal and ventral striatum. *Seminars in Neuroscience, 4*(2), 119–127. DOI: 10.1016/1044-5765(92)90010-Y

Rodríguez, J. J., Noristani, H. N., & Verkhratsky, A. (2012). The serotonergic system in ageing and Alzheimer's disease. *Progress in Neurobiology, 99*(1), 15–30. DOI: 10.1016/j.pneurobio.2012.06.010

Roeper, J. (2013). Dissecting the diversity of midbrain dopamine neurons. *Trends in Neurosciences*, *36*(6), 336–342. DOI: 10.1016/j.tins.2013.03.003

Saliminejad, K., Khorram Khorshid, H. R., Soleymani Fard, S., & Ghaffari, S. H. (2019). An overview of microRNAs: Biology, functions, therapeutics, and analysis methods. *Journal of Cellular Physiology*, *234*(5), 5451–5465. DOI: 10.1002/jcp.27486

Sara, S. J. (1985). Noradrenergic modulation of selective attention: Its role in memory retrieval. *Annals of the New York Academy of Sciences*, *444*(1), 178–193. DOI: 10.1111/j.1749-6632.1985.tb37588.x

Schneider-Garces, N. J., Gordon, B. A., & Brumback-Peltz, C. R. (2010). Span, CRUNCH, and beyond: Working memory capacity and the aging brain. *Journal of Cognitive Neuroscience*, *22*(4), 655–669. DOI: 10.1162/jocn.2009.21230

Schulz, J., Takousis, P., Wohlers, I., Itua, I. O. G., Dobricic, V., Rücker, G., Binder, H., Middleton, L., Ioannidis, J. P. A., Perneczky, R., & Bertram, L. (2019). Meta-analyses identify differentially expressed microRNAs in Parkinson's disease. *Annals of Neurology*, *85*(6), 835–851. DOI: 10.1002/ana.25490

Schwartz, J. C. (1975). Histamine as a transmitter in brain. *Life Sciences*, *17*(4), 503–517. DOI: 10.1016/0024-3205(75)90083-1

Selvam, S., & Ayyavoo, V. (2024). Biomarkers in neurodegenerative diseases: A broad overview. *Exploration of Neuroprotective Therapy*, *4*(2), 162–181. DOI: 10.37349/ent.2024.00075

Seyedabadi, M., Fakhfouri, G., Ramezani, V., Mehr, S. E., & Rahimian, R. (2014). The role of serotonin in memory: Interactions with neurotransmitters and downstream signaling. *Experimental Brain Research*, *232*(3), 723–738. DOI: 10.1007/s00221-013-3818-4

Sheffler, Z. M., Reddy, V., & Pillarisetty, L. S. (2025). Physiology, neurotransmitters. In *StatPearls*. StatPearls Publishing. https://www.ncbi.nlm.nih.gov/books/NBK539894/

Shi, J., Xie, J., Li, Z., He, X., Wei, P., Sander, J. W., & Zhao, G. (2025). The role of neuroinflammation and network anomalies in drug-resistant epilepsy. *Neuroscience Bulletin*, *41*(4), 881–905. DOI: 10.1007/s12264-025-01348-w

Shohamy, D., & Adcock, R. A. (2010). Dopamine and adaptive memory. *Trends in Cognitive Sciences*, *14*(10), 464–472. DOI: 10.1016/j.tics.2010.08.002

Silverberg, B., Shah, S. D., Haymond, M. W., & Cryer, P. E. (1978). Norepinephrine: Hormone and neurotransmitter in man. *American Journal of Physiology. Endocrinology and Metabolism*, *234*(3), E252–E256. DOI: 10.1152/ajpendo.1978.234.3.E252

Singaram, C., Ashraf, W., Gaumnitz, E. A., Torbey, C., Sengupta, A., Pfeiffer, R., & Quigley, E. M. M. (1995). Dopaminergic defect of enteric nervous system in Parkinson's disease patients with chronic constipation. *Lancet*, *346*(8979), 861–864. DOI: 10.1016/s0140-6736(95)92707-7

Song, J., Cho, E., Lee, H., Lee, S., Kim, S., & Kim, J. (2025). Development of neurodegenerative disease diagnosis and monitoring from traditional to digital biomarkers. *Biosensors (Basel), 15*(2), 102. Advance online publication. DOI: 10.3390/bios15020102

Speranza, L., di Porzio, U., Viggiano, D., de Donato, A., & Volpicelli, F. (2021). Dopamine: The neuromodulator of long-term synaptic plasticity, reward and movement control. *Cells, 10*(4), 735. Advance online publication. DOI: 10.3390/cells10040735

Stockmeier, C. A. (2003). Involvement of serotonin in depression: Evidence from postmortem and imaging studies of serotonin receptors and the serotonin transporter. *Journal of Psychiatric Research, 37*(5), 357–373. DOI: 10.1016/S0022-3956(03)00050-5

Südhof, T. C. (2008). Neurotransmitters release. In Lajtha, A., & Sershen, H. (Eds.), Handbook of experimental pharmacology. Springer. DOI: 10.1007/978-3-540-74805-2_1

Szabadi, E. (2013). Functional neuroanatomy of the central noradrenergic system. *Journal of Psychopharmacology (Oxford, England), 27*(8), 659–693. DOI: 10.1177/0269881113490326

Tang, F., Hartz, A. M. S., & Bauer, B. (2017). Drug-resistant epilepsy: Multiple hypotheses, few answers. *Frontiers in Neurology, 8*, 301. Advance online publication. DOI: 10.3389/fneur.2017.00301

Teleanu, R. I., Niculescu, A.-G., Roza, E., Vladâcenco, O., Grumezescu, A. M., & Teleanu, D. M. (2022). Neurotransmitters—Key factors in neurological and neurodegenerative disorders of the central nervous system. *International Journal of Molecular Sciences, 23*(11), 5954. Advance online publication. DOI: 10.3390/ijms23115954

Tian, Y. (2024). The role of dopamine neurotransmitters in neurological diseases: New sight. *International Journal of Molecular Sciences, 25*(14), 7529. Advance online publication. DOI: 10.3390/ijms25147529

Tobin, M. K., Musaraca, K., Disouky, A., Shetti, A., Bheri, A., Honer, W. G., & Lazarov, O. (2019). Human hippocampal neurogenesis persists in aged adults and Alzheimer's disease patients. *Cell Stem Cell, 24*(6), 974–982. DOI: 10.1016/j.stem.2019.05.003

Varvel, N. H., Neher, J. J., Bosch, A., Wang, W., Ransohoff, R. M., Miller, R. J., & Dingledine, R. (2016). Infiltrating monocytes promote brain inflammation and exacerbate neuronal damage after status epilepticus. *Proceedings of the National Academy of Sciences of the United States of America, 113*(38), E5665–E5674. DOI: 10.1073/pnas.1604263113

Vezzani, A., Di Sapia, R., Kebede, V., Balosso, S., & Ravizza, T. (2023). Neuroimmunology of status epilepticus. *Epilepsy & Behavior, 140*, 109095. Advance online publication. DOI: 10.1016/j.yebeh.2023.109095

Vezzani, A., Ravizza, T., Bedner, P., Aronica, E., Steinhäuser, C., & Boison, D. (2022). Astrocytes in the initiation and progression of epilepsy. *Nature Reviews. Neurology, 18*(12), 707–723. DOI: 10.1038/s41582-022-00727-5

Voorn, P., Kalsbeek, A., Jorritsma-Byham, B., & Groenewegen, H. J. (1988). The pre-and postnatal development of the dopaminergic cell groups in the ventral mesencephalon and the dopaminergic innervation of the striatum of the rat. *Neuroscience*, *25*(3), 857–887. DOI: 10.1016/0306-4522(88)90041-3

Vu, L. T., & Bowser, R. (2017). Fluid-based biomarkers for amyotrophic lateral sclerosis. *Neurotherapeutics; the Journal of the American Society for Experimental NeuroTherapeutics*, *14*(1), 119–134. DOI: 10.1007/s13311-016-0503-x

Wada, H., Yamatodani, A., Inagaki, N., Itowi, N., Wang, N. P., & Fukui, H. (1988). Histaminergic neuron system and its function. In *Advances in experimental medicine and biology* (Vol. 236, pp. 459–466). Springer. DOI: 10.1007/978-1-4757-5971-6_27

Wang, L. P., Li, F., Wang, D., Xie, K., Wang, D., Shen, X., & Tsien, J. Z. (2011). NMDA receptors in dopaminergic neurons are crucial for habit learning. *Neuron*, *72*(6), 1055–1066. DOI: 10.1016/j.neuron.2011.10.019

Wang, Q., Geng, Y., Li, X., Hao, Y., & Huang, S. (2025). The progress of cognitive dysfunction impairment caused by temporal lobe epilepsy. *Journal of Molecular Neuroscience*, *75*(1), 81. Advance online publication. DOI: 10.1007/s12031-025-02365-0

Weissberg, I., Wood, L., Kaminsky, L., Vazquez, O., Milikovsky, D. Z., Alexander, A., & Friedman, A. (2015). Albumin induces excitatory synaptogenesis through astrocytic TGF-β/ALK5 signaling in a model of acquired epilepsy following blood-brain barrier dysfunction. *Neurobiology of Disease*, *78*, 115–125. DOI: 10.1016/j.nbd.2015.02.029

Witt, J. A., Meschede, C., & Helmstaedter, C. (2020). Reader response: Antiepileptic drugs are not independently associated with cognitive dysfunction. *Neurology*, *95*(23), 1069. DOI: 10.1212/WNL.0000000000009061

Wu, C., & Sun, D. (2015). GABA receptors in brain development, function, and injury. *Metabolic Brain Disease*, *30*(2), 367–379. DOI: 10.1007/s11011-014-9596-8

Yang, T., Velagapudi, R., & Terrando, N. (2020). Neuroinflammation after surgery: From mechanisms to therapeutic targets. *Nature Immunology*, *21*(11), 1319–1327. DOI: 10.1038/s41590-020-00812-1

Yu, C., Deng, X. J., & Xu, D. (2023). Microglia in epilepsy. *Neurobiology of Disease*, *185*, 106249. Advance online publication. DOI: 10.1016/j.nbd.2023.106249

Yu, J., Zhang, Y., Yao, H., Zhang, Z., Yang, X., Zhu, W., & Xu, J. (2024). ERβ activation improves nonylphenol-induced depression and neurotransmitter secretion disruption via the TPH2/5-HT pathways. *Ecotoxicology and Environmental Safety*, *280*, 116521. Advance online publication. DOI: 10.1016/j.ecoenv.2024.116521

Yuan, H., & Silberstein, S. D. (2018). Histamine and migraine. *Headache*, *58*(1), 184–193. DOI: 10.1111/head.13164

Zhou, Y., & Danbolt, N. C. (2014). Glutamate as a neurotransmitter in the healthy brain. *Journal of Neural Transmission (Vienna, Austria)*, *121*(8), 799–817. DOI: 10.1007/s00702-014-1180-8

Chapter 2
Improved Method of Identification of Leakage of Cerebrospinal Fluid (CSF) and Brain–Blood Barrier (BBB):
Using Artificial Intelligence for Medical Practices

Soobia Saeed
https://orcid.org/0009-0006-9399-7090
Taylor's University, Malaysia

Mohsin Qadeer
https://orcid.org/0000-0001-7509-6885
Jinnah Medical and Dental College, Pakistan

ABSTRACT

One of the most complex organs in the body is the human brain, which is composed of numerous neuronal networks that maintain processes such as homeostasis, cognition, and emotions. The purpose of this research is to detect brain cancer cells and leakage of CSF due to a breach of the BBB. We proposed two phases: the first is based on chemical testing to target the cancer cells in the brain using the UHPLC, which shows the presence of cancer and diagnoses the leakage symptoms of the CSF. The second phase is based on the hybrid k-mean cluster and Hidden Markov Model (HMM), namely kCHMM. In the first phase, we used UHPLC with immunotoxin antibodies. In the second phase, we used the hybrid k-mean cluster hidden Markov model (kCHMM) technique. The efficiency of the proposed datasets that we received after implementation of the kCHMM model is 0.9984.

DOI: 10.4018/979-8-3373-4627-4.ch002

INTRODUCTION

Cancers, particularly those of the nervous system, are frequently thought to be fatal; yet, neither the cellular and molecular mechanisms nor the underlying causes are entirely understood. Although there is an abundance of knowledge about the many forms of brain tumors today, the process by which they spread and endanger other sections of the brain is still poorly understood. The research proposal is based on a longitudinal prospective strategy to gather information on cerebrospinal fluid (CSF) leakage in the case of brain cancer present in the brain and the numerous secreted proteins and enzymes contained to be accountable for the breach of the blood-brain barrier (Erickson et.al, 2018). A large sample of data is being gathered for this qualitative investigation using cohort studies and logical reasoning. We collect the brain fluid (CSF) flowing from cancer patients. The leakage frequently happens at the level of the spine, especially close to the base of the brain, where the thoracic spine and the cardiothoracic connection are located. First, we characterize the various proteins and enzymes present in the CSF using CT scan studies, and then we locate the foci where the released products enter the blood-brain barrier (Whitehead et.al, 2023; Johnson et.al, 2011; Prastawa et.al, 2003). We specifically examine proteins and enzymes using high-pressure liquid chromatography (HPLC) (Zhuge et.al, 2017; Saeed et.al, 2017; Martínez-Más et.al, 2019). These samples were tested by the University of Calgary lab, located at the Hotchkiss Brain Institute, which is under the authority of the Research Institute of the Cumming School of Medicine, University of Calgary, Alberta, Canada.

The blood-brain interfaces in the brain highlight the importance of brain barriers as mediators of neuroimmune communication (neurotransmitters) and regulators of neurological function (Min, R., 2008; Saeed et.al, 2020). As neuroscience has progressed, it has become increasingly clear that the brain-brain barrier (BBB) serves as a two-way (bidirectional) communication barrier between the brain and the rest of the body (Machhale et.al, 2015; Saeed et.al, 2022; Chen et.al, 2018). It is also possible to estimate newly emerging CNS locations that are exposed to chemicals and blood-borne immune compounds, as well as significant brain homologous interfaces and pathogenic functions (Song et.al, 2020; Saeed et.al, 2020; Zhang et.al, 2007). The research in this series focuses on a novel aspect of how the brain interface functions, with particular attention paid to mechanisms that control barrier integrity and transporter activities, the subsequent effects of neurovascular injury, peripheral organ infection or damage, and the removal of pathogenic proteins (Prosser et.al, 2011; Kumari et.al, 2018; El-Baz et.al, 2011; Stoffel et.al, 2022). In diseases like Alzheimer's disease, multiple sclerosis, dead fetus/cerebral and adult hypoxic/ischemic injury, brain injury, malignant infections, and acute lung injury, the novel pathways demonstrate how brain dysfunction can produce neuroinflammation and CNS damage (Saeed and Hashim, 2023; Saeed, 2022). The brain interfaces may be useful therapeutic targets in and of themselves for a number of central nervous system diseases associated with immunological dyshomeostasis. Contrarily, we discovered that aberrant lymphatic entrance into the ventricles as well as brain exposure to antibodies are both made easier by blood-CSF barrier failure (Ludwig et.al, 2021; Saeed et.al, 2022; Poortmans et.al, 2020).

We first identify a blood-brain barrier substance that may invade extracellular space in the brain through endothelial cells at sites without the brain blood barrier (BBB), and it may also travel through an interstitial fluid (ISF) from sites to adjacent brain parenchyma without the BBB. The resulting samples of CSF leaks that occur at the time of blood-brain barrier break due to growing cancer cells also focus on identifying the stage of cancer as well (Murthy et.al, 2021).

We also know that brain tumors are one of the major issues that have claimed the lives of many people in recent years. The brain tumor can be efficiently treated if it is classified at an early stage. However, brain tumor classification requires multiple algorithms (Jung et.al, 2016; Saeed et.al, 2022). For this purpose, weight-based classification algorithms are often used; however, they have lower classification accuracy. In this research, a brain tumor classification system based on the HMM is described, which improves classification accuracy. The efficiency of the HMM classifier in terms of transition matrix and voxel is simulated using MATLAB (Chung et.al, 2016; Silva, 2016; Dansereau, 2019).

Based on Figure 1, the classification method of HMM represents the state of the voxel in terms of HMM. The HMM approach for calculating the lesion and non-lesion values of the tumour and CSF through voxel is discussed in this study (Varatharaj, et.al, 2017; Strazielle and Ghersi, 2013). To track the classification of the brain tumour tissue through time, the 3D spatial segmentation algorithm is repeated for each individual time point (Dritsas et.al, 2018; Raja and Nirmala, 2019). Improvements can be achieved when selecting the tissue classes for the current scan by taking the results of earlier and later 3D segmentations into account. The goal of this study is to develop a novel temporal strategy for the 4D categorization of brain cancer CT scan images by combining probabilistic reasoning over space and time. The temporal model consists of a dynamic Bayesian network, in particular the HMM, sensor models, and image-based transitions (Sedghi et.al, 2021; Naughton et.al, 2018; Erickson et.al, 2018). The author made the supposition that all potential lesion and non-lesion values for brain tumours and CSF, as well as each voxel's lesion status, were included in the 4D imaging data. The classifying and segmenting lesions over time problems can be implemented as an HMM, where Et denotes the MR signal intensity at each voxel and Xt denotes the visible or non-visible state of the lesion or non-lesion system (Niranjana & Chatterjee, 2021; Rother et.al, 2004; Altaf et.al, 2016; Kinaci, et.al, 2018).

Figure 1. Working procedure of HMM

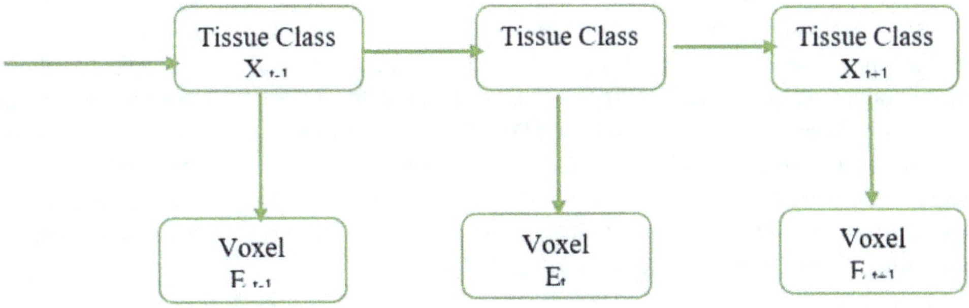

The rest of the section is sequenced as per the following guidelines: This study (i) is the first to demonstrate that blood-brain interfaces in the brain highlight the importance of brain barriers as mediators of neuroimmune communication (neurotransmitters) and regulators of neurological function. (ii) To check the breakage of BBB through CSF and identify the symptoms of different kinds of cancer. (iii) Implement the hidden Markov model to identify the brain tumor and CSF leakage through the BBB. The following subsection describes the proposed work in this research. Section II mentioned the proposed method, including clinical and CT scans of brain tumors. This

section describes how to target the cancer cell through UHPLC and identify the brain cancer cell through HMM. Section IV mentioned the results and discussion. Section V mentioned the conclusion and future work.

PROPOSED METHOD

The proposed two new techniques used in this research are based on the detection of brain cancer cells and leakage of CSF due to the breach of the BBB. In this research, we proposed two phases. The first is based on chemical testing to target cancer cells in the brain using the UHPLC. The second phase is based on a hybrid k-mean cluster and the Hidden Markov Model (HMM), namely kCHMM. In the first phase, we used UHPLC with immuno-toxin antibodies. Immuno-toxin antibodies were used with UHPLC with a C18 column and carbon chains bonded to the silica particles inside the column to identify the cancer cell in Universiti Teknologi Malaysia (UTM), Faculty of Science, under the supervision of Prof. Dr. Naweed. I. Syed (PhD. Neuroscience) and Dr. Mohsin Qadeer (Neurosurgeon) also provide his assistant in this research as guidance as per his field of expertise. Samples were provided by Prof. Dr. Abdul Sattar Hashim. He is a neurosurgeon as well as he is from that institute of Neurospinal Cancer Care Institute (NCCI). In the second phase, we used the hybrid k-mean cluster hidden Markov model (kCHMM) technique that we have developed, which consists of two main components, including the k-mean cluster and the hidden Markov model approach, which are implemented in CT scan images as illustrated in Figure 3. The suggested methods are based on CT scan implementations that are sufficient for classifying all different types of brain cancer CT scan images. Another characteristic used in this study to build the Markov chain outside the cancer cell's border is the iterated conditional maximizing mode. In order to increase the accuracy of the images used to detect brain cancer cells, these steps carry out activities like labelling the datasets and preparing the images for algorithms for regression and classification for training. The HMM and the k-mean clustering algorithm are the two components of the HMM and k-mean clustering algorithm techniques that we have proposed. These steps enhance and reconstruct images, as well as connect the likelihood of the trained dataset's images with the statistical confidence interval (d), with the use of the iterated conditional maximizing mode (ICMM). The ICMM arranges the generated images using statistical confidence intervals to give the same sequence form as the two aforementioned techniques, which combine the range of the HMM's stated probability. The k-mean cluster is where the information used to categories trained datasets is eventually kept. The suggested technique is thoroughly explained in the subsection that follows.

Figure 2. Proposed method of identifying brain cancer cell and CSF leakage

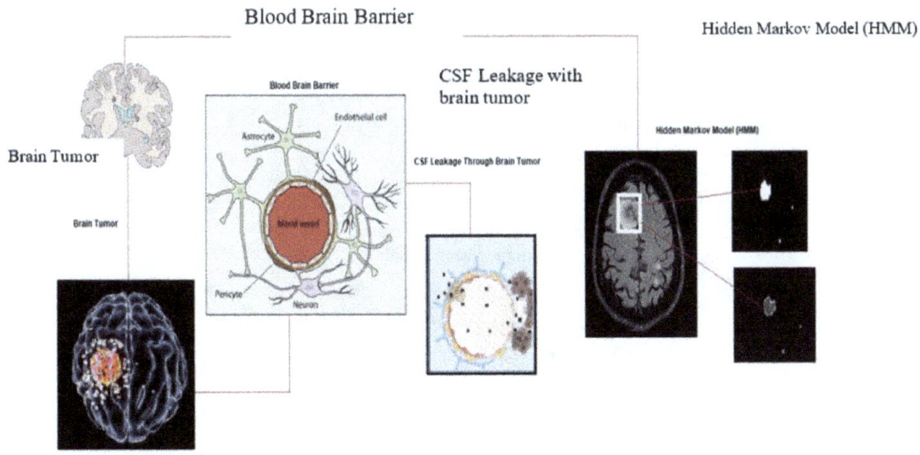

Figure 3. Proposed methodology of brain cancer and CSF leakage due to breakage of BBB

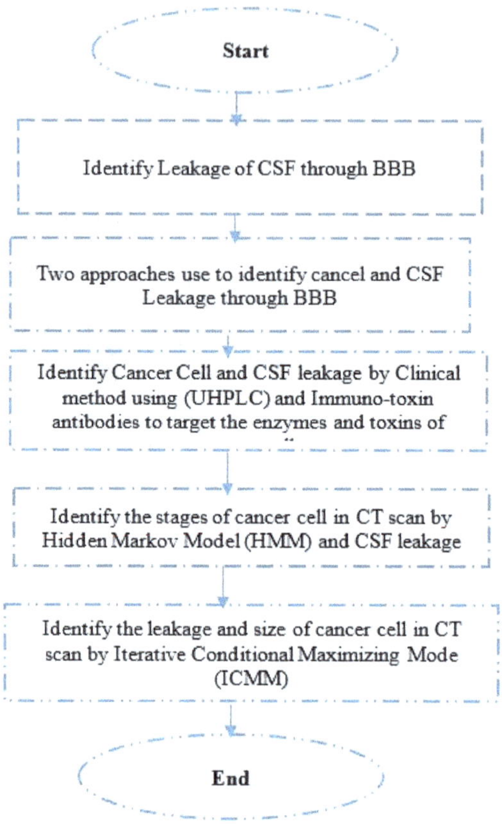

DATASETS AND PREPARATION

The Cumming School of Medicine Lab at the University of Calgary in Canada provided the original images used in this study to assess the enhanced performance of CSF and brain cancer cell classification in original and CT scans sample. It is carried out at the Cumming School of Medicine Lab of the University of Calgary, Toronto, Canada, using human brain samples gathered at the Neurospinal & Cancer Care Institute (NCCI) and Medicare Cardiac and General Hospital (MCGH). We appreciate the helpful hand of all of these three organizations in this research and prompt the research publication after finding the concluding experimental results. The Cumming School of Medicine Lab specializes in neuroscience and related fields. In this stage, an empirical analysis is conducted in order to assess the effectiveness of the proposed technique in relation to the main objective of the method. This research introduces brain cancer and CSF CT scan datasets using the Light Field Toolkit and incorporates the raw data improved by Dansereau (2019) at Stanford University at the URL https://Vincentqyw/Depth-Estimation-Light-Field/.

CSF with brain cancer cell images and the raw data are available at https://Vincentqyw/Depth -Estimation-Light-Field/. Lytro Illum software tools were used to improve the accuracy and quality of images using the spatial and intensity resolution of these datasets. Spatial resolution describes the size of an image in terms of column and row pixels (Dansereau and Wetzstein, 2019). Improved LFD consists of 5000 CT scan images, including male, female, age, and type of cancer datasets. These datasets contain 2800 male images and 2200 female images. The 14 shifted viewpoints, which can be utilized for a number of purposes, are recreated using external standardized light fields that are extracted using the Lytro command-line tools. The Lytro light field software application is generally believed to improve the accuracy of CT scan datasets that can provide improved LFD datasets.

DATA COLLECTION

The data were extracted from the Cumming School of Medicine Lab, University of Calgary, Canada. The information obtained included gender, size of cancer, age factor, and BBB breach cases due to cancer development in the brain. The Statistical Package for Social Science (SPSS) was used for data evaluation and analysis. The data were expressed as an analysis of the mean. Median, range, and percentage. There were 5000 total CT scans of patients we used in this research, including 2200 female and 2800 male cancer cases, during the study period. Few cases were resolved due to minor or initial recovery once diagnosed, but many cases were reported for serious conditions and chances of death due to brain cancer and continuous leakage of CSF as shown in Figure.4. The details of the demographics shown in Table 1 are given below:

Table 1. Demographic profile of patient's data

Gender	Calculation of SPSS
Male	2200 (23%)
Female	2800(29%)
Range	20-45 years old (median 26)
Brain Cancer: (M)	1200 (09%)
Brain Cancer: (F)	1600 (12%)
Brain Cancer with CSF leakage (M)	600(70%)
Brain Cancer with CSF leakage (F)	300(20%)
Breach of BBB through Brain Cancer (M)	200(21%)
Breach of BBB through Brain Cancer (F)	200(19%)
Duration of Hospitalization (Average)	20 days (range 8-25)

Figure 4: Demographic position of Brain Cancer patients

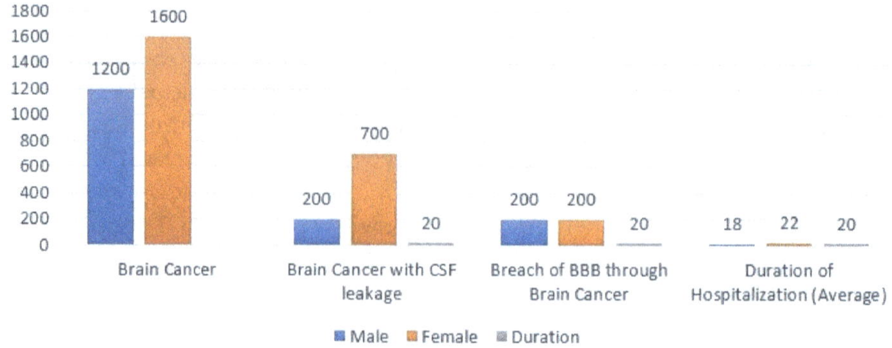

CLINICAL METHOD PREPARATION

The University of Calgary's Human Care and Use Committee oversees all study protocols involving CSF leakage, and it conducts them in accordance with the standards set forth by the blood-brain interfaces, which are paradigm-shifting and necessitate an improvement in our methodology. Immunological reactions are controlled by brain-immune system communication pathways, which are frequently triggered by immune system signals. These signals are mostly represented by pro-inflammatory cytokines and come from auxiliary immune cells such as monocytes and macrophages. In this frame of work, we proposed a method after investigating the history of the cancer patient and finding the actual situation of the disease: either the spinal leakage of the patient is an injury, or the cancer patient's injury is contained in the actual tumor or immune system. We investigate the patient records and check the dura-plexus to see if the search fluid is accurate or not. Furthermore, which type of cancer is sustained in the body is one of the most important things to relate to our research.

PREPARATION OF TESTING SAMPLES

Using immuno-toxin antibodies and UHPLC with a C-18 column (a C18 column is a reverse-phase HPLC column with carbon chains connected to the silica particles inside the column), we analyze the BBB. The C18 shows the number of carbon atoms in each chain, which in this case totals 18 carbon atoms per chain. Chimeric proteins called immunotoxins (IT) are created specifically to target and destroy cancer cells. These compounds are made up of two main components: a receptor-binding moiety, typically an antibody (the name comes from the term "immuno-toxin"). This moiety is focused on a particular receptor that is expressed on the cell membrane. The second component of IT is typically the toxin's catalytic component, an enzyme that is in charge of the lethality the toxin causes. In order to introduce harmful elements into the cell, immunotoxin uses the specificity of the antibodies produced on the cell membrane against

their intended target molecules. UHPLC is used together with a C-18 column (a C18 column is a reverse-phase HPLC column containing carbon chains attached to the silica particles inside the column) and antibodies against immunotoxin, such as immunotoxin. These investigations are carried out to identify cancer cells and BBB breaches. The C18 indicates the length of the carbon chains, which in this case have a total of 18 carbon atoms.

IDENTIFY THE BRAIN CANCER THROUGH HIDDEN MARKOV MODEL USING PATIENT CT-SCAN

The Hidden Markov Model (HMM) classifier uses the spatial method of HMM to categories the CSF fluid and size of cancer cells in a CT scan of the brain. HMM segments the enhanced CT scan images into datasets using probabilistic reasoning over time and space. In this part, the k-mean clustering approach also has a significant impact. In terms of classification, the classes of datasets are stored in cluster form using the k mean. The HMM approach was chosen in order to classify CSF fluid and brain cancer cells sequentially employing CT scan images, especially CSF fluid. The internal factor of the images, which cannot be seen immediately, is what drives the HMM analysis and observation events. The suggested HMM method builds a Markov chain and distributes the likelihood of the image's initial state being viewed. Since HMM is an excellent method for locating fluid in images, this section defines the transition state of HMM. This section uses the Iterative Conditional Maximizing Mode (ICMM) to increase the probability range from the previous section by joining the probabilities in a sequence of distances based on the iteration condition.

Calculating the observed data led to an evident classification of the CSF fluid in the image since the fluid leaks in one direction and the cancer cells have spread throughout the brain. An iterated maximizing mode that locates the fluid or cancer cell's border throughout the image's development is used to categories the region of the fluid or cancer cell. In this study, cancer cell CT scan images were employed in the HMM classifier technique, and the K-mean clustering algorithm was applied to improve the accuracy of the images. K-mean finds the hidden information in the CT scan image datasets by assigning objects to the closest centroids using the Euclidean distance as a measure of closeness. The k-mean cluster stores the datasets of CT scan images, identifies the object class at a position around the centroid, and restructures the images following object class categorization. This process is performed until all object-class close points have been identified. This method aims to improve the accuracy of the images, and the feature vectors statistically consider the HMM of enhanced CT scan image datasets. With iterative conditional mode (ICM), HMM provides conditional transition probabilities on the states of neighboring blocks in both horizontal and vertical orientations. This method extracts the hidden data from the dataset's noisy images. Additionally, HMM uses Voxel (a volume element of the 2D pixel extension) with enhanced CT scan datasets for 4D pictures. This illustrates how a cancer cell or CSF fluid can be classified in an isolated position in an image using HMM. The presence or absence of either a cancer cell or fluid is indicated by a number value. Over time, an HMM classifier can show difficulty in segmenting and tracing the presence of cancer cells or fluid. By utilizing the two transition states S = (S1, S2) in such a way that S1 shows the presence of cancer cells or fluid and S2 shows their absence, this technique carries out the main contributions of this research section and offers a better solution to check for their presence and absence. One of these

two states is chosen as the starting point for the technique, which then moves smoothly from one state to the next and outputs the probabilities of sequencing. These probabilities are applied to the Iterative Conditional Maximizing Mode (ICMM) condition and correspond to either the first state or the second state. The Markov chain moved with a certain probability to the following state, S2, if it existed in state S1. With each of the provided images from the CT scan datasets, the Markov transition matrix is initially detected during the HMM procedure. This method was applied to the images for ICMM to show the size of the tumor or range of fluid when the probability was combined to classify the shape, size, and CSF fluid or cancer cell as t, t + d, t + 2d, t + 3d..., t + nd. The distance, or d, in this situation indicates the presence of a cancer cell or a fluid state. This transition stage displays the likelihood that the specified state "t" will apply the ICMM strategy (maximum or minimum values successively, depending on the state condition). The ICMM builds datasets of images to estimate the ideal coefficients, enabling the selection of less noticeable images after connecting the probabilities to one another with the transition matrix variable. The ICMM extends the empirical probability of the image datasets with ease and is computationally fast. It produces the signed distance map from the mask together with centered posterior probability. Accurate values are calculated after applying the ICMM to the images, and both the preliminary and final outputs clearly show the cancer cell and the flow of CSF fluid in the location in the CT scan images. When the condition of the transition matrix is used, the HMM approach generates novel results, such as the potential state of a voxel that has classified a fluid or cancer cell. By employing HMM to obtain accurate results, the suggested HMM approach for categorizing all sorts of images in the voxel state considerably improved the datasets as shown in Figure.5.

Figure 5. CT scan sample signaling result of brain cancer cell and CSF leakage due to breach of BBB

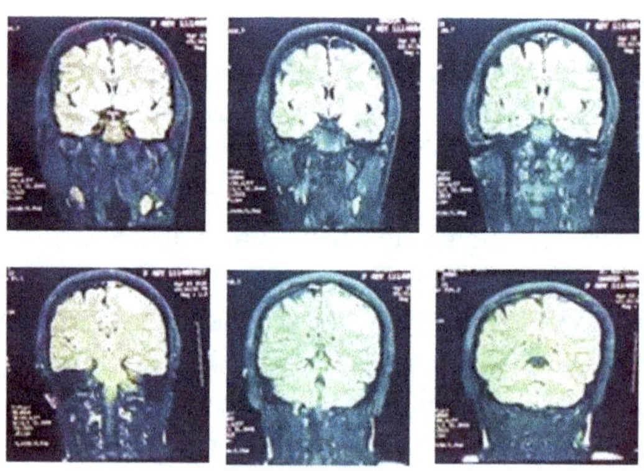

(a) (b) (c)

RESULTS

The location of the CSF is determined by using a Markov probability chain using the most up-to-date diagnostic imaging and specialized four-dimensional therapy software (HMM) to directly target the cancer cell in the brain. This precise technique is used to identify cancer cells, the location of CSF in CT scans, and damaged brain tissues that are present close to both benign and malignant brain tumors, such as high-grade gliomas or gliomas. Benign brain tumors include acoustic neuromas, meningiomas, pituitary adenomas, pineal tumors, craniopharyngiomas, chordomas, and low-grade glial and gliomas tumors. In this study, we use a hybrid HMM and k-mean clustering method to focus on brain cancer cells and CSF.

Results of applying HMM and k-mean clustering to categories the locations of cancer cells on CT scan pictures Figures 4 and 5, which depict the cancer cells and range of CSF fluid in the brain, present the findings of proposed datasets using a hybrid of HMM and k-mean clustering. To determine the current condition of the cancer cell or CSF fluid with potential values of presence and absence, the HMM for object classification takes into account each state of a voxel in CT scan image datasets. For instance, using the transition matrix of the two states, it is possible to replicate how HMM is used for tracking segmentation through time and space. Figure 6 and Figure7 shows the CT scan picture values at time t to be D1 = 0.9984, size, with an implied probability of (t - 1). At the time, the voxel was recognized as having a cancer cell size and CSF fluid leak range. The posterior distribution of the HMM is used to compute the two transition stages, which are represented by a filtering technique. The first shows how to calculate distance, while the other presents the pixel brightness of both pixels as a P (Xt/Xt+1). Table 1 displays the accuracy ratings for classifying the pixel intensity values at time (t + 1) using the pixel intensity state for both cancer cells and brain CSF fluid leaks. Instead of utilizing HMM, ICMM is employed to extract the hidden data from the CT scan images in the enhanced dataset. The ICMM builds datasets of images to estimate the ideal coefficients, permitting the choice of less obvious probabilities after linking the probabilities to one another with the transition matrix variable. In order to show how well cancer cells and CSF may be seen in CT scan images once the data from the images has been retrieved, the simulated results of ICMM are shown in the figure below. The efficiency of datasets and the precision of suggested CT scan brain cancer cell datasets are both shown in Table 2.

Figure 6. Results of ICMM over HMM classification of datasets of cancer cell and CSF

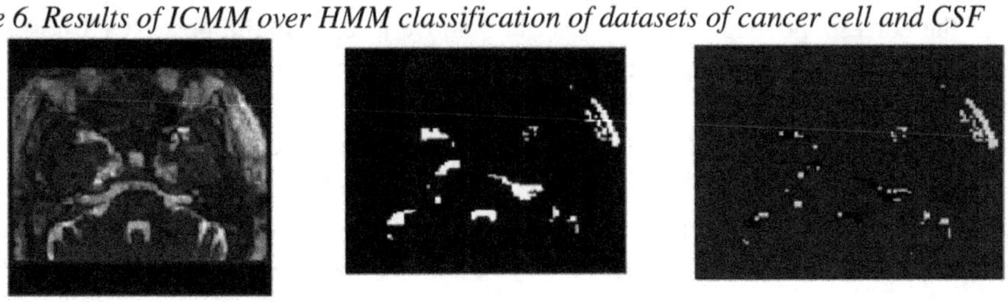

Original Image of datasets of cancer cell and CSF leakage | Hmm Classify Result | ICMM with HMM Result

Figure 7. Brain Cancer cell extracted through kCHMM

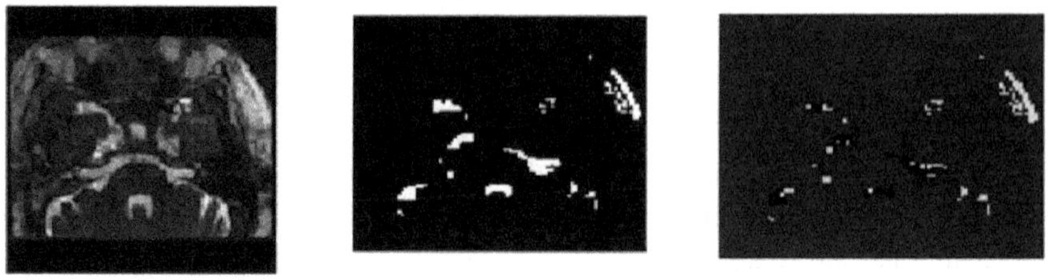

Original Image of datasets of cancer cell and CSF leakage | Hmm Classify Result | ICMM with HMM Result

Table 2. AccuracyofHMM Results over the improved datasets

Image	**Accuracy Values**
Datasets of CT scan Image	0.9984

DISCUSSION

The proposed research is to collect data related to detecting of a brain cancer cell using for finding the surgery cases of a variety of cancer-type patients for finding in CSF, including enzymes and toxin in cancer cell evaluation. Whereas only relevant sample data is to be collected; these are constructed based on deductive reasoning and cohort studies. Although the implementation strategies are based on patient case histories and their CT scans, the data that appears in this investigation should be considered directional. First, although samples of patient data were collected at the NCCI and MGCH and tested by a school of Cuming lab in Canada due to the availability of all comfort tools and equipment, this rules out the presumption that statistical inferences should be interpreted causally. Second, despite the implementation of some of the correspondence methods described above to choose the best NCCI hospital and sample evaluation, key variable distributions, including age at initial diagnosis, gender, race, and marital status at diagnosis, as well as the year of initial diagnosis, were the same as those mentioned in the case studies. Finally, survival analyses were based on statistical comparisons of the prevalence of cancer surgery patients for all potential causes, only for specific cancer diseases and their surgeries, which are diagnosed by utilizing the UHPLC technique to identify the cancer cell availability and diagnose the symptoms of CSF leakage through BBB breakage. The second part of this research is related to the HMM and k-mean clustering techniques that we used to identify cancer cells and CSF leakage in the brain through the datasets of CT scans. The proposed techniques provide better results with CT scan images, as CSF and cancer cells are clearly visible. This will help physicians easily identify cancer cells and CSF inside the brain and diagnose the tumor in its early stages, which might save someone's life. The aim of this research

is to develop a unique model in terms of improved classification to classify cancer cells and CSF leaks in a brain tumor's initial phase. These parameters classify brain cancer, cancer cell size, and the location of CSF inside the brain as well.

CONCLUSION

Brain cancer, CSF leakage, and breach of the BBB through any type of brain cancer are increasing day by day, increasing morbidity and mortality in developing countries. The purpose of this research is to detect brain cancer cells and leakage of CSF due to a breach of the BBB. We proposed a novel technique to identify the cancer cells and target these cells through chemical testing to target the cancer cells in the brain using UHPLC, which shows the presence of cancer and diagnoses the leakage symptoms of CSF. The hybrid technique of k-mean cluster and hidden Markov model (HMM), namely kCHMM, is also used in this research to detect the size, location, and presence of cancer cells in the brain. These datasets contain 2800 male images and 2200 female images, including brain cancer cell (M) at 23%, brain cancer cell (F) at 29%, brain cancer with CSF leakage (M) at 12%, brain cancer with CSF leakage (F) at 30%, brain cancer with CSF leakage (M) at 30%, brain cancer with CSF leakage (F) at 74%, breach of BBB through brain cancer with CSF leakage (M) at 21%, and breach of BBB through brain cancer with CSF leakage (F) at 11%. The efficiency of the proposed datasets that we received after the implementation of the kCHMM model is 0.9984. With concerted efforts, the safety of our brain cancer patients can be achieved through the proposed techniques.

Ethical Statement

The Cumming School of Medicine Lab, University of Calgary and other two hospital allow the authors to use these patients sample data in their research as the authors receive the signed written informed consent of patients regarding the publication of their medical data in the journal article.

Abbreviation

NCCI: National Cancer Care Institute; MGCH: Medicare Cardiac and General Hospital; HMM: Hidden Markov Model; BBB: Blood Brain Barrier; CSF: Cerebrospinal Fluid

ACKNOWLEDGMENTS

This work was supported by the Department of Neurosurgery, Faculty of Surgery, NCCI, Medicare hospital, Karachi, Pakistan and the Cumming School of Medicine Lab, University of Calgary, Canada.

REFERENCES

Altaf, I., Vohra, A. H., & Shams, S. (2016). Management of cerebrospinal fluid leak following posterior cranial fossa surgery. *Pakistan Journal of Medical Sciences*, *32*(6), 1439.

Chen, D. Y., Chen, C. C., Crawford, J. R., & Wang, S. G. (2018). Tumor-related epilepsy: Epidemiology, pathogenesis and management. *Journal of Neuro-Oncology*, *139*(1), 13–21. DOI: 10.1007/s11060-018-2862-0

Chung, E. J., Kim, G. W., Cho, B. K., Park, H. S., & Rho, Y. S. (2016). Pattern of lymph node metastasis in hypopharyngeal squamous cell carcinoma and indications for level VI lymph node dissection. *Head & Neck*, *38*(S1), E1969–E1973. DOI: 10.1002/hed.24361

Dansereau, D. G., Girod, B., & Wetzstein, G. (2019). LiFF: Light field features in scale and depth. In *Proceedings of the IEEE/CVF Conference on Computer Vision and Pattern Recognition* (pp. 8042-8051). DOI: 10.1109/CVPR.2019.00823

Dritsas, E., Trigka, M., Gerolymatos, P., & Sioutas, S. (2018). Trajectory clustering and k-NN for robust privacy preserving spatiotemporal databases. *Algorithms*, *11*(12), 207. DOI: 10.3390/a11120207

El-Baz, A. S., Acharya, R., Mirmehdi, M., & Suri, J. S. (Eds.). (2011). *Multi-Modality State-of-the-Art Medical Image Segmentation and Registration Methodologies* (Vol. 1). Springer Science & Business Media.

Erickson, M. A., Nicolazzo, J. A., & Banks, W. A. (2018). Commentary on the 2018 Named Series on blood-brain interfaces: Roles of neuroimmunomodulation in health and disease. *Brain, Behavior, and Immunity*, *74*, 3–6. DOI: 10.1016/j.bbi.2018.08.016

Erickson, M. A., Nicolazzo, J. A., & Banks, W. A. (2018). Commentary on the 2018 Named Series on blood-brain interfaces: Roles of neuroimmunomodulation in health and disease. *Brain, Behavior, and Immunity*, *74*, 3–6. DOI: 10.1016/j.bbi.2018.08.016

Johnson, R. C., Kalb, S. R., & Barr, J. R. (2011). Toxin analysis using mass spectrometry. In *Microbial Forensics* (pp. 405–420). Academic Press. DOI: 10.1016/B978-0-12-382006-8.00024-4

Jung, H., Law, A., Grunblatt, E., Wang, L. L., Kusano, A., Mejino, J. L.Jr, & Whipple, M. E. (2016). Development of a novel markov chain model for the prediction of head and neck squamous cell carcinoma dissemination. [). American Medical Informatics Association.]. *AMIA ... Annual Symposium Proceedings - AMIA Symposium. AMIA Symposium*, *2016*, 1832.

Kinaci, A., Algra, A., Heuts, S., O'Donnell, D., van der Zwan, A., & van Doormaal, T. (2018). Effectiveness of dural sealants in prevention of cerebrospinal fluid leakage after craniotomy: A systematic review. *World Neurosurgery, 118*, 368–376. DOI: 10.1016/j.wneu.2018.06.196

Kumari, N., & Saxena, S. (2018, March). Review of brain tumor segmentation and classification. In *2018 International conference on current trends towards converging technologies (ICCTCT)* (pp. 1-6). IEEE. DOI: 10.1109/ICCTCT.2018.8551004

Ludwig, R., Pouymayou, B., Balermpas, P., & Unkelbach, J. (2021). A hidden Markov model for lymphatic tumor progression in the head and neck. *Scientific Reports, 11*(1), 12261. DOI: 10.1038/s41598-021-91544-1

Machhale, K., Nandpuru, H. B., Kapur, V., & Kosta, L. (2015, May). MRI brain cancer classification using hybrid classifier (SVM-KNN). In *2015 International Conference on Industrial Instrumentation and Control (ICIC)* (pp. 60-65). IEEE. DOI: 10.1109/IIC.2015.7150592

Martínez-Más, J., Bueno-Crespo, A., Khazendar, S., Remezal-Solano, M., Martínez-Cendán, J. P., Jassim, S., Du, H., Al Assam, H., Bourne, T., & Timmerman, D. (2019). Evaluation of machine learning methods with Fourier Transform features for classifying ovarian tumors based on ultrasound images. *PLoS One, 14*(7), e0219388. DOI: 10.1371/journal.pone.0219388

Min, R. (2008). *Adaptive KNN classification based on Laplacian Eigenmaps and kernel mixtures*. Technical report, University of Toronto.

Murthy, V., Maitre, P., Kannan, S., Panigrahi, G., Krishnatry, R., Bakshi, G., Prakash, G., Pal, M., Menon, S., Phurailatpam, R., Mokal, S., Chaurasiya, D., Popat, P., Sable, N., Agarwal, A., Rangarajan, V., Joshi, A., Noronha, V., Prabhash, K., & Mahantshetty, U. (2021). Prostate-only versus whole-pelvic radiation therapy in high-risk and very high-risk prostate cancer (POP-RT): Outcomes from phase III randomized controlled trial. *Journal of Clinical Oncology, 39*(11), 1234–1242. DOI: 10.1200/JCO.20.03282

Naughton, M. J., Case, L. D., Peiffer, A., Chan, M., Stieber, V., Moore, D., Falchuk, S., Piephoff, J., Edenfield, W., Giguere, J., Loghin, M., Shaw, E. G., & Rapp, S. R. (2018). Quality of life of irradiated brain tumor survivors treated with donepezil or placebo: Results of the WFU CCOP research base protocol 91105. *Neuro-Oncology Practice, 5*(2), 114–121. DOI: 10.1093/nop/npx016

Niranjana, G., & Chatterjee, D. (2021). Security and privacy issues in biomedical AI systems and potential solutions. In *Handbook of Artificial Intelligence in Biomedical Engineering* (pp. 289–309). Apple Academic Press. DOI: 10.1201/9781003045564-13

Poortmans, P. M., Weltens, C., Fortpied, C., Kirkove, C., Peignaux-Casasnovas, K., Budach, V., van der Leij, F., Vonk, E., Weidner, N., Rivera, S., van Tienhoven, G., Fourquet, A., Noel, G., Valli, M., Guckenberger, M., Koiter, E., Racadot, S., Abdah-Bortnyak, R., Van Limbergen, E. F., & Bartelink, H. (2020). Internal mammary and medial supraclavicular lymph node chain irradiation in stage I–III breast cancer (EORTC 22922/10925): 15-year results of a randomised, phase 3 trial. *The Lancet. Oncology, 21*(12), 1602–1610. DOI: 10.1016/S1470-2045(20)30472-1

Prastawa, M., Bullitt, E., Moon, N., Van Leemput, K., & Gerig, G. (2003). Automatic brain tumor segmentation by subject specific modification of atlas priors1. *Academic Radiology*, *10*(12), 1341–1348. DOI: 10.1016/S1076-6332(03)00506-3

Prosser, J. D., Vender, J. R., & Solares, C. A. (2011). Traumatic cerebrospinal fluid leaks. *Otolaryngologic Clinics of North America*, *44*(4), 857–873. DOI: 10.1016/j.otc.2011.06.007

Raja, S. G., & Nirmala, K. (2019). Detection of brain tumor using K-nearest neighbor (KNN) based classification model and self-organizing map (SOM) algorithm. [IJITEE]. *International Journal of Innovative Technology and Exploring Engineering*, *8*(8).

Rother, C., Kolmogorov, V., & Blake, A. (2004). GrabCut" interactive foreground extraction using iterated graph cuts. [TOG]. *ACM Transactions on Graphics*, *23*(3), 309–314. DOI: 10.1145/1015706.1015720

Saeed, S. (2022). A Systematic Mapping Study of Tumor Cell Released by Enzymes and Toxins. *Clinical Cancer Investigation Journal*, *11*(5), 1–5. DOI: 10.51847/wpdou0F3Sc

Saeed, S., & Abdul, S. M. H. (2023). A Systematic Mapping Study of detection of Tumor Cell Targeted by Enzymes though Cerebrospinal Fluid. *Clinical Cancer Investigation Journal*, *12*(1), 1–5. DOI: 10.51847/VqorizLQM3

Saeed, S., Abdullah, A., Jhanjhi, N. Z., Naqvi, M., & Khan, A. (2020). Comparison analysis of multidimensional segmentation using medical health-care information. In *Machine Learning for Healthcare* (pp. 81–94). Chapman and Hall/CRC. DOI: 10.1201/9780429330131-7

Saeed, S., Abdullah, A., Jhanjhi, N. Z., Naqvi, M., & Khan, A. (2020). Comparison analysis of multidimensional segmentation using medical health-care information. In *Machine Learning for Healthcare* (pp. 81–94). Chapman and Hall/CRC. DOI: 10.1201/9780429330131-7

Saeed, S., Haron, H., Jhanjhi, N. Z., Naqvi, M., Alhumyani, H. A., & Masud, M. (2022). Improve correlation matrix of discrete fourier transformation technique for finding the missing values of mri images. *Mathematical Biosciences and Engineering*, *19*(9), 9039–9059. DOI: 10.3934/mbe.2022420

Saeed, S., Haroon, H. B., Naqvi, M., Jhanjhi, N. Z., Ahmad, M., & Gaur, L. (2022). A systematic mapping study of low-grade tumor of brain cancer and csf fluid detecting approaches and parameters. *Approaches and applications of deep learning in virtual medical care*, 236-259.

Saeed, S., Shaikh, A., Memon, M. A., Saleem, M. Q., & Naqvi, S. M. R. (2017). Assessment of Brain Tumor Due to the Usage of MATLAB Performance [JMIHI]. *Journal of Medical Imaging and Health Informatics*, *7*(6), 1454–1460. DOI: 10.1166/jmihi.2017.2187

Sedghi, A., O'Donnell, L. J., Kapur, T., Learned-Miller, E., Mousavi, P., & Wells, W. M.III. (2021). Image registration: Maximum likelihood, minimum entropy and deep learning. *Medical Image Analysis*, *69*, 101939. DOI: 10.1016/j.media.2020.101939

Silva, A. (2016). *Light field processor: a lytro illum imaging application* (Master's thesis, ISCTE-Instituto Universitario de Lisboa (Portugal)).

Song, Y., Adobah, B., Qu, J., & Liu, C. (2020). Segmentation of ordinary images and medical images with an adaptive Hidden Markov model and Viterbi algorithm. *Current Signal Transduction Therapy*, *15*(2), 109–123. DOI: 10.2174/1574362413666181109113834

Soobia, S., Afnizanfaizal, A., & Jhanjhi, N. Z. (2022). Hybrid graph cut hidden Markov model of k-mean cluster technique. *CMC-Computers. Materials & Continua*, *72*(1), 1–15.

Stoffel, R., Quilliam, M. A., Hardt, N., Fridstrom, A., & Witting, M. (2022). N-Alkylpyridinium sulfonates for retention time indexing in reversed-phase-liquid chromatography-mass spectrometry–based metabolomics. *Analytical and Bioanalytical Chemistry*, *414*(25), 1–12. DOI: 10.1007/s00216-021-03828-0

Strazielle, N., & Ghersi-Egea, J. F. (2013). Physiology of blood–brain interfaces in relation to brain disposition of small compounds and macromolecules. *Molecular Pharmaceutics*, *10*(5), 1473–1491. DOI: 10.1021/mp300518e

Varatharaj, A., & Galea, I. (2017). The blood-brain barrier in systemic inflammation. *Brain, Behavior, and Immunity*, *60*, 1–12. DOI: 10.1016/j.bbi.2016.03.010

Whitehead, H. D., Hayes, K. L., Swartz, J. A., Prete, E., Robison-Taylor, L., Mackesy-Amiti, M. E., & Lieberman, M. (2023). Validated method for the analysis of 22 illicit drugs and their metabolites via liquid chromatography tandem mass spectrometry (LC-MS/MS) in illicit drug samples collected in Chicago, IL. *Forensic Chemistry (Amsterdam, Netherlands)*, *33*, 100475. DOI: 10.1016/j.forc.2023.100475

Zhang, Y., Matuszewski, B. J., Shark, L. K., & Moore, C. J. (2007, July). A novel medical image segmentation method using dynamic programming. In *International Conference on Medical Information Visualisation-BioMedical Visualisation (MediVis 2007)* (pp. 69-74). IEEE. DOI: 10.1109/MEDIVIS.2007.2

Zhuge, Y., Krauze, A. V., Ning, H., Cheng, J. Y., Arora, B. C., Camphausen, K., & Miller, R. W. (2017). Brain tumor segmentation using holistically nested neural networks in MRI images. *Medical Physics*, *44*(10), 5234–5243. DOI: 10.1002/mp.12481

Chapter 3
Medical Nanoparticles: Breakthroughs in Diagnostics and Targeted Therapies

Saloua Mabsor-Zgandaoui
https://orcid.org/0009-0006-4601-9059
Ibn Tofail University, Morocco

Khawla Rachmoune
https://orcid.org/0009-0001-6483-1060
Cadi Ayyad University, Marrakech, Morocco

Hassane Boulmane
Sidi Mohamed Ben Abdellah University, Morocco

Hafssa Dakir
https://orcid.org/0009-0006-7097-2894
Mohammed VI University of Health and Science (UM6SS), Casablanca, Morocco

Ilham Aftais
https://orcid.org/0000-0002-9609-7411
Ibn Tofail University, Morocco

Kawtar Ettayri
Jiangsu University, China

Youssef Ait Hamdan
Cadi Ayyad University, Morocco

Youness Zgandaoui
Ibn Tofail University, Morocco

Adnane Moutaouakkil
https://orcid.org/0000-0002-1762-881X
National Centre for Nuclear Energy, Science and Technology (CNESTEN), Rabat, Morocco

ABSTRACT

Nanoparticles have emerged as pivotal components in medical applications, particularly in diagnostics, imaging and targeted therapy. Various types of nanoparticles facilitate precise therapeutic targeting while minimizing systemic side effects. Recent advancements in surface functionalization techniques have significantly improved nanoparticle stability and reduced immunogenicity, allowing for enhanced specificity in cellular targeting. Future directions in this field may include the exploration of smart nanoparticles capable of sequential drug delivery in response to real-time biomarkers and the development of biocompatible coatings that ensure prolonged stability.

DOI: 10.4018/979-8-3373-4627-4.ch003

INTRODUCTION

Nanoparticles (NPs) are a key and revolutionary component of modern medicine, contributing to major advances in the fields of diagnostics, targeted therapies and even regenerative medicine (Raheem et al. 2023). Their nanometric dimensions and unique physico-chemical properties make them ideal for providing innovative solutions to complex medical problems such as cancer, neurodegenerative diseases, infections, metabolic disorders and inflammatory pathologies. Versatility and adaptability make them essential tools for pushing back the limits of conventional treatments (Liu et al. 2021).

In the diagnostic field, NPs have revolutionized disease detection and monitoring, dramatically increasing the sensitivity, precision and response time of biosensors. Nanomaterials such as fluorescent NPs, quantum dots, nanorobots and metal-organic frameworks enable the early and precise diagnosis of biomarkers, even at extremely low concentrations. Innovative technologies such as these enable rapid, accurate and sometimes non-invasive diagnostics, crucial for diagnosing cancers, viral diseases, immune disorders or toxic residues in organisms. In addition, they enable real-time monitoring of treatment progress (Bobo et al. 2016).

NPs have become the vectors of choice for the delivery of therapeutic compounds including drugs, genes, proteins and vaccines in targeted therapies. This focused approach can minimize the systemic side-effects often associated with drugs, while boosting therapeutic effect. Recent technological advancements in the operationalization of NPs include the sophisticated use for molecular engineering to reinforce their specific characteristics. NPs adapt to the targeted cellular environment, interact with their specific receptors and liberate their therapeutical charge in a controlled manner, sometimes activated by external impulses (light, heat or pH) (Yetisgin et al. 2020). Advances such as these open up new possibilities in the treatment of drug-resistant cancers, genetic diseases, and chronic infections, as well as in the development of RNA vaccines such as those used against COVID-19. Besides diagnostics and therapy, NPs also play a role in regenerative medicine, contributing to tissue repair or bone regeneration through nanostructured biomaterials. In fact, they are used in integrated approaches combining medical imaging and therapy, as in the field of theranostics, where a single nanoparticle can detect a disease and provide a treatment at the identical time (Gurunathan et al. 2018).

This chapter explored in depth the key role of NPs in the advancement of precise medicine, examining their mechanisms of action, their diverse categories, their current applications and their potential for integrating into current clinical practice. Highlighting the opportunities and challenges of this emerging technology, we aimed to prove how it may transform healthcare paradigms. As nanomedicine research advances rapidly, it is poised to be a major breakthrough in improving diagnosis, treatment and, more broadly, quality of life for patients across a wide range of pathologies.

NANOPARTICLES IN DIAGNOSTICS

Fluorescent nanomaterials are water-soluble molecular aggregates made up of several to hundreds of atoms. They were extremely efficient at biosensing due to their great biocompatibility and strong anti-polymerization capabilities (Chen et al., 2018; Lopes et al., 2022), DNA, peptides, proteins, small molecule ligands, and polymers are examples of common MNCs templates (Ou

et al., 2018). Among these, DNA templated MNCs (DNA-MNCs) have been widely employed in biosensors to detect a variety of targets, including nucleic acids, metal ions, tiny biomolecules, and proteins (Li et al., 2015). DNA-MNCs has provided for in situ synthesis under relatively mild preparation conditions, a regulated operation process, adjustable fluorescence emission, and the possibility of linking DNA templates with aptamers, all of which have been advantageous for their use as aptasensors. As well as DNA-MNCs, gold NPs (AuNPs) and silver NPs (AgNPs) are commonly utilized as probes. Fluorescence-based aptasensors used strong surface plasmon resonance (SPR) to amplify fluorescence signals through interactions with fluorescent molecules near their surface. Other nanomaterials, including carbon dots (CDs), quantum dots (QDs), and metal-organic frameworks (MOFs), provide further advantages. CDs and QDs provide photostability and adjustable fluorescence, whereas MOFs have a porous structure and a large surface area for target binding, strengthening sensitivity and specificity in biosensing applications (Liang et al., 2021).

Detection of Cancer Biomarkers

Chen and colleagues developed a unique detection approach that uses a hairpin DNA probe containing cytosine bases to generate a C-Ag+-C structure in the presence of silver ions (Figure 1). In its closed condition, the probe quenches fluorescence by keeping a fluorophore and quencher close together. When IFN-γ binds to its aptamer, it releases a single-stranded DNA (P1). This causes a catalytic hairpin assembly (CHA) reaction, unfolding the probe and displacing Ag+ ions. These ions are detected when they interact with QDs and calcein, with increasing Ag+ concentrations resulting in lower fluorescence. Furthermore, ink-jet printed test strips clearly reveal Ag+ ion diffusion distance, which correlates with IFN-γ levels. This dual-mode technique combines fluorescence and visual detection to provide accurate, instrument-free proof-of-concept testing (Fan et al., 2018).

Figure 1. Schematic of the homogeneous analysis of IFN-γ in tuberculosis patients using CER and CHA (Chen et al. 2023)

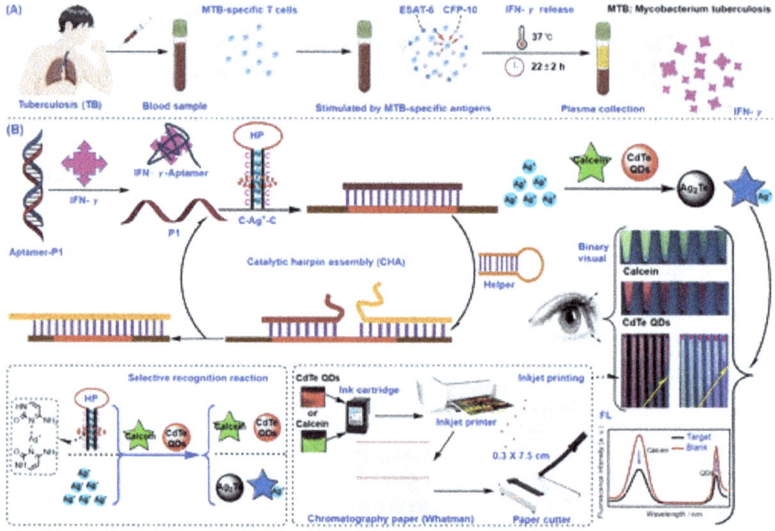

Qiu and co-workers designed an innovative paper-based analytical device (PAD) for visual fluorescence detection of carcinoembryonic antigen (CEA) using QDs (CdTe/CdSe QDs) and glucose oxidase (GOD) (Figure 2) (Qiu et al., 2017). The detection method employs mesoporous silica NPs (MSNs) gated with a DNA aptamer that specifically targets CEA. When MSNs connect to CEA, glucose within them is released, causing a reaction that quenches the QDs' fluorescence. This change in fluorescence can be visually observed with a smartphone or quantitatively evaluated with a spectrometer, enabling for sensitive and specific CEA detection in the linear range of 0.05 to 20 ng/mL (Qiu et al., 2017).

Figure 2. PAD for CEA detection via aptamer-gated MSNs with enzymatic amplification (Qiu, Shu, & Tang, 2017)

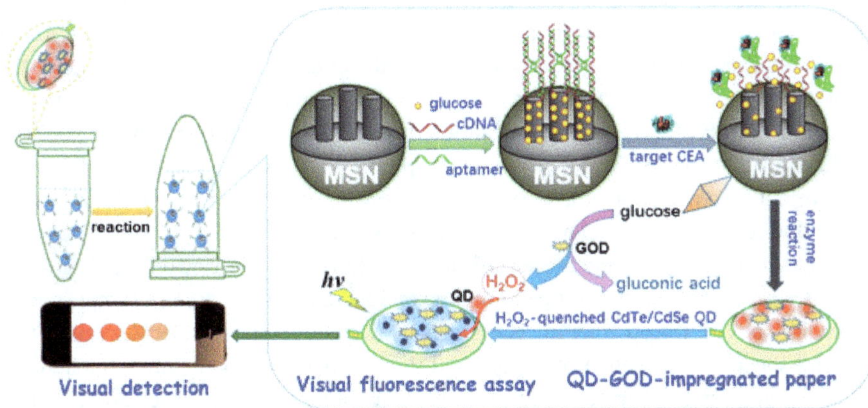

Detection of Cancer Cells

Song's team designed a DNA-based cytosensor for detecting several cancer cell types by using MSNs functionalized with QDs as a signal amplification platform (Figure 3). The detection mechanism is based on the particular interaction between aptamer-functionalized MSNs/QDs and target cancer cells such as MCF-7, HL-60, and K562 cell lines. The aptamers bind specifically to these cells, maintaining the fluorescence signal from the QDs, confirming the presence of cancer cells. Non-target cells show low fluorescence due to a lack of binding, (Liang et al., 2016).

Figure 3. Cytosensor fabrication and assembly on PADs (Liang et al., 2016)

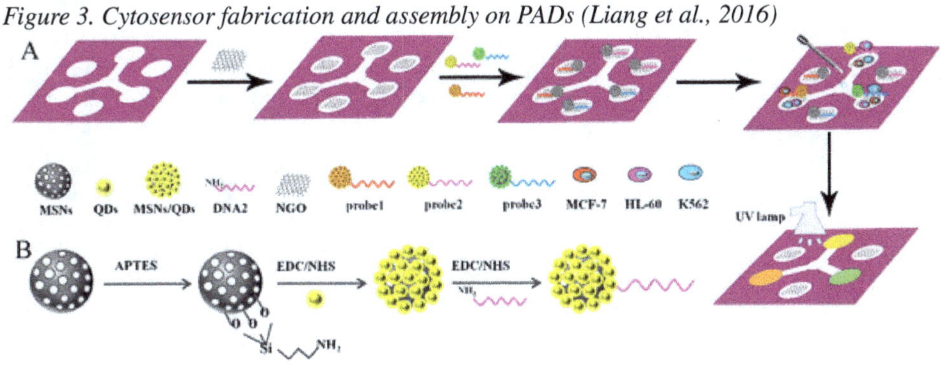

Detection of Antibiotic Residues and Drug-Resistant Infections

β-lactam antibiotics, including Ampicillin (AMPI), have been widely used in medicine and agriculture to treat harmful microorganisms (Yang et al., 2021). However, the misuse and reliance on these medicines in both human treatment and farm animal care has led to the rise of antibiotic-resistant bacterial species. As a result, the clinical appearance of difficult-to-treat drug-resistant infections (DRIs) has increased the risk of medical costs for customers and patients (Yang et al., 2021). Furthermore, leftover antibiotics have been identified in meat, poultry, fish, and milk, which can cause allergic responses, respiratory issues, and seizures. As a result, it is more important than ever to identify these medications quickly and precisely in order to avoid the global development of antimicrobial resistance (Barton, 2000).

Initially, a biotin-labelled aptamer specific to ampicillin is immobilized on streptavidin-coated magnetic beads, leveraging the strong biotin-streptavidin interaction. When a sample containing ampicillin is supplied, the aptamer binds exclusively to the ampicillin molecules due to the high affinity and specificity provided by its unusual three-dimensional structure, which allows for hydrogen bonding and electrostatic interactions. This binding event causes a conformational shift in the aptamer, allowing it to release a previously hybridized single-stranded DNA (ssDNA) activator (Figure 4). This released ssDNA acts as a critical activator for the CRISPR/Cas12a system, which includes the Cas12a enzyme and a guide RNA (gRNA). The ssDNA activator induces the Cas12a enzyme's trans-cleavage activity. Next, the activated Cas12a enzyme cleaves a fluorescent reporter probe tagged with both a fluorophore (Cy3) and a quencher (BHQ-2). Under typical conditions, fluorescence is prevented by the near proximity of the fluorophore and quencher. However, when the Cas12a enzyme cleaves the fluorophore, it separates from the quencher, resulting in a considerable increase in fluorescence emissions. The intensity of the produced fluorescence, which can be detected and measured with a microplate reader, corresponds directly to the concentration of ampicillin in the sample.

Figure 4. CRISPR/Cas12a aptasensor for AMPI detection showing fluorescence response (Yee et al., 2023)

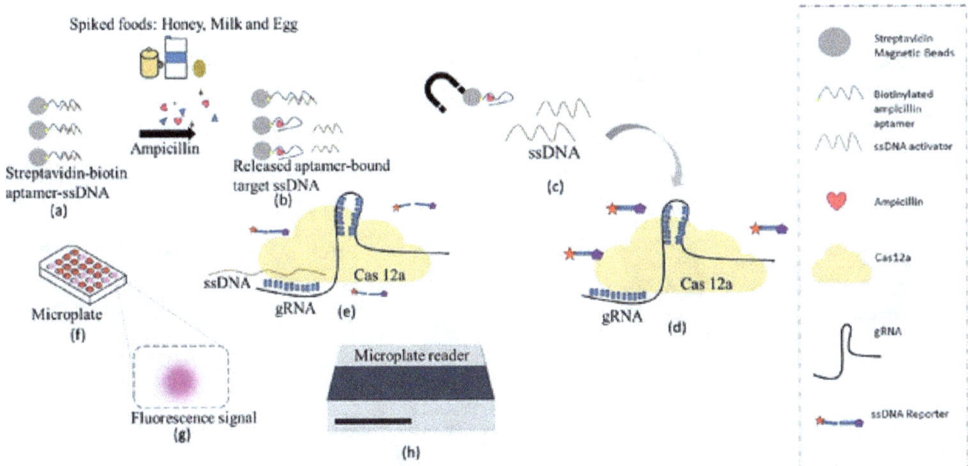

Chen et al. (2023) developed a novel sandwich-type electrochemical aptasensor for the simultaneous detection of cardiac biomarkers, specifically cardiac troponin I (cTnI) and myoglobin (Myo), which are critical indicators of acute myocardial infarction (AMI) (Figure 5). The sensor utilizes aptamers single-stranded DNA or RNA molecules selected for their high specificity and strong binding affinity to recognize cTnI and Myo. These aptamers are immobilized on a carbonized zirconium-based metal-organic framework (Zr-MOF) modified electrode, further decorated with coralloid-like gold (CAu) to enhance surface area and electrochemical signal sensitivity. Upon introducing a sample, the biomarkers bind to their respective capture aptamers, forming an aptamer-biomarker complex. Signal amplification is achieved by introducing polydopamine (PDA) spheres decorated with gold NPs (Au) and metal ions (Pb^{2+} and Cu^{2+}), which bind to the captured biomarkers, forming a sandwich-like structure. The electrochemical signal generated by the Pb^{2+} and Cu^{2+} ions is detected using differential pulse voltammetry (DPV), allowing for the quantification of cTnI and Myo concentrations. This aptasensor's high specificity, signal amplification, and the sensitivity of DPV offer an efficient and reliable platform for early AMI diagnosis, highlighting the potential of aptasensors in clinical applications (Chen et al., 2023).

Figure 5. The fabrication steps of (A) CAu/CC/SPCE, (B) Apt-label (TrO6-label+S232-label), and (C) the aptasensor for Myo+cTnI simultaneous (Chen et al. 2023)

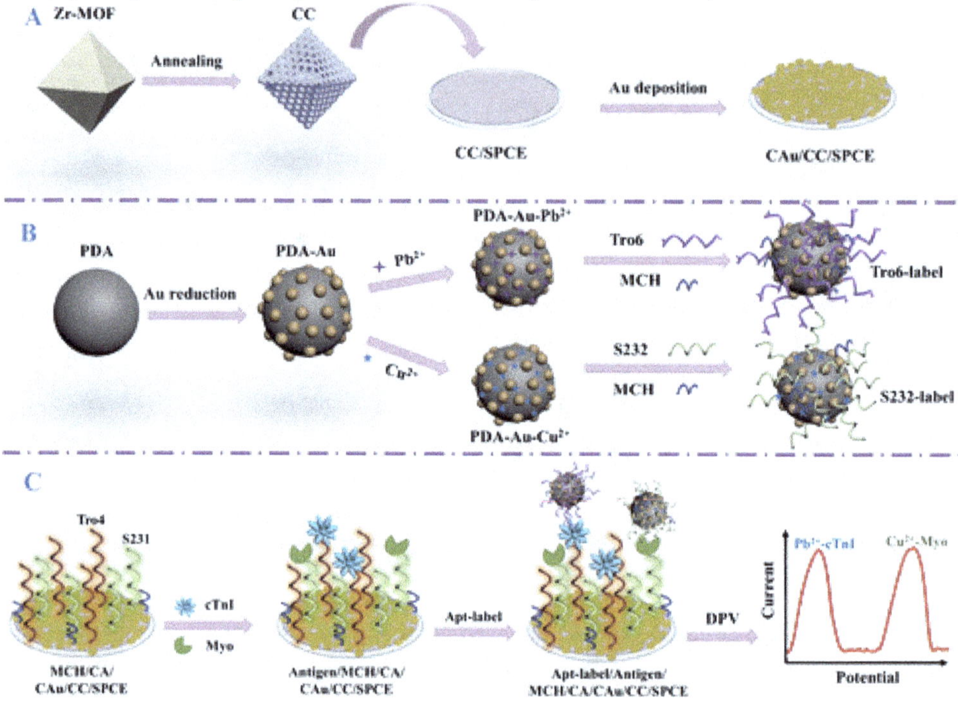

MicroRNAs (miRNAs) are small, non-coding RNA molecules typically about 20-24 nucleotides long that play crucial roles in regulating gene expression. They function by binding to complementary sequences on target messenger RNAs (mRNAs), leading to mRNA degradation or inhibition of translation, thereby controlling various biological processes such as development, differentiation, proliferation, and apoptosis. Aberrant expression of miRNAs is associated with numerous diseases, including cancer, making miRNAs important biomarkers for disease diagnosis and prognosis (Lin et al., 2022).

Liu et al. (2021) developed a novel distance-based biosensor for miRNA detection, leveraging the CRISPR/Cas12a system and a target-triggered strand displacement amplification (SDA) reaction to achieve high sensitivity and visual quantification (Feng et al., 2023). The process begins with the target miRNA hybridizing with a designed DNA probe to form a DNA/RNA hybrid, which serves as a template for the SDA reaction. During SDA, a DNA polymerase extends and displaces the DNA probe, producing double-stranded DNA (dsDNA), which activates the CRISPR/Cas12a system. When complexed with a guide RNA (gRNA) specific to the dsDNA, Cas12a is activated upon binding and triggers its collateral cleavage activity. This activity cleaves a specially designed single-stranded DNA (ssDNA) linker attached to magnetic beads, releasing trypsin into the solution. The released trypsin then hydrolyzes gelatin pre-coated on a filter paper, reducing its viscosity and allowing a dye solution to move along a cotton thread. The distance the solution travels on the cotton thread creates a visible signal that is directly proportional to the miRNA concentration, providing a quantifiable, visual output. The biosensor's performance

was optimized by adjusting reagent concentrations and reaction times to maximize sensitivity and specificity, and its efficacy was validated using synthetic miRNA-let-7a, serum samples, and cell lysates (Yang et al., 2021).

Dengue virus (DENV) is a mosquito-borne pathogen responsible for dengue fever, a significant global health concern characterized by symptoms ranging from mild fever to severe hemorrhagic conditions. Early detection of DENV is crucial for timely medical intervention and effective outbreak management. A smartphone-based wireless pocket sensor for DENV detection employs an innovative mechanism to achieve rapid and sensitive detection. The process begins with the synthesis of zinc oxide (ZnO)-NPs through a chemical method, chosen for their superior electrochemical properties and biocompatibility, which enhance the sensor's sensitivity (Hasan et al., 2024).

These NPs are functionalized to immobilize a DNA aptamer specific to the dengue antigen by modifying their surface to create aptamer-binding sites. Upon introducing a sample containing the dengue antigen, the antigen binds to the immobilized aptamer, inducing a change in the electrochemical properties of the ZnO-NPs. This change is measured using cyclic voltammetry, and the resulting electrochemical data is transmitted wirelessly to a smartphone application for processing and display. The sensor's performance is optimized by fine-tuning detection parameters such as temperature and time, achieving detection of dengue antigen concentrations as low as 0.1 µg/mL within 20 seconds and demonstrating a linear response across a range of concentrations. Stability and selectivity are validated using human serum samples, ensuring minimal interference from other proteins and reliable functionality over weeks. This pocket sensor showcases exceptional portability, accessibility, and efficiency, establishing it as a promising tool for point-of-care applications and public health management in dengue-prone regions, (Chen et al., 2018) .

NANOPARTICLES IN TARGETED THERAPY

NPs are versatile vectors for the targeted delivery of therapeutic agents, transforming the field of targeted therapy. Their nanometric size (1-100 nm) enables enhanced permeability and retention (EPR effect) in pathological areas such as tumours or inflamed tissues, making them particularly successful in the treatment of a wide variety of diseases. By encapsulating drugs, ribonucleic acids, deoxyribonucleic acids, monoclonal antibodies, peptides or receptor-specific proteins. Several NPs give improved biodisponibility, reduced systemic toxicity and controlled release of active ingredients (Gavas et al., 2021).

Advances in nanotechnology have revolutionized the design of NPs, enabling their functionalization with specific targeting ligands. This innovation significantly enhances the precision with which NPs interact with targeted cellular receptors or specific microenvironments. Such functionalization is particularly advantageous in addressing challenges like tumour acidity or elevated enzymatic activity, allowing for more effective and localized therapeutic interventions. The applications of NPs in targeted therapy span diverse fields, including cancer treatment, neurodegenerative diseases, gene therapy, immunotherapy, and cardiovascular conditions. These advancements highlight their potential to overcome the limitations associated with conventional drug delivery systems. There is a wide variety of NPs used in targeted therapy, including polymeric, liposomal, inorganic, biomimetic and hybrid NPs, each with their specific characteristics adapted to specific applications (Yetisgin et al., 2020).

Polymeric NPs (PNPs)

Solid or hollow nanometric particles, typically ranging from 10 to 100 nm, made from natural, semi-synthetic, or synthetic polymers. These nanoscale structures play a central role in the controlled release of active ingredients, including drugs, peptides, genes, or other therapeutic agents. They can exist as solid matrices, where active substances are uniformly dispersed, or as hollow cavities encapsulating therapeutic compounds. This category of nanostructures is particularly important in targeted therapy due to its compositional diversity and versatile applications. Based on the type of polymer used, these systems are generally classified as natural, synthetic, or stimuli-responsive. Their structural flexibility allows for the creation of delivery platforms tailored to meet specific therapeutic requirements. Natural polymers, such as albumin, collagen, alginate, cellulose, and chitosan (CS), are derived from renewable biological resources. They are well-known for their biocompatibility and biodegradability, making them ideal for sensitive applications like the encapsulation of vaccines or biomolecules. For instance, CS, with its cationic properties, enhances the delivery of RNA and other hydrophilic agents, while alginate is frequently employed in the formation of gels for encapsulating cells or drugs (Seyedi et al., 2022).

Synthetic polymers, such as PLGA (poly (lactic-co-glycolic acid)), PEG (polyethylene glycol), and PCL (polycaprolactone), are valued for their enhanced chemical stability and advanced customization options. PLGA, widely utilized, enables sustained release of active compounds, while PEG improves the pharmacokinetics of NPs by extending their circulatory half-life. These polymers are particularly suited for applications in cancer therapy and immunotherapy, where precision is critical. Stimuli-responsive polymers represent a significant technological advancement. These polymers can react to stimuli such as pH, temperature, enzymatic activity, or external triggers like magnetic fields or light, enabling controlled and targeted drug release. For instance, pH-sensitive polymers utilize the acidic tumour microenvironment to trigger the release of encapsulated agents, while thermo-sensitive polymers are employed in localized hyperthermic treatments. Such intelligent systems are particularly well-suited for addressing complex conditions like cancer (Mai et al., 2018).

PNPs have been applied across various medical fields. In chemotherapy, they enable prolonged and targeted delivery of anticancer agents, reducing systemic side effects. For instance, paclitaxel-loaded PLGA-NPs have shown enhanced efficacy against solid tumours. Similarly, in gene therapy, CS nanospheres carrying siRNA have been designed to specifically target genes implicated in neurodegenerative diseases. PEGylated nanocapsules containing monoclonal antibodies have demonstrated effectiveness in immunotherapy, particularly in treating resistant cancers (Suk et al., 2016). Furthermore, alginate NPs are employed in tissue regeneration to encapsulate stem cells, thereby promoting bone and cartilage repair. Several PNPs have been approved for clinical use or are currently undergoing evaluation. Examples include albumin-bound paclitaxel NPs, is used for breast cancer treatment. A liposomal formulation of irinotecan, has proven effective against metastatic pancreatic cancer. Also, a polymeric nanoparticle encapsulating paclitaxel, is approved for the treatment of solid tumours, highlighting the significant clinical impact of nanotechnologies (Wang et al., 2023).

Polymeric nanostructures possess unique characteristics that make them particularly suitable for therapeutic applications. Their tuneable composition and intrinsic properties offer significant advantages in drug delivery and in minimizing side effects. Notably, their biocompatibility ensures excellent compatibility with biological tissues, reducing the risk of adverse reaction (Calzoni et

al., 2019). Additionally, these nanostructures excel in protecting active ingredients by shielding encapsulated molecules from enzymatic or chemical degradation, making them ideal for sustained therapies. They also enable controlled release, facilitating slow and targeted delivery of active agents, which enhances therapeutic efficacy. Furthermore, their design can be tailored for both active and passive targeting, allowing precise interaction with diseased cells or tissues while minimizing off-target effects. Lastly, their structural versatility, stemming from customizable compositions and preparation methods, allows adaptation to meet diverse therapeutic requirements.

PNPs present exciting opportunities in drug delivery and tissue engineering due to their unique properties. However, their development faces various challenges that must be addressed to optimize their applications. Some natural polymers, like alginate, may degrade prematurely, thereby reducing their efficacy in certain applications. Synthetic polymers such as PLGA, while chemically stable, can sometimes induce immune responses, potentially compromising clinical tolerance. The large-scale production of PNPs, particularly those made from synthetic polymers, remains costly. processes involved in the synthesis and formulation of PNPs are often complex and require rigorous optimization. Striking a balance between stability, biodegradability, and low toxicity continues to be a challenge for widespread adoption. Certain formulations are unsuitable for complex physiological environments or specific targeted treatments (Agrahari et al., 2019).

Despite these challenges, ongoing technological advancements and continuous research aim to overcome these limitations and maximize their therapeutic potential. To summarize the key points and provide a comparative overview, the Table 1 outlines the main categories of PNPs, their properties, preparation methods, therapeutic applications, advantages, and limitations.

Table 1. Comparison of main categories of PNPs: Properties, preparation methods, applications, advantages and limitations

Category	Properties	Preparation Methods	Therapeutic Applications	Advantages	Limitations
Natural Polymers	High biocompatibility, biodegradable; prone to premature degradation	Ionic gelation, nano-precipitation	Drug delivery, tissue regeneration, vaccine encapsulation	Excellent biocompatibility	Limited stability in certain physiological conditions
Synthetic Polymers	Precisely controlled physicochemical properties; may trigger immune response	Solvent evaporation, spray drying	Chemotherapy, gene therapy, targeted drug delivery	Tunable properties for specific needs	Potential immunogenicity and higher production cost
Stimuli-Responsive Polymers	Responsive to specific stimuli (e.g., pH, temperature, enzymes)	Various methods (controlled radical polymerization, self-assembly)	Targeted and controlled drug delivery	High specificity for the target environment	Dependence on environmental factors

Liposomal NPs (LNPs)

LNPs are spherical structures composed of one or more lipid bilayers surrounding an aqueous core. These bilayers are primarily formed from phospholipids, the main constituents of biological membranes, often supplemented with sterols such as cholesterol to enhance stability. This unique architecture allows liposomes to encapsulate both hydrophilic agents within their aqueous core

and hydrophobic agents within the lipid bilayer, making them highly versatile for therapeutic and diagnostic applications. Based on their structure, liposomes can be categorized into two main types: unilamellar vesicles (UV), containing a single lipid bilayer (including small UV, and large UV), and multilamellar vesicles (MLV), which are composed of multiple concentric lipid bilayers, each enclosing aqueous compartment. Additionally, liposome composition can be customized to include functional components such as polymers (PEGylated liposomes), antibodies (immunoliposomes), or peptides, thereby enhancing their ability to target specific cellular receptors (Mabsor-Zgandaoui et al. 2026).

LNPs encompass several distinct types, each designed to address specific therapeutic challenges. Classical liposomes, composed solely of phospholipids and cholesterol, provide basic drug encapsulation but face limitations due to their short circulatory half-life caused by rapid clearance by the reticuloendothelial system (RES) (Klyachko et al., 2020). PEGylated liposomes, or stealth liposomes, overcome this drawback by incorporating polyethylene glycol (PEG) on their surface, significantly extending their circulatory half-life and enhancing their effectiveness in oncology applications. Immunoliposomes, functionalized with antibodies or antibody fragments, enable precise active targeting of pathological cells, such as cancer cells. Stimuli-responsive liposomes are designed to release their payload in response to external stimuli or internal stimuli, offering significant potential for controlled drug delivery. Finally, cationic liposomes, characterized by their positive charge, are primarily used in gene therapy as they interact with nucleic acids to form stable complexes known as lipoplexes (Klyachko et al., 2020).

LNPs have revolutionized the medical field due to their remarkable ability to effectively deliver therapeutic agents. Their biocompatibility, structural versatility, and capability for targeted delivery have established them as essential tools in advancing innovative treatments across diverse applications. In oncology, liposomal formulations such as PEGylated Doxil® have been widely used to deliver anticancer agents like doxorubicin, leveraging the enhanced permeability and retention (EPR) effect to achieve higher tumour accumulation and reduced systemic toxicity. Similarly, in gene therapy, cationic liposomes play a crucial role in transporting genetic materials, such as siRNA and plasmids, enabling targeted and efficient treatment of genetic and infectious diseases (Taléns-Visconti et al., 2022). In the management of cardiovascular diseases, liposomes encapsulating thrombolytic agents, like tissue plasminogen activator (tPA), have demonstrated improved targeting of vascular obstructions, thereby enhancing therapeutic efficacy while minimizing systemic side effects. In vaccinology, liposomes serve as delivery vectors for antigens, significantly boosting immunogenicity. A notable example is their use in mRNA vaccines, where they protect and efficiently deliver mRNA to target cells, as seen in the development of modern vaccine platforms. Additionally, in the treatment of infectious diseases, liposomal formulations of antibiotics, such as amphotericin B, offer a dual advantage of reduced toxicity and enhanced therapeutic performance, proving critical in managing severe systemic infections. These multifaceted applications underscore the transformative potential of LNPs in addressing complex medical challenges and improving patient outcomes (Groll et al., 2019).

Inorganic NPs (INPs)

INPs are composed of non-organic materials, including pure metals such as gold and silver, metal oxides like iron oxide and titanium dioxide, as well as carbon-based structures such as nanotubes and fullerenes. These NPs can be engineered into various shapes, including spherical,

tubular, cubic, or mesoporous forms. Surface modifications are frequently applied to enhance their stability, enable targeted tissue delivery, or facilitate the transport of active biomolecules (Bayda et al., 2018).

INPs, valued for their remarkable properties such as chemical stability and unique optical or magnetic behaviours, are central to advancements in nanomedicine. These NPs find extensive use in various fields, including medical imaging and targeted therapies. This category encompasses a wide array of materials, each defined by its specific composition and functionalities. Metallic NPs such as gold (Au), silver (Ag), and platinum are renowned for their stability and biocompatibility, making them suitable for biological applications. Metal oxides, including iron oxide, titanium dioxide, and zinc oxide (ZnO), stand out due to their magnetic and photocatalytic capabilities. Semiconductor nanocrystals, also known as quantum dots, such as cadmium selenide, cadmium telluride, and zinc sulfide, are prized for their outstanding optical and electronic features. Carbon-based nanostructures, like nanotubes and fullerene, exhibit exceptional mechanical strength and electrical conductivity. Lastly, silica NPs, whether in amorphous or mesoporous forms, serve as highly adaptable platforms for drug delivery and surface engineering. Through their diverse properties and functions, INPs offer immense potential for innovation in biomedical applications (Bayda et al., 2018).

INPs have already demonstrated their potential in various clinical contexts. Several innovative formulations have been approved or are under evaluation for applications ranging from diagnostic imaging to targeted therapy. These advancements highlight their growing significance in modern medicine. INPs are distinguished by their unique properties, making them highly suitable for a wide range of medical applications. Their rigid structure and chemical stability provide superior performance in demanding biological environments. Additionally, their ability to interact with optical, magnetic, or biological signals offers remarkable versatility. Key characteristics and advantages of these NPs include plasmon resonance, enabling light absorption and scattering for optical imaging and photothermal therapy, magnetic properties, such as superparamagnetic, for MRI and hyperthermia; long-lasting fluorescence for extended imaging with quantum dots; adjustable biocompatibility through chemical surface modification, chemical stability, ensuring resistance to biological degradation; encapsulation capability for both hydrophilic and hydrophobic drugs; and ease of functionalization, allowing for the addition of ligands or antibodies for specific targeting (Jiao et al., 2018).

Biomimetic NPs (BNPs)

BNPs are nanoscale structures enveloped in cellular membranes, enabling them to mimic the biological behaviour of natural cells. The cellular coating provides these NPs with the ability to evade immune detection by masking their identity, allowing them to circulate in the body for extended periods. These NPs can be fabricated using various core materials, including polymeric, lipid-based, or inorganic NPs, which are subsequently coated with membranes derived from specific cell types such as erythrocytes, platelets, or tumour cells (Gavas et al., 2021).

NPs coated with erythrocyte membranes are among the most studied biomimetic types. The membrane coating inhibits phagocytosis and ensures prolonged circulation within the bloodstream. Similarly, platelet membrane-coated NPs are designed to target vascular injuries and inflammatory sites, exploiting the natural adhesion properties of platelets to enhance therapeutic precision. NPs cloaked in tumour cell membranes are particularly effective for cancer treatments, as they allow

for specific targeting of cancer cells and improved delivery of anticancer therapies. Another important category includes macrophage membrane-coated NPs, which are developed to combat infections and inflammation by utilizing the immune-modulating properties of macrophages to enhance treatment efficacy (Shrestha et al., 2019).

BNPs offer several significant advantages, making them highly promising for medical and technological applications. Their prolonged circulation time in the bloodstream results from the incorporation of cell membrane properties, which help evade immune system detection and enhance stability. These NPs also exhibit precise targeting capabilities by leveraging the biological characteristics of cell membranes to bind specifically to target cells or tissues, improving treatment accuracy. Additionally, their hybrid design, combining synthetic cores with biological membranes, ensures increased biocompatibility, thereby reducing toxicity and minimizing side effects. Inspired by nature's evolutionary solutions, BNPs incorporate features such as adaptability, robustness, energy efficiency, and self-repair capabilities, making them versatile for complex environments while maintaining high reliability and functionality (Issaka and Amu-Darko, 2024).

The limitations and challenges of BNPs include their intricate production processes, as extracting and integrating biological materials require advanced techniques. Stability is another concern, as biological components may degrade under physiological conditions, compromising functionality. Additionally, achieving consistent and reproducible production remains a significant obstacle, affecting clinical reliability. The high costs associated with these advanced materials and methods further restrict large-scale applications. Despite their promise in cancer therapy, gaps in understanding their mechanisms and optimizing their design for broader therapeutic use remain critical hurdles (Issaka and Amu-Darko, 2024).

NANOPARTICLES IN COMBINATION THERAPIES

Synergy with Immunotherapy and Radiotherapy

Cancer, an intricate multifactorial disease, is characterized by unopposed proliferation and dissemination of malignant cells in the host. Besides side effects due to therapeutic window and anticancer drug inventory, tumor cell heterogeneity causes serious problems, for instance, radio-resistance and anticancer drug resistance (Shrestha, Tang, and Romero 2019). For instance, tumor cells cultured in vitro with various conventional chemotherapeutics exhibited resistance rates of 65–70%, making the therapeutic efficacy much more complex (Shrestha et al., 2019). As such, it is possible to improve the selective administration of therapeutic agents and utilize nanocarriers such as liposomes, carbon nanotubes, PNPs, quantum dots, dendrimers and MNPs to decrease systemic cytotoxicity and improve clinical efficacy through novel nanomedicine. (Gurunathan et al., 2018), for instance, noted a 50% reduction in cytotoxicity in healthy cells as well as a 45% increase in the therapeutic index of anticancer agents when AuNPs were used. For immunotherapy, on the other hand, NPs have emerged as an adjunct to enhance of cancer synergy between immunotherapy and radiation therapy (Jin and Zhao 2020).

Several recent studies have demonstrated that NPs exert promising efficacy of immunotherapy and radiation therapy in tumor cells by selectively targeting to tumor cells, improving the active principal stability, and prolonging its half-life. Combining NPs with immunotherapeutic agents versus monotherapy has been shown to increase tumor remission rates by almost 30% (Qiu et al.,

2017). NPs combined with siRNAs, including EGFR and PD-L1 targeting siRNAs, significantly reduce glioblastoma growth and the survival rate of mice is improved by 40% (Erel-Akbaba et al., 2019). Additionally, CPV virus-based viral NPs have also been shown to stimulate the immune system and halt tumor growth by 35% when used with radiation therapy. Dynamic X-ray radiotherapeutic NPs are another variant (Z/high atomic number NPs modify radiotherapy by improved X-ray absorption). One such NP is NBTXR3, a hafnium-based NP that functions as a radiosensitizer by accelerating cell death and DNA damage, leading to a 60% increase in tumor control compared to radiotherapy alone. However, nMOFs with photosensitizing ligands enhance the DNA damage brought on by radiation by generating reactive oxygen species (ROS) and improving the oxygenation of hypoxic tumors (Mabsor-Zgandaoui et al. 2024), achieving a 25% improvement in radiation efficacy in preclinical trials (Hagan et al., 2020).

Co-Delivery Systems for Multiple Drugs

The co-administration of many medications based on NPs has emerged as a promising approach to cancer treatment. As noted Bostami et al. (2022), studies have shown that nanoparticle-mediated drug delivery can significantly improve drug accumulation in tumor tissues (Bostami et al., 2022). For instance, liposome-based nanotechnologies, solid NPs, and polymeric micelles have been developed to regulate the spatiotemporal distribution of medications, achieving up to a 4-fold increase in drug delivery efficiency compared to free drug administration (Table 2). The use of nanotransporters that carry the active ingredients of various medications is an effective way to treat cancer while preventing undesirable side effects, with reported reductions in systemic toxicity by 35% to 60% in some clinical trials (Fumoto and Nishida, 2020).

Table 2. Lipid and polymer-based NPs

Type	Key Component	Indication	Approval Date	Company	Reference
Lipid-based	PEGylated liposomal doxorubicin	Metastatic cancer, HIV-KS	FDA: 1995, EMA: 1996	Janssen-Cilag	(Franco et al., 2018)
	Liposomal cytarabine	Lymphomatous meningitis	FDA: 1999	Skye Pharma	(Yan et al., 2018)
	PEGylated liposomal irinotecan	Pancreatic cancer	FDA: 2015	Merrimack	(Franco et al., 2018)
	Liposomal paclitaxel	Breast cancer, NSCLC	China: 2006	Luye Pharma	(Zhou et al., 2021)
	Daunorubicin + cytarabine	Acute myeloid leukemia	FDA: 2017, EMA: 2018	Jazz Pharmaceuticals	(Krauss et al., 2019)
Polymer-based	Paclitaxel micellar	Breast, gastric cancer, NSCLC	South Korea: 2007	Samyang	(Kim and Shin, 2010)
	Leuprolide acetate + polymer	Prostate cancer	FDA: 2002	Tolmar	(Bobo et al., 2016)

There are two main categories of nanotransporters: inorganic and organic. Among inorganic nanotransporters, AuNPs are extensively studied for their biocompatibility and versatility. Ma et al. (2017), reported that AuNPs loaded with doxorubicin (DOX) or siRNA targeting the ASCL1 gene have demonstrated a 65% increase in tumor cell apoptosis compared to conventional DOX

treatments (Table 3) (Ma et al., 2017). Iron NPs, which are superparamagnetic, are employed in thermal therapy or targeted tumor therapy. As described by Chen (2010), their use has shown a 45% improvement in therapeutic precision, but Gwili et al. (2021) and Li et al. (2022), emphasized concerns regarding their interaction with antioxidant mechanisms, potentially leading to increased cytotoxicity (Chen, 2010; Gwili et al., 2021; Li et al., 2022). Silica mesoporous NPs (MSNs) are also noteworthy due to their high surface area and volume, which enable effective drug encapsulation and chemical modification. Protón et al. (2020), found that MSNs loaded with microRNA and DOX improved therapeutic efficacy by 40%, with a 50% reduction in systemic toxicity compared to free DOX administration, although Tian (2018) observed side effects such as endothelial lesions and thrombosis in 10%-15% of cases (Table 3) (Pontón et al., 2020). Copper NPs (CuNPs) have shown strong utherapeutic potential due to their redox activity and influence on oxidative stress, cell morphology, and apoptosis. In preclinical studies, CuNPs, when combined with folic acid, reduced tumor size by 55% while maintaining minimal cytotoxic effects on healthy cells. Despite these promising results, stressed that CuNPs require extensive toxicological studies and clinical trials before regulatory approval (Zhuang et al., 2022).

Organic nanotransporters, including polymeric micelles, nano-emulsions, liposomes, and dendrimers, provide chemical flexibility to enhance the biodistribution of therapeutic drugs. Liposomes, capable of carrying both hydrophilic and lipophilic drugs within their lipid bilayer, have demonstrated up to a 5-fold increase in drug delivery efficiency in tumor models, with a 30%-40% reduction in off-target effects. Similarly, lipid nano-emulsions address solubility and encapsulation challenges for hydrophobic drugs. These systems are characterized by high physical stability and strong targeting capabilities, resulting in an average 70% increase in drug accumulation in tumor vessels compared to conventional delivery methods (Table 2) (Fumoto and Nishida, 2020).

Polymers such as polymeric micelles have also shown significant promise. Liu et al. (2021), demonstrated that these systems can co-transport hydrophilic and lipophilic drugs, achieving controlled release with minimal toxicity (Liu et al., 2021). Similarly, nanogels offer precise control over drug release, responding to stimuli like pH, redox, and temperature. Cubosomes, auto-assembled from cubic lipid phases, further enhance drug release efficiency and anti-cancer effectiveness, but their application is limited by particle size inconsistencies that may affect delivery efficiency (Wang et al., 2011).

Table 3. Protein and INPs

Type	Key Component	Indication	Approval date	Reference
Protein-drug conjugate	PEGylated L-asparaginase	Acute lymphoblastic leukemia	FDA: 1994	(Bobo et al., 2016)
Protein-based	Albumin-bound paclitaxel	Metastatic breast and lung cancer	FDA: 2005, EMA: 2008	(Al-Hajeili, et al., 2014)
Inorganic	Hafnium oxide	Squamous cell carcinoma	EMA: 2019	(Krauss et al. 2019)
	Iron oxide	Glioblastoma, prostate cancer	FDA: 2010, EMA: 2013	(Drummond et al. 2006)

Innovations like Theragnostic NPs Integrating Therapy and Diagnostics in a Single Platform

Nanomedicine demonstrates promising developments in the simultaneous delivery of therapeutic and diagnostic (theragnostic) chemicals. This approach is particularly advantageous as it enables non-invasive disease detection and treatment while providing real-time tracking of drug release and biodistribution, improving the precision of therapeutic interventions (Raheem et al. 2023). For instance, MNPs equipped with imaging agents like gadolinium or radioactive isotopes have demonstrated an enhancement of 50%-60% in MRI contrast efficiency while simultaneously enabling targeted drug delivery, which can improve tumor accumulation by up to 45%. Similarly, silica-based NPs functionalized with fluorescent dyes have shown a twofold increase in imaging sensitivity and a 30%-40% reduction in systemic side effects when delivering chemotherapeutics (Gwili et al., 2021).

Moreover, QDs and up-conversion NPs have emerged as potent theragnostic tools, offering exceptional optical properties for deep tissue imaging while delivering anticancer drugs. Studies indicate that QDs conjugated with doxorubicin achieve tumor-specific targeting with a 40% improvement in drug efficacy compared to free drugs, highlighting their potential for enhanced treatment outcomes. Carbon-based NPs, such as graphene oxide, have further demonstrated versatility, with a reported 50%-60% increase in the therapeutic index of encapsulated agents due to their high surface area and functionalization potential (Parveen et al., 2024). Despite their immense promise, the clinical translation of these systems faces challenges, including the optimization of size, shape, surface charge, and biocompatibility, as well as issues related to large-scale production and economic feasibility (Carrese et al., 2022).

CHALLENGES AND LIMITATIONS

Biocompatibility and Long-Term Safety Concerns

NPs hold great promise for a variety of medical applications, particularly cancer treatment. However, their clinical integration has encountered considerable obstacles, mainly linked to biosafety issues. Studies have shown that the safety of nanoparticle-based therapies is a major concern, with less than 10% of emerging nanomedicines having received clinical approval. The potential toxicological profile of NPs, which could lead to oxidative stress and inflammation, is a crucial issue (Mendes et al., 2021). Oxidative stress, mainly caused by the production of ROS, is linked to significant tissue damage (Mabsor-Zgandaoui et al. 2025). Moreover, inflammatory responses could exacerbate adverse effects, contributing to potential damage in patients. Once administered, NPs are generally metabolized in the liver and kidneys, with elimination via the kidneys or bile. However, non-biodegradable NPs can accumulate in the body over time and cause long-term organ damage, including physical obstructions to microcirculation and cellular dysfunction. This has raised serious concerns about the long-term safety of these materials and called for the development of biodegradable, biocompatible nanocarriers that can mitigate these risks (Xu et al., 2022).

Challenges in Scaling Up Production and Maintaining Reproducibility

One of the biggest challenges in the clinical application of nanomedicine is the difficulty of increasing production while maintaining reproducibility. In research, NPs have often been developed in the laboratory under highly controlled conditions. Yet when it came to industrial-scale production, these conditions were difficult to reproduce. Variability in the size, shape and surface properties of NPs can occur during mass production, which can have an impact on their efficacy and safety (Sia et al., 2022). Furthermore, the lack of standardized methods for characterizing NPs has exacerbated this problem. This lack of standardization has made it difficult to ensure the quality and consistency of nanoparticle-based therapies. The development of robust manufacturing protocols and analytical methods to characterize NPs was essential to meet these challenges. Advances in materials science and nanotechnology have enabled progress in this area, but achieving the level of consistency required for clinical applications remains a major hurdle (Jiang et al., 2021).

Regulatory Hurdles and Ethical Considerations

In a world where not only, technical challenges but also regulatory hurdles and ethical considerations hampered the widespread use of NPs in medicine, the approval process for nanoparticle-based drugs was complex. The approval process for nanoparticle-based drugs was complex, as regulators had to carefully assess their safety and efficacy. The lack of standardized protocols for assessing NPs safety further complicated the approval process. Although frameworks for drug approval existed, they often failed to consider the unique properties of NPs, such as their capacity to accumulate in specific tissues or to cross biological barriers (Sia et al., 2022). It was therefore necessary to develop new guidelines tailored to nanoparticle-based therapeutics, which should address concerns such as toxicity, biodegradability and potential long-term effects. Ethics issues have also arisen, particularly with regard to the possibility of NPs crossing the blood-brain barrier and affecting the central nervous system. These required a thorough ethical review, ensuring that patient safety was paramount while encouraging innovation in nanomedicine (Pei et al., 2023).

Prospects of Nanomedicine in Cancer Treatment

Nanomedicine offers great promise for the diagnosis and treatment of cancer, particularly solid tumors. The tumor microenvironment (TME) has a crucial role to play in determining the efficacy of nanomedicines, as tumors often express specific receptors or ligands that NPs can target. By engineering NPs to specifically target these receptors, it has been possible to precisely deliver drugs directly to the tumor site. This has facilitated early detection and improved treatment accuracy, enabling healthcare providers to design personalized treatment plans (Xu et al., 2022). The integration of diagnostic and therapeutic functions in NPs, often referred to as theragnostic, has enabled cancer to be monitored and treated in real time. In addition, the ability of NPs to simultaneously carry multiple therapeutic agents such as chemotherapeutic drugs, genes and antibodies has further enhanced their potential in personalized cancer treatment. However, the tumor microenvironment remains a major challenge, as its heterogeneity could hamper the efficacy of nanoparticle-based treatments (J. Yang et al., 2022).

FUTURE DIRECTIONS AND PROSPECTS FOR NANOMEDICINE

The future of nanoparticle-based therapies is promising, thanks to constant advances in materials science, nanotechnology and biomedical engineering. Future research aimed to develop multifunctional NPs capable of playing an integrated diagnostic and therapeutic role, thus enhancing precision medicine approaches. These NPs could be designed to interact with patient-specific biomarkers, enabling the targeted delivery of therapies tailored to individual molecular profiles. In addition, targeting the tumor microenvironment remains a priority, as it offers the potential to overcome immunosuppression and improve patient outcomes by enhancing the immune system's ability to fight cancer (Thorat et al., 2020). Emerging therapeutic modalities such as RNA interference, gene editing and cellular therapies would be facilitated by NPs, further advancing the field (Swaminathan et al., 2021). Significant translational hurdles and regulatory challenges remain, though, requiring ongoing collaboration between researchers, clinicians, regulators and industry partners to establish standardized safety protocols and facilitate widespread clinical adoption of nanomedicines (Đorđević et al., 2022).

The field of nanomedicine is poised to revolutionize healthcare through innovations that harness precision, personalization, and integration with emerging technologies. In the case of personalized nanomedicine, one of the most promising avenues is the development driven by AI. AI enables the rapid design and optimization of nanomaterials tailored to individual patients' needs, leveraging vast datasets that include genomic, proteomic, and clinical information. According to recent studies, these AI-driven frameworks can predict the most effective nanoparticle formulations for targeted drug delivery, minimizing off-target effects and maximizing therapeutic outcomes (Mazumdar et al., 2024). By integrating AI with high-throughput screening and computational modeling, nanomedicine can advance toward precise, patient-specific treatments, particularly in areas where traditional therapies have limitations. The synthesis of these technologies creates an ecosystem where the therapeutic landscape evolves continually, driven by patient-specific insights and feedback (Mazi et al., 2023).

Personalized Nanomedicine with AI-driven Design for Precise Applications

Recent advancements in nanomedicine emphasize the transformative potential of AI in optimizing therapies through highly personalized approaches. Leveraging sophisticated algorithms, AI processes complex biological data including genetic profiles, disease biomarkers, and environmental factors to design NPs tailored to individual treatment needs. In oncology, AI demonstrates exceptional capability in identifying tumor-specific molecular targets, enabling the precise delivery of therapeutic NPs to malignant cells while sparing healthy tissues (Moingeon et al., 2022). This precision enhances the efficacy of cancer treatments, reduces adverse effects, and improves patients' quality of life. Beyond drug delivery, AI applications extend to improving diagnostic accuracy and monitoring tumor progression.

In infectious diseases, AI-driven platforms exhibit remarkable adaptability by dynamically modifying nanoparticle configurations to counteract pathogen resistance, fostering a responsive approach to antimicrobial therapy (Moingeon et al., 2022). These platforms also show promise in developing nanomaterials for vaccine delivery, improving stability and enhancing immune responses. Another key application of AI is predictive modeling, which is revolutionizing drug

response optimization. By accurately forecasting therapeutic outcomes, AI reduces reliance on conventional trial-and-error methods, enabling efficient dosage adjustments and personalized treatment protocols (Smith et al., 2023). As computational power advances and real-world data integration deepens, AI-driven nanoparticle design is poised to achieve unprecedented precision. This convergence of AI and nanomedicine heralds a new era in healthcare, defined by personalized, adaptive, and highly effective therapeutic solutions.

Integration with Wearable Diagnostics for Continuous Monitoring

Advances in wearable technologies are revolutionizing the integration of nanomedicine with diagnostic systems, marking a transformative leap in healthcare. Modern wearables equipped with advanced biosensors enable continuous real-time monitoring of physiological and biochemical parameters. When synchronized with nanomedicine, these devices create an intelligent feedback loop, enhancing diagnostic accuracy and therapeutic precision. For example, wearables that detect inflammation markers can trigger the controlled release of anti-inflammatory drugs from NPs, enabling prompt and targeted treatment of autoimmune flares (Mazumdar et al., 2024). Innovations such as multi-analyte sensors, capable of detecting multiple biomarkers simultaneously, have significantly enhanced the capabilities of wearable technologies, enabling comprehensive monitoring for chronic diseases. The integration of wearables into treatment protocols facilitates early detection of critical events, such as myocardial infarction or stroke, by continuously tracking relevant biomarkers and enabling immediate therapeutic responses.

These advancements also extend to fields like sports medicine, where wearables integrated with nanomedical interventions monitor and address injuries while optimizing athletic performance. This synergy ushers in a new era of proactive healthcare, where real-time data drives timely and targeted interventions, reducing hospitalizations and improving long-term health outcomes. By continuously updating patient health metrics, these devices not only support personalized care but also contribute to an adaptive healthcare ecosystem that evolves with individual needs (Tan et al., 2023).

CONCLUSION

In summary, NPs are becoming key tools in the progression of contemporary healthcare, thanks to their specific physico-chemical properties and their wide-ranging applications, from advanced diagnostics to targeting therapies. They make possible the solution of complex medical challenges, while reducing side effects and improving treatment efficacy. Though obstacles relating to their toxicity, biodegradability and clinical implementation remain, ongoing research is opening up promising new prospects. By blending innovation and scientific rigor, nanomedicine is set to transform healthcare research paradigms over the years to come, and provide new solutions to global medical challenges.

REFERENCES

Agrahari, V., Burnouf, P. A., Burnouf, T., & Agrahari, V. (2019). Nanoformulation properties, characterization, and behavior in complex biological matrices: Challenges and opportunities for brain-targeted drug delivery applications and enhanced translational potential. *Advanced Drug Delivery Reviews*, *141*, 101–122. DOI: 10.1016/j.addr.2019.02.008

Al-Hajeili, M., Azmi, A. S., & Choi, M. (2014). Nab-paclitaxel: Potential for the treatment of advanced pancreatic cancer. *OncoTargets and Therapy*, *7*, 187–192. DOI: 10.2147/OTT.S40705

Barton, M. D. (2000). Antibiotic use in animal feed and its impact on human health. *Nutrition Research Reviews*, *13*(2), 279–299. DOI: 10.1079/095442200108729106

Bayda, S., Hadla, M., Palazzolo, S., Riello, P., Corona, G., Toffoli, G., & Rizzolio, F. (2018). Inorganic nanoparticles for cancer therapy: A transition from lab to clinic. *Current Medicinal Chemistry*, *25*(34), 4269–4303. DOI: 10.2174/0929867325666171229141156

Bobo, D., Robinson, K. J., Islam, J., Thurecht, K. J., & Corrie, S. R. (2016). Nanoparticle-based medicines: A review of FDA-approved materials and clinical trials to date. *Pharmaceutical Research*, *33*(10), 2373–2387. DOI: 10.1007/s11095-016-1958-5

Bostami, R. D. A., Abuwatfa, W. H., & Husseini, G. A. (2022). Recent advances in nanoparticle-based co-delivery systems for cancer therapy. *Nanomaterials*, *12*(15), Article 2672. DOI: 10.3390/nano12152672

Calzoni, E., Cesaretti, A., Polchi, A., Di Michele, A., Tancini, B., & Emiliani, C. (2019). Biocompatible polymer nanoparticles for drug delivery applications in cancer and neurodegenerative disorder therapies. *Journal of Functional Biomaterials*, *10*(1), Article 4. DOI: 10.3390/jfb10010004

Carrese, B., Sanità, G., & Lamberti, A. (2022). Nanoparticles design for theranostic approach in cancer disease. *Cancers*, *14*(19), Article 4654. DOI: 10.3390/cancers14194654

Chen, K., Zhao, H., Wang, Z., Zhou, F., & Lan, M. (2023). Sandwich-type electrochemical aptasensor based on polydopamine-Au-metal ions as signal label and coralloid Au-conductive carbon architecture-modified electrode for the simultaneous detection of cardiac troponin I and myoglobin. *Sensors and Actuators B: Chemical*, *390*. *Sensors and Actuators. B, Chemical, 134044*, 134044. Advance online publication. DOI: 10.1016/j.snb.2023.134044

Chen, P., Li, M., Peng, W., Liu, T., Huang, J., & Ying, B. (2023). Multiple signal amplification and selective recognition reactions-assisted homogeneous binary visual aptasensor of tuberculosis interferon γ in clinical samples. *Sensors and Actuators B: Chemical*, *376*. *Sensors and Actuators. B, Chemical, 132997*, 132997. Advance online publication. DOI: 10.1016/j.snb.2022.132997

Chen, Y., Phipps, M. L., Werner, J. H., Chakraborty, S., & Martinez, J. S. (2018). DNA templated metal nanoclusters: From emergent properties to unique applications. *Accounts of Chemical Research*, *51*(11), 2756–2763. DOI: 10.1021/acs.accounts.8b00366

Chen, Z. G. (2010). Small-molecule delivery by nanoparticles for anticancer therapy. *Trends in Molecular Medicine*, *16*(12), 594–602. DOI: 10.1016/j.molmed.2010.08.001

Đorđević, S., Gonzalez, M. M., Conejos-Sánchez, I., Carreira, B., Pozzi, S., Acúrcio, R. C., Satchi-Fainaro, R., Florindo, H. F., & Vicent, M. J. (2022). Current hurdles to the translation of nanomedicines from bench to the clinic. *Drug Delivery and Translational Research*, *12*(3), 500–525. DOI: 10.1007/s13346-021-01024-2

Drummond, D. C., Noble, C. O., Guo, Z., Hong, K., Park, J. W., & Kirpotin, D. B. (2006). Development of a highly active nanoliposomal irinotecan using a novel intraliposomal stabilization strategy. *Cancer Research*, *66*(6), 3271–3277. DOI: 10.1158/0008-5472.CAN-05-4007

Erel-Akbaba, G., Carvalho, L. A., Tian, T., Zinter, M., Akbaba, H., Obeid, P. J., Chiocca, E. A., Weissleder, R., Kantarci, A. G., & Tannous, B. A. (2019). Radiation-induced targeted nanoparticle-based gene delivery for brain tumor therapy. *ACS Nano*, *13*(4), 4028–4040. DOI: 10.1021/acsnano.8b08177

Fan, J., Wang, S., Zhang, X., Chen, W., Li, Y., Yang, P., Cao, Z., Wang, Y., Lu, W., & Ju, D. (2018). Quantum dots elicit hepatotoxicity through lysosome-dependent autophagy activation and reactive oxygen species production. *ACS Biomaterials Science & Engineering*, *4*(4), 1418–1427. DOI: 10.1021/acsbiomaterials.7b00824

Feng, S., Chen, H., Hu, Z., Wu, T., & Liu, Z. (2023). Ultrasensitive detection of miRNA via CRISPR/Cas12a coupled with strand displacement amplification reaction. *ACS Applied Materials & Interfaces*, *15*(24), 28933–28940. DOI: 10.1021/acsami.3c03399

Franco, Y. L., Vaidya, T. R., & Ait-Oudhia, S. (2018). Anticancer and cardio-protective effects of liposomal doxorubicin in the treatment of breast cancer. *Breast Cancer: Targets and Therapy*, *10*, 131–141. DOI: 10.2147/BCTT.S170239

Fumoto, S., & Nishida, K. (2020). Co-delivery systems of multiple drugs using nanotechnology for future cancer therapy. *Chemical and Pharmaceutical Bulletin*, *68*(7), 583–591. DOI: 10.1248/cpb.c20-00008

Gavas, S., Quazi, S., & Karpiński, T. M. (2021). Nanoparticles for cancer therapy: Current progress and challenges. *Nanoscale Research Letters*, *16*(1), Article 173. DOI: 10.1186/s11671-021-03628-6

Groll, A. H., Rijnders, B. J. A., Walsh, T. J., Adler-Moore, J., Lewis, R. E., & Brüggemann, R. J. M. (2019). Clinical pharmacokinetics, pharmacodynamics, safety and efficacy of liposomal amphotericin B. *Clinical Infectious Diseases*, *68*(Supplement_4), S260–S274. DOI: 10.1093/cid/ciz076

Mabsor-Zgandaoui, S., Rachmoune, K., Aftais, I., Elamrani, F. E., Amradi, I., El Housseini, A., Hamdan, Y. A., Zgandaoui, Y., Iddar, A., El Mzibri, M., Moutaouakkil, A., El Hessni, A., & Mesfioui, A. (2026). Biomedical Polymers: Foundations and Future Innovations in Medicine. In Erişen, D., Khan, F., Chang, C., & Yan, K. (Eds.), *Biomedical Applications and Toxicity of Polymers, Nanoparticles, Biomaterials, and Metal Ions* (pp. 1–30). IGI Global Scientific Publishing., DOI: 10.4018/979-8-3373-0055-9.ch001

Gurunathan, S., Kang, M. H., Qasim, M., & Kim, J. H. (2018). Nanoparticle-mediated combination therapy: Two-in-one approach for cancer. *International Journal of Molecular Sciences*, *19*(10), Article 3264. DOI: 10.3390/ijms19103264

Gwili, N., Jones, S. J., Al Amri, W., Carr, I. M., Harris, S., Hogan, B. V., Hughes, W. E., & others. (2021). Transcriptome profiles of stem-like cells from primary breast cancers allow identification of ITGA7 as a predictive marker of chemotherapy response. *British Journal of Cancer*, *125*(7), 983–993. DOI: 10.1038/s41416-021-01484-w

Hagan, C. T., Mi, Y., Knape, N. M., & Wang, A. Z. (2020). Enhancing combined immunotherapy and radiotherapy through nanomedicine. *Bioconjugate Chemistry*, *31*(5), 1253–1262. DOI: 10.1021/acs.bioconjchem.0c00520

Hasan, M. R., Sharma, P., Singh, S., & Narang, J. (2024). Smartphone-integrated wireless portable potentiostat to develop 5th-generation dengue pocket aptasensor toward portronicx-approach. *ACS Applied Bio Materials*, *7*(4), 2299–2308. DOI: 10.1021/acsabm.3c01299

Issaka, E., & Amu-Darko, J. N. O. (2024). Biomimetic nanoparticles for cancer therapy: A review of recent advances, applications, and bottlenecks. *. *Biomedical Materials & Devices*. Advance online publication. DOI: 10.1007/s44174-024-00179-z

Jiang, W., Wang, Y., Wargo, J. A., Lang, F. F., & Kim, B. Y. S. (2021). Considerations for designing preclinical cancer immune nanomedicine studies. *Nature Nanotechnology*, *16*(1), 6–15. DOI: 10.1038/s41565-020-00817-9

Jiao, M., Zhang, P., Meng, J., Li, Y., Liu, C., Luo, X., & Gao, M. (2018). Recent advancements in biocompatible inorganic nanoparticles towards biomedical applications. *Biomaterials Science*, *6*(4), 726–745. DOI: 10.1039/C7BM01020F

Jin, J., & Zhao, Q. (2020). Engineering nanoparticles to reprogram radiotherapy and immunotherapy: Recent advances and future challenges. *Journal of Nanobiotechnology*, *18*(1), Article 74. DOI: 10.1186/s12951-020-00629-y

Kim, J., & Shin, S. (2010). Cost-effectiveness of Genexol-PM for treating metastatic breast cancer. *Journal of Breast Cancer*, *13*(1), 104–110. DOI: 10.4048/jbc.2010.13.1.104

Klyachko, N. L., Arzt, C. J., Li, S. M., Gololobova, O. A., & Batrakova, E. V. (2020). Extracellular vesicle-based therapeutics: Preclinical and clinical investigations. *Pharmaceutics*, *12*(12), Article 1171. DOI: 10.3390/pharmaceutics12121171

Krauss, A. C., Gao, X., Li, L., Manning, M. L., Patel, P., Fu, W., Janoria, K. G., Gieser, D. A., & Bateman, D. A. (2019). FDA approval summary: (Daunorubicin and cytarabine) liposome for injection for the treatment of adults with high-risk acute myeloid leukemia. *Clinical Cancer Research*, *25*(9), 2685–2690. DOI: 10.1158/1078-0432.CCR-18-2990

Li, C., Meng, Y., Wang, S., Qian, M., Wang, J., Lu, W., & Huang, R. (2015). Mesoporous carbon nanospheres featured fluorescent aptasensor for multiple diagnosis of cancer in vitro and in vivo. *ACS Nano*, *9*(12), 12096–12103. DOI: 10.1021/acsnano.5b05137

Li, S., Yang, Y., Wang, S., Gao, Y., Song, Z., Chen, L., & Chen, Z. (2022). Advances in metal graphitic nanocapsules for biomedicine. *Exploration*, *2*(4), Article 20210223. DOI: 10.1002/EXP.20210223

Liang, L., Su, M., Li, L., Lan, F., Yang, G., Ge, S., Yu, J., & Song, X. (2016). Aptamer-based fluorescent and visual biosensor for multiplexed monitoring of cancer cells in microfluidic paper-based analytical devices. *Sensors and Actuators B: Chemical*, *229*, 347–354. DOI: 10.1016/j.snb.2016.01.137

Liang, N., Hu, X., Li, W., Mwakosya, A. W., Guo, Z., Xu, Y., Huang, X., Li, Z., Zhang, X., Zou, X., & Shi, J. (2021). Fluorescence and colorimetric dual-mode sensor for visual detection of malathion in cabbage based on carbon quantum dots and gold nanoparticles. *Food Chemistry*, *343*. *Food Chemistry, 128494*, 128494. Advance online publication. DOI: 10.1016/j.foodchem.2020.128494 PMID: 33162257

Lin, Q., Han, G., Fang, X., Chen, H., Weng, W., & Kong, J. (2022). Programmable analysis of microRNAs by *Thermus thermophilus* Argonaute-assisted exponential isothermal amplification for multiplex detection (TEAM). *Analytical Chemistry*, *94*(32), 11290–11297. DOI: 10.1021/acs.analchem.2c01945

Liu, G., Yang, L., Chen, G., Xu, F., Yang, F., Yu, H., Li, L., Dong, X., Han, J., Cao, C., Qi, J., Su, J., Xu, X., Li, X., & Li, B. (2021). A review on drug delivery system for tumor therapy. *Frontiers in Pharmacology*, *12*. *Frontiers in Pharmacology, 735446*, 735446. Advance online publication. DOI: 10.3389/fphar.2021.735446 PMID: 34675807

Lopes, R. C. F. G., Rocha, B. G. M., Maçôas, E. M. S., Marques, E. F., & Martinho, J. M. G. (2022). Combining metal nanoclusters and carbon nanomaterials: Opportunities and challenges in advanced nanohybrids. *Advances in Colloid and Interface Science*, *304*. *Advances in Colloid and Interface Science, 102667*, 102667. Advance online publication. DOI: 10.1016/j.cis.2022.102667 PMID: 35462268

Ma, H., Du, X., Zhang, S., Wang, Q., Yin, Y., Qiu, X., Da, P., Yue, H., Wu, H., & Xu, F. (2017). Achaete-scute complex homologue-1 promotes development of laryngocarcinoma via facilitating the epithelial-mesenchymal transformation. *Tumor Biology*, *39*(6). DOI: 10.1177/1010428317705752

Mabsor-Zgandaoui, S., Moussaif, A., El Hessni, A., Mesfioui, A., El Mzibri, M., Iddar, A., & Moutaouakkil, A. (2024). Ionising and ultraviolet radiation induce the secretion of melanin in *Tetrahymena pyriformis*. *. *The International Journal of Environmental Studies*. Advance online publication. DOI: 10.1080/00207233.2024.2412455

Mabsor-Zgandaoui, S., Rachmoune, K., El Hessni, A., El Mzibri, M., Iddar, A., & Moutaouakkil, A. (2025). Effect of hydrogen peroxide pre-treatment on enhancing the cellular resistance of *Tetrahymena pyriformis* exposed to ionizing radiation. *Toxicological & Environmental Chemistry*, *107*(2), 294–309. DOI: 10.1080/02772248.2025.2460804

Mai, B. T., Fernandes, S., Balakrishnan, P. B., & Pellegrino, T. (2018). Nanosystems based on magnetic nanoparticles and thermo- or pH-responsive polymers: An update and future perspectives. *Accounts of Chemical Research*, *51*(5), 999–1013. DOI: 10.1021/acs.accounts.7b00549

I Mazi, S., Hassen, A. M., Alrashed, F. A., Benslimane, F. M., & Mohamed, N. A. (2023). Artificial intelligence-nanomedicine interface: Today's theory tomorrow's technology. *Archives of Clinical and Biomedical Research*, *7*(6), 555–563. DOI: 10.26502/acbr.50170379

Mazumdar, H., Reza Khondakar, K., Das, S., Halder, A., & Kaushik, A. (2024). Artificial intelligence for personalized nanomedicine: From material selection to patient outcomes. *Expert Opinion on Drug Delivery*, *21*(7), 995–1012. DOI: 10.1080/17425247.2024.2440618

Mendes, B. B., Sousa, D. P., Conniot, J., & Conde, J. (2021). Nanomedicine-based strategies to target and modulate the tumor microenvironment. *Trends in Cancer*, *7*(9), 847–862. DOI: 10.1016/j.trecan.2021.05.001

Moingeon, P., Kuenemann, M., & Guedj, M. (2022). Artificial intelligence-enhanced drug design and development: Toward a computational precision medicine. *Drug Discovery Today*, *27*(1), 215–222. DOI: 10.1016/j.drudis.2021.09.006

Ou, G., Zhao, J., Chen, P., Xiong, C., Dong, F., Li, B., & Feng, X. (2018). Fabrication and application of noble metal nanoclusters as optical sensors for toxic metal ions. *Analytical and Bioanalytical Chemistry*, *410*(10), 2483–2496. DOI: 10.1007/s00216-017-0808-6

Parveen, S., Abira, R., Paikray, S., Sahoo, L., Tripathy, N. S., & Dilnawaz, F. (2024). Recent advancement of nanotheranostics in cancer applications. *Current Drug Delivery*, *21*(5), 673–689. DOI: 10.2174/0115672018307617240514092110

Pei, Z., Lei, H., & Cheng, L. (2023). Bioactive inorganic nanomaterials for cancer theranostics. *Chemical Society Reviews*, *52*(6), 2031–2081. DOI: 10.1039/D2CS00352J

Pontón, I., Martí del Rio, A., Gómez Gómez, M., & Sánchez-García, D. (2020). Preparation and applications of organo-silica hybrid mesoporous silica nanoparticles for the co-delivery of drugs and nucleic acids. *Nanomaterials*, *10*(12), Article 2466. DOI: 10.3390/nano10122466

Qiu, H., Min, Y., Rodgers, Z., Zhang, L., & Wang, A. Z. (2017). Nanomedicine approaches to improve cancer immunotherapy. *Wiley Interdisciplinary Reviews: Nanomedicine and Nanobiotechnology*, *9*(5), Article e1456. DOI: 10.1002/wnan.1456

Qiu, Z., Shu, J., & Tang, D. (2017). Bioresponsive release system for visual fluorescence detection of carcinoembryonic antigen from mesoporous silica nanocontainers mediated optical color on quantum dot-enzyme-impregnated paper. *Analytical Chemistry*, *89*(9), 5152–5160. DOI: 10.1021/acs.analchem.7b00989

Raheem, M. A., Rahim, M. A., Gul, I., Zhong, X., Xiao, C., Zhang, H., Wei, J., He, Q., Hassan, M., Zhang, C. Y., Yu, D., Pandey, V., Du, K., Wang, R., Han, S., Han, Y., & Qin, P. (2023). Advances in nanoparticles-based approaches in cancer theranostics. *OpenNano*, *10*. *Article, 100152*, 100152. Advance online publication. DOI: 10.1016/j.onano.2023.100152

Seyedi, F., Torabizadeh, S. A., & Naeimi, A. (2022). Radioprotective effect of a novel and green bio-nanohybrid, chitosan/silver/cobalt complex, based on *Ferulago angulate* plant. *Biotechnology and Applied Biochemistry*, *69*(4), 1567–1575. DOI: 10.1002/bab.2228

Shrestha, B., Tang, L., & Romero, G. (2019). Nanoparticles-mediated combination therapies for cancer treatment. *Advanced Therapeutics*, *2*(11), Article 1900076. DOI: 10.1002/adtp.201900076

Sia, C. S., Lim, H. P., Tey, B. T., Goh, B. H., & Low, L. E. (2022). Stimuli-responsive nanoassemblies for targeted delivery against tumor and its microenvironment. *Biochimica et Biophysica Acta - Reviews on Cancer*, *1877*(5), Article 188779. DOI: 10.1016/j.bbcan.2022.188779

Smith, I. T., Zhang, E., Yildirim, Y. A., Campos, M. A., Abdel-Mottaleb, M., Yildirim, B., Ramezani, Z., & others. (2023). Nanomedicine and nanobiotechnology applications of magnetoelectric nanoparticles. *Wiley Interdisciplinary Reviews: Nanomedicine and Nanobiotechnology*, *15*(3), Article e1849. DOI: 10.1002/wnan.1849

Suk, J. S., Xu, Q., Kim, N., Hanes, J., & Ensign, L. M. (2016). PEGylation as a strategy for improving nanoparticle-based drug and gene delivery. *Advanced Drug Delivery Reviews*, *99*(Pt A), 28–51. DOI: 10.1016/j.addr.2015.09.012

Swaminathan, G., Shigna, A., Kumar, A., Byroju, V. V., Durgempudi, V. R., & Kumar, L. D. (2021). RNA interference and nanotechnology: A promising alliance for next generation cancer therapeutics. *Frontiers in Nanotechnology*, *3*. *Frontiers in Nanotechnology, 694838*, 694838. Advance online publication. DOI: 10.3389/fnano.2021.694838

Taléns-Visconti, R., Díez-Sales, O., de Julián-Ortiz, J. V., & Nácher, A. (2022). Nanoliposomes in cancer therapy: Marketed products and current clinical trials. *International Journal of Molecular Sciences*, *23*(8), Article 4249. DOI: 10.3390/ijms23084249

Tan, P., Chen, X., Zhang, H., Wei, Q., & Luo, K. (2023). Artificial intelligence aids in development of nanomedicines for cancer management. *Seminars in Cancer Biology*, *89*, 61–75. DOI: 10.1016/j.semcancer.2023.01.005

Thorat, N. D., Townley, H. E., Patil, R. M., Tofail, S. A. M., & Bauer, J. (2020). Comprehensive approach of hybrid nanoplatforms in drug delivery and theranostics to combat cancer. *Drug Discovery Today*, *25*(7), 1245–1252. DOI: 10.1016/j.drudis.2020.04.018

Wang, H., Zhao, Y., Wu, Y., Hu, Y. L., Nan, K., Nie, G., & Chen, H. (2011). Enhanced anti-tumor efficacy by co-delivery of doxorubicin and paclitaxel with amphiphilic methoxy PEG-PLGA copolymer nanoparticles. *Biomaterials*, *32*(32), 8281–8290. DOI: 10.1016/j.biomaterials.2011.07.032

Wang, Y., Yang, Y., Zheng, X., Shi, J., Zhong, L., Duan, X., & Zhu, Y. (2023). Application of iron oxide nanoparticles in the diagnosis and treatment of leukemia. *Frontiers in Pharmacology*, *14*. *Frontiers in Pharmacology, 1177068*, 1177068. Advance online publication. DOI: 10.3389/fphar.2023.1177068 PMID: 37063276

Xu, Y., Xiong, J., Sun, X., & Gao, H. (2022). Targeted nanomedicines remodeling immunosuppressive tumor microenvironment for enhanced cancer immunotherapy. *Acta Pharmaceutica Sinica B*, *12*(11), 4327–4347. DOI: 10.1016/j.apsb.2022.11.001

Yan, G., Li, A., Zhang, A., Sun, Y., & Liu, J. (2018). Polymer-based nanocarriers for co-delivery and combination of diverse therapies against cancers. *Nanomaterials*, *8*(2), Article 85. DOI: 10.3390/nano8020085

Yang, B., Fang, D., Lv, Q., Wang, Z., & Liu, Y. (2021). Targeted therapeutic strategies in the battle against pathogenic bacteria. *Frontiers in Pharmacology*, *12*. *Frontiers in Pharmacology, 673239*, 673239. Advance online publication. DOI: 10.3389/fphar.2021.673239 PMID: 34054548

Yang, J., Wang, X., Wang, B., Park, K., Wooley, K., & Zhang, S. (2022). Challenging the fundamental conjectures in nanoparticle drug delivery for chemotherapy treatment of solid cancers. *Advanced Drug Delivery Reviews*, *189*. *Advanced Drug Delivery Reviews, 114525*, 114525. Advance online publication. DOI: 10.1016/j.addr.2022.114525 PMID: 36100142

Yee, B. J., Shafiqah, N. F., Mohd-Naim, N. F., & Ahmed, M. U. (2023). A CRISPR/Cas12a-based fluorescence aptasensor for the rapid and sensitive detection of ampicillin. *International Journal of Biological Macromolecules*, *242*(Pt 3), Article 125211. DOI: 10.1016/j.ijbiomac.2023.125211

Yetisgin, A. A., Cetinel, S., Zuvin, M., Kosar, A., & Kutlu, O. (2020). Therapeutic nanoparticles and their targeted delivery applications. *Molecules*, *25*(9), Article 2193. DOI: 10.3390/molecules25092193

Zhou, H., Yan, J., Chen, W., Yang, J., Liu, M., Zhang, Y., Shen, X., Ma, Y., Hu, X., Wang, Y., Du, K., & Li, G. (2021). Population pharmacokinetics and exposure–safety relationship of paclitaxel liposome in patients with non-small cell lung cancer. *Frontiers in Oncology*, *10*. *Frontiers in Oncology, 1731*, 1731. Advance online publication. DOI: 10.3389/fonc.2020.01731 PMID: 33614470

Zhuang, X., Kang, Y., Zhao, L., & Guo, S. (2022). Design and synthesis of copper nanoparticles for the treatment of human esophageal cancer: Introducing a novel chemotherapeutic supplement. *Journal of Experimental Nanoscience*, *17*(1), 274–284. DOI: 10.1080/17458080.2022.2065264

Chapter 4
Iron Oxide Nanoparticles as Potential Nano-Based Neurotherapeutic Agents for Neurodegenerative Disorders:
Current Perspectives

Ghadha Ibrahim Fouad
https://orcid.org/0000-0003-3665-3153
Department of Therapeutic Chemistry, Pharmaceutical Industries and Drug Research Institute, Egypt

Hanan Farouk Aly
https://orcid.org/0000-0003-3642-1571
Department of Therapeutic Chemistry, Pharmaceutical Industries and Drug Research Institute, Egypt

Mah Zaki Rizk
Department of Therapeutic Chemistry, Pharmaceutical Industries and Drug Research Institute, Egypt

ABSTRACT

Neurodegenerative diseases including Alzheimer's disease, Parkinson's disease, multiple sclerosis, amyotrophic lateral sclerosis, and Huntington's disease exerts a socio-economic burden and affecting a high percentage of population. Traditional medications of neurodegenerative disorders are asymptomatic and reliefs pain without halting progression of neuronal damage. Recently, nanotechnology is regarded as a very promising therapeutic approach for the prevention and treatment of several disorders, through enabling targeted and direct drug-delivery of active and therapeutic molecules to cross the Blood Brain Barrier in different neuropathological situations. The application of nanotechnology in neurology is a promising field and presenting a new horizon for treatment and diagnosis (Neurotheranostics) of neurodegenerative disorders.

DOI: 10.4018/979-8-3373-4627-4.ch004

This review investigated the nano-based neurotherapeutics to manage CNS disorders. This review focuses on the recent application of iron oxide nanoparticles to act as drug carriers or as detection agents of brain disorders.

INTRODUCTION

Neurodegenerative disorders are chronic progressive diseases of central nervous system (CNS) with unknown etiology and unrevealed mechanism of pathogenesis (Miller et al. 2012; Kimura 2016; Altowaijri et al. 2017). Moreover, neurodegenerative disorders are complex multifactorial disorders occurred due to involvement of both genetic and environmental factors (Armstrong 2013; Sanchez-Mut et al. 2016). Neuroinflammation occurs as result of excessive production of pro-inflammatory mediators, excessive oxidative stress, and reduction in antioxidant defense mechanisms (Sorto-Gomez et al. 2016; Elsheikh et al. 2025). Alzheimer disease (AD) is the most common neurodegenerative disorder that affects neurocognitive function and accounts for 60%–70% of dementia cases in the elderly populations (Alzheimer Association 2016). AD is a proteinopathy characterized by modified protein processing and featured by specific neuropathological markers of Aβ-plaques, tau-laden neurofibrillary tangles (Baker et al. 2018). Parkinson's disease (PD) is the second most common neurodegenerative disorder that affects aged community (Rajabally & Martey 2011; Pringsheim et al. 2014) and is characterized by dopaminergic neuronal loss in substantia nigra region and neurotoxic accumulation of the protein α-synuclein into Lewy bodies (Braak et al. 2003). Multiple sclerosis (MS) is a chronic, disabling, and demyelinating neuro-inflammatory disease, that has an autoimmune component (Escribano et al. 2017); through being involved in immune attacks on myelin sheath, the primary component of white matter in CNS (Miller et al. 2012). MS onset is more common in young adults, and the disease has a female predominance (Amato et al. 2017). Amyotrophic lateral sclerosis (ALS) is another complex neurodegenerative disease involving moto-neuron cell death (Stampfli et al. 2018). Huntington disease (HD) is a progressive neurodegenerative disorder identified by motor, cognitive, and neuropsychiatric signs. HD results in motor deficits, such as gait disruption and muscle wasting (Manfré et al. 2017).

The strategy of "one alteration, one disease, and one drug" does not seem to work well for these multifactorial neurodegenerative disorders. Conventional treatments cannot achieve satisfactory therapeutic outputs due to the impact of several physiological factors and the multifactorial nature of the neurodegenerative disease. Currently available traditional drugs merely delay disease onset or alleviate symptoms (Abbott 2011; Ojha and Kumar 2018). For example, L-DOPA, a drug used to manage PD, ameliorated the PD symptoms without retardation of progression of neurodegeneration (Cranwell-Bruce 2010), in addition, the use of these drugs is accompanied with several adverse effects such as extreme emotional sensitivity, compulsive behaviour, gastrointestinal irritability and depression (Kaushik et al. 2018). There are several reasons that contribute to the lack of effectiveness of CNS drugs such as the continuous chronic neuroinflammation (Volkman and Ofen 2017), the absence of diagnostic biomarkers available for CNS disorders (Borai et al. 2017; Ojha and Kumar 2018), that enable early detection of the disease before manifestation of symptoms (Rojas et al. 2015). Moreover, long time, about10 years, is required for clinical trial and approval phases of CNS drugs to observe their efficacy on disease

progression (Kaitin 2010). Therefore, future research should focus on identifying mechanisms responsible for pathophysiology of CNS disorders (Ajetunmobi et al. 2014).

Nano-based neurotheranostics or nanotheranostic application to treat/detect neurodegenerative disorders is an innovative approach that utilizes nanoparticles (NPs) to overcome the selective permeability of the BBB. The term "theranostics" means a single structure that combines diagnosis and therapy, whereas "neurotheranostics" refers to the nervous system. This strategy of nano-neuro-theranostics will contribute to the development of nano-theranostic agents that are capable of establishing neurotherapeutic agents or nano-imaging agents for rapid diagnosis of CNS disorders (Kevadiya et al. 2019). Several nano-based applications demonstrated minimal cytotoxicity in pre-clinical experiments and could be developed to act as nano-based neurotheranostic agents through enabling early diagnosis and treatment of AD (Harilal et al. 2019).

To manage CNS disorders, nano-based approaches could serve both diagnostic and therapeutic potential at the same time (Kang et al. 2018); in other words, to act as nanotheranostic agents that combine diagnostic and therapeutic platforms. Therefore, it is essential to develop innovative delivery systems carrying diagnostic reagents or therapeutic active molecules for CNS disorders (Kang et al. 2018). In addition, it is required to understand the underlying mechanisms of the brain functions, as well as to uncover the pathological pathways of neurodegenerative disorders (Hassan and Singh 2014). Nanotheranostic -based approaches could encounter these neurotherapeutic challenges and provide a novel platform for development of nanodrugs and diagnostic agents of CNS disorders (Ojha and Kumar 2018; Gidwani and Singh 2014). Moreover, the use of nanomedicine as therapeutic approaches for neurodegenerative disorders will enable the discovery of novel biomarkers (Kang et al. 2018).

The brain is the most challenging targets for nanoparticles (NPs) because of the presence of physiological barriers such as blood-brain barrier (BBB) that limit the entry of most CNS-targeting drugs (Teleanu et al. 2019). NPs are regarded as molecular Trojan horses to carry therapeutic active molecules and drugs through the BBB (Schlachetzki et al. 2004). Several types of NPs have been studied for drug delivery to the CNS, however, inorganic NPs (silica, gold, iron, etc.) was more adaptable through being easily functionalized in shape, size, and surface coating (Saraiva et al., 2016). Different NPs demonstrated anti-amyloidogenic potential neuroprotective activity such as graphene NPs, superparamagnetic iron-oxide nanoparticles (SPIONPs), and cerium oxide NPs (Mahmoudi et al. 2012; Hegazy et al. 2017; Luo et al., 2020); cerium oxide NPs showed higher inhibitory activity of α-synuclein than L-DOPA and can be employed as nanodrugs for PD (Kaushik et al. 2018).

NANOSCALE-BASED DELIVERY OF NUTRACEUTICALS

Bioactive dietary compounds are used as alternative therapeutic approaches to treat different neurological disorders to improve the quality of life of patients (Altowaijri et al. 2017). These phytochemicals demonstrate neuroprotective potential through exerting anti-inflammatory and anti-oxidative activities (Borai et al. 2017; Labuschagne and Blaauw 2018). However, after oral administration, these compounds are subjected to the digestion and metabolism that renders them inactive (Jiménez-Aguilar et al. 2011; Xiao et al. 2017). In addition, most phytochemicals are

poorly absorbed and unable to cross the lipid membranes of the cells, that finally resulting in reduced bioavailability and decreased therapeutic efficiency (Kumar and Sharma 2018).

Nanoceuticals are designed natural compounds with biological activities or nutraceuticals based on a nano-scale approach. Recently, there is a great interest to develop an optimized drug delivery platform to deliver nanoceuticals, denoting that nano-carriers provoked no or minimal cytotoxicity (Kakkar et al. 2018; Martínez-Ballesta et al. 2018). Several factors influence the delivery of nutraceuticals such as solubility, biocompatibility, bioavailability, biodistribution, toxicity, and biological interaction with biomolecules (Odeh et al. 2014; Rao et al. 2016). For instance, IONPs is capable of inducing structural degenerative alterations and elevated iron contents in the brain tissues and disrupted the BBB integrity and permeability (Elsheikh et al. 2025). Najafabadi et al. (2018) demonstrated that superparamagnetic iron-oxide nanoparticles (SPIONPs) ameliorated the cerebral biodistribution of quercetin. Nanoparticles (NPs) could be used to ensure a sustainable and controlled treatment by allowing the release of active therapeutic phytochemicals or drugs in a slow and controlled manner (Xiao et al. 2017; Martínez-Ballesta et al. 2018).

NPs confer the loaded phytochemicals the biostability during processing, keeping the bioactivity through encapsulation, and controlled release to improve the bioavailability and biodistribution (Radhakrishnan et al. 2016). The neuroprotective potential of "biodegradable and poorly bioavailable" curcumin was improved by being loaded within NPs to cross BBB (Elbialy et al. 2019). Clinically, there are several nanoscale-phytochemicals therapeutics such as Abraxane (Albumin-coated paclitaxel) and Daunoxome (liposomal daunorubicin) (Siddiqui et al. 2015). In addition, Resveratrol (RSV) has been encapsulated to increase half-life of RSV and to favor its biological activity (Summerlin et al. 2015). For instance, Wang et al. (2018) used magnetic RSV Liposomes as a novel Platform for Magnetic Resonance Imaging (MRI), using iron oxide NPs, to treat PD. Recently, Sallem et al. (2019) developed a novel nano-hybrids of superparamagnetic iron oxide NPs (SPIONs) and RSV that could be used for further therapeutic application in neurological disorders.

IRON OXIDE NANOPARTICLES (IONPS)

Iron Oxide Nanoparticles (IONPs) are promising multifunctional NPs to be used in the field of nanotheranostics due to their magnetic properties, high biocompatibility, ease of surface engineering, and minimal cytotoxicity (Kunzmann et al., 2011; Paik et al., 2015). Iron oxides are benign, non-toxic, and highly biocompatible compounds that could be incorporated in the *in vivo* metabolic activities (Ling and Hyeon 2013). There are several biomedical applications of IONPs such as MRI contrast agent (CAs), cell labeling, hyperthermia, magnetic separation of cells or molecules, and drug delivery system (Pan et al. 2012; Arami et al. 2015; Manjili et al. 2016). Moreover, IONPs can be used in the clinical diagnosis of neuroinflammation (Farrell et al. 2013); IONPs-labelled monocytes could facilitate the clinical therapeutics *via* targeting monocyte recruitment in the inflammation (Engberink et al. 2010). From our point of view, IONPs could be regarded as ideal nanotheranostic agents that combine the therapy and diagnosis in one package through combining drug delivery of therapeutic molecules or as imagining tool such as MRI. Some IONPs are undergoing clinical trials (Thanh et al. 2012; Bobo et al. 2016),

for example, Feridex® (ferumoxides) "dextran-coated IONPs" is approved as an imaging contrast agent for the detection of hepatic injury (Bulte 2009).

MAGNETIC IRON OXIDE NANOPARTICLES (MIONPS)

Brain cells are more sensitive to magnetic NPs (MNPs) (Laurent et al. 2012), subjecting MNPs to an external magnetic field increase brain uptake of MNPs and enhance the BBB permeability, demonstrating the potential application of MNPs for diagnostic and therapeutic purposes (Kiyatkin et al. 2009; Raut et al. 2010). The use of magnetic iron oxide NPs (MIONPs), in the form of magnetite (Fe_3O_4) and maghemite (γ-Fe_2O_3), is common (Vikram et al. 2015). Their use is eco-safe and favorable in theranostics applications due to their stability, biocompatibility, and hyper-parametric characteristics (Mody et al. 2010). The magnetic property of IONPs enables the use of MIONPs as "magnetic vectors" that can be controlled by magnetic fields to direct them towards a specific location "targeted drug delivery", or as magnetic contrast agents in MRI for diagnostic purposes, or as agents for hyperthermia using a high-frequency magnetic field (Arruebo et al. 2007). Moreover, superparamagnetic iron oxide (SPIONPs) and ultra-small superparamagnetic iron oxide (USPIO) are used as MRI CAs in targeted drug delivery (Busquets et al., 2014; Dulińska-Litewka et al. 2019; Thomas et al. 2016). SPIONPs are excellent contrast media for molecular imaging, thus the use of SPIONPs-labeled provides simple, rapid, and economic diagnostic approaches (Burtea et al. 2011). In addition, USPIONPs are regarded as promising theranostic agents in different CNS disorders (Mahmoudi et al. 2011). Functionalized USPIONPs could be employed in various in vitro applications including the determination of antibody concentration and enzymatic activity in aqueous suspensions, MRI visualization of cells, and detection of specific biomolecules by histochemistry (Burtea et al. 2011). USPIONPs could be used to understand the underlying pathological mechanisms of CNS disorders, as in the case of multiple sclerosis (MS); USPIONPs enhanced brain MRI and demonstrated a clinically relevant pattern of MS (Vellinga et al. 2008). Moreover, it was demonstrated that T2-weighted MRI presented a strong biomarker potential in transgenic ALS mouse model (Evans et al. 2014).

MIONPs can be synthesized by physicochemical method or by green-chemical method, the first method demonstrated several defects such as the being lengthy, expensive, severe and toxic, in addition to, it required severe reaction conditions and the low output of products, on the other hand, the green synthesis method represented an economic, simple, rapid and safe method (Prasad et al. 2017). Furthermore, green synthesis enabled the synthesis of biocompatible, stable, economic (cost-effective), and eco-friendly NPs using natural compounds instead of organic chemical substances (Fahmy 2019). For example, Nosrati et al. (2018) developed an innovative method to synthetize biocompatible AA-IONPs that demonstrated their potential theranostic use in cellular labeling or drug delivery.

THE LIMITATIONS AND POTENTIAL TOXICITY OF IONPS

The extensive use of IONPs raised several issues regarding the biosafety, long-term distribution, clearance, the biological interactions, and cytotoxicity (Feng et al. 2018). The biological use of "IONPs" is contradictory and requires further investigations. A study by Jain et al. (2008)

investigated the alterations in the iron levels in serum and tissue in rats for a period of three weeks after intravenous administration of MIONPs and demonstrated that the use MIONPs for is safe, as MIONPs did not result in long-term alterations in the hepatic enzymes or enhanced oxidative stress. In addition, a study by Fahmy (2019) demonstrated the antioxidant impact of green-synthesized MIONPs, introduced intravenously to rats, in different organs and revealed the safety of these NPs. Several nano-based applications demonstrated minimal cytotoxicity in pre-clinical experiments and could be developed to act as theranostic agents through enabling early diagnosis and treatment of neurological disorders such as AD (Harilal et al. 2019).

On the other hand, the use of IONPs could result in oxidative stress and toxicity (Shen et al. 2011; Soenen et al. 2012); the released iron ions from IONPs might lead to iron deposition, oxidative injury, pathological protein aggregation, and genotoxicity in different cells including neural cells (Chinde and Grover, 2017; Yarjanli et al., 2017). For example, a single intravenous injection of 10 nm maghemite to rats could result in, renal toxicity, hepatotoxicity, and pulmonary toxicity, whereas there is no apparent toxicity in brain and heart (Hanini et al. 2011). Another study by Reddy et al. (2017) demonstrated the oxidative potential of IONPs in female rats after 28 days of oral administration of 30, 300, and 1000 mg/kg and found that IONPs deposited in different organs (liver, kidneys, and brain) and triggered oxidative stress. Moreover, several animal studies suggested a possible existing links between neurodegenerative disorders and NPs (Feng et al. 2015), it was demonstrated that administration of NPs in the early phase of development, could result in harmful effect on the fetus, directly or indirectly (Siddiqui et al. 2013). For example, MIONPs can result in neuronal loss in the chicken embryo (Patel et al. 2017). SPIONPs may introduce toxic effects through their interactions with biomolecules such as DNA, nucleus, and mitochondria (Hsieh et al. 2015; Patil et al. 2018).

The decreased biodegradation of NPs may result in their accumulation in the target tissue and subsequent cytotoxicity, in addition to inducing oxidative stress (Feng et al. 2015). Moreover, metal-based NPs tend to accumulate in the brain, as these NPs are hard to metabolize (Niu et al. 2019) and could result in neural damage and microglial activation (Wong et al. 2012; Yarjanli et al. 2017). Nano-neurotoxicity might be more challenging, as neurons are incapable of regeneration (von Bohlen and Halbach 2015); moreover, the nano-scale size of NPs facilitates their accessibility to the brain and subsequent accumulation in neurons and glia (Asharani et al. 2009) and finally affecting both the morphology and function of the brain. Therefore, several studies investigated the neurotoxic potential of NPs and showed that the administration of NPs could result in disruption of BBB, increased membrane permeability, signaling pathway activation, oxidative stress neuroinflammation, and neurodegeneration (Xia et al. 2009; Tang et al. 2009; Ma et al. 2010; Hirst et al. 2013). From this perspective, the systemic evaluation of neurotoxicity of NPs is a mandatory requirement to avoid neuronal degeneration (Feng et al. 2015) and to design a biosafe and multifunctional NPs. In addition, clinical evaluation of the risk/benefit ratio of nanomedicines or nanovaccines and defining the dose required and the route of administration are essential steps to facilitate the clinical application of NPs-based treatment.

In addition, to enhance the concentration of therapeutic molecules in the brain, "nose to brain method" or "intranasal pathway " was applied to avoid the deactivation of active molecules by gastric enzymes (Amanzadeh et al. 2019). For instance, olfactory pathways is one of the non-invasive and alternative pathways that used to deliver drugs and/or NPs to CNS, Sancini et al. (2016) demonstrated that pulmonary administration of synthesized NPs was effective in reducing amyloid-β (Aβ) in the brain of AD-mice. Further research is required to study this possible

route of administration to treat different CNS disorders. However, the administration of bare IONPs through intratracheal instillation resulted in inflammation and a reduction in the level of intracellular reduced glutathione in the cells of bronchoalveolar lavage (BAL) fluid, whereas the intratracheal instillation of surface coated IONPs demonstrated no toxicity (Cho et al. 2009). Therapeutic agents could be delivered from the olfactory mucosa to the brain through the olfactory pathway (Khan et al. 2017). In a previous study, sulforaphane was loaded on IONPs and administrated intranasally to Cisplatin-neurotoxicated rats and mitigated the chemodrug-induced neurotoxicity on behavioural, biochemical, and histopathological aspects (Ibrahim Fouad et al. 2022). Therefore, it was suggested that administration of lower doses of the IONPs could be of minimal or no toxicity and mild adverse effects (Masselli and Gualdi 2012).

However, these concerns might be related to the variation in the physicochemical properties of IONPs such as size, shape, and surface coating, or to the experimental factors such as animal models, administration route, the exposure time, the type of tissue, and quantification techniques (Kumar et al. 2011; Aliakbari et al. 2018). The physicochemical features of IONPs is a relevant factor in the determination of the pharmacokinetics, the biological interactions, and the destiny of IONPs; IONPs, larger than 100 nm-sized, are accumulated in the liver and spleen through macrophage phagocytosis, whereas IONPs, smaller than 10 nm-sized, are cleared through the kidney (Kumar et al. 2011; Arami et al. 2015). Moreover, the limited biodistribution of IONPs is linked to the active clearance mechanism (Valdiglesias et al. 2016; Albanese et al. 2012). After getting into the body, blood proteins are adsorbed on the surface of the IONPs "opsonization process", followed by recognition and uptake by macrophages, eventually resulting in their clearance from the body (Gustafson et al. 2015). Accordingly, keeping "iron homeostasis" could inhibit the induced oxidative stress of IONPs-released free iron ions; to ferritin can bind to these iron ions to maintain the iron store (Arami et al. 2015). Therefore, further research is required to elucidate the behaviour of IONPs with different physicochemical characteristics including their distribution, degradation, toxicity, and clearance (Feng et al. 2018)[REMOVED HYPERLINK FIELD].

SURFACE COATING OF IONPS

Uncoated "bare" IONPs demonstrated cytotoxicity that might be attributed to the "the colloidal instability" as these unstable NPs tend to form aggregates that are biodegraded slowly and pose a potential toxicity (Berry et al. 2004). Thus, application of surface-engineering approaches can modulate the *in vivo* application of IONPs and facilitate their theranostic use in CNS disorders (Ojha and Kumar 2018). IONPs have a wide surface area that can be functionalized to enable a high number of functional groups to bind to different molecules for diagnostic imaging or therapeutic activity (Peng et al. 2011). The surface coating of IONPs will balance the intermolecular interaction between the biological molecules and the surface of IONPs (Nosrati et al. 2019). Moreover, the toxicity of IONPs relies on charge of the surface, and the type of coating, in addition to the size and concentration of NPs (Yarjanli et al. 2017).

Various coating materials, either natural or synthetic, were used to increase the stability, improve the pharmacokinetics, promote the bioavailability, and prevent opsonization (anti-fouling) of bare IONPs (Feng et al. 2018). The coating materials that adsorb onto the IONPs should be non-expensive, biocompatible, and non-toxic, such as polyethylene glycol (PEG), dextran, Pluronic, and amino acids (AAs) (El-Boubbou et al. 2018; Ebrahiminezhad et al. 2012). PEG

polymer is a very common coating material that stabilizes IONPs through steric hindrance and decreasing macrophage uptake and elimination of the IONPs (Jokerst et al. 2011), PEGylated-IONPs demonstrated non-fouling potential *via* minimizing binding with opsonin proteins in the blood, coating the surface charge of the IONPs, and subsequently enhancing their hydrophilicity (Arami et al. 2015). The low dispersibility of the IONPs in hydrophilic solvents is a critical issue for cargo loading and delivery. Recently, MIONPs-functionalized with amino or carboxylic acid groups have shown ameliorated dispersibility. Oligosaccharides-coated MIONPs were explored as a nanocarrier for targeting brain tumors that facilitated the non-invasive imaging of cancer cells through MRI for improved theranostics application (Vashist et al. 2023).

Multiple administrations of IONPs could represent a limitation through demonstrating accelerated blood clearance (ABC) and increased pharmacokinetics of NPs that finally results in clearance of NPs through the mononuclear phagocytic system (MPS), as shown in the PEGylated IONPs (Feng et al. 2018). Moreover, PEGylated-MIONPs showed improved bioavailability and biocompatibility (Hadjipanayis et al. 2010); this could result in additional physicochemical properties, such as magneto-optical/ electrical/ or thermal properties (Kang et al. 2018). To enhance the hydrophobicity of IONPs and their passive crossing of BBB, IONPS could be coated with the natural chitosan (CS) polymer, the positively charged CS directs the CS-IONPs towards the negatively charged cellular membranes (Arias et al. 2018) and renders the CS-NPs system as a novel drug delivery approach that is safe, biocompatible and hydrophobic. The drawback of CS to act as efficient coating material is that their solubility, at physiological pH, could be decreased by the partial protonation of its amino groups (Prabaharan 2008). To overcome this limitation, Veiseh et al. (2009) introduced the "co-polymer" coating of IONPs with both CS and PEG. These CS-PEG-IONPs demonstrated a strong potential of passively crossing BBB, through the strong binding activity cationic of CS, the high lipophilic potential of PEG, and the hydrodynamic size of NPs. In addition, other modifications such as the O-carboxymethyl CS (Zhu et al. 2005) and carboxymethyl starch-CS (Saikia et al. 2015) could be applied to enhance the potential of MIONPs. Moreover, intraperitoneal administration of silica coated-MIONPs facilitates the penetration of the BBB (Kim et al. 2006).

Surface coating of SPIONPs enables NPs to cross the BBB through facilitating their cellular uptake (Champagne et al. 2018). Moreover, their supermagnetic nature enhances their penetration in brain *via* hyperthermia through magnetic heating-induced BBB permeability (Chertok et al. 2010; Tabatabaei et al. 2015). The percentage of SPIONPs that attain the CNS has ranged from 17-30% according to rodent studies (Dan et al. 2013). SPIONPs with several surface-coatings demonstrated extensive biomedical applications including diagnostic approaches, drug/gene delivery, MRI, DNA detection, inhibiting the microglial cells, and targeting Aβ in the brain (Barreto et al. 2011; Hasany et al. 2012; Glat et al. 2013). SPIONPs are characterized by their small size, reduced toxicity, magnetic field-directed drug delivery, high magnetic nature, biocompatibility, the high ratio of spin polarization, and good conductivity (Yew et al. 2018; Amanzadeh et al. 2019).

TARGETED DRUG DELIVERY (TDD)

The strategy of targeted-drug delivery (TDD) relies on the use of nanocarriers to deliver directly the active therapeutic molecules, at pharmacological concentration, to specific targets, resulting in improving their therapeutic index (Kumar and Sharma, 2018), TDD could contribute

to the development of more accessible and effective novel therapeutics with no or minimal adverse effects (Kaushik et al. 2018). Applying a drug delivery system comprising both hydrophilic and hydrophobic components improves the solubility of a poorly soluble drug and facilitates their delivery to the brain (Feng et al. 2015). The "Nanotherapeutics" aimed to improve TDD to damaged neuronal regions to enable controlled, direct, and sustainable treatment (Spuch et al. 2012). TDD allows the therapeutic agent to passively cross the biological barriers (e.g. BBB) and to be concentrated in specific tissues of interest while reducing its systemic distribution in other tissues, and thus avoiding its side effects (Durán et al., 2008). Functionalized small-sized IONPs could act as effective nano-vehicles for drug/gene delivery with minimal cytotoxicity (Wu et al. 2015). In addition, using coating materials such as PEG could increase the circulation time of IONPs with hydrophobic surface (Zhu et al. 2012). Therefore, IONPs are regarded as promising candidates for nano-based therapeutic approaches for neurodegenerative disorders and brain tumors, though their ability to cross BBB (Wu et al. 2015). Moreover, the application of a functionalized magnetic field (FMF), or a field function (FF), instead of constant magnetic fields, was used to avoid accumulation of NPs (Tehrani et al. 2014 a, b).

Magnetic drug targeting (MDT) is an innovative technique that utilizes drug-loaded magnets (Magnetic vehicles or magnetizable NPs) to enhance "magnetic localization" of therapeutic agents, through applying a magnetic field gradient to concentrate them at a specific location (Amin et al. 2017). MDT is a bio-safe delivery system that decreases systemic biodistribution of therapeutic agents and increases its concentration at the target site (Polyak and Friedman 2009). SPIONPs-based TDD could be regarded as ideal nanotheranostics application through enabling the magnetic targeting that allows the retention of NPs in the target tissue longer (Arruebo et al. 2007) and allowing the nano-imaging and detection of Aβ plaques in transgenic mice (Sillerud et al. 2013). Magnetic targeting cell delivery (MTCD) is a recent approach that depends on the magnetic cell labeling and subjecting the region of interest to an external magnet (Connell et al. 2015; Silva et al. 2017). The cells are labeled with magnetizable NPs such as SPIONPs; MRI detects SPIONPs-labelled cells (Barrow et al. 2018; Hour et al. 2020). Magnetic field-subjected IONPs can be used as MDT vehicles in aqueous suspensions for drug delivery (Marcu et al. 2013).

NANO-NEURO-THERANOSTICS APPLICATIONS OF IONPS

Citric acid (CA)-functionalized MIONPs (CA-MIONPs) are stable, highly biocompatible, and pH-sensitive vehicles that enhance TDD at low pH values (Semkina et al. 2015). Moreover, Osmotin-loaded MIONPs, under electromagnetic field, demonstrated neuroprotective potential in Aβ-induced AD in mice; through reducing amyloid deposition and hyperphosphorylation of tau protein and finally improving the memory function (Amin et al. 2017). In addition, several studies could contribute to the development of multifunctional agents for AD; for instance, Yang et al. (2011a) synthesized MNPs labelled with antibodies against Aβ-40 and Aβ-42 (anti-Aβ antibody), these conjugated MNPs could be used as a diagnostic tool for AD to estimate low-concentration Aβs through immuno-magnetic reduction (IMR) assay. Moreover, the immobilization of the "Aβ mAb clone BAM10" to near-infrared fluorescent MNPs, for the detection of Aβ- by MRI and fluorescence imaging, inhibit the Aβ40 fibrillation kinetics and decreased the Aβ40-induced cytotoxicity *in vitro* (Skaat et al. 2013). Moreover, anti-biofouling polymer polyethylene glycol-block-allyl glycidyl ether (PEG-b-AGE) coated MIONPs could detect Aβ-peptides and

tau protein in CSF- and serum-mimicking samples, with high specificity and sensitivity (Li et al. 2019). In addition, Kouyoumdjian et al. (2013) reported a biomimetic approach applying SIO-glyconNPs to facilitate the detection of Aβ, *in vitro* and *ex vivo*, using different techniques including ELISA, gel electrophoresis, and transmission electron microscopy (TEM). These NPs showed no toxicity and reduced Aβ-induced cytotoxicity, demonstrating their potential use in for nanodiagnostics and nano-imaging of Aβ plaques.

IONPs could be used as nanotherapeutics of PD; oleic acid-coated MIONPs were employed as nanocarriers for both short hairpin RNA (shRNA) and nerve growth factor (NGF) demonstrated a neurorestorative potential in PD-model *in vitro* and *in vivo* and anti-apoptotic activity, as well as downregulated the expression of α-synuclein (Niu et al. 2017). Moreover, combining NGF and quercetin with SIONPs promoted neurogenesis and increased the complexity of the neuronal branching trees *in vitro* (Katebi et al. 2019). Moreover, USPIONPs can monitor the "cellular infiltration" and the neuroinflammation in white matter (WM) in MS, thus USPIONPs-MRI could be a diagnostic tool for MS (Gidwani et al. 2013). Bioactive molecules such as berberine, resveratrol and sulforaphane loaded on IONPs exhibited therapeutic activities and remyelinating potential in cuprizone-induced rat model of MS (Ibrahim Fouad et al. 2023; 2025; El-Sayed et al. 2025). Combining nerve growth factor (NGF) and quercetin with SMIONPs enhanced neurite outgrowth and stimulated the complexity of the neuronal branching trees in PC12 cells, as potential therapeutics for neurodegenerative disorders (Katebi et al., 2019).

Moreover, Combination of stem cells and NPs could provide novel platforms for treatment of CNS disorders and promoting neuronal differentiation of stem cells into neurons (Sibov et al. 2014; Stephanopoulos et al. 2014; Misra et al. 2016). A study by Tiwari et al. (2013) demonstrated that curcumin-encapsulated PLGA NPs induced neural stem cells (NSC) proliferation, enhanced neurogenesis and improved neurocognitive function, through upregulating the genes required for the NSC proliferation and differentiation, in AD-rats. Accordingly, curcumin magnetic nanoparticles (Cur-MNPs) -diameter <100 nm- enabled the non-invasive diagnosis of AD using MRI; Cur-MNPs were co-localized with Aβ-plaques in the mouse brains using immunohistochemical examination (Cheng et al. 2015). In addition, Cur-IONPs could be used as "a drug nanocarrier" that can pass across BBB, or as a contrast agent (CA) in MRI (Elbialy et al. 2019); in other words, Cur-IONPs could be used as biosafe "nanotheranostic" agents.

Dextran-coated IONPs (Dex-IO NPs) can enhance the therapeutic effects of human MSCs in a murine model of PD through promoting the differentiation of MSCs to dopaminergic neurons (Chung et al. 2018). Moreover, transplanting MNP-labeled human ventral mesencephalic NSC (hVM1) cells into the striatum of the PD-rat, facilitates the monitoring of MNPs (50 and 100 nm) up to 5 months after transplantation at different time points (Ramos-Gómez et al. 2015). MRI enabled us to visualize the transplanted stem cells and to trace their migration into the CNS of animals models (Canzi et al. 2012). For instance, the signal in the brain of both Wobbler mice (the model of spontaneous motor neuron degeneration) and control mice became hypo-intense, after receiving SPION loaded-amniotic fluid cells (hAFCs), demonstrating the efficacy of SPION to evaluate stem cells-based treatment for ALS (Bigini et al. 2012). Moraes et al. (2012) demonstrated the nanotherapeutics activity of SPION-labeled MSC in a rat model of Huntington's disease (HD) and found that transplantation of MSC reduced the number of damaged neurons, through provoking the expression of FGF-2 in the striatum. Moreover, this study utilized SPION to track MSC. *In vivo* tracing of "SPION-conjugated MSC" suggested migration from the site of injection to the damaged striatum.

Several studies used "SPION-labeling" in stem cell research (Niemeyer et al., 2010; Zhu et al., 2007; Moraes et al., 2012), confirming the SPION biosafety and viability maintenance 3 to 7 days after labeling, even using high concentrations of SPION (Moraes et al., 2012). Thereby, further research is required to understand the migratory dynamics of transplanted stem cells to promote clinical transplantation approaches (Moraes et al., 2012). In addition, conjugated amyloid oligomer-specific scFv antibody (W20) to SPIONs "W20-SPIONs" is non-toxic, stable, and could be used to MRI CA, that is capable of crossing BBB, to differentiate PD and HD from negative control Tg mice. W20-SPIONs could be used as nanodiagnostics for early detection of PD and HD (Liu et al., 2019). Therefore, W20-SPIONs could represent an ideal nanotheranostic agent that combines therapeutic and diagnostic functions.

CONCLUSION

This review highlighted the nanotheranostic role of iron oxide NPs by combining the nanotherapeutic potential and the nanodiagnostics potential in a single platform. IONPs could represent nanotheranostic agents for treating or detecting neurodegenerative disorders such as AD, PD. IONPs could be used as drug carriers to deliver neurotherapeutic agents to neurodegeneration regions or as diagnostic agents for MRI and nano-imaging of the brain and neural cells. Further research is required to understand the behavior of these NPs to interact with neural cells and to cross BBB; this will contribute to the establishment of nano-based therapeutic/detecting agents for future clinical applications. Moreover, synthesizing multifunctional, safe, and biocompatible IONPs will be essential to enhance brain localization, to target specific neural regions, or to track NPs to understand their pharmacokinetics in CNS. Therefore, developing a nano-based neurotheranostic platform that can deal with BBB alterations in CNS disorders is essential, this platform will provide a therapeutic potential or a diagnostic accuracy to trace the pathological stages of the disease or to determine the efficiency of drugs. More research is required to improve TDD and therapeutic efficacy, and to enhance sensitivity and specificity of non-invasive imaging. Moreover, the safety of IONPs should be carefully estimated before their clinical applications, and approaches should be acclaimed to reduce the toxic potential of IONPs. Therefore, it would be essential to conduct research concerned with exploring the underlying mechanism of neurotoxicity as well as to synthesize safer IONPs.

REFERENCES

Abbott, A. (2011). Novartis to shut brain research facility. *Nature*, *480*(7376), 161–162. DOI: 10.1038/480161a PMID: 22158218

Ajetunmobi, A., Prina-Mello, A., Volkov, Y., Corvin, A., & Tropea, D. (2014). Nanotechnologies for the study of the central nervous system. *Progress in Neurobiology*, *123*, 18–36. DOI: 10.1016/j.pneurobio.2014.09.004 PMID: 25291406

Albanese, A., Tang, P. S., & Chan, W. C. (2012). The effect of nanoparticle size, shape, and surface chemistry on biological systems. *Annual Review of Biomedical Engineering*, *14*(1), 1–16. DOI: 10.1146/annurev-bioeng-071811-150124 PMID: 22524388

Aliakbari, M., Mohammadian, E., & Esmaeili, A. (2018). Pahlevanneshan, Z. Differential effect of polyvinylpyrrolidone-coated superparamagnetic iron oxide nanoparticles on BT-474 human breast cancer cell viability. *Toxicology In Vitro*.

Altowaijri, G., Fryman, A., & Yadav, V. (2017). Dietary interventions and multiple sclerosis. *Current Neurology and Neuroscience Reports*, *17*(3), 28. Advance online publication. DOI: 10.1007/s11910-017-0732-3 PMID: 28317084

Alzheimer Association. (2016). Alzheimer's disease facts and figures. *Alzheimer's & Dementia*, *12*, 1–80. PMID: 27570871

Amanzadeh, E., Esmaeili, A., Abadi, R. E. N., Kazemipour, N., Pahlevanneshan, Z., & Beheshti, S. (2019). Quercetin conjugated with superparamagnetic iron oxide nanoparticles improves learning and memory better than free quercetin via interacting with proteins involved in LTP. *Scientific Reports*, *9*(1), 1–19. DOI: 10.1038/s41598-019-43345-w PMID: 31053743

Amato, M. P., Derfuss, T., & Hemmer, B.. (2017, January 6). Environmental modifiable risk factors for multiple sclerosis: Report from the 2016 ECTRIMS focused workshop. *MSJ*, *1352458516686847*. Advance online publication. DOI: 10.1177/1352458516686847 PMID: 28671487

Amin, F. U., Hoshiar, A. K., Do, T. D., Noh, Y., Shah, S. A., Khan, M. S., Yoon, J., & Kim, M. O. (2017). Osmotin-loaded magnetic nanoparticles with electromagnetic guidance for the treatment of Alzheimer's disease. *Nanoscale*, *9*(30), 10619–10632. DOI: 10.1039/C7NR00772H PMID: 28534925

Arami, H., Khandhar, A., Liggitt, D., & Krishnan, K. M. (2015). *In vivo* delivery, pharmacokinetics, biodistribution and toxicity of iron oxide nanoparticles. *Chemical Society Reviews*, *44*(23), 8576–8607. DOI: 10.1039/C5CS00541H PMID: 26390044

Arias, L. S., Pessan, J. P., Vieira, A. P. M., Lima, T. M. T. D., Delbem, A. C. B., & Monteiro, D. R. (2018). Iron oxide nanoparticles for biomedical applications: A perspective on synthesis, drugs, antimicrobial activity, and toxicity. *Antibiotics (Basel, Switzerland)*, *7*(2), 46. DOI: 10.3390/antibiotics7020046 PMID: 29890753

Armstrong, R. A. (2013). What causes Alzheimer's disease? *Folia Neuropathologica*, *51*, 169–188. DOI: 10.5114/fn.2013.37702 PMID: 24114635

Arruebo, M., Fernández-Pacheco, R., Ibarra, M. R., & Santamaría, J. (2007). Magnetic nanoparticles for drug delivery. *Nano Today*, *2*(3), 22–32. DOI: 10.1016/S1748-0132(07)70084-1

Asharani, P. V., Hande, M. P., & Valiyaveettil, S. (2009). Valiyaveettil S. Anti-proliferative activity of silver nanoparticles. *BMC Cell Biology*, *10*(1), 65. DOI: 10.1186/1471-2121-10-65 PMID: 19761582

Baker, S. K., Chen, Z. L., Norris, E. H., Revenko, A. S., MacLeod, A. R., & Strickland, S. (2018). Blood-derived plasminogen drives brain inflammation and plaque deposition in a mouse model of Alzheimer's disease. *Proceedings of the National Academy of Sciences of the United States of America*, *115*(41), 9687–9696. DOI: 10.1073/pnas.1811172115 PMID: 30254165

Barreto, A., Santiago, V. R., Mazzetto, S. E., Denardin, J. C., Lavín, R., Mele, G., Ribeiro, M. E. N. P., Vieira, I. G. P., Gonçalves, T., Ricardo, N. M. P. S., & Fechine, P. B. A. (2011). Magnetic nanoparticles for a new drug delivery system to control quercetin releasing for cancer chemotherapy. *Journal of Nanoparticle Research*, *13*(12), 6545–6553. DOI: 10.1007/s11051-011-0559-9

Barrow, M., Taylor, A., Fuentes-Caparrós, A. M., Sharkey, J., Daniels, L. M., Mandal, P., Park, B. K., Murray, P., Rosseinsky, M. J., & Adams, D. J. (2018). SPIONs for cell labelling and tracking using MRI: Magnetite or maghemite? *Biomaterials Science*, *6*(1), 101–106. DOI: 10.1039/C7BM00515F PMID: 29188240

Berry, C. C., Wells, S., Charles, S., Aitchison, G., & Curtis, A. S. (2004). Cell response to dextran-derivatised iron oxide nanoparticles post internalisation. *Biomaterials*, *25*(23), 5405–5413. DOI: 10.1016/j.biomaterials.2003.12.046 PMID: 15130725

Bigini, P., Diana, V., Barbera, S., Fumagalli, E., Micotti, E., Sitia, L., Paladini, A., Bisighini, C., De Grada, L., Coloca, L., Colombo, L., Manca, P., Bossolasco, P., Malvestiti, F., Fiordaliso, F., Forloni, G., Morbidelli, M., Salmona, M., Giardino, D., & Cova, L. (2012). Longitudinal tracking of human fetal cells labeled with super paramagnetic iron oxide nanoparticles in the brain of mice with motor neuron disease. *PLoS One*, *7*(2), e32326. DOI: 10.1371/journal.pone.0032326 PMID: 22384217

Bobo, D., Robinson, K. J., Islam, J., Turecht, K. J., & Corrie, S. R. (2016). Nanoparticle-Based Medicines: A Review of FDA-Approved Materials and Clinical Trials to Date. *Pharmaceutical Research*, *33*(10), 2373–2387. DOI: 10.1007/s11095-016-1958-5 PMID: 27299311

Borai, I. H., Ezz, M. K., Rizk, M. Z., Aly, H. F., El-Sherbiny, M., Matloub, A. A., & Fouad, G. I. (2017). Therapeutic impact of grape leaves polyphenols on certain biochemical and neurological markers in AlCl3-induced Alzheimer's disease. *Biomedicine and Pharmacotherapy*, *93*, 837–851. DOI: 10.1016/j.biopha.2017.07.038 PMID: 28715867

Braak, H., Del Tredici, K., Rub, U., de Vos, R. A., Jansen Steur, E. N., & Braak, E. (2003). Staging of brain pathology related to sporadic Parkinson's disease. *Neurobiology of Aging*, *24*(2), 197–211. DOI: 10.1016/S0197-4580(02)00065-9 PMID: 12498954

Bulte, J. W. (2009). *In vivo* MRI cell tracking: Clinical studies. *AJR. American Journal of Roentgenology*, *193*(2), 314–325. DOI: 10.2214/AJR.09.3107 PMID: 19620426

Burtea, C., Laurent, S., Mahieu, I., Larbanoix, L., Roch, A., Port, M., Rousseaux, O., Ballet, S., Murariu, O., Toubeau, G., Corot, C., Vander Elst, L., & Muller, R. N. (2011). *In vitro* biomedical applications of functionalized iron oxide nanoparticles, including those not related to magnetic properties. *Contrast Media & Molecular Imaging*, *6*(4), 236–250. DOI: 10.1002/cmmi.423 PMID: 21861284

Busquets, M. A., Sabate, R., & Estelrich, J. (2014). Potential applications of magnetic particles to detect and treat Alzheimer's disease. *Nanoscale Research Letters*, *9*(1), 538. DOI: 10.1186/1556-276X-9-538 PMID: 25288921

Canzi, L., Castellaneta, V., Navone, S., Nava, S., Dossena, M., Zucca, I., Mennini, T., Bigini, P., & Parati, E. A. (2012). Human skeletal muscle stem cell antiinflammatory activity ameliorates clinical outcome in amyotrophic lateral sclerosis *models. Molecular Medicine (Cambridge, Mass.)*, *18*(3), 401–411. DOI: 10.2119/molmed.2011.00123 PMID: 22076467

Champagne, P.-O., Westwick, H., Bouthillier, A., & Sawan, M. (2018). Colloidal stability of superparamagnetic iron oxide nanoparticles in the central nervous system: A review. *Nanomedicine (London)*, *13*(11), 1385–1400. DOI: 10.2217/nnm-2018-0021 PMID: 29949472

Cheng, K. K., Chan, P. S., Fan, S., Kwan, S. M., Yeung, K. L., Wáng, Y.-X. J., Chow, A. H. L., Wu, E. X., & Baum, L. (2015). Curcumin-conjugated magnetic nanoparticles for detecting amyloid plaques in Alzheimer's disease mice using magnetic resonance imaging (MRI). *Biomaterials*, *44*, 155–172. DOI: 10.1016/j.biomaterials.2014.12.005 PMID: 25617135

Chertok, B., David, A. E., & Yang, V. C. (2010). Polyethyleneimine-modified iron oxide nanoparticles for brain tumor drug delivery using magnetic targeting and intra-carotid administration. *Biomaterials*, *31*(24), 6317–6324. DOI: 10.1016/j.biomaterials.2010.04.043 PMID: 20494439

Chinde, S., & Grover, P. (2017). Toxicological assessment of nano and micron-sized tungsten oxide after 28days repeated oral administration to Wistar rats. *Mutation Research*, *819*, 1–13. DOI: 10.1016/j.mrgentox.2017.05.003 PMID: 28622824

Cho, W. S., Cho, M., Kim, S. R., Choi, M., Lee, J. Y., Han, B. S., Park, S. N., Yu, M. K., Jon, S., & Jeong, J. (2009). Pulmonary toxicity and kinetic study of Cy5. 5-conjugated superparamagnetic iron oxide nanoparticles by optical imaging. *Toxicology and Applied Pharmacology*, *239*(1), 106–115. DOI: 10.1016/j.taap.2009.05.026 PMID: 19520096

Chung, T. H., Hsu, S. C., Wu, S. H., Hsiao, J. K., Lin, C. P., Yao, M., & Huang, D.-M. (2018). Dextran-coated iron oxide nanoparticle-improved therapeutic effects of human mesenchymal stem cells in a mouse model of Parkinson's disease. *Nanoscale*, *10*(6), 2998–3007. DOI: 10.1039/C7NR06976F PMID: 29372743

Connell, J. J., Patrick, P. S., Yu, Y., Lythgoe, M. F., & Kalber, T. L. (2015). Advanced cell therapies: Targeting, tracking and actuation of cells with magnetic particles. *Regenerative Medicine*, *10*(6), 757–772. DOI: 10.2217/rme.15.36 PMID: 26390317

Cranwell-Bruce, L. A. (2010). Drugs for Parkinson's disease. *Medsurg Nursing*, *19*, 347. PMID: 21337993

Dan, M., Cochran, D. B., Yokel, R. A., & Dziubla, T. D. (2013). Binding, Transcytosis and Biodistribution of Anti-PECAM−1 Iron Oxide Nanoparticles for Brain-Targeted Delivery. *PLoS One*, *8*(11), e81051. DOI: 10.1371/journal.pone.0081051 PMID: 24278373

Dulińska-Litewka, J., Łazarczyk, A., Hałubiec, P., Szafranski, O., Karnas, K., & Karewicz, A. (2019). Superparamagnetic iron oxide nanoparticles-current and prospective medical applications. *Materials (Basel)*, *12*(4), E617. DOI: 10.3390/ma12040617 PMID: 30791358

Durán, J. D., Arias, J. L., Gallardo, V., & Delgado, A. V. (2008). Magnetic colloids as drug vehicles. *Journal of Pharmaceutical Sciences*, *97*(8), 2948–2983. DOI: 10.1002/jps.21249 PMID: 18064669

Ebrahiminezhad, A., Ghasemi, Y., Rasoul-Amini, S., Barar, J., & Davaran, S. (2012). Impact of amino-acid coating on the synthesis and characteristics of iron-oxide nanoparticles (IONs). *Bulletin of the Korean Chemical Society*, *33*(12), 3957–3962. DOI: 10.5012/bkcs.2012.33.12.3957

El-Boubbou, K. (2018). Magnetic iron oxide nanoparticles as drug carriers: Clinical relevance. *Nanomedicine (London)*, *13*(8), 953–971. DOI: 10.2217/nnm-2017-0336 PMID: 29376469

El-Sayed, S. A., Fouad, G. I., Rizk, M. Z., Beherei, H. H., & Mabrouk, M. (2025). Comparative neuroprotective potential of nanoformulated and free resveratrol against cuprizone-induced demyelination in rats. *Molecular Neurobiology*, *62*(3), 2710–2725. DOI: 10.1007/s12035-024-04415-x PMID: 39152208

Elbialy, N. S., Aboushoushah, S. F., & Alshammari, W. W. (2019). Long-term biodistribution and toxicity of curcumin capped iron oxide nanoparticles after single-dose administration in mice. *Life Sciences*, *230*, 76–83. DOI: 10.1016/j.lfs.2019.05.048 PMID: 31128136

Elsheikh, A. A., Abd-Almotaleb, N. A., Ahmed, M. M., & Khayal, E. E. S. (2025). IONPs-induced

Engberink, R., van der Pol, S., Walczak, P., van der Toorn, A., Viergever, M., Dijkstra, C., Bulte, J., de Vries, H., & Blezer, E. (2010). Magnetic resonance imaging of monocytes labeled with ultrasmall superparamagnetic particles of iron oxide using magnetoelectroporation in an animal model of multiple sclerosis. *Molecular Imaging*, *9*(5), 268–277. DOI: 10.2310/7290.2010.00016 PMID: 20868627

Escribano, B. M., Medina-Fernández, F. J., Aguilar-Luque, M., Agüera, E., Feijoo, M., Garcia-Maceira, F. I., Lillo, R., Vieyra-Reyes, P., Giraldo, A. I., Luque, E., Drucker-Colín, R., & Túnez, I. (2017). Lipopolysaccharide binding protein and oxidative stressin a multiple sclerosis model. *Neurotherapeutics; the Journal of the American Society for Experimental NeuroTherapeutics*, *14*(1), 199–211. DOI: 10.1007/s13311-016-0480-0 PMID: 27718209

Evans, M. C., Serres, S., Khrapitchev, A. A., Stolp, H. B., Anthony, D. C., Talbot, K., Turner, M. R., & Sibson, N. R. (2014). T(2)-weighted MRI detects presymptomatic pathology in the SOD1 mouse model of ALS. *Journal of Cerebral Blood Flow and Metabolism*, *34*(5), 785–793. DOI: 10.1038/jcbfm.2014.19 PMID: 24496176

Fahmy, H. M. (2019). Oxidative Impact of Carob Leaf Extract–Synthesized Iron Oxide Magnetic Nanoparticles on the Kidney, Liver, Testis, and Spleen of Wistar Rats. *BioNanoScience*, •••, 1–8.

Farrell, B. T., Hamilton, B. E., Dósa, E., Rimely, E., Nasseri, M., Gahramanov, S., Lacy, C. A., Frenkel, E. P., Doolittle, N. D., Jacobs, P. M., & Neuwelt, E. A. (2013). Using iron oxide nanoparticles to diagnose CNS inflammatory diseases and PCNSL. *Neurology*, *81*(3), 256–263. DOI: 10.1212/WNL.0b013e31829bfd8f PMID: 23771486

Feng, Q., Liu, Y., Huang, J., Chen, K., Huang, J., & Xiao, K. (2018). Uptake, distribution, clearance, and toxicity of iron oxide nanoparticles with different sizes and coatings. *Scientific Reports*, *8*(1), 1–13. DOI: 10.1038/s41598-018-19628-z PMID: 29391477

Gidwani, M., & Singh, A. V. (2013). Nanoparticle enabled drug delivery across the blood brain barrier: In vivo and in vitro models, opportunities and challenges. *Current Pharmaceutical Biotechnology*, *14*(14), 1201–1212. DOI: 10.2174/1389201015666140508122558 PMID: 24809717

Gidwani M, Singh AV (2014) Nanoparticle enabled drug delivery across the blood brain barrier: in vivo and in vitro models, opportunities and challenges. Curr Pharmaceut Biotechnol 14:1201e12.

Glat, M., Skaat, H., Menkes-Caspi, N., Margel, S., & Stern, E. A. (2013). Age-dependent effects of microglial inhibition in vivo on Alzheimer's disease neuropathology using bioactive-conjugated iron oxide nanoparticles. *Journal of Nanobiotechnology*, *11*(1), 32. DOI: 10.1186/1477-3155-11-32 PMID: 24059692

Gustafson, H. H., Holt-Casper, D., Grainger, D. W., Ghandehari, H., & Grainger, D. (2015). Nanoparticle Uptake: Te Phagocyte Problem HHS Public Access. *Nano Today*, *10*(4), 487–510. DOI: 10.1016/j.nantod.2015.06.006 PMID: 26640510

Hadjipanayis, C. G., Machaidze, R., Kaluzova, M., Wang, L., Schuette, A. J., Chen, H., Wu, X., & Mao, H. (2010). EGFRvIII antibody-conjugated iron oxide nanoparticles for magnetic resonance imaging-guided convectionenhanced delivery and targeted therapy of glioblastoma. *Cancer Research*, *70*(15), 6303–6312. DOI: 10.1158/0008-5472.CAN-10-1022 PMID: 20647323

Hanini, A, & Schmitt, A, Kacem k, Chau F, Ammar S, Gavard J. (2011). Evaluation of iron oxide nanoparticle biocompatibility. *International Journal of Nanomedicine*, *6*, 787. PMID: 21589646

Harilal, S., Jose, J., Parambi, D. G. T., Kumar, R., Mathew, G. E., Uddin, M., Kim, H., & Mathew, B. (2019). Advancements in nanotherapeutics for Alzheimer's disease: Current perspectives. *The Journal of Pharmacy and Pharmacology*, *71*(9), 1370–1383. DOI: 10.1111/jphp.13132 PMID: 31304982

Hasany, S., Ahmed, I., Rajan, J., & Rehman, A. (2012). Systematic review of the preparation techniques of iron oxide magnetic nanoparticles. *J NANOSCI NANOTECHNO*, *2*, 148–158. DOI: 10.5923/j.nn.20120206.01

Hassan S, Singh AV (2014) Biophysicochemical perspective of nanoparticle compatibility: a critically ignored parameter in nanomedicine. J Nanosci Nanotechnol;14:402e14.

Hegazy, M. A. E., Maklad, H. M., Abd Elmonsif, D. A., Elnozhy, F. Y., Alqubiea, M. A., Alenezi, F. A., Al abbas, O. M., & Al abbas, M. M. (2017). The possible role of cerium oxide (CeO_2) nanoparticles in prevention of neurobehavioral and neurochemical changes in 6-hydroxydopamine-induced parkinsonian disease. *Alexandria Journal of Medicine*, *53*(4), 351–360. DOI: 10.1016/j.ajme.2016.12.006

Hirst, S. M., Karakoti, A., Singh, S., Self, W., Tyler, R., Seal, S., & Reilly, C. M. (2013). Biodistribution and in vivo antioxidant effects of cerium oxide nanoparticles in mice. *Environmental Toxicology*, *28*(2), 107–118. DOI: 10.1002/tox.20704 PMID: 21618676

Hour, F. Q., Moghadam, A. J., Shakeri-Zadeh, A., Bakhtiyari, M., Shabani, R., & Mehdizadeh, M. (2020). Magnetic targeted delivery of the SPIONs-labeled mesenchymal stem cells derived from human Wharton's jelly in Alzheimer's rat models. *Journal of Controlled Release*, *321*, 430–441. DOI: 10.1016/j.jconrel.2020.02.035 PMID: 32097673

Hsieh, H. C., Chen, C.-M., Hsieh, W.-Y., Chen, C.-Y., Liu, C.-C., & Lin, F.-H. (2015). ROS-induced toxicity: Exposure of 3T3, RAW264. 7, and MCF7 cells to superparamagnetic iron oxide nanoparticles results in cell death by mitochondria-dependent apoptosis. *Journal of Nanoparticle Research*, *17*(2), 71. DOI: 10.1007/s11051-015-2886-8

Ibrahim Fouad, G., El-Sayed, S. A., Mabrouk, M., Ahmed, K. A., & Beherei, H. H. (2022). Neuroprotective potential of intranasally delivered sulforaphane-loaded iron oxide nanoparticles against cisplatin-induced neurotoxicity. *Neurotoxicity Research*, *40*(5), 1479–1498. DOI: 10.1007/s12640-022-00555-x PMID: 35969308

Ibrahim Fouad, G., El-Sayed, S. A., Mabrouk, M., Ahmed, K. A., & Beherei, H. H. (2022). Neuroprotective potential of intranasally delivered sulforaphane-loaded iron oxide nanoparticles against cisplatin-induced neurotoxicity. *Neurotoxicity Research*, *40*(5), 1479–1498. DOI: 10.1007/s12640-022-00555-x PMID: 35969308

Ibrahim Fouad, G., Mabrouk, M., El-Sayed, S. A., Abdelhameed, M. F., Rizk, M. Z., & Beherei, H. H. (2025). Berberine-loaded iron oxide nanoparticles alleviate cuprizone-induced astrocytic reactivity in a rat model of multiple sclerosis. *Biometals*, *38*(1), 203–229. DOI: 10.1007/s10534-024-00648-4 PMID: 39543075

Ibrahim Fouad, G., Mabrouk, M., El-Sayed, S. A., Rizk, M. Z., & Beherei, H. H. (2023). Neurotherapeutic efficacy of loaded sulforaphane on iron oxide nanoparticles against cuprizone-induced neurotoxicity: Role of MMP-9 and S100β. *Toxicology Mechanisms and Methods*, *33*(6), 463–479. DOI: 10.1080/15376516.2023.2177219 PMID: 36775846

Jain, T. K., Reddy, M. K., Morales, M. A., Leslie-Pelecky, D. L., & Labhasetwar, V. (2008). Biodistribution, clearance, and biocompatibility of iron oxide magnetic nanoparticles in rats. *Molecular Pharmaceutics*, *5*(2), 316–327. DOI: 10.1021/mp7001285 PMID: 18217714

Jiménez-Aguilar, D. M., Ortega-Regules, A. E., Lozada-Ramírez, J. D., Pérez-Pérez, M. C. I., Vernon-Cartere, E. J., & Welti-Chanesa, J. (2011). Color, and chemical stability of spray-dried blueberry extract using mesquite gum as wall material. *Journal of Food Composition and Analysis*, *24*(6), 889–894. DOI: 10.1016/j.jfca.2011.04.012

Jokerst, J. V., Lobovkina, T., Zare, R. N., & Gambhir, S. S. (2011). Nanoparticle PEGylation for imaging and therapy. *Nanomedicine (London)*, *6*(4), 715–728. DOI: 10.2217/nnm.11.19 PMID: 21718180

Kaitin, K. (2010). Deconstructing the drug development process: The new face of innovation. *Clinical Pharmacology and Therapeutics*, *87*(3), 356–361. DOI: 10.1038/clpt.2009.293 PMID: 20130565

Kakkar, V., Kumar, M., & Saini, K. (2018). Nanoceuticals governance and market review. *Environmental Chemistry Letters*, *16*(4), 1293–1300. DOI: 10.1007/s10311-018-0754-3

Kang, Y. J., Cutler, E. G., & Cho, H. (2018). Therapeutic nanoplatforms and delivery strategies for neurological disorders. *Nano Convergence*, *5*(1), 1–15. DOI: 10.1186/s40580-018-0168-8 PMID: 30499047

Katebi, S., Esmaeili, A., Ghaedi, K., & Zarrabi, A. (2019). Superparamagnetic iron oxide nanoparticles combined with NGF and quercetin promote neuronal branching morphogenesis of PC12 cells. *International Journal of Nanomedicine*, *14*, 2157–2169. DOI: 10.2147/IJN.S191878 PMID: 30992663

Katebi, S., Esmaeili, A., Ghaedi, K., & Zarrabi, A. (2019). Superparamagnetic iron oxide nanoparticles combined with NGF and quercetin promote neuronal branching morphogenesis of PC12 cells. *International Journal of Nanomedicine*, *14*, 2157–2169. DOI: 10.2147/IJN.S191878 PMID: 30992663

Kaushik, A. C., Bharadwaj, S., Kumar, S., & Wei, D. Q. (2018). Nano-particle mediated inhibition of Parkinson's disease using computational biology approach. *Scientific Reports*, *8*(1), 1–8. DOI: 10.1038/s41598-018-27580-1 PMID: 29907754

Kevadiya, B. D., Ottemann, B. M., Thomas, M. B., Mukadam, I., Nigam, S., McMillan, J., Gorantla, S., Bronich, T. K., Edagwa, B., & Gendelman, H. E. (2019). Neurotheranostics as personalized medicines. *Advanced Drug Delivery Reviews*, *148*, 252–289. DOI: 10.1016/j.addr.2018.10.011 PMID: 30421721

Khan, A. R., Liu, M., Khan, M. W., & Zhai, G. (2017). Progress in brain targeting drug delivery system by nasal route. *Journal of Controlled Release*, *268*, 364–389. DOI: 10.1016/j.jconrel.2017.09.001 PMID: 28887135

Kim, J. S., Yoon, T. J., Yu, K. N., Kim, B. G., Park, S. J., Kim, H. W., Lee, K. H., Park, S. B., Lee, J.-K., & Cho, M. H. (2006). Toxicity and tissue distribution of magnetic nanoparticles in mice. *Toxicological Sciences*, *89*(1), 338–347. DOI: 10.1093/toxsci/kfj027 PMID: 16237191

Kimura, N. (2016). Diabetes mellitus induces Alzheimer's disease pathology: Histopathological evidence from animal models. *International Journal of Molecular Sciences*, *17*(4), 503. Advance online publication. DOI: 10.3390/ijms17040503 PMID: 27058526

Kiyatkin, E. A., & Sharma, H. S. (2009). Permeability of the blood-brain barrier depends on brain temperature. *Neuroscience*, *161*(3), 926–939. DOI: 10.1016/j.neuroscience.2009.04.004 PMID: 19362131

Kouyoumdjian, H., Zhu, D. C., El-Dakdouki, M. H., Lorenz, K., Chen, J., Li, W., & Huang, X. (2013). Glyconanoparticle aided detection of β-amyloid by magnetic resonance imaging and attenuation of β-amyloid induced cytotoxicity. *ACS Chemical Neuroscience*, *4*(4), 575–584. DOI: 10.1021/cn3002015 PMID: 23590250

Kumar, A., Pandey, A. K., Singh, S. S., Shanker, R., & Dhawan, A. (2011). Cellular uptake and mutagenic potential of metal oxide nanoparticles in bacterial cells. *Chemosphere*, *83*(8), 1124–1132. DOI: 10.1016/j.chemosphere.2011.01.025 PMID: 21310462

Kumar, R., & Sharma, M. (2018). Herbal nanomedicine interactions to enhance pharmacokinetics, pharmaco-dynamics, and therapeutic index for better bioavailability and biocompatibility of herbal formulations. *J Mater Nanosci*, *5*(1), 35–58.

Kunzmann, A., Andersson, B., Vogt, C., Feliu, N., Ye, F., Gabrielsson, S., Toprak, M. S., Buerki-Thurnherr, T., Laurent, S., Vahter, M., Krug, H., Muhammed, M., Scheynius, A., & Fadeel, B. (2011). Efficient internalization of silica-coated iron oxide nanoparticles of different sizes by primary human macrophages and dendritic cells. *Toxicology and Applied Pharmacology*, *253*(2), 81–93. DOI: 10.1016/j.taap.2011.03.011 PMID: 21435349

Labuschagne, I. L., & Blaauw, R. (2018). An anti-inflammatory approach to the dietary management of multiple sclerosis: A condensed review. *The South African Journal of Clinical Nutrition: SAJCN: the Official Journal of the South African Society of Parenteral and Enteral Nutrition and the Association for Dietetics in South Africa*, *31*(3), 67–73. DOI: 10.1080/16070658.2018.1465652

Laurent, S., Burtea, C., Thirifays, C., Häfeli, U. O., & Mahmoudi, M. (2012). Crucial ignored parameters on nanotoxicology: The importance of toxicity assay modifications and "cell vision". *PLoS One*, *7*(1), e29997. DOI: 10.1371/journal.pone.0029997 PMID: 22253854

Li, Y., Lim, E., Field, T., Wu, H., & Mao, H. (2019). Improving sensitivity and specificity of amyloid-β peptide and tau protein detection with anti-biofouling magnetic nanoparticles for liquid biopsy of Alzheimer's disease. *ACS Biomaterials Science & Engineering*, *5*(7), 3595–3605. DOI: 10.1021/acsbiomaterials.9b00086 PMID: 33405741

Ling, D., & Hyeon, T. (2013). Chemical design of biocompatible iron oxide nanoparticles for medical applications. *Small*, *9*(9-10), 1450–1466. DOI: 10.1002/smll.201202111 PMID: 23233377

Liu, X. G., Lu, S., Liu, D. Q., Zhang, L., Zhang, L. X., Yu, X. L., & Liu, R. T. (2019). ScFv-conjugated superparamagnetic iron oxide nanoparticles for MRI-based diagnosis in transgenic mouse models of Parkinson's and Huntington's diseases. *Brain Research*, *1707*, 141–153. DOI: 10.1016/j.brainres.2018.11.034 PMID: 30481502

Luo, S., Ma, C., Zhu, M. Q., Ju, W. N., Yang, Y., & Wang, X. (2020). Application of Iron Oxide Nanoparticles in the Diagnosis and Treatment of Neurodegenerative Diseases With Emphasis on Alzheimer's Disease. *Frontiers in Cellular Neuroscience*, *14*, 14. DOI: 10.3389/fncel.2020.00021 PMID: 32184709

Ma, L. L., Liu, J., Li, N., Wang, J., Duan, Y., Yan, J., Liu, H., Wang, H., & Hong, F. (2010). Oxidative stress in the brain of mice caused by translocated nanoparticulate TiO2 delivered to the abdominal cavity. *Biomaterials*, *31*(1), 99–105. DOI: 10.1016/j.biomaterials.2009.09.028 PMID: 19783296

Mahmoudi, M., Akhavan, O., Ghavami, M., Rezaee, F., & Ghiasi, S. M. (2012). Graphene oxide strongly inhibits amyloid beta fbrillation. *Nanoscale*, *4*(23), 7322–7325. DOI: 10.1039/c2nr31657a PMID: 23079862

Mahmoudi, M., Sant, S., Wang, B., Laurent, S., & Sen, T. (2011). Superparamagnetic iron oxide nanoparticles (SPIONs): Development, surface modification and applications in chemotherapy. *Advanced Drug Delivery Reviews*, *63*(1-2), 24–46. DOI: 10.1016/j.addr.2010.05.006 PMID: 20685224

Manfré, G., Clemensson, E. K. H., Kyriakou, E. I., Clemensson, L. E., van der Harst, J. E., Homberg, J. R., & Nguyen, H. P. (2017). The BACHD Rat Model of Huntington Disease Shows Specific Deficits in a Test Battery of Motor Function. *Frontiers in Behavioral Neuroscience*, *11*, 218. DOI: 10.3389/fnbeh.2017.00218 PMID: 29163089

Manjili, H. K., Ma'mani, L., Tavaddod, S., Mashhadikhan, M., Shafiee, A., & Naderi-Manesh, H. (2016). D, L-sulforaphane loaded Fe3O4@ gold core shell nanoparticles: A potential sulforaphane delivery system. *PLoS One*, *11*(3). PMID: 26982588

Marcu, A., Pop, S., Dumitrache, F., Mocanu, M., Niculite, C. M., Gherghiceanu, M., Lungu, C. P., Fleaca, C., Ianchis, R., Barbut, A., Grigoriu, C., & Morjan, I. (2013). Magnetic iron oxide nanoparticles as drug delivery system in breast cancer. *Applied Surface Science*, *281*, 60–65. DOI: 10.1016/j.apsusc.2013.02.072

Martínez-Ballesta, MCarment, et al. (2018) Nanoparticles and controlled delivery for bioactive compounds: Outlining challenges for new "Smart-foods" for health. Foods 7.5: 72.

Masselli, G., & Gualdi, G. (2012). MR imaging of the small bowel. *Radiology*, *264*(2), 333–348. DOI: 10.1148/radiol.12111658 PMID: 22821694

Miller, D. H., Chard, D. T., & Ciccarelli, O. (2012). Clinically isolated syndromes. *Lancet Neurology*, *11*(2), 157–169. DOI: 10.1016/S1474-4422(11)70274-5 PMID: 22265211

Misra, S., Chopra, K., Saikia, U. N., Sinha, V. R., Sehgal, R., Modi, M., & Medhi, B. (2016). Effect of mesenchymal stem cells and galantamine nanoparticles in rat model of Alzheimer's disease. *Regenerative Medicine*, *11*(7), 629–646. DOI: 10.2217/rme-2016-0032 PMID: 27582416

Mody, V. V., Siwale, R., Singh, A., & Mody, H. R. (2010). Introduction to metallic nanoparticles. *Journal of Pharmacy & Bioallied Sciences*, *2*(4), 282–289. DOI: 10.4103/0975-7406.72127 PMID: 21180459

Moraes, L., Vasconcelos-dos-Santos, A., Santana, F. C., Godoy, M. A., Rosado-de-Castro, P. H., Jasmin, , Azevedo-Pereira, R. L., Cintra, W. M., Gasparetto, E. L., Santiago, M. F., & Mendez-Otero, R. (2012). Neuroprotective effects and magnetic resonance imaging of mesenchymal stem cells labeled with SPION in a rat model of Huntington's disease. *Stem Cell Research*, *9*(2), 143–155. DOI: 10.1016/j.scr.2012.05.005 PMID: 22742973

Najafabadi, R. E., Kazemipour, N., Esmaeili, A., Beheshti, S., & Nazif, S. (2018). Using superparamagnetic iron oxide nanoparticles to enhance bioavailability of quercetin in the intact rat brain. *BMC Pharmacology & Toxicology*, *19*(1), 59. DOI: 10.1186/s40360-018-0249-7 PMID: 30253803

Niemeyer, M., Oostendorp, R. A., Kremer, M., Hippauf, S., Jacobs, V. R., Baurecht, H., Ludwig, G., Piontek, G., Bekker-Ruz, V., Timmer, S., Rummeny, E. J., Kiechle, M., & Beer, A. J. (2010). Non-invasive tracking of human haemopoietic CD34+ stem cells in vivo in immunodeficient mice by using magnetic resonance imaging. *European Radiology*, *20*(9), 2184–2193. DOI: 10.1007/s00330-010-1773-z PMID: 20393719

Niu, S., Zhang, L. K., Zhang, L., Zhuang, S., Zhan, X., Chen, W., Du, S., Yin, L., You, R., Li, C.-H., & Guan, Y.-Q. (2017). Inhibition by multifunctional magnetic nanoparticles loaded with alpha-synuclein RNAi plasmid in a Parkinson's disease model. *Theranostics*, *7*(2), 344–356. DOI: 10.7150/thno.16562 PMID: 28042339

Niu, X., Chen, J., & Gao, J. (2019). Nanocarriers as a powerful vehicle to overcome blood-brain barrier in treating neurodegenerative diseases: Focus on recent advances. *Asian Journal of Pharmaceutical Sciences*, *14*(5), 480–496. DOI: 10.1016/j.ajps.2018.09.005 PMID: 32104476

Nosrati, H., Salehiabar, M., Attari, E., Davaran, S., Danafar, H., & Manjili, H. K. (2018). Green and one-pot surface coating of iron oxide magnetic nanoparticles with natural amino acids and biocompatibility investigation. *Applied Organometallic Chemistry*, *32*(2), e4069. DOI: 10.1002/aoc.4069

Odeh, F., Al-Jaber, H., & Khater, D. (2014). Nanoflora—how nanotechnology enhanced the use of active phytochemicals. In *Application of Nanotechnology in Drug Delivery*. InTech. DOI: 10.5772/58704

Ojha, S., & Kumar, B. (2018). A review on nanotechnology based innovations in diagnosis and treatment of multiple sclerosis. *JCI*, *4*(2), 56–64. DOI: 10.1016/j.jocit.2017.12.001

Paik, S. Y. R., Kim, J. S., Shin, S. J., & Ko, S. (2015). Characterization, quantification, and determination of the toxicity of iron oxide nanoparticles to the bone marrow cells. *International Journal of Molecular Sciences*, *16*(9), 22243–22257. DOI: 10.3390/ijms160922243 PMID: 26389886

Pan, Y., Du, X., Zhao, F., & Xu, B. (2012). Magnetic nanoparticles for the manipulation of proteins and cells. *Chemical Society Reviews*, *44*(7), 8576–8607. DOI: 10.1039/c2cs15315g PMID: 22318454

Patel, S., Jana, S., Chetty, R., Thakore, S., Singh, M., & Devkar, R. (2017). Toxicity evaluation of magnetic iron oxide nanoparticles reveals neuronal loss in chicken embryo. *Drug and Chemical Toxicology*, *27*, 1–8. PMID: 29281933

Patil, R. M., Thorat, N. D., Shete, P. B., Bedge, P. A., Gavde, S., Joshi, M. G., Tofail, S. A. M., & Bohara, R. A. (2018). Comprehensive cytotoxicity studies of superparamagnetic iron oxide nanoparticles. *Biochemistry and Biophysics Reports*, *13*, 63–72. DOI: 10.1016/j.bbrep.2017.12.002 PMID: 29349357

Peng, X., Chen, H., Huang, J., Mao, H., & Shin, D. M. (2011). *Targeted magnetic iron oxide nanoparticles for tumor imaging and therapy Biomedical Engineering—From Theory to Applications*. InTech.

Polyak, B., & Friedman, G. (2009). Magnetic targeting for site-specific drug delivery: Applications and clinical potential. *Expert Opinion on Drug Delivery*, *6*(1), 53–70. DOI: 10.1517/17425240802662795 PMID: 19236208

Prabaharan, M. (2008). Review paper: Chitosan derivatives as promising materials for controlled drug delivery. *Journal of Biomaterials Applications*, *23*(1), 5–36. DOI: 10.1177/0885328208091562 PMID: 18593819

Prasad, C., Yuvaraja, G., & Venkateswarlu, P. (2017). Biogenic synthesis of Fe3O4 magnetic nanoparticles using Pisum sativum peels extract and its effect on magnetic and methyl orange dye degradation studies. *Journal of Magnetism and Magnetic Materials*, *424*, 376–381. DOI: 10.1016/j.jmmm.2016.10.084

Pringsheim, T., Jette, N., Frolkis, A., & Steeves, T. D. (2014). The prevalence of Parkinson's disease: A systematic review and meta-analysis. *Movement Disorders*, *29*(13), 1583–1590. DOI: 10.1002/mds.25945 PMID: 24976103

Radhakrishnan, R., Kulhari, H., Pooja, D., Gudem, S., Bhargava, S., Shukla, R., & Sistla, R. (2016). Encapsulation of biophenolic phytochemical EGCG within lipid nanoparticles enhances its stability and cytotoxicity against cancer. *Chemistry and Physics of Lipids*, *198*, 51–60. DOI: 10.1016/j.chemphyslip.2016.05.006 PMID: 27234272

Rajabally, Y. A., & Martey, J. (2011). Neuropathy in Parkinson disease: Prevalence and determinants. *Neurology*, *77*(22), 1947–1950. DOI: 10.1212/WNL.0b013e31823a0ee4 PMID: 22049200

Ramos-Gómez, M., Seiz, E. G., & Martinez-Serrano, A. (2015). Optimization of the magnetic labeling of human neural stem cells and MRI visualization in the hemiparkinsonian rat brain. *Journal of Nanobiotechnology*, *13*(1), 20. DOI: 10.1186/s12951-015-0078-4 PMID: 25890124

Rao, P. V., Nallappan, D., Madhavi, K., Rahman, S., Jun Wei, L., & Gan, S. H. (2016). Phytochemicals and biogenic metallic nanoparticles as anticancer agents. *Oxidative Medicine and Cellular Longevity*, *2016*(1), 3685671. DOI: 10.1155/2016/3685671 PMID: 27057273

Raut, S. L., Kirthivasan, B., Bommana, M. M., Squillante, E., & Sadoqi, M. (2010). The formulation, characterization and in vivo evaluation of a magnetic carrier for brain delivery of NIR dye. *Nanotechnology*, *21*(39), 395102. DOI: 10.1088/0957-4484/21/39/395102 PMID: 20820096

Reddy, U. A., Prabhakar, P. V., & Mahboob, M. (2017). Biomarkers of oxidative stress for *in vivo* assessment of toxicological effects of iron oxide nanoparticles. *Saudi Journal of Biological Sciences*, *24*(6), 1172–1180. DOI: 10.1016/j.sjbs.2015.09.029 PMID: 28855809

Rojas, J. I., Patrucco, L., Miguez, J., Besada, C., & Cristiano, E. (2015). Brain atrophy in radiologically isolated syndromes. *Journal of Neuroimaging*, *25*(1), 68–71. DOI: 10.1111/jon.12182 PMID: 25307993

Saikia, C., Hussain, A., Ramteke, A., Sharma, H. K., & Maji, T. K. (2015). Carboxymethyl starch-chitosan-coated iron oxide magnetic nanoparticles for controlled delivery of isoniazid. *Journal of Microencapsulation*, *32*(1), 29–39. DOI: 10.3109/02652048.2014.940015 PMID: 25090597

Sallem, F., Haji, R., Vervandier-Fasseur, D., Nury, T., Maurizi, L., Boudon, J., Lizard, G., & Millot, N. (2019). Elaboration of Trans-Resveratrol Derivative-Loaded Superparamagnetic Iron Oxide Nanoparticles for Glioma Treatment. *Nanomaterials (Basel, Switzerland)*, *9*(2), 287. DOI: 10.3390/nano9020287 PMID: 30781702

Sanchez-Mut, J. V., Heyn, H., Vidal, E., Moran, S., Sayols, S., Delgado-Morales, R., Schultz, M. D., Ansoleaga, B., Garcia-Esparcia, P., Pons-Espinal, M., de Lagran, M. M., Dopazo, J., Rabano, A., Avila, J., Dierssen, M., Lott, I., Ferrer, I., Ecker, J. R., & Esteller, M. (2016). Human DNA methylomes of neurodegenerative diseases show common epigenomic patterns. *Translational Psychiatry*, *6*(1), e718. DOI: 10.1038/tp.2015.214 PMID: 26784972

Sancini, G., Dal Magro, R., Ornaghi, F., Balducci, C., Forloni, G., Gobbi, M., Salmona, M., & Re, F. (2016). Pulmonary administration of functionalized nanoparticles significantly reduces beta-amyloid in the brain of an Alzheimer's disease murine model. *Nano Research*, *9*(7), 2190–2201. DOI: 10.1007/s12274-016-1108-8

Saraiva, C., Praça, C., Ferreira, R., Santos, T., Ferreira, L., & Bernardino, L. (2016). Nanoparticle-mediated brain drug delivery: Overcoming blood–brain barrier to treat neurodegenerative diseases. *Journal of Controlled Release*, *235*, 34–47. DOI: 10.1016/j.jconrel.2016.05.044 PMID: 27208862

Schlachetzki, F., Zhang, Y., Boado, R. J., & Pardridge, W. M. (2004). Gene therapy of the brain Te trans-vascular approach. *Neurology*, *62*(8), 1275–1281. DOI: 10.1212/01.WNL.0000120551.38463.D9 PMID: 15111662

Semkina, A., Abakumov, M., Grinenko, N., Abakumov, A., Skorikov, A., Mironova, E., Davydova, G., Majouga, A. G., Nukolova, N., Kabanov, A., & Chekhonin, V. (2015). Core–shell–corona doxorubicin-loaded superparamagnetic Fe3O4 nanoparticles for cancer theranostics. *Colloids and Surfaces. B, Biointerfaces*, *136*, 1073–1080. DOI: 10.1016/j.colsurfb.2015.11.009 PMID: 26595387

Shen, C. C., Wang, C. C., Liao, M. H., & Jan, T. R. (2011). A single exposure to iron oxide nanoparticles attenuates antigen-specific antibody production and T-cell reactivity in ovalbumin-sensitized BALB/c mice. *International Journal of Nanomedicine*, *6*, 1229. PMID: 21753874

Sibov, T. T., Pavon, L. F., Miyaki, L. A., Mamani, J. B., Nucci, L. P., Alvarim, L. T., & Gamarra, L. (2014). Umbilical cord mesenchymal stem cells labeled with multimodal iron oxide nanoparticles with fluorescent and magnetic properties: Application for *in vivo* cell tracking. *International Journal of Nanomedicine*, *9*, 337. PMID: 24531365

Siddiqui, M. A., Alhadlaq, H. A., Ahmad, J., Al-Khedhairy, A. A., Musarrat, J., & Ahamed, M. (2013). Copper oxide nanoparticles induced mitochondria mediated apoptosis in human hepatocarcinoma cells. *PLoS One*, *8*(8), e69534. DOI: 10.1371/journal.pone.0069534 PMID: 23940521

Sillerud, L. O., Solberg, N. O., Chamberlain, R., Orlando, R. A., Heidrich, J. E., Brown, D. C., Brady, C. I., Vander Jagt, T. A., Garwood, M., & Vander Jagt, D. L. (2013). SPION-enhanced magnetic resonance imaging of Alzheimer's disease plaques in AbetaPP/PS-1 transgenic mouse brain. *Journal of Alzheimer's Disease*, *34*(2), 349–365. DOI: 10.3233/JAD-121171 PMID: 23229079

Silva, L. H., Cruz, F. F., Morales, M. M., Weiss, D. J., & Rocco, P. R. M. (2017). Magnetic targeting as a strategy to enhance therapeutic effects of mesenchymal stromal cells. *Stem Cell Research & Therapy*, *8*(1), 58. DOI: 10.1186/s13287-017-0523-4 PMID: 28279201

Skaat, H., Corem-Slakmon, E., Grinberg, I., Last, D., Goez, D., & Mardor, Y.. (2013). Antibody-conjugated, dual-modal, near-infrared fluorescent iron oxide nanoparticles for antiamyloidgenic activity and specific detection of amyloid-beta fibrils. *International Journal of Nanomedicine*, *8*, 4063–4076. DOI: 10.2147/IJN.S52833 PMID: 24194640

Soenen, S. J., De Cuyper, M., De Smedt, S. C., & Braeckmans, K. (2012) Investigating the toxic effects of iron oxide nanoparticles. In Methods in enzymology. Academic Press 509: 195–224 DOI: 10.1016/B978-0-12-391858-1.00011-3

Sorto-Gomez, TE, Ortiz, GG, & Pacheco-Moises, FP, Torres- Sanchez ED, Ramirez-Ramirez V, Macias-Islas MA, De La Rosa AC, Velázquez-Brizuela IE. (2016). Effect of fish oil on glutathione redox system in multiple sclerosis. *American Journal of Neurodegenerative Disease*, *5*(2), 145–151. PMID: 27335704

Spuch, C., Saida, O., & Navarro, C. (2012). Advances in the treatment of neurodegenerative disorders employing nanoparticles. *Recent Patents on Drug Delivery & Formulation*, *6*(1), 2–18. DOI: 10.2174/187221112799219125 PMID: 22272933

Stampfli, P., Sommer, S., & Czell, D.. (2018). Investigation of neurodegenerative processes in amyotrophic lateral sclerosis using white matter fiber density. *Clinical Neuroradiology*, *2*, 1–11. PMID: 29460142

Stephanopoulos, N., Freeman, R., North, H. A., Sur, S., Jeong, S. J., Tantakitti, F., & Stupp, S. I. (2014). Bioactive DNA-peptide nanotubes enhance the differentiation of neural stem cells into neurons. *Nano Letters*, *15*(1), 603–609. DOI: 10.1021/nl504079q PMID: 25546084

Summerlin, N., Soo, E., Thakur, S., Qu, Z., Jambhrunkar, S., & Popat, A. (2015). Resveratrol nanoformulations: Challenges and opportunities. *International Journal of Pharmaceutics*, *479*(2), 282–290. DOI: 10.1016/j.ijpharm.2015.01.003 PMID: 25572692

Tabatabaei, S. N., Girouard, H., Carret, A. S., & Martel, S. (2015). Remote control of the permeability of the blood–brain barrier by magnetic heating of nanoparticles: A proof of concept for brain drug delivery. *Journal of Controlled Release*, *206*, 49–57. DOI: 10.1016/j.jconrel.2015.02.027 PMID: 25724273

Tang, J. L., Xiong, L., Wang, S., Wang, J., Liu, L., Li, J., Yuan, F., & Xi, T. (2009). Distribution, translocation and accumulation of silver nanoparticles in rats. *Journal of Nanoscience and Nanotechnology*, *9*(8), 4924–4932. DOI: 10.1166/jnn.2009.1269 PMID: 19928170

Tehrani, M. D., Yoon, J. H., Kim, M. O., & Yoon, J. (2014). [a]) A novel scheme for nanoparticle steering in blood vessels using a functionalized magnetic field. *IEEE Transactions on Biomedical Engineering*, *62*(1), 303–313. DOI: 10.1109/TBME.2014.2351234 PMID: 25163053

Tehrani, M. D., Yoon, J. H., Kim, M. O., & Yoon, J. (2014). [b]) A novel electromagnetic actuation system for magnetic nanoparticle guidance in blood vessels. *IEEE Transactions on Magnetics*, *50*(7), 1–12. DOI: 10.1109/TMAG.2014.2307271

Teleanu, D. M., Negut, I., Grumezescu, V., Grumezescu, A. M., & Teleanu, R. I. (2019). Nanomaterials for drug delivery to the central nervous system. *Nanomaterials (Basel, Switzerland)*, *9*(3), E371. DOI: 10.3390/nano9030371 PMID: 30841578

Thanh, N. T. (2012). *Magnetic nanoparticles: from fabrication to clinical applications*. CRC press. DOI: 10.1201/b11760

Thomas, G., Demoisson, F., Chassagnon, R., Popova, E., & Millot, N. (2016). One-step continuous synthesis of functionalized magnetite nanoflowers. *Nanotechnology*, *27*(13), 135604. DOI: 10.1088/0957-4484/27/13/135604 PMID: 26900748

Tiwari, S. K., Agarwal, S., Seth, B., Yadav, A., Nair, S., Bhatnagar, P., & Patel, D. K. (2013). Curcumin-loaded nanoparticles potently induce adult neurogenesis and reverse cognitive deficits in Alzheimer's disease model *via* canonical Wnt/β-catenin pathway. *ACS Nano*, *8*(1), 76–103. DOI: 10.1021/nn405077y PMID: 24467380

Valdiglesias, V., Fernández-Bertólez, N., Kiliç, G., Costa, C., Costa, S., Fraga, S., Bessa, M. J., Pásaro, E., Teixeira, J. P., & Laffon, B. (2016). Are iron oxide nanoparticles safe? Current knowledge and future perspectives. *Journal of Trace Elements in Medicine and Biology*, *38*, 53–63. DOI: 10.1016/j.jtemb.2016.03.017 PMID: 27056797

Vashist, A., Manickam, P., Raymond, A. D., Arias, A. Y., Kolishetti, N., Vashist, A., Arias, E., & Nair, M. (2023). Recent advances in nanotherapeutics for neurological disorders. *ACS Applied Bio Materials*, *6*(7), 2614–2621. DOI: 10.1021/acsabm.3c00254 PMID: 37368486

Veiseh, O., Sun, C., Fang, C., Bhattarai, N., Gunn, J., Kievit, F., Du, K., Pullar, B., Lee, D., Ellenbogen, R. G., Olson, J., & Zhang, M. (2009). Specific targeting of brain tumors with an optical/magnetic resonance imaging nanoprobe across the blood-brain barrier. *Cancer Research*, *69*(15), 6200–6207. DOI: 10.1158/0008-5472.CAN-09-1157 PMID: 19638572

Vellinga, M. M., Oude Engberink, R. D., Seewann, A., Pouwels, P. J., Wattjes, M. P., van der Pol, S. M. A., Pering, C., Polman, C. H., de Vries, H. E., Geurts, J. J. G., & Barkhof, F. (2008). Pluriformity of inflammation in multiple sclerosis shown by ultra-small iron oxide particle enhancement. *Brain*, *131*(3), 800–807. DOI: 10.1093/brain/awn009 PMID: 18245785

Vikram, S., Dhakshnamoorthy, M., Vasanthakumari, R., Rajamani, A. R., Rangarajan, M., & Tsuzuki, T. (2015). Tuning the magnetic properties of iron oxide nanoparticles by a room-temperature air-atmosphere (RTAA) co-precipitation method. *Journal of Nanoscience and Nanotechnology*, *15*(5), 3870–3878. DOI: 10.1166/jnn.2015.9544 PMID: 26505017

Volkman, R., & Ofen, D. (2017). Concise Review: Mesenchymal Stem Cells in Neurodegenerative Diseases. Stem Cells von Bohlen and Halbach O (2007) Immunohistological markers for staging neurogenesis in adult hippocampus. *Cell and Tissue Research*, *329*(3), 409–420.

Wang, N., Jin, X., Guo, D., Tong, G., & Zhu, X. (2017). Iron chelation nanoparticles with delayed saturation as an effective therapy for Parkinson disease. *Biomacromolecules*, *18*(2), 461–474. DOI: 10.1021/acs.biomac.6b01547 PMID: 27989126

Wong, H. L., Wu, X. Y., & Bendayan, R. (2012). Nanotechnological advances for the delivery of CNS therapeutics. *Advanced Drug Delivery Reviews*, *64*(7), 686–700. DOI: 10.1016/j.addr.2011.10.007 PMID: 22100125

Wu, W., Wu, Z., Yu, T., Jiang, C., & Kim, W. S. (2015). Recent progress on magnetic iron oxide nanoparticles: Synthesis, surface functional strategies and biomedical applications. *Science and Technology of Advanced Materials*, *16*(2), 023501. DOI: 10.1088/1468-6996/16/2/023501 PMID: 27877761

Xia, T., Li, N., & Nel, A. E. (2009). Potential health impact of nanoparticles. *Annual Review of Public Health*, *30*(1), 137–150. DOI: 10.1146/annurev.publhealth.031308.100155 PMID: 19705557

Xiao, J., Cao, Y., & Huang, Q. (2017). Edible Nanoencapsulation Vehicles for Oral Delivery of Phytochemicals: A Perspective Paper. *Journal of Agricultural and Food Chemistry*, *65*(32), 6727–6735. DOI: 10.1021/acs.jafc.7b02128 PMID: 28737908

Yang, C. C., Yang, S. Y., Chieh, J. J., Horng, H. E., Hong, C. Y., Yang, H. C., Chen, K. H., Shih, B. Y., Chen, T.-F., & Chiu, M.-J. (2011). Biofunctionalized magnetic nanoparticles for specifically detecting biomarkers of Alzheimer's disease *in* vitro. *ACS Chemical Neuroscience*, *2*(9), 500–505. DOI: 10.1021/cn200028j PMID: 22860173

Yarjanli, Z., Ghaedi, K., Esmaeili, A., Rahgozar, S., & Zarrabi, A. (2017). Iron oxide nanoparticles may damage to the neural tissue through iron accumulation, oxidative stress and protein aggregation. *BMC Neuroscience*, *18*(1), 51. DOI: 10.1186/s12868-017-0369-9 PMID: 28651647

Yarjanli, Z., Ghaedi, K., Esmaeili, A., Rahgozar, S., & Zarrabi, A. (2017). Iron oxide nanoparticles may damage to the neural tissue through iron accumulation, oxidative stress, and protein aggregation. *BMC Neuroscience*, *18*(1), 51. DOI: 10.1186/s12868-017-0369-9 PMID: 28651647

Yew, Y. P., (2018). Green biosynthesis of superparamagnetic magnetite Fe3O4 nanoparticles and biomedical applications in targeted anticancer drug delivery system: A review. *Arabian Journal of Chemistry*. Advance online publication. DOI: 10.1016/j.arabjc.2018.04.013

Zhu, A., Chan-Park, M. B., Dai, S., & Li, L. (2005). The aggregation behavior of O-carboxymethylchitosan in dilute aqueous solution. *Colloids and Surfaces. B, Biointerfaces*, *43*(3-4), 143–149. DOI: 10.1016/j.colsurfb.2005.04.009 PMID: 15941653

Zhu, C. L., Liu, L. B., Yang, Q., Lv, F. T., & Wang, S. (2012). Watersoluble conjugated polymers for imaging, diagnosis, and therapy. *Chemical Reviews*, *112*(8), 4687–4735. DOI: 10.1021/cr200263w PMID: 22670807

Zhu W, Li X, Tang Z, Zhu S, Qi J, Wei L, Lei H (2007) Superparamagnetic iron oxide labeling of neural stem cells and 4.7 T MRI tracking in vivo and in vitro. J HUAZHONG U SCI-MED, 27(1), 107-110.

Chapter 5
Activation of Enzymes by Radiation:
A Frontier for the Discovery of Neuroprotective Drugs

Saloua Mabsor-Zgandaoui
https://orcid.org/0009-0006-4601-9059
Department of Biology, Ibn Tofail University, Kenitra, Morocco

Hassane Boulmane
Sidi Mohamed Ben Abdellah University, Morocco

Khawla Rachmoune
https://orcid.org/0009-0001-6483-1060
Cadi Ayyad University, Marrakech, Morocco

Youness Zgandaoui
Department of Biology, Ibn Tofail University, Kenitra, Morocco

ABSTRACT

While radiation is often viewed solely as a damaging agent, emerging research suggests that certain doses and types of radiation may activate endogenous protective enzymes involved in cellular repair, redox balance, and inflammation modulation. This chapter explores the under-investigated concept of radiation-induced enzymatic activation in the central nervous system, positioning it as a potential gateway for neuroprotective drug development. We examine the paradoxical role of low-dose ionizing radiation and how it stimulates beneficial responses such as Nrf2 pathway activation, increased antioxidant enzyme expression, and DNA repair enzyme upregulation. The chapter discusses the concept of radiation hormesis and how pre-conditioning the brain with controlled exposures may prime neuroprotective pathways.

DOI: 10.4018/979-8-3373-4627-4.ch005

INTRODUCTION

Ionising radiation has long been considered purely noxious, with biological effects directly proportional to the dose received. Based on the linear no-threshold (LNT) model, this traditional view assumes that even the lowest doses of radiation carry an inherent risk, with cumulative exposure increasing the risk of DNA damage, mutations and carcinogenesis. However, new scientific evidence is challenging this paradigm, highlighting a complex and dose-dependent relationship between radiation and biological systems. In particular, studies on low-dose ionising radiation (LDIR), generally defined as exposures below 0.5 gray (Gy), have revealed a surprising range of adaptive cellular responses that may have beneficial effects, particularly in non-cancerous tissues such as the nervous system (Wojcik & Zölzer, 2024).

This adaptive phenomenon, often referred to as radiation hormesis, suggests that low levels of stress caused by sublethal doses of IR can stimulate protective pathways that improve cellular resilience and survival (Mabsor-Zgandaoui et al., 2025). Rather than inducing apoptosis or cytotoxicity, low doses appear to prepare cells through moderate oxidative signalling, prompting them to upregulate antioxidant enzymes, strengthen DNA repair mechanisms, modulate inflammatory responses and improve metabolic flexibility. These responses are neither random nor fortuitous, but are part of a conserved biological programme designed to restore homeostasis and defend against future insults in a preventive manner. In recent years, this radiation-induced adaptation has been increasingly studied in the context of neurobiology, where the balance between oxidative damage and endogenous defense mechanisms plays a key role in the progression of age-related neurodegenerative diseases, (Liu et al., 2025).

The central nervous system (CNS) is particularly vulnerable to oxidative stress due to its high oxygen consumption, high lipid content and limited capacity for regeneration. These pathophysiological characteristics are often accompanied by an accumulation of reactive oxygen species (ROS), oxidized proteins and lipids, as well as pro-inflammatory mediators, all of which contribute to the progressive loss of neuronal structure and function. As such, strategies aimed at strengthening endogenous antioxidant defenses and correcting redox imbalances have attracted considerable interest in the search for effective neuroprotective therapies, (Dash et al., 2025).

LDIR has emerged as a new approach to neuroprotection, capable of triggering the activation of a specific set of adaptive enzymes and signalling pathways that protect against oxidative damage. At the heart of this response is the Nrf2-Keap1 axis, a key regulator of redox homeostasis. When activated by moderate oxidative signals, Nrf2 translocates to the nucleus and initiates the transcription of a wide range of cytoprotective genes, (Ngo & Duennwald, 2022).

Beyond activating antioxidant pathways, LDIR also influences immune and inflammatory responses, with evidence showing downregulation of NF-κB signalling and decreased expression of pro-inflammatory cytokines such as TNF-α and IL-1β. Furthermore, LDIR enhances the recruitment and activity of DNA repair enzymes such as PARP1, OGG1, and APE1, thereby contributing to the genomic stability of neurons exposed to oxidative stress. In in vitro and in vivo models, these coordinated effects translate into measurable improvements in cell viability, synaptic plasticity, and cognitive function, particularly when LDIR is used as a preconditioning stimulus prior to more damaging events, (Ngo & Duennwald, 2022).

It is important to note that these results have sparked interest in the translational potential of radiation-induced enzyme activation, not only as a research tool but also as a potential therapeutic adjuvant in the management of neurodegenerative diseases. A number of preclinical studies have

demonstrated that combining LDIR with pharmacological activators of Nrf2, such as resveratrol, curcumin or sulforaphane, can produce synergistic neuroprotective effects. Furthermore, early clinical data suggest that very low doses of radiation targeting the brain are well tolerated and may even improve cognitive function in patients with mild to moderate Alzheimer's disease, although these interventions remain experimental and need to be validated by rigorous trials, (Ngo & Duennwald, 2022).

This chapter aims to give a full overview of the adaptive enzymatic responses triggered by low-dose IR, with a special focus on their neuroprotective implications. It'll explore the molecular and cellular mechanisms involved, including the activation of redox-sensitive transcription factors and the modulation of immune and DNA repair pathways. Experimental data from in vitro models, animal studies, and early clinical trials in humans will be reviewed, highlighting both the potential and limitations of this approach. Finally, the chapter will discuss future directions for translational research, including the development of pharmacological mimetics, the optimization of dose fractionation protocols, and integration with precision medicine strategies.

LDIR: SHIFTING AGGRESSION TOWARD BENEFICIAL ADAPTATION

The conventional view that all irradiation is deleterious is now being reassessed (Jankovic et al., 2021). Numerous studies have shown that, at sublethal doses (typically below 0.5 Gy), radiation can trigger endogenous defense mechanisms (Hussien, 2023). Exposure to low doses (~0.1–0.3 Gy), for example, leads to a slight elevation in the generation of ROS, acting as an adaptive signal (Rozhko et al., 2019; Mabsor-Zgandaoui et al., 2025). Indeed, this "radiation hormesis" phenomenon implies that, at low doses, radiation stimulates cell survival responses rather than death mechanisms (Bondy, 2023). A narrow therapeutic window is nevertheless observed: the "priming" threshold (~0.05-0.5 Gy) is critical; beyond this, the effect changes from protective to cytotoxic, underlining the need for very precise dose adjustment for safe clinical use (Le Reun & Foray, 2023a; Mabsor-Zgandaoui et al., 2025b).

Activation of a Survival Program Under Low Doses of Radiation

To illustrate this paradigm shift, several in vitro studies have exposed cells to low-dose radiation (< 0.5 Gy), revealing that, under such conditions, cells preferentially activate defense pathways rather than death programs. By way of illustration, Pre-irradiation at 0.1 Gy induces a transient ~20 % increase in ROS within two hours, sufficient to activate pro-survival kinases (e.g. ERK1/2) and stimulate glutathione synthesis (Sun et al., 2022a). As a result, the cell mobilizes several complementary responses:

- Antioxidant defense is enhanced, as glutathione (GSH) production increases and glutathione-S-transferase (GST) activity is stimulated (Hernández Estévez & Rodríguez Hernández, 2020).
- The DNA repair process is strengthened, leading to a rapid accumulation of repair enzymes, such as PARP1, OGG1 and 53BP1, to correct DNA breaks, whether single- or double-stranded (Kong et al., 2020a).

- Modulation of inflammation down-regulates the NF-κB pathway, thereby lowering the synthesis of pro-inflammatory cytokines such as TNF-α and IL-1β. For example, immune cells exposed to 0.5-0.7 Gy secrete significantly less IL-1β. This is due to reduced translocation of the RelA subunit (NF-κB) to the nucleus (Lödermann et al., 2012).

These coordinated adjustments lead to improved tolerance to secondary stress. In so-called "priming" protocols, an increase in cell viability is generally observed after a second shock. For example, pretreatment with 0.5 Gy can increase neuronal resistance to a subsequent higher dose (Betlazar et al., 2016). In vivo studies confirm these trends. Low-dose pre-irradiated animals subsequently show greater neuronal and glial survival in the face of oxidative stress. In this sense, LDIR priming is a vector of optimism for strengthening neuronal resilience in the face of possible future aggression.

Figure 1. Modelling intracellular enzyme activation mechanisms under the effect of low doses of ionizing radiation

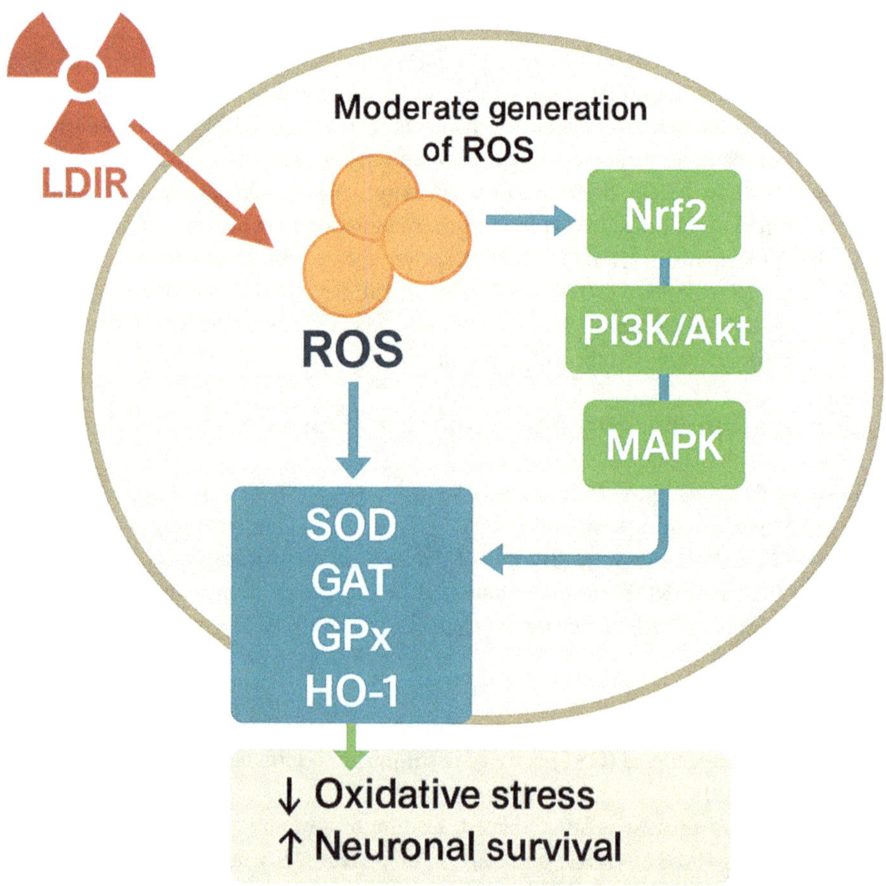

Figure 1 shows the major cellular mechanisms involved after exposure to low doses of ionising radiation (LDIR). It sheds light on how LIR exposure affects cells, showing a moderate increase in reactive oxygen species (ROS), the involvement of key signalling pathways (Nrf2, PI3K/Akt, MAPK), and the subsequent activation of antioxidant enzymes to promote neuroprotection.

The Nrf2-Keap1 Pathway, at the Heart of Redox Homeostasis

The transcription factor Nrf2 is critical for the antioxidant defense and is a key player in the antioxidant process. At rest, the Nrf2–Keap1 complex in the cytosol binds, promoting the proteasomal degradation of Nrf2. Upon prolonged moderate oxidative stress ($\leq$ 0.5 Gy of irradiation), modifications of the cysteines of Keap1 liberate Nrf2 from its anchorage (Ulasov et al., 2022). The latter then migrates into the nucleus and binds to the Antioxidant Response Elements (ARE) of the genome, activating a dozen cytoprotective genes (Raghunath et al., 2018). Induced enzymes include:

- Heme oxygenase-1 (HO-1): heme is catabolized into biliverdin, iron and CO, with an anti-inflammatory effect (de Oliveira et al., 2022).
- Glutathione-S-transferases (GST): enzymes catalyze the conjugation of GSH to electrophiles, facilitating detoxification (Behrens et al., 2019).
- superoxide dismutase (SOD) and catalase: these two enzymes respectively neutralize superoxide anions and hydrogen peroxide, which are oxygenated free radicals. They form the body's first line of antioxidant defense (Jomova et al., 2024).
- DNA repair enzymes, such as OGG1, APE1, Rad4 and PARP, are capable of detecting and correcting oxidative damage to DNA strands. This helps limit mutations (Kong et al., 2020b).

ROS levels are rapidly restored to normal by the coordinated induction of these genes (typically within a few hours), and long-term cell survival potential is restored. In summary, the central role played by the Nrf2-Keap1 pathway in the restoration of redox homeostasis after LDIR has been demonstrated, and the protection of neurons against the accumulation of oxidative stress has been demonstrated.

The low-dose radiation adaptive response depends on the transient induction of a limited number of critical enzymes. Table 1 summarizes the principal enzymes, their subcellular distribution, their specific antioxidant functions, and the effects that are observed following moderate exposure to LDIR.

Table 1. Major antioxidant enzymes activated by low-dose radiation in neuronal cells

Enzyme	Intracellular Location	Function	Change upon LDIR
SOD	Cytoplasm	ROS detoxification	Increased activity
Catalase	Mitochondria	ROS detoxification	Increased activity
GPx	Nucleus	ROS detoxification	Increased activity
HO-1	Cytoplasm	ROS detoxification	Increased expression
NOS	Cytoplasm	Nitric oxide regulation	Increased activity

Transient Enzyme Induction and Neuroprotection

The most notable consequence of this adaptive response is the overexpression of cytoprotective enzymes. A few hours after a single low-dose exposure, the following are generally observed:

- HO-1: a 2- to 3-fold increase in its protein expression can be observed (de Oliveira et al., 2022).
- GSH and other GSH conjugates strongly increase enzymatic activity, enhancing toxic elimination (Behrens et al., 2019).
- SOD, catalase, GPx: these antioxidant substances increase their detoxification capacity by around 50-60% (Jomova et al., 2024).
- DNA repairers (OGG1, APE1, Rad4 and PARP) were recruited. Convergence on lesions was observed to be twice as fast as in non-primed cells (Kong et al., 2020b).

These changes do not last forever (between 48 hours and a few days), and create a protective effect during which neurons and brain cells are more resistant to future stress (Lau et al., 2021; McDonald et al., 2010). In vivo, this effect translates into improved functional parameters, as demonstrated by experiments carried out on pre-conditioned mice: better synaptic plasticity and preservation of spatial memory in cognitive tests were observed. In other words, post-LDIR enzyme enhancement translates into tangible neuronal protection.

ADAPTIVE ENZYMES AND NEUROPROTECTION IN NEURODEGENERATIVE CONTEXTS

Neurodegenerative disorders, including Alzheimer's, Parkinson's, and amyotrophic lateral sclerosis, typically present with chronic oxidative stress and ongoing neuroinflammation. Diseased neurons are overloaded with free radicals and accumulated DNA and lipid damage (Teleanu et al., 2022). Biomarkers such as 8-oxo-2'-deoxyguanosine, which shows damage to mitochondrial or nuclear DNA, and malondialdehyde, which comes from lipid peroxidation. These biomarkers are much higher in the plasma or cerebrospinal fluid of affected patients (Buccellato et al., 2021). This signature of oxidative stress is behind the hypothesis that neurodegeneration may be slowed by stimulation of Nrf2 and associated enzymes. Indeed, when the Nrf2-Keap1

complex is activated, it reduces oxidative damage and inflammation in neurons. In practice, activating this adaptive process would mean reducing retrogenic oxidative damage (8 oxo-dG, MDA...) and accelerating DNA repair, which could slow the progression of clinical symptoms (Chakkittukandiyil et al., 2022).

Oxidative Stress and Inflammation: Clinical Targets

In the context of Alzheimer's disease, both the cerebral cortex and the hippocampus show an accumulation of oxidative lesions. For example, levels of 8 oxo-dG in circulating DNA are significantly higher in Alzheimer's patients than in healthy subjects (Peña-Bautista et al., 2019). Similarly, in Parkinson's patients, MDA concentration is increased (up to +30-+40% compared with controls), indicating persistent peroxidation of neuronal membranes (Tamtaji et al., 2019). These biomarkers offer quantifiable targets: their normalization, thanks to activation of the Nrf2 pathway, correlates with a reduction in neuronal damage. Indeed, in analogy with other pathological models, Nrf2 enhancement would induce a decrease in inflammatory cytokines (TNF-α, IL-1β) and oxidation products, thus helping to preserve cellular integrity (Sadrkhanloo et al., 2022).

Experimental Evidence of Neuroprotection by LDIR

Numerous experimental studies illustrate the protective effect of low doses. For example, using an Alzheimer's disease mouse model (5xFAD), repeated moderate irradiation reduced synaptic loss and improved spatial memory compared to untreated animals (Kim et al., 2020). Other experiments showed that the number of activated microglia (marker Iba1+) decreased significantly after exposure to the LDIR head (0,063Gy) (Hladik et al., 2019). Preconditioning neuronal cultures with TNF-α has been shown to confer neuroprotection in vitro by reducing apoptosis and dampening TNF-α-mediated inflammatory signaling when exposed to oxidative stress (Saha et al., 2009). In parallel, low-dose radiation or redox-based preconditioning has been associated with prolonged HO-1 induction and increased GST activity, confirming that antioxidant and reparative enzyme responses also contribute to cellular resilience (Holcombe & Weavers, 2022).

Studies on rodent models point to similar conclusions: for example, mice showed no measurable cognitive deficits and performed normally on behavioural testing of spatial recognition up to 12 months post-irradiation if exposed to ^28Si ion radiation at 0.2 Gy (Minnier et al., 2021). In addition, we did not observe any signs of chronic inflammation or long-term toxicity. These data are of particular promise for translational research because they suggest that low-dose radiotherapy may offer important reductions in neurodegenerative disease markers and symptom burden, which could lead to new interventions in the prioritization of cancer care as prevention or palliation.

A number of intracellular signalling cascades are triggered by ROS production induced by LDIR. Figure 2 demonstrates that these molecular cascades, including Nrf2/ARE, PI3K/Akt/mTOR, and ERK/MAPK, can be activated, leading to enzymatic induction that promotes neuronal cell protection (Sun et al., 2022b; Zhang et al., 2024).

Figure 2. Intracellular signalling pathways involved in neuroprotection after exposure to low doses of radiation

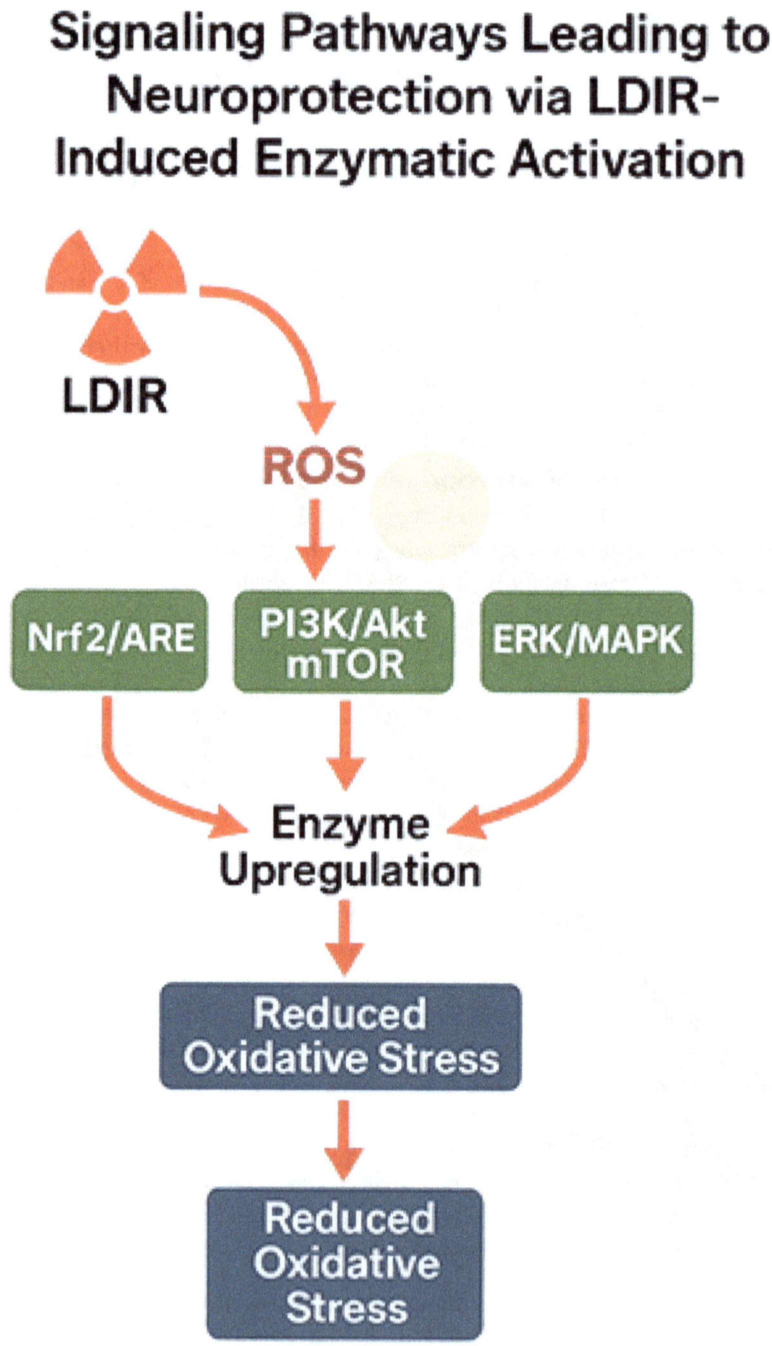

Therapeutic Perspectives: Combinations and Challenges

These experimental results suggest the combination of LDIR with pharmacological therapies. Natural or synthetic compounds capable of activating the Nrf2 transcription factor could potentially enhance the adaptive effect of radiation. For example, preclinical work suggests that a Nrf2 agonist co-administered with 0.3 Gy increases HO-1 expression and neuronal resistance more than 0.3 Gy alone (Kim A et al., 2023). Similarly, small clinical trials have reported improved cognitive scores (MMSE) in AD patients after a single session of LDIR (~0.5 Gy), with no significant adverse effects (Chung & Chung, 2021). The idea is to generate an additive synergy between LDIR (initial stimulus) and pharmacological Nrf2 activators to maximize enrichment of protective enzymes.

However, several challenges remain, the main one being long-term safety. According to the LNT model, even very low doses present a proportional carcinogenic risk. However, the neuroprotective benefits of this model are limited to areas where the risk is not clearly documented. The aim is therefore to demonstrate that occasional exposure to levels of 0.1 to 0.5 Gy (i.e. a few tenths of a Sievert) does not significantly increase tumour risk over the long term (Wilson et al., 2024). We should also think about other practical limitations, namely defining the irradiation protocol (dose, fractionation, targeted volume) and choosing pharmacological treatments as well. The goal is to obtain the right timing of LDIR with medication, to maximize their synergies but not to significantly increase overall toxicity (Le Reun & Foray, 2023b). Therefore, it is necessary to carry out more pilot clinical studies and in vivo studies to explore and optimize these parameters and to demonstrate that such a neuroprotective approach is feasible (Kim, D. Y. et al., 2023).

The adaptive mechanisms observed after low-dose radiation promise new possibilities for drug development, especially for multifactorial diseases like neurodegenerative disorders. The following figure summarizes the connection between LDIR-induced enzyme activation, correction of redox balance and neuroprotection, and potential therapeutic applications. Benefits and hurdles to be overcome for future clinical transposition are also presented in Figure 3.

Figure 3. Pharmacological perspectives of LDIR-induced enzyme activation in neurodegenerative diseases

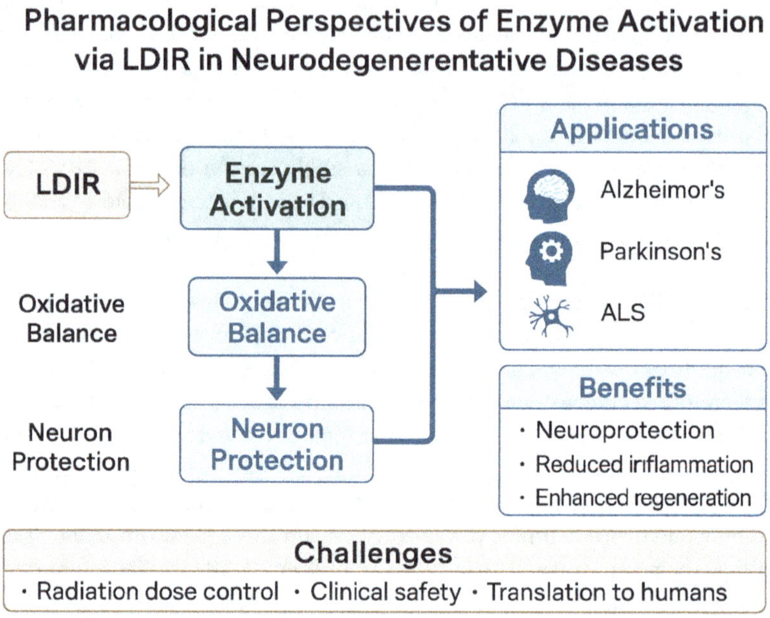

RADIATION HORMESIS AND NEURAL PRE-CONDITIONING

Concept and Evidence of Hormesis

Hormesis refers to a biphasic biological response to exposure to a stressor, such as IR, in which low doses trigger beneficial effects while high doses cause damage. This notion, inherited from Paracelsus' famous maxim that "the dose makes the poison", has been progressively integrated into the field of radiobiology, notably through the work of Calabrese and Feinendegen (Tsatsakis et al., 2018; Agathokleous et Calabrese., 2022). Radiation hormesis challenges the LNT model traditionally used to assess radiation risks. The LNT model assumes that no level of radiation is totally safe, even at very low doses, whereas the hormesis model argues that low doses may induce protective adaptive mechanisms, notably via the activation of DNA repair systems, antioxidant pathways and modulated immune responses (Laurier et al., 2023).

Studies in animals have shown that sub-toxic exposures to doses of 0.1 to 0.5 Gy can activate endogenous antioxidant pathways, such as increased catalase, glutathione peroxidase (GPx) and superoxide dismutase (SOD). For instance, in mice, exposure to 250 mGy significantly induces brain antioxidant enzymes and improves neuronal survival (Olufunmilayo et al., 2023). Genetic models, such as Drosophila melanogaster expressing an Alzheimer phenotype, have also con-

firmed improved cognitive function and reduced amyloid protein aggregation after exposure to low-dose radiation (Malta et al., 2024).

Further studies have shown that this type of exposure can also enhance the immune response by stimulating T lymphocytes, reducing pro-inflammatory cytokines such as TNF-α or IL-6, and promoting the production of neuronal growth factors such as BDNF (JIN et al., 2019). In addition, some studies have demonstrated moderate activation of the p53 pathway, enabling efficient repair of DNA damage without triggering the massive apoptosis observed at high doses (Honeywell et al., 2023; Wang et al., 2023). This adaptive response also appears to involve the regulation of heat shock proteins (HSPs), known for their role in protein folding and cell protection (Hu et al., 2023).

Moreover, it has been observed that chronic exposure to very low doses can induce a memory effect, or adaptive response, whereby cells previously exposed to a minimal dose react more effectively to a higher dose administered subsequently (Guéguen et al., 2019). This cellular memory is of particular interest in the context of radiation protection of the central nervous system, particularly in the event of radiotherapy or accidental exposure (Srivastava et al., 2023). However, although preclinical results are promising, the transposition of these observations to humans still requires rigorous investigations to assess their safety, reproducibility and biological limits.

Brain Pre-Conditioning with Sub-Toxic Irradiation

Cerebral pre-conditioning by sub-toxic irradiation is an innovative experimental strategy aimed at exposing neural tissue to low doses of radiation to trigger a protective adaptive response to subsequent more severe stresses, such as hypoxia, inflammation or major oxidative stresses. This approach is inspired by the hormesis principle, according to which a moderate dose of a stressor can induce beneficial cellular defense mechanisms (Holcombe et Weavers., 2022).

Activation of the Nrf2 pathway is one of the main molecular mechanisms involved in this response. This pathway regulates the transcription of numerous genes encoding antioxidant enzymes, including HO-1, NQO1 (NAD(P)H quinone dehydrogenase 1), GCLC (glutamate cysteine ligase catalytic subunit) and GCLM (glutamate cysteine ligase modifier subunit), which are involved in glutathione (GSH) synthesis (He et al., 2020). Nrf2 promotion leads to improvements in redox metabolism, reduced neuronal apoptosis and modulation of the inflammatory response, notably through inhibition of the NF-κB and MAPK pathways (Pant et al., 2024).

In addition, further studies have demonstrated stimulation of neurogenesis in the hippocampus following repeated exposure to low doses of radiation, accompanied by an improvement in cognitive function in rodents (McNerlin et al., 2022). Regulation of stress proteins such as HSP70 (heat shock protein 70) and Bcl-2 was also observed, suggesting a limitation of classical apoptotic cascades (Srinivasan et al., 2018). Pre-conditioning might thus represent a complementary approach to preventing or slowing down certain chronic neurological pathologies, provided that exposure protocols are rigorously defined and controlled (Dash et al., 2024).

However, despite the encouraging results obtained in vivo, the clinical applicability of this approach remains limited by the lack of human clinical trials and by ethical and regulatory concerns linked to voluntary exposure to radiation, even at low doses. A detailed understanding of the underlying molecular mechanisms, as well as the identification of tolerance thresholds, therefore, remains a crucial step for the eventual transposition of radiative pre-conditioning to the therapeutic field (Zhou et al., 2021).

Ethical and Practical Considerations

Although experimental results have been encouraging, the clinical application of low-level radiation brain preconditioning raises major ethical and practical concerns. The brain, which is particularly sensitive to IR, may suffer functional alterations, mutations or an increased risk of long-term pathologies, even at low doses. Any therapeutic use outside oncology therefore requires extremely rigorous safety protocols. The lack of scientific consensus on a safety threshold, combined with high inter-individual variability - influenced by genetic, epigenetic or environmental factors - complicates the establishment of standardized clinical recommendations. Furthermore, radiation protection bodies such as the ICRP and NCRP do not yet officially recognize the principle of hormesis, due to a lack of robust clinical evidence (Kovalchuk et Kolb., 2017; Lau et al., 2022).

A further critical point lies in the benefit/risk dilemma: while animal data are promising, the beneficial potential in humans remains hypothetical in the absence of well-controlled clinical trials. Using this approach in vulnerable populations (neurological patients, children) also raises major ethical issues: informed consent, application of the precautionary principle, and medical liability (Gangwal et Lavecchia., 2025).

At the same time, logistical obstacles remain high cost of irradiation equipment, need for specialized personnel and precise control of administered doses. In the face of these challenges, research must focus on identifying biomarkers of individual sensitivity, optimizing minimum effective doses, and comparing them with alternative non-radiation strategies, such as pharmacological activation of the Nrf2 pathway (Swartz et al., 2020). In short, although brain preconditioning with low-level radiation offers innovative therapeutic prospects, its clinical application can only be envisaged in the light of solid scientific evidence and in strict compliance with fundamental ethical principles.

TRANSLATIONAL POTENTIAL AND PHARMACOLOGICAL EXPLOITATION

Mimicking Radiation-Induced Enzymatic Activity

Pharmacological mimetics of the induced enzymatic response are one of the most promising avenues of research for exploiting the beneficial effects of radiation preconditioning. A strategic class of therapeutic agents are compounds capable of activating the Nrf2 pathway. Among them, several natural compounds such as curcumin, quercetin, sulforaphane and resveratrol have demonstrated their ability to induce Nrf2 translocation in the nucleus and activate the expression of antioxidant and cytoprotective genes (Ginés et al., 2017).

Research has shown that pharmacological activation of Nrf2 results in neuronal protection like that induced by low-dose radiation, including up-regulation of HO-1, restoration of intracellular glutathione and reduction of mitochondrial oxidative stress. Additional agents such as direct HO-1 inducers (like cobalt protoporphyrin) or glutathione modulators (N-acetylcysteine, alpha-lipoic acid) are also being studied in the context of neuroprotection (Wang et al., 2021).

Synergistic Approaches

Another emerging area of translational research is the synergistic approach combining controlled low-dose irradiation with concomitant or sequential administration of pharmacological compounds activating the same cellular protection pathways. This strategy aims to maximize neuroprotection by reinforcing the endogenous adaptive mechanisms triggered by hormesis. For example, a recent study showed that the combination of resveratrol - a natural polyphenol known for its antioxidant properties - with 0.3 Gy of sub-toxic irradiation in a mouse model of cerebral ischemia significantly improved neuronal survival, reduced inflammation and promoted motor recovery (Wang et al., 2021).

Such combination therapies could also prove relevant in the early treatment of neurodegenerative diseases such as Alzheimer's or Parkinson's, by simultaneously targeting several pathogenic mechanisms such as oxidative stress, chronic inflammation and the accumulation of toxic proteins. Identifying optimal therapeutic windows, as well as adapting doses and timing of administration according to each patient's genetic and biochemical profile, would make it possible to design personalized treatments that are more effective and better tolerated. Such approaches could eventually form part of precision medicine protocols combining physical and molecular interventions (Gao et al., 2024).

Future Research and Clinical Outlook

Although experimental advances have been made, several hurdles remain before radiation preconditioning and its pharmacological mimetics can be translated into clinical therapy. The main challenge lies in the complexity of transposing results obtained in animals to humans, not least because of metabolic, anatomical and immunological differences. Moreover, few clinical trials have been conducted to date to assess the effect of low-dose radiation on human neuronal tissue in a therapeutic setting (Ji et al., 2023).

Research should focus on standardized in vivo studies in different species, and on the development of 3D models or "organs on a chip" that faithfully reproduce human brain physiology. In addition, high-throughput screening of compounds mimicking the hormone response could accelerate the discovery of new neuroprotectants. Finally, a better understanding of the spatio-temporal dynamics of the molecular mechanisms activated by low doses is essential to optimize therapeutic windows and minimize risks (Maoz., 2021).

In parallel, the integration of multi-omics approaches (transcriptomics, proteomics, metabolomics) will enable us to identify precise molecular signatures associated with radiation-induced neuroprotection. This data could not only shed light on the signaling pathways involved but also provide the basis for the development of biomarkers predictive of therapeutic response. In the long term, combining these tools with artificial intelligence could lead to clinical decision support algorithms, facilitating the individualization of low-dose treatments in a safe, personalized setting (Chen et al., 2023).

CONCLUSION

LDIR is challenging the conventional view of radiation as exclusively harmful. Growing evidence suggests that LDIR can activate adaptive cellular responses that promote neuroprotection, particularly through redox signalling pathways such as Nrf2-Keap1, and enhance DNA repair and anti-inflammatory mechanisms. These transient enzymatic inductions increase neuronal resilience and may delay the progression of neurodegenerative diseases such as Alzheimer's and Parkinson's. While preclinical studies offer promising prospects, their translation into the clinical setting remains limited by ethical considerations, regulatory frameworks, and the need for standardised protocols. Nevertheless, the combination of LDIR with pharmacological agents targeting similar protective pathways represents an interesting therapeutic avenue. Future research should focus on clarifying dose-response relationships, identifying biomarkers of sensitivity, and developing safe and personalised strategies. Ultimately, understanding and exploiting radiation-induced hormesis could open up new perspectives in the management of neurodegenerative diseases and brain resilience.

REFERENCES

Agathokleous, E., & Calabrese, E. J. (2022). Editorial overview: Hormesis and dose-response. *Current Opinion in Toxicology*, *30*, 100343. DOI: 10.1016/j.cotox.2022.03.004

Behrens, K. A., Jania, L. A., Snouwaert, J. N., Nguyen, M. T., Moy, S. S., Tikunov, A. P., Macdonald, J. M., & Koller, B. H. (2019). Beyond detoxification: Pleiotropic functions of multiple glutathione S-transferase isoforms protect mice against a toxic electrophile. *PLoS One*, *14*(11), e0225449. DOI: 10.1371/journal.pone.0225449 PMID: 31747445

Betlazar, C., Middleton, R. J., Banati, R. B., & Liu, G. J. (2016). The impact of high and low dose ionising radiation on the central nervous system. *Redox Biology*, *9*, 144–156. DOI: 10.1016/j.redox.2016.08.002 PMID: 27544883

Bondy, S. C. (2023). The Hormesis Concept: Strengths and Shortcomings. Biomolecules 2023, Vol. 13, Page 1512, 13(10), 1512.

Buccellato, F. R., D'Anca, M., Galimberti, D., Fenoglio, C., & Scarpini, E. (2021). Role of Oxidative Damage in Alzheimer's Disease and Neurodegeneration: From Pathogenic Mechanisms to Biomarker Discovery. Antioxidants 2021, Vol. 10, Page 1353, 10(9), 1353.

Chakkittukandiyil, A., Sajini, D. V., Karuppaiah, A., & Selvaraj, D. (2022). The principal molecular mechanisms behind the activation of Keap1/Nrf2/ARE pathway leading to neuroprotective action in Parkinson's disease. *Neurochemistry International*, *156*, 105325. DOI: 10.1016/j.neuint.2022.105325 PMID: 35278519

Chen, C., Wang, J., Pan, D., Wang, X., Xu, Y., Yan, J., Wang, L., Yang, X., Yang, M., & Liu, G. P. (2023). Applications of multi-omics analysis in human diseases. *MedComm*, *4*(4), e315. DOI: 10.1002/mco2.315 PMID: 37533767

Chung, M., & Chung, W. K. (2021). Clinical approach of low-dose whole-brain ionizing radiation treatment in Alzheimer's disease dementia patients. *Journal of Alzheimer's Disease*, *80*(3), 941–947. DOI: 10.3233/JAD-210042 PMID: 33612549

Dash, U. C., Bhol, N. K., Swain, S. K., Samal, R. R., Nayak, P. K., Raina, V., Panda, S. K., Kerry, R. G., Duttaroy, A. K., & Jena, A. B. (2025). Oxidative stress and inflammation in the pathogenesis of neurological disorders: Mechanisms and implications. *Acta Pharmaceutica Sinica. B*, *15*(1), 15–34. DOI: 10.1016/j.apsb.2024.10.004 PMID: 40041912

De Oliveira, J., Denadai, M. B., & Costa, D. L. (2022). Crosstalk between Heme Oxygenase-1 and Iron Metabolism in Macrophages: Implications for the Modulation of Inflammation and Immunity. Antioxidants 2022, Vol. 11, Page 861, 11(5), 861.

Gangwal, A., & Lavecchia, A. (2025). Artificial intelligence in preclinical research: Enhancing digital twins and organ-on-chip to reduce animal testing. *Drug Discovery Today*, *30*(5), 104360. DOI: 10.1016/j.drudis.2025.104360 PMID: 40252989

Gao, W., Jing, S., He, C., Saberi, H., Sharma, H. S., Han, F., & Chen, L. (2024). Advancements in Neurodegenerative Diseases: Pathogenesis and Novel Neurorestorative Interventions. *Journal of Neurorestoratology*, •••, 100176.

Ginés, C., Cuesta, S., Kireev, R., García, C., Rancan, L., Paredes, S. D., Vara, E., & Tresguerres, J. A. (2017). Protective effect of resveratrol against inflammation, oxidative stress and apoptosis in pancreas of aged SAMP8 mice. *Experimental Gerontology*, *90*, 61–70. DOI: 10.1016/j.exger.2017.01.021 PMID: 28130161

Guéguen, Y., Bontemps, A., & Ebrahimian, T. G. (2019). Adaptive responses to low doses of radiation or chemicals: Their cellular and molecular mechanisms. *Cellular and Molecular Life Sciences: CMLS*, *76*(7), 1255–1273. DOI: 10.1007/s00018-018-2987-5 PMID: 30535789

He, F., Ru, X., & Wen, T. (2020). NRF2, a transcription factor for stress response and beyond. *International Journal of Molecular Sciences*, *21*(13), 4777. DOI: 10.3390/ijms21134777 PMID: 32640524

Hernández Estévez, I., & Rodríguez Hernández, M. (2020). Plant Glutathione S-transferases: An overview. *Plant Gene*, *23*, 100233. DOI: 10.1016/j.plgene.2020.100233

Hladik, D., Dalke, C., Von Toerne, C., Hauck, S. M., Azimzadeh, O., Philipp, J., Ung, M. C., Schlattl, H., Rößler, U., Graw, J., Atkinson, M. J., & Tapio, S. (2019). Creb signaling mediates dose-dependent radiation response in the murine hippocampus two years after total body exposure. *Journal of Proteome Research*, 337–345. PMID: 31657930

Holcombe, J., & Weavers, H. (2022). The role of preconditioning in the development of resilience: Mechanistic insights. *Current Opinion in Toxicology*, *30*, 100338. DOI: 10.1016/j.cotox.2022.02.011

Holcombe, J., & Weavers, H. (2022). The role of preconditioning in the development of resilience: Mechanistic insights. *Current Opinion in Toxicology*, *30*, 100338. DOI: 10.1016/j.cotox.2022.02.011

Honeywell, M. E., Isidor, M. S., Harper, N. W., Fontana, R. E., Cruz-Gordillo, P., Porto, S. A., . . . Lee, M. J. (2023). p53 controls choice between apoptotic and non-apoptotic death following DNA damage. bioRxiv.

Hu, C., Yang, J., Qi, Z., Wu, H., Wang, B., Zou, F., Mei, H., Liu, J., Wang, W., & Liu, Q. (2022). Heat shock proteins: Biological functions, pathological roles, and therapeutic opportunities. *MedComm*, *3*(3), e161. DOI: 10.1002/mco2.161 PMID: 35928554

Hussien, S. M. (2023). Radio-adaptive Response Induced by Low-dose Ionizing Radiation in Innate Immunity for Radiotherapy. *Health Physics*, *124*(3), 166–174. DOI: 10.1097/HP.0000000000001649 PMID: 36719932

Jankovic, A., Zakic, T., Milicic, M., Unic-Stojanovic, D., Kalezic, A., Korac, A., Jovic, M., & Korac, B. (2021). Effects of remote ischaemic preconditioning on the internal thoracic artery nitric oxide synthase isoforms in patients undergoing coronary artery bypass grafting. *Antioxidants*, *10*(12), 1910. DOI: 10.3390/antiox10121910 PMID: 34943013

Ji, S., Xiong, M., Chen, H., Liu, Y., Zhou, L., Hong, Y., Wang, M., Wang, C., Fu, X., & Sun, X. (2023). Cellular rejuvenation: Molecular mechanisms and potential therapeutic interventions for diseases. *Signal Transduction and Targeted Therapy*, *8*(1), 116. DOI: 10.1038/s41392-023-01343-5 PMID: 36918530

Jin, Y., Sun, L. H., Yang, W., Cui, R. J., & Xu, S. B. (2019). The role of BDNF in the neuro-immune axis regulation of mood disorders. *Frontiers in Neurology*, *10*, 515. DOI: 10.3389/fneur.2019.00515 PMID: 31231295

Jomova, K., Alomar, S. Y., Alwasel, S. H., Nepovimova, E., Kuca, K., & Valko, M. (2024). Several lines of antioxidant defense against oxidative stress: antioxidant enzymes, nanomaterials with multiple enzyme-mimicking activities, and low-molecular-weight antioxidants. Archives of Toxicology 2024 98:5, 98(5), 1323–1367.

Kim, A., Lee, J., Moon, H., Kim, C., Yoo, M. Y., Park, W. Y., Kim, W. D., & Seo, Y. S. (2023). The effects of low-dose radiation therapy in patients with mild-to-moderate Alzheimer's dementia: An interim analysis of a pilot study. *Radiation Oncology Journal*, *41*(2), 89–97. DOI: 10.3857/roj.2023.00052 PMID: 37403351

Kim, D. Y., Kim, J. S., Seo, Y. S., Park, W. Y., Kim, B. H., Hong, E. H., Kim, J. Y., Cho, S. J., Rhee, H. Y., Kim, A., Kim, K. Y., Oh, D. J., & Chung, W. K. (2023). Evaluation of Efficacy and Safety Using Low Dose Radiation Therapy with Alzheimer's Disease: A Protocol for Multicenter Phase II Clinical Trial. *Journal of Alzheimer's Disease*, *95*(3), 1263–1272. DOI: 10.3233/JAD-230241 PMID: 37638435

Kim, S., Nam, Y., Kim, C., Lee, H., Hong, S., Kim, H. S., Shin, S. J., Park, Y. H., Mai, H. N., Oh, S. M., Kim, K. S., Yoo, D. H., Chung, W. K., Chung, H., & Moon, M. (2020). Neuroprotective and Anti-Inflammatory Effects of Low–Moderate Dose Ionizing Radiation in Models of Alzheimer's Disease. International Journal of Molecular Sciences 2020, Vol. 21, Page 3678, 21(10), 3678.

Kong, M., Beckwitt, E. C., & Van Houten, B. (2020a). Dynamic action of DNA repair proteins as revealed by single molecule techniques: Seeing is believing. *DNA Repair*, *93*, 102909. DOI: 10.1016/j.dnarep.2020.102909 PMID: 33087275

Kong, M., Beckwitt, E. C., & Van Houten, B. (2020b). Dynamic action of DNA repair proteins as revealed by single molecule techniques: Seeing is believing. *DNA Repair*, *93*, 102909. DOI: 10.1016/j.dnarep.2020.102909 PMID: 33087275

Kovalchuk, A., & Kolb, B. (2017). Low dose radiation effects on the brain–from mechanisms and behavioral outcomes to mitigation strategies. *Cell Cycle (Georgetown, Tex.)*, *16*(13), 1266–1270. DOI: 10.1080/15384101.2017.1320003 PMID: 28656797

Lau, Y. S., Chew, M. T., Alqahtani, A., Jones, B., Hill, M. A., Nisbet, A., & Bradley, D. A. (2021). Low Dose Ionising Radiation-Induced Hormesis: Therapeutic Implications to Human Health. Applied Sciences 2021, Vol. 11, Page 8909, 11(19), 8909.

Lau, Y. S., Chew, M. T., Alqahtani, A., Jones, B., Hill, M. A., Nisbet, A., & Bradley, D. A. (2021). Low dose ionising radiation-induced hormesis: Therapeutic implications to human health. *Applied Sciences (Basel, Switzerland)*, *11*(19), 8909. DOI: 10.3390/app11198909

Laurier, D., Billarand, Y., Klokov, D., & Leuraud, K. (2023). The scientific basis for the use of the linear no-threshold (LNT) model at low doses and dose rates in radiological protection. *Journal of Radiological Protection*, *43*(2), 024003. DOI: 10.1088/1361-6498/acdfd7 PMID: 37339605

Le Reun, E., & Foray, N. (2023a). Low-Dose Radiation Therapy (LDRT) against Cancer and Inflammatory or Degenerative Diseases: Three Parallel Stories with a Common Molecular Mechanism Involving the Nucleoshuttling of the ATM Protein? Cancers 2023, Vol. 15, Page 1482, 15(5), 1482.

Le Reun, E., & Foray, N. (2023b). Low-Dose Radiation Therapy (LDRT) against Cancer and Inflammatory or Degenerative Diseases: Three Parallel Stories with a Common Molecular Mechanism Involving the Nucleoshuttling of the ATM Protein? Cancers 2023, Vol. 15, Page 1482, 15(5), 1482.

Liu, S., Liu, J., Wang, Y., Deng, F., Deng, Z. (2025). Oxidative Stress: Signaling Pathways, Biological Functions, and Disease. MedComm (2020). 1;6(7): e70268. .DOI: 10.1002/mco2.70268

Lödermann, B., Wunderlich, R., Frey, S., Schorn, C., Stangl, S., Rödel, F., Keilholz, L., Fietkau, R., Gaipl, U. S., & Frey, B. (2012). Low dose ionising radiation leads to a NF-κB dependent decreased secretion of active IL-1β by activated macrophages with a discontinuous dose-dependency. *International Journal of Radiation Biology*, *88*(10), 727–734. DOI: 10.3109/09553002.2012.689464 PMID: 22545750

Mabsor-Zgandaoui, S., Moussaif, A., El Hessni, A., Mesfioui, A., El Mzibri, M., Iddar, A., & Moutaouakkil, A. (2025a). Ionising and Ultraviolet Radiation Induce the Secretion of Melanin in Tetrahymena Pyriformis. *The International Journal of Environmental Studies*, *82*(1), 1–14. https://doi.org/10.1080/00207233.2024.2412455

Mabsor-Zgandaoui, S., Rachmoune, K., El Hessni, A., El Mzibri, M., Iddar, A., & Moutaouakkil, A. (2025b). Effect of Hydrogen Peroxide Pre-Treatment on Enhancing the Cellular Resistance of Tetrahymena Pyriformis Exposed to Ionizing Radiation. *Toxicological and Environmental Chemistry*, *107*(2), 294–309. DOI: 10.1080/02772248.2025.2460804

Mabsor-Zgandaoui, S., Rachmoune, K., El Hessni, A., El Mzibri, M., Iddar, A., & Moutaouakkil, A. (2025). Effect of Hydrogen Peroxide Pre-Treatment on Enhancing the Cellular Resistance of *Tetrahymena Pyriformis* Exposed to Ionizing Radiation. *Toxicological and Environmental Chemistry*, *107*(2), 294–309. DOI: 10.1080/02772248.2025.2460804

Malta, S. M., Rodrigues, T. S., Silva, M. H., Marquez, A. S., Ferreira, R. B., do Prado Mascarenhas, F. N. A., Zanon, R. G., Bernardes, L. M. M., Batista, L. L., da Silva, M. N. T., de Oliveira Santos, D., Santos, A. C. C., Mendes-Silva, A. P., Spindola, F. S., & Ueira-Vieira, C. (2024). Brazilian kefir fraction mitigates the Alzheimer-like phenotype in Drosophila melanogaster with β-amyloid overexpression model. *Scientific Reports*, *14*(1), 25474. DOI: 10.1038/s41598-024-76601-9 PMID: 39461991

Maoz, B. M. (2021). Brain-on-a-Chip: Characterizing the next generation of advanced in vitro platforms for modeling the central nervous system. *APL Bioengineering*, *5*(3), 030902. DOI: 10.1063/5.0055812 PMID: 34368601

McDonald, J. T., Kim, K., Norris, A. J., Vlashi, E., Phillips, T. M., Lagadec, C., Della Donna, L., Ratikan, J., Szelag, H., Hlatky, L., & McBride, W. H. (2010). Ionizing radiation activates the Nrf2 antioxidant response. *Cancer Research*, *70*(21), 8886–8895. DOI: 10.1158/0008-5472.CAN-10-0171 PMID: 20940400

McNerlin, C., Guan, F., Bronk, L., Lei, K., Grosshans, D., Young, D. W., Gaber, M. W., & Maletic-Savatic, M. (2022). Targeting hippocampal neurogenesis to protect astronauts' cognition and mood from decline due to space radiation effects. *Life Sciences in Space Research*, *35*, 170–179. DOI: 10.1016/j.lssr.2022.07.007 PMID: 36336363

Minnier, J., Emmett, M. R., Perez, R., Ding, L. H., Barnette, B. L., Larios, R. E., Hong, C., Hwang, T. H., Yu, Y., Fallgren, C. M., Story, M. D., Weil, M. M., & Raber, J. (2021). Associations between lipids in selected brain regions, plasma miRNA, and behavioral and cognitive measures following 28Si ion irradiation. *Scientific Reports*, *11*(1), 1–30. DOI: 10.1038/s41598-021-93869-3 PMID: 34290258

Ngo V, Duennwald ML. (2022) Nrf2 and Oxidative Stress: A General Overview of Mechanisms and Implications in Human Disease. Antioxidants (Basel). 27;11(12):2345. .DOI: 10.3390/antiox11122345

Olufunmilayo, E. O., Gerke-Duncan, M. B., & Holsinger, R. D. (2023). Oxidative stress and antioxidants in neurodegenerative disorders. *Antioxidants*, *12*(2), 517. DOI: 10.3390/antiox12020517 PMID: 36830075

Pant, T., Uche, N., Juric, M., Zielonka, J., & Bai, X. (2024). Regulation of immunomodulatory networks by Nrf2-activation in immune cells: Redox control and therapeutic potential in inflammatory diseases. *Redox Biology*, *70*, 103077. DOI: 10.1016/j.redox.2024.103077 PMID: 38359749

Peña-Bautista, C., Tirle, T., López-Nogueroles, M., Vento, M., Baquero, M., & Cháfer-Pericás, C. (2019). Oxidative Damage of DNA as Early Marker of Alzheimer's Disease. International Journal of Molecular Sciences 2019, Vol. 20, Page 6136, 20(24), 6136.

Raghunath, A., Sundarraj, K., Nagarajan, R., Arfuso, F., Bian, J., Kumar, A. P., Sethi, G., & Perumal, E. (2018). Antioxidant response elements: Discovery, classes, regulation and potential applications. *Redox Biology*, *17*, 297–314. DOI: 10.1016/j.redox.2018.05.002 PMID: 29775961

Rozhko, T. V., Nogovitsyna, E. I., Badun, G. A., Lukyanchuk, A. N., & Kudryasheva, N. S. (2019). Reactive Oxygen Species and low-dose effects of tritium on bacterial cells. *Journal of Environmental Radioactivity*, *208–209*, 106035. DOI: 10.1016/j.jenvrad.2019.106035 PMID: 31499317

Sadrkhanloo, M., Entezari, M., Orouei, S., Zabolian, A., Mirzaie, A., Maghsoudloo, A., Raesi, R., Asadi, N., Hashemi, M., Zarrabi, A., Khan, H., Mirzaei, S., & Samarghandian, S. (2022). Targeting Nrf2 in ischemia-reperfusion alleviation: From signaling networks to therapeutic targeting. *Life Sciences*, *300*, 120561. DOI: 10.1016/j.lfs.2022.120561 PMID: 35460707

Saha, R. N., Ghosh, A., Palencia, C. A., Fung, Y. K., Dudek, S. M., & Pahan, K. (2009). TNF-α Preconditioning Protects Neurons via Neuron-Specific Up-Regulation of CREB-Binding Protein. *The Journal of Immunology : Official Journal of the American Association of Immunologists*, *183*(3), 2068–2078. DOI: 10.4049/jimmunol.0801892 PMID: 19596989

Srinivasan, S. R., Cesa, L. C., Li, X., Julien, O., Zhuang, M., Shao, H., Chung, J., Maillard, I., Wells, J. A., Duckett, C. S., & Gestwicki, J. E. (2018). Heat shock protein 70 (Hsp70) suppresses RIP1-dependent apoptotic and necroptotic cascades. *Molecular Cancer Research*, *16*(1), 58–68. DOI: 10.1158/1541-7786.MCR-17-0408 PMID: 28970360

Srivastava, T., Chirikova, E., Birk, S., Xiong, F., Benzouak, T., Liu, J. Y., Villeneuve, P. J., & Zablotska, L. B. (2023). Exposure to ionizing radiation and risk of dementia: A systematic review and meta-analysis. *Radiation Research*, *199*(5), 490–505. DOI: 10.1667/RADE-22-00153.1 PMID: 37293601

Sun, Y., Yang, Y. M., Hu, Y. Y., Ouyang, L., Sun, Z. H., Yin, X. F., Li, N., He, Q. Y., & Wang, Y. (2022a). Inhibition of nuclear deacetylase Sirtuin-1 induces mitochondrial acetylation and calcium overload leading to cell death. *Redox Biology*, *53*, 53. DOI: 10.1016/j.redox.2022.102334 PMID: 35636016

Sun, Y., Yang, Y. M., Hu, Y. Y., Ouyang, L., Sun, Z. H., Yin, X. F., Li, N., He, Q. Y., & Wang, Y. (2022b). Inhibition of nuclear deacetylase Sirtuin-1 induces mitochondrial acetylation and calcium overload leading to cell death. *Redox Biology*, *53*, 102334. DOI: 10.1016/j.redox.2022.102334 PMID: 35636016

Swartz, H. M., Flood, A. B., Singh, V. K., & Swarts, S. G. (2020). Scientific and logistical considerations when screening for radiation risks by using biodosimetry based on biological effects of radiation rather than dose: The need for prior measurements of homogeneity and distribution of dose. *Health Physics*, *119*(1), 72–82. DOI: 10.1097/HP.0000000000001244 PMID: 32175928

Tamtaji, O. R., Taghizadeh, M., Daneshvar Kakhaki, R., Kouchaki, E., Bahmani, F., Borzabadi, S., Oryan, S., Mafi, A., & Asemi, Z. (2019). Clinical and metabolic response to probiotic administration in people with Parkinson's disease: A randomized, double-blind, placebo-controlled trial. *Clinical Nutrition (Edinburgh, Lothian)*, *38*(3), 1031–1035. DOI: 10.1016/j.clnu.2018.05.018 PMID: 29891223

Teleanu, D. M., Niculescu, A. G., Lungu, I. I., Radu, C. I., Vladâcenco, O., Roza, E., Costăchescu, B., Grumezescu, A. M., & Teleanu, R. I. (2022). An Overview of Oxidative Stress, Neuroinflammation, and neurodegenerative diseases. International Journal of Molecular Sciences 2022, Vol. 23, Page 5938, 23(11), 5938.

Tsatsakis, A. M., Vassilopoulou, L., Kovatsi, L., Tsitsimpikou, C., Karamanou, M., Leon, G., Liesivuori, J., Hayes, A. W., & Spandidos, D. A. (2018). The dose response principle from philosophy to modern toxicology: The impact of ancient philosophy and medicine in modern toxicology science. *Toxicology Reports*, *5*, 1107–1113. DOI: 10.1016/j.toxrep.2018.10.001 PMID: 30450285

Ulasov, A. V., Rosenkranz, A. A., Georgiev, G. P., & Sobolev, A. S. (2022). Nrf2/Keap1/ARE signaling: Towards specific regulation. *Life Sciences*, *291*, 120111. DOI: 10.1016/j.lfs.2021.120111 PMID: 34732330

Wang, H., Guo, M., Wei, H., & Chen, Y. (2023). Targeting p53 pathways: Mechanisms, structures and advances in therapy. *Signal Transduction and Targeted Therapy*, *8*(1), 92. DOI: 10.1038/s41392-023-01347-1 PMID: 36859359

Wang, Y., Gao, L., Chen, J., Li, Q., Huo, L., Wang, Y., Wang, H., & Du, J. (2021). Pharmacological modulation of Nrf2/HO-1 signaling pathway as a therapeutic target of Parkinson's disease. *Frontiers in Pharmacology*, *12*, 757161. DOI: 10.3389/fphar.2021.757161 PMID: 34887759

Wilson, C., Adams, G. G., Patel, P., Windham, K., Ennis, C., & Caffrey, E. (2024). A Review of Recent Low-dose Research and Recommendations for Moving Forward. *Health Physics*, *126*(6), 386–396. DOI: 10.1097/HP.0000000000001808 PMID: 38568156

Wojcik, A., & Zölzer, F. (2024). The scientific nature of the linear no-threshold (LNT) model used in the system of radiological protection. *Radiation and Environmental Biophysics*, *63*(4), 483–489. DOI: 10.1007/s00411-024-01092-1 PMID: 39222266

Zhang, G., Liang, Z., Wang, Y., Zhang, Z., & Hoi, P. M. (2024). Tetramethylpyrazine Analogue T-006 Protects Neuronal and Endothelial Cells Against Oxidative Stress via PI3K/AKT/mTOR and Nrf2 Signaling. Antioxidants 2024, Vol. 13, Page 1272, 13(10), 1272.

Zhou, T., Yuan, Z., Weng, J., Pei, D., Du, X., He, C., & Lai, P. (2021). Challenges and advances in clinical applications of mesenchymal stromal cells. *Journal of Hematology & Oncology*, *14*(1), 1–24. DOI: 10.1186/s13045-021-01037-x PMID: 33579329

Chapter 6
In Silico Identification of Multi-Target Ligands for Neurodegenerative Disorders

Ajay Sharma
https://orcid.org/0000-0001-6620-4805
Lovely Professional University, India

Isha Batra
Lovely Professional University, India

Arun Malik
Lovely Professional University, India

ABSTRACT

Neurodegenerative disorders such as Alzheimer's disease, Parkinson's disease, Huntington's disease, and Amyotrophic Lateral Sclerosis present a growing global health burden due to their progressive nature, complex etiologies, and lack of effective disease-modifying therapies. Traditional drug discovery approaches that rely on single-target interventions have largely failed to yield successful treatments, primarily due to the multifaceted and overlapping pathological mechanisms involved, which range from protein misfolding and oxidative stress to neuroinflammation and synaptic dysfunction. This chapter explores the emerging paradigm of multi-target drug discovery, emphasizing the use of in silico techniques to identify ligands capable of modulating multiple disease-relevant targets such as β-secretase (BACE1), acetylcholinesterase (AChE), tau protein, NMDA receptors, MAO-B, and α-synuclein. The author has outline a comprehensive computational pipeline that integrates ligand-based and structure-based drug design approaches, including QSAR modeling, pharmacophore mapping, molecular docking.

DOI: 10.4018/979-8-3373-4627-4.ch006

INTRODUCTION

Background on Neurodegenerative Disorders

Neurodegenerative disorders (ND) is a heterogeneous group of chronic, progressive diseases characterized by the gradual and irreversible loss of structure or function of neurons, eventually leading to cognitive, motor, and functional impairments. Among the most prevalent neurodegenerative diseases are Alzheimer disease (AD), Parkinson disease (PD), Huntington disease (HD), and Amyotrophic Lateral Sclerosis (ALS). Each of these conditions presents distinct clinical features, yet they share several overlapping molecular and cellular mechanisms that underline their progression. One of the hallmark pathological features of many neurodegenerative diseases is protein misfolding and aggregation. For example, in an AD, the extracellular amyloid-beta plaques and intracellular tau tangles are widely recognized as central to the disease process. PD is marked by the accumulation of alpha-synuclein in the form of Lewy bodies. The mutant huntingtin protein aggregates in HD and TDP-43 inclusions in ALS point to a common theme of proteostasis failure. Other critical pathological mechanisms include oxidative stress, which results from the overproduction of reactive oxygen species (ROS), and neuroinflammation, mediated by the persistent activation of microglia and astrocytes. These events contribute to synaptic dysfunction, mitochondrial impairment, and neuronal death. The disturbances in neurotransmitter signaling, impaired autophagy, and genetic factors often exacerbate the progression of these disorders. Given their complex etiology and multifactorial nature, effective treatment of ND remains an urgent and unmet medical challenge. The are some challenges in the drug discovery process related to the neurodegenerative disease. The next section works on and highlights and works on the some of the challenges related to the neurodegenerative disease like AD, Parkinson(Cummings, 2017; De Pedro-Cuesta et al., 2015; Levy, 2007).

Challenges in Drug Discovery

Despite significant research efforts over the past few decades, the discovery of effective therapeutics for neurodegenerative diseases has been largely unsuccessful. Most existing pharmacological interventions are symptomatic rather than disease-modifying, offering only temporary relief without halting, reversing neuronal degeneration. A major challenge lies in the "single-target" approach traditionally employed in drug discovery. This reductionist model focuses on modulating a single molecular target, under the assumption that correcting one key pathway can mitigate disease progression. There are several dysregulated targets and interconnected pathways in neurodegenerative diseases. As a consequence, there is no guarantee that targeting a particular molecule will lead to beneficial therapeutic effects and may even cause unintended side effects or compensatory mechanisms, (Kumar & Sharma, 2023; Sharma, Kala, et al., 2021, 2024). The development and identification of multi-target ligands that may affect several disease-relevant sites has attracted a lot of attention from researchers as a potential solution to this limitation. This field is known as polypharmacology. In diseases where several factors combine to cause disease, this method may have a more holistic and synergistic effect on therapy. For complex diseases like Alzheimer's and Parkinson's, where blocking important signaling pathways and enzymes twice or even three times may improve outcomes, the shift to multi-target drug development is

very beneficial(Cummings, 2017; De Pedro-Cuesta et al., 2015; Josephs et al., 2009; Kovacs, 2018; Zádori et al., 2011).

Figure 1. Challenges in drug discovery

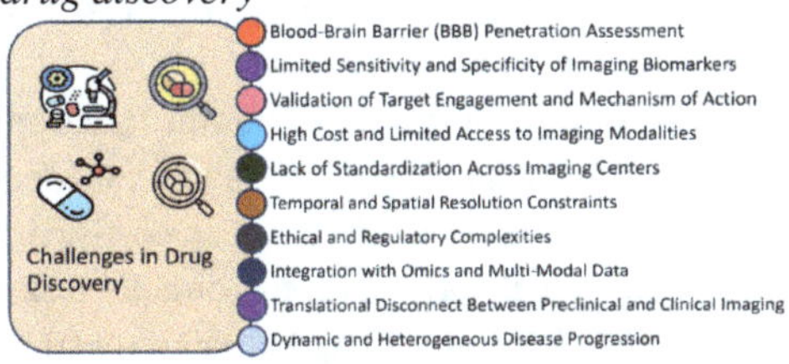

Despite its unique challenges, neuroimaging holds great promise for revolutionizing central nervous system (CNS) medication development. Collaborative efforts including neuroscientists, imaging experts, physicians, and computer modelers are necessary to tackle technology limitations, prohibitive costs, biomarker validation, and data integration. Personalized neurodegenerative disease treatments and multi-target therapeutics will be increasingly guided by standardized and improving imaging technology. Understanding brain function, disease progression, and treatment efficacy in neurodegenerative diseases has been greatly advanced by neuroimaging, which has now become an integral part of translational neuroscience. Integrating neuroimaging techniques such as fMRI, PET, SPECT, and MRI into the process of developing drugs for diseases affecting the central nervous system (CNS) presents several significant challenges, despite the fact that these approaches provide unparalleled insights into the structure and function of the brain. The inherent complexity of brain disorders, together with regulatory subtleties, technological limitations, and biological considerations, all contribute to these challenges(Enciu et al., 2011; Nguyen et al., 2021; Tăuţan et al., 2021).

Blood-Brain Barrier (BBB) Penetration Assessment

Protecting the brain while severely limiting medication delivery, the blood-brain barrier is one of the most basic obstacles in neurotherapeutics. For neuroimaging-based drug discovery, ensuring that candidate compounds or imaging probes can cross the BBB in sufficient quantities is critical. Neuroimaging techniques can quantify drug delivery and distribution, yet accurately interpreting BBB penetration remains a challenge due to inter-patient variability, regional differences in BBB permeability, and dynamic changes due to pathology or aging. Imaging biomarkers that can non-invasively assess BBB integrity (e.g., dynamic contrast-enhanced MRI) are still evolving and may lack standardization(Heifetz, 2020; Sweeney et al., 2018, 2019).

Limited Sensitivity and Specificity of Imaging Biomarkers

Imaging biomarkers are crucial for visualizing drug-target engagement, disease progression, and therapeutic effects. Many neuroimaging biomarkers lack sufficient sensitivity or specificity to reliably detect early pathological changes or subtle drug effects. For example, in Alzheimer's disease, amyloid PET imaging has been revolutionary, but amyloid burden does not always cor-

relate with clinical symptoms, leading to challenges in interpreting therapeutic efficacy. The tau imaging agents are still under development, and imaging synaptic density or neuroinflammation is complicated by overlapping signals and non-specific tracer binding.

Validation of Target Engagement and Mechanism of Action

One of the major hurdles in CNS drug discovery is the confirmation that a drug interacts with its intended target in the brain. Neuroimaging provides indirect evidence of target engagement, yet developing reliable PET tracers for every new target is costly, time-consuming, and often technically infeasible. The imaging signal may not always directly reflect functional engagement or downstream effects. A drug may bind to its target but fail to exert a therapeutic effect due to pathway redundancy, compensatory mechanisms, or insufficient dosing, issues not easily captured through imaging alone.

High Cost and Limited Access to Imaging Modalities

Neuroimaging studies, particularly those involving PET or high-resolution MRI, are expensive and resource intensive. The development of radioligands for PET imaging requires specialized facilities, radiochemistry expertise, and compliance with radioactive material handling regulations. These financial and logistical barriers limit the scalability of neuroimaging in early-stage drug discovery, especially for academic labs and smaller biotech firms. Limited access to imaging infrastructure restricts large scale, multi-center studies that are essential for validating imaging endpoints across populations.

Lack of Standardization Across Imaging Centers

In multicenter clinical trials, variability in scanner types, imaging protocols, data acquisition parameters, and preprocessing pipelines introduces significant heterogeneity, reducing the reliability and reproducibility of imaging data. Even slight differences in resolution, contrast settings, or reconstruction algorithms can affect the quantification of biomarkers. Standardized protocols (e.g., ADNI, HARMONI) help, but harmonization across centers remains an ongoing challenge, making it difficult to pool imaging data for large-scale drug efficacy analysis.

Temporal and Spatial Resolution Constraints

While neuroimaging provides non-invasive access to the brain, current modalities are limited by temporal and spatial resolution. PET imaging, for example, offers high sensitivity but poor temporal resolution. On the other hand, fMRI has high temporal but modest spatial resolution and is prone to noise and motion artifacts. These limitations impact the ability to monitor rapid pharmacokinetic and pharmacodynamic responses, especially when evaluating early drug effects, short-lived interactions.

Ethical and Regulatory Complexities

The use of advanced imaging in drug trials raises ethical and regulatory considerations, particularly for vulnerable populations such as patients with cognitive decline psychiatric conditions. The administration of radioactive tracers, contrast agents, or repeated scanning also poses safety concerns. The imaging endpoints used in regulatory filings must undergo rigorous validation to be accepted as surrogate markers for clinical efficacy. The absence of a standardized framework for imaging biomarker qualification hampers regulatory approval and delays translation from bench to bedside.

Integration with Omics and Multi-Modal Data

In the era of systems biology, drug discovery is increasingly reliant on integrated multi-modal datasets, including genomics, proteomics, transcriptomics. The interconnection of neuroimaging data with molecular profiles is technically challenging due to mismatched scales, data dimensionality, and statistical complexities. Efforts such as imaging genetics aim to link brain phenotypes with genetic risk, but building predictive models that can guide drug discovery requires large, well-annotated datasets and advanced machine learning pipelines, which are still under active development.

Translational Disconnect Between Preclinical and Clinical Imaging

Animal models are widely used in early drug discovery, and preclinical imaging (e.g., small animal MRI, micro-PET) is common. A translational gap often exists between animal imaging findings and human outcomes. Differences in brain anatomy, drug metabolism, and tracer pharmacokinetics limit the direct applicability of preclinical imaging data to clinical scenarios. Bridging this translational gap requires better cross species imaging biomarkers, improved animal models, and sophisticated computational frameworks for data interpretation.

Dynamic and Heterogeneous Disease Progression

Neurodegenerative diseases are inherently heterogeneous, both in terms of clinical presentation and progression patterns. Imaging findings may differ substantially between patients, even within the same diagnostic category. This heterogeneity complicates the use of neuroimaging as a universal readout for drug response, as not all patients will exhibit the same trajectory of biomarker changes. Stratification of patients based on imaging subtypes or disease stages is essential but requires large-scale, longitudinal imaging datasets, which are costly and difficult to maintain.

Role of In Silico Methods

The current section has discussed the role of the Insilco method in neuroimaging drug design, in silico approaches encompassing computational modeling, virtual screening, machine learning, and systems biology have emerged as indispensable tools in modern drug discovery. These methods offer significant advantages in terms of efficiency, scalability, and cost-effectiveness compared to traditional experimental approaches. Simulating molecular interactions and predicting

pharmacological properties, in silico techniques can rapidly identify promising candidates from a large chemical library, online database (Drug Bank), dramatically narrowing down the number of compounds that need to be synthesized and tested in vitro or in vivo. In silico workflows enable the rational design of multi-target ligands by predicting compound-target interactions across multiple proteins. Virtual screening, molecular docking, and pharmacophore modeling are widely used to identify lead compounds that exhibit favorable binding affinities to more than one therapeutic target. In addition, computational ADMET (Absorption, Distribution, Metabolism, Excretion, and Toxicity) prediction tools allow for the early removal of molecules with less-than-ideal drug-like properties, making late-stage failures less likely. Researchers may now more successfully navigate the complexities of neurodegenerative illnesses thanks to the amalgamation and usage of in silico techniques into medication development. By assisting with target selection, ligand design, and early-stage validation, computational tools speed up and improve the success rate of discovering multi-target medicines(Heifetz, 2020; Sweeney et al., 2018; Tautermann, 2020).

PATHOPHYSIOLOGY AND DRUG TARGETS IN NEURODEGENERATION

Here the author has focus on neurodegenerative illnesses, which cause memory loss, cognitive impairment, motor control issues, and other symptoms as brain cells (neurons) progressively deteriorate and die. These diseases usually get worse over time and currently have no complete cure. One major cause is the build-up of abnormal proteins in the brain. For example, in Alzheimer's, clumps of amyloid and tangled tau proteins disrupt brain function. In Parkinson's, another protein called α-synuclein builds up. These harmful proteins stop brain cells from working properly and may spread damage to nearby cells. One of the other factors is that brain cells need a lot of energy to survive. When their mitochondria (the "power plants" of cells) stop working well, energy production drops, and harmful molecules called free radicals increase, causing further damage. Too much activity of brain signals like glutamate can also overexcite and kill neurons. On top of that, the brain's immune cells (microglia) sometimes overreact, causing inflammation that worsens cell death. Current drugs mostly help with symptoms. For example, Alzheimer's treatments boost memory-related chemicals, and Parkinson's drugs replace lost dopamine. However, newer research is targeting the root causes, like stopping abnormal proteins from forming, improving cell energy, reducing inflammation, or even using gene therapy to correct faulty genes. Diseases involve many different problems at once, doctors believe that future treatments will need to target several pathways together slowing or even stopping the disease, not just easing the symptoms, (Berdigaliyev & Aljofan, 2020; Gupta et al., 2020; Mohan et al., 2021; Sadybekov & Katritch, 2023a).

Key Factor in the Neuro Degenerative Disease

Neurodegenerative diseases are driven by diverse but often converging molecular and cellular dysfunctions. Several key proteins and pathways have been identified as critical contributors to disease onset and progression, offering viable therapeutic targets for drug discovery. Among these, β-Secretase (BACE1), Acetylcholinesterase (AChE), Tau protein, N-Methyl-D-Aspartate

(NMDA) receptors, Monoamine oxidase-B (MAO-B), and α-synuclein are prominently involved across various neurodegenerative disorders.

β-Secretase (BACE1) plays a central role in the amyloidogenic pathway implicated in Alzheimer's disease (AD). It initiates the cleavage of amyloid precursor protein (APP) to produce amyloid-beta (Aβ) peptides, which aggregate to form neurotoxic plaques. Inhibiting BACE1 has been considered a promising strategy for reducing Aβ load, although challenges related to selectivity and off-target effects persist. Acetylcholinesterase (AChE) is another classical target in AD therapy. It degrades the neurotransmitter acetylcholine (ACh), whose levels are notably decreased in AD patients. AChE inhibitors, such as donepezil and rivastigmine, aim to enhance cholinergic transmission and improve cognitive function, albeit temporarily.

Tau protein, when hyperphosphorylated, forms neurofibrillary tangles a hallmark of AD and other tauopathies. Tau-related pathology is closely linked to cytoskeletal instability and neuronal degeneration. Modulating tau phosphorylation or promoting its clearance is an active area of therapeutic investigation. NMDA receptors are involved in synaptic plasticity and memory. However, excessive NMDA receptor activation leads to excitotoxicity, a key driver of neuronal death in AD, Huntington's disease (HD), and Amyotrophic Lateral Sclerosis (ALS). NMDA antagonists such as memantine aim to regulate glutamatergic signaling and prevent excitotoxic damage. Monoamine oxidase-B (MAO-B) is responsible for the catabolism of dopamine in the brain and is upregulated in Parkinson's disease (PD). When it comes to alleviating symptoms of motor disorders and assisting in the maintenance of dopaminergic function, MAO-B inhibitors like rasagiline and selegiline are beneficial therapies. In Parkinson's disease (PD), the protein α-synuclein, which is present in neurons prior to their synapse formation, forms aggregates that result in the formation of Lewy bodies. As a result of the formation of these aggregates, mitochondrial activity is hindered, which in turn leads to oxidative stress and impairs the functioning of the cell. When it comes to treatment, the ways that are used to target α-synuclein include immunotherapy approaches, boosting clearance, and reducing aggregation. Taking all of these targets into consideration demonstrates how complex neurodegenerative diseases are at the molecular level. Additionally, it lays the framework for the development of novel medications that are capable of modulating many pathogenic pathways simultaneously (Berdigaliyev & Aljofan, 2020; Khanna, 2012; Lavé et al., 2007).

Rationale for Multi-Target Approach

The traditional *"one disease–one target–one drug"* model is increasingly insufficient in addressing the multifactorial nature of neurodegenerative diseases. Disorders such as AD and PD are not caused by a single defective gene or protein but result from a complex interplay of genetic, molecular, and environmental factors. This complexity calls for a paradigm shift toward multi-target drug discovery.

Interconnected and overlapping pathways are determinants that influence the pathophysiology of disease. An example of this phenomenon is the development of amyloid, which exacerbates oxidative stress, thus intensifying tau hyperphosphorylation and neuroinflammation. Mitochondrial dysfunction may exacerbate α-synuclein aggregation, so establishing a detrimental loop. Focusing just on a single component often yields inadequate therapeutic advantages or transient relief, since compensatory mechanisms may diminish the therapy's efficacy over time. The objective of a multi-target approach is to generate therapeutic synergy by the creation of ligands

that engage with two or more relevant targets. A medication that inhibits both BACE1 and AChE may simultaneously reduce amyloid accumulation and enhance cholinergic function, hence providing superior cognitive benefits. Dual inhibitors of MAO-B and AChE may be advantageous in addressing both motor and cognitive symptoms related to Parkinson's disease (PD). Pharmaceuticals that engage several targets may reduce the likelihood of therapy failure and resistance, while also enhancing their efficacy. By concurrently affecting several nodes within the disease network, such pharmaceuticals diminish the probability of adaptive responses, a prevalent element that impedes the efficacy of single-target therapies. By consolidating therapeutic benefits into a single molecule, multi-target approaches may streamline treatment protocols. This may enhance patient adherence and decrease the incidence of drug-drug interactions. The intricate molecular nature of neurodegenerative illnesses, the interconnectedness of pathogenic mechanisms, and the need for more robust and enduring therapeutic effects are driving the pursuit of multi-target ligands in neurodegeneration therapy. The rational design and evaluation of these compounds, to be covered in subsequent parts, is greatly enhanced by the integration of in silico approaches, which are essential to the process, (Ramsay et al., 2016; Van Der Schyf, 2011; Wang et al., 2015).

COMPUTATIONAL DRUG DISCOVERY PIPELINE

When it comes to the modern age of pharmaceutical research, computational drug discovery pipelines have emerged as a crucial facilitator in the process of expediting the identification, optimization, and validation of candidate compounds. It is necessary to develop multi-target ligands for neurodegenerative illnesses, which are characterized by various sources and converging pathogenic pathways. This may be accomplished via the use of a high-throughput, inexpensive, and systematic design strategy, which is supported by in silico approaches. This may be attributed to the fact that neurodegenerative diseases often share similar pathogenic mechanisms. In this section, a full study of the computational technique is presented, with a particular emphasis on three essential pillars: ligand-based drug design (LBDD), structure-based drug design (SBDD), and ADMET/toxicity prediction. The use of these approaches makes it possible to identify viable candidates at an early stage, especially those that display positive biological activity and attractive pharmacokinetic features(Dar et al., 2020; Ramsay et al., 2016; Wu et al., 2019).

Figure 2.

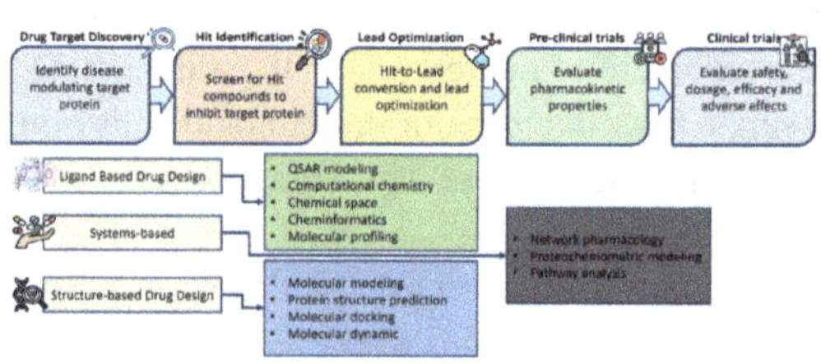

Ligand-Based Drug Design (LBDD)

Ligand-Based Drug Design (LBDD) is a fundamental technique in computational pharmacology, particularly effective when the three-dimensional structure of the target protein is unknown or unavailable. Instead of relying on target structure, LBDD uses knowledge derived from known active ligands to predict or design new compounds with similar or improved bioactivity(Budd Haeberlein & Harris, 2015; de la Fuente et al., 2023; Harrington et al., 2023).

Quantitative Structure-Activity Relationship (QSAR) Models

QSAR is a well-established technique used to correlate chemical structure with biological activity using mathematical models(Budd Haeberlein & Harris, 2015). These models are constructed using a set of molecular descriptors that quantitatively represent properties such as:

- Hydrophobicity (e.g., logP)
- Electronic distribution (e.g., HOMO-LUMO gap)
- Steric effects
- Topological indices
- Molecular weight and shape

A typical QSAR workflow includes:

Figure 3.

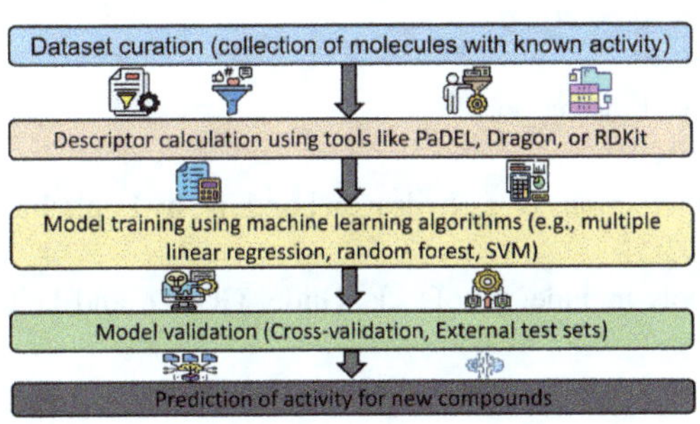

QSAR models are particularly useful for high-throughput screening of large chemical libraries and for prioritizing compounds before resource-intensive synthesis or testing. Multi-target QSAR (mt-QSAR) models are being increasingly used to predict the activity of compounds across multiple neurodegenerative targets (e.g., BACE1, AChE, MAO-B) simultaneously(Van Der Schyf, 2011; Wang et al., 2015).

Pharmacophore Modeling

A pharmacophore is defined as the ensemble of steric and electronic features necessary to ensure optimal interactions with a specific biological target. The pharmacophore modeling involves:

- Identifying common features among active compounds
- Defining their spatial relationships
- Using this model to screen chemical databases for new molecules with matching features

There are two types of pharmacophore modeling:

- Ligand-based pharmacophore (LBP): Derived from a series of active ligands
- Structure-based pharmacophore (SBP): Derived from the 3D structure of a ligand bound to its target

Software tools like Ligand Scout, PHASE, and Discovery Studio, AutoDock etc. allow users to generate and validate pharmacophore models. In the context of neurodegeneration, pharmacophore modeling can be particularly effective in identifying molecules capable of interacting with shared structural motifs across multiple targets (e.g., dual AChE/MAO-B inhibitors).

Structure-Based Drug Design (SBDD)

When the three-dimensional structure of the target is available (X-ray crystallography, NMR, or cryo-EM), Structure-Based Drug Design (SBDD) becomes a powerful tool. SBDD is used to identify novel molecules that fit precisely into the binding site of a target protein and optimize existing compounds for better efficacy and selectivity.

Molecular Docking

Molecular docking simulates the interaction between a ligand and its target protein(Khanna, 2012; Wang et al., 2015), predicting:

- The most favorable binding pose
- The binding affinity
- Key molecular interactions (e.g., hydrogen bonding, hydrophobic contacts)

Popular docking tools include AutoDock, Glide, GOLD, and DOCK. A typical docking process involves:

1. Preparing the protein (Removing water, adding hydrogens, Defining the binding site)
2. Ligand preparation (Energy minimization, Tautomer generation)
3. Docking simulation
4. Scoring and ranking based on binding energies or scoring functions

In the context of neurodegenerative diseases, docking is a technique that may be used in the setting of neurodegenerative illnesses to locate compounds that are capable of simultaneously binding to the active sites of enzymes such as BACE1 and AChE. In addition, docking is helpful in lead optimization, which instructs medicinal chemists on how to change chemical structures in order to achieve higher levels of efficacy.

Virtual Screening Workflows

Virtual screening involves evaluating large compound libraries against target structures to identify hits. It can be divided into:

- Structure-based virtual screening (SBVS): Uses docking algorithms to screen compounds based on fit to the target binding site.
- Ligand-based virtual screening (LBVS): Screens compounds based on similarity to known actives

The general workflow includes:

- Compound library preparation (e.g., from ZINC, PubChem, Enamine)
- Screening using high throughput docking or pharmacophore filters
- Post-screening filtering using ADMET or toxicity predictions

Virtual screening is particularly beneficial in multi-target drug discovery, as it can be configured to identify molecules that perform well across several docking simulations with different proteins.

Binding Site Analysis

Accurate identification and characterization of binding sites is crucial for SBDD. Tools such as SiteMap (Schrödinger), FTMap, and CASTp allow researchers to:

- Visualize binding pockets
- Evaluate pocket druggability
- Identify cryptic or allosteric sites

In multi-target ligand design, identifying overlapping or structurally similar binding pockets on different targets (e.g., cholinesterases and monoamine oxidases) can facilitate the design of broad-spectrum inhibitors. Binding site flexibility (induced fit) is also considered via molecular dynamics simulations.

ADMET and Toxicity Prediction

The majority of drug candidates fail in late-stage development due to poor pharmacokinetic properties or unexpected toxicity. To reduce these failures, in silico ADMET (Absorption, Distribution, Metabolism, Excretion, and Toxicity) profiling is integrated into the early phases of drug discovery(Gupta et al., 2020; Lavé et al., 2007; Wang et al., 2015). There are several tools for early-stage drug-likeness filtering, several computational platforms are available for assessing drug-likeness and pharmacokinetic behavior:

- **SwissADME:** Calculates properties like Lipinski's Rule of Five, solubility, lipophilicity (logP), and topological polar surface area (TPSA)

- **pkCSM:** Uses graph-based signatures to predict ADMET properties, including intestinal absorption and CYP450 metabolism.
- **ADMETlab 2.0:** Offers a suite of predictive models for physicochemical, toxicological, and pharmacokinetic properties.

For CNS drugs, specific emphasis is placed on properties such as:

- Molecular weight (< 500 Da)
- LogP (\~2–4)
- TPSA (< 90 Å^2 for BBB penetration)

These tools allow for the filtering of large compound libraries, prioritizing those with favorable profiles for further testing. Prediction of BBB permeability, hepatotoxicity, and other toxicities poses a significant challenge in neurotherapeutic design. In silico prediction tools help, assess a compound likelihood to cross the BBB based on physicochemical properties and molecular descriptors. Models using support vector machines, decision trees, and deep learning networks have been trained to predict BBB penetration with reasonable accuracy.

Other toxicity endpoints predicted include:

- **Hepatotoxicity:** e.g., Elevation of liver enzymes, mitochondrial dysfunction
- **Cardiotoxicity:** e.g., hERG channel inhibition
- **Mutagenicity and carcinogenicity:** Using Ame's test predictions and structural alerts
- **CYP450 inhibition:** Predicting drug-drug interactions

Integrating these predictive tools early in the discovery process reduces attrition rates, ensures better safety profiles, saves time and cost. The computational drug discovery pipeline has revolutionized the landscape of therapeutic development for complex diseases, such as neurodegeneration. By seamlessly integrating ligand-based, structure-based techniques with in silico ADMET, toxicity prediction, researchers can identify promising multi-target ligands with higher confidence, efficiency, and precision. Ligand-based methods such as QSAR, pharmacophore modeling enable rapid screening and activity prediction without structural knowledge of the target. Structure-based methods including molecular docking and virtual screening, offer atomic-level insights that drive rational design. ADMET profiling ensures that only the most viable candidates progress to experimental validation. This multi-tiered computational approach not only accelerates the drug discovery cycle but also paves the way for more personalized and mechanism-informed therapeutic interventions in neurodegenerative disorders. Artificial intelligence, big data, and systems biology continue to evolve, the synergy between computational and experimental methods will only deepen, redefining the future of precision neuropharmacology.

MULTI-TARGET LIGAND IDENTIFICATION STRATEGIES

Neurodegenerative disorders such as Alzheimer's disease, Parkinson's disease, and Huntington's disease involve complex, multifactorial pathologies. These conditions typically involve the dysregulation of several interconnected biological pathways and molecular targets. A single-target

therapies often fail to provide sufficient clinical benefit. Multi-target ligand identification has emerged as a promising strategy to address this complexity by identifying or designing compounds capable of modulating multiple disease-relevant targets simultaneously. The section explores the key strategies involved in identifying such ligands, including data curation, target prediction, network pharmacology, multi-target QSAR modeling, multi-target molecular docking, using a mix of detailed explanations, tabular formats, and concise summaries for clarity(Ramsay et al., 2016; Van Der Schyf, 2011).

Data Preparation and Curation

Accurate and comprehensive data are the foundation of any computational drug discovery effort. The quality of input data directly influences the reliability of model predictions, target identification, and virtual screening outcomes(Armstrong et al., 2020; de la Fuente et al., 2023; Hou et al., 2019).

Ligand Databases

These databases provide extensive chemical information, including molecular structure, activity data, and drug-like properties:

Table 1.

Database	Description	Key Features
ChEMBL	Curated bioactivity database from literature	Contains IC50, EC50, and Ki values for over 2 million compounds across ~12,000 targets
ZINC	Free database of commercially available compounds	Contains over 230 million purchasable molecules with 3D structures
PubChem	Public repository of chemical compounds	Provides molecular descriptors, bioassay data, and drug-likeness filters

Protein/Target Databases

These repositories provide target structures, annotations, and sequence data required for docking, pharmacophore mapping, and binding site analysis:

Table 2.

Database	Description	Applications
PDB (Protein Data Bank)	3D structures of biomolecules	Used for molecular docking and structure-based drug design
UniProt	Protein sequences and functional data	Useful for target annotation and biological relevance
BindingDB	Measured binding affinities	Provides ligand-target binding constants useful for QSAR training sets

Key Points

- Ensure data normalization (e.g., same units for activity values).
- Remove duplicates, salts, and stereoisomers when preparing ligand libraries.
- Use drug-likeness filters (Lipinski's, Veber's rules) to enhance screening quality.

Target Fishing and Network Pharmacology

The process of identifying possible therapeutic targets is a key part of the design process for multi-target compounds. This technique, which is sometimes referred to as target fishing, is aided by computational tools that come from the fields of chemo genomics and network pharmacology, (Budd Haeberlein & Harris, 2015; Khanna, 2012; Van Der Schyf, 2011).

Table 3.

Approach	Description	Tools
Ligand-based	Predicts targets based on chemical similarity to known ligands	SEA (Similarity Ensemble Approach), Swiss Target Prediction
Structure-based	Compares query compounds with known active site structures	Reverse docking via INVDOCK, Pharm Mapper
Machine learning-based	Uses molecular descriptors and activity labels to classify targets	DeepDTnet, Chem-Prot

Network Pharmacology Concepts

Network pharmacology leverages systems biology to understand how ligands interact across biological pathways and disease networks. It focuses on the various factors like:

- Mapping relationships among diseases, genes, proteins, and drugs.
- Analyzing pathway crosstalk and feedback mechanisms.
- Predicting off-target effects and drug repurposing potential.

Workflow for Network Pharmacology in Neurodegeneration:

- Collect disease genes (e.g., DisGeNET, OMIM)
- Identify interacting proteins (STRING, BioGRID)
- Overlay drug-target data (DrugBank or ChEMBL)
- Construct pathway map (KEGG, Reactome)
- Analyze hub nodes and bottlenecks to prioritize multi-targets.

Table 4.

Component	Example Tool	Purpose
Disease-gene associations	DisGeNET	Identify genes associated with Alzheimer's or Parkinson's
Protein interaction networks	STRING	Visualize direct/indirect interactions among proteins
Drug-pathway interactions	STITCH	Link small molecules to pathways and diseases

Multi-Target QSAR Modeling

Multi-target QSAR models, which are also known as quantitative structure-activity relationship models, are models that are intended to predict the biological activity of a molecule across a number of targets simultaneously. These models are also known as qualitative structure-activity relationship models. When compared to the traditional single-target QSAR approach, the multi-target QSAR method requires the use of certain machine learning frameworks that are capable of doing multi-label classification or regression. This is in contrast to the single-target QSAR method (Berdigaliyev & Aljofan, 2020; Gupta et al., 2020; Mohan et al., 2021; Tautermann, 2020).

Molecular Descriptors and Fingerprints

- Descriptors: topological, electronic, geometric, physicochemical
- Fingerprints: ECFP (Morgan), MACCS, RDKit

Multi-Label Machine Learning Algorithms

Table 5.

Algorithm	Description	Application
Random Forest (RF)	Ensemble-based decision trees for multi-label outputs	Good baseline, handles nonlinear patterns
Support Vector Machine (SVM)	Margin maximization, adapted for multi-target classification	Requires careful kernel tuning
XGBoost	Gradient boosting handles high-dimensional descriptors well	Effective for sparse data
Deep Learning (DNN, CNN)	Learns complex patterns from molecular graphs or SMILES	Useful for large datasets with diverse targets

Statistical Validation Techniques

Table 6.

Metric	Purpose
Accuracy	Percentage of correctly predicted labels
F1 Score (micro/macro)	Balance between precision and recall
Area under ROC curve (AUC)	Evaluates model performance across thresholds
Y-randomization	Checks for overfitting
Cross-validation (k-fold)	Ensures model generalization

Advantages

- Reduces computational costs compared to separate QSAR models.
- Identifies molecules with balanced multi-target activity.
- Enables activity prediction on unknown targets if trained well.

Molecular Docking for Multiple Targets

Molecular docking plays a pivotal role in virtual screening and lead optimization for multi-target drug discovery. Molecular docking is an essential component in the process of virtual screening and lead optimization for the purpose of multi-target drug development. The interaction between a tiny molecule (the ligand) and one or more protein targets is simulated by this method, which also estimates the binding affinities and interaction patterns of the ligand(Berdigaliyev & Aljofan, 2020; Enciu et al., 2011; Gupta et al., 2020; Sadybekov & Katritch, 2023a; Sweeney et al., 2019). Included in the following list are some of the docking strategies that may be used for multi-target screening:

Sequential Docking

- Ligands are docked one target at a time.
- Allows focused analysis on specific target combinations (e.g., AChE + MAO-B).
- Computationally less expensive than parallel strategies.

Parallel Docking

- Ligands are docked against all selected targets simultaneously.
- Suitable for large-scale screening.
- Enables ranking of ligands by cumulative binding score.

Table 7.

Strategy	Pros	Cons
Sequential	Focused, interpretable	Slower if many targets
Parallel	Scalable, high-throughput	May miss nuances in binding orientation

Scoring Function Consensus

Multiple docking programs and scoring functions (e.g., GlideScore, ChemScore, AutoDock Vina score) often give varying results. Consensus scoring involves:

- Using multiple scoring functions
- Ranking compounds by average or majority rank
- Improving prediction reliability

Table 8.

Scoring Function	Key Feature	Software
GlideScore	Empirical, protein-ligand complementarity	Schrodinger Glide
AutoDock Vina Score	A hybrid of empirical and knowledge-based	AutoDock Vina
ChemScore	Focuses on hydrogen bonds, metal coordination	GOLD

Post-Docking Analysis

- Interaction profiling: Identify H-bonds, π-π stacking, salt bridges.
- Binding poses clustering: Evaluate binding conformation consistency.
- Selectivity analysis: Compare differential binding energy across targets.

The creation of multi-target ligands marks a big step forward in the fight against the complex pathologies that are associated with neurodegenerative disorders. Computational strategies have enabled researchers to design, screen, and optimize compounds that interact with multiple proteins involved in overlapping disease mechanisms. This chapter highlighted critical strategies in the multi-target ligand discovery pipeline, including:

- Curated, high-quality ligand and target datasets (ChEMBL, ZINC, PDB).
- Target fishing and network pharmacology approach to prioritize disease-relevant pathways.
- Machine learning-driven multi-target QSAR modeling for activity prediction across multiple targets.
- Molecular docking workflows with sequential, parallel, and consensus scoring to evaluate compound binding potential.

These strategies reduce the need for costly experimental iterations, allow for early de-risking of compounds, and provide a robust foundation for rational drug design. As datasets grow and AI-driven platforms evolve, the in-silico identification of multi-target ligands will continue to accelerate the development of safer, more effective neurotherapeutics.

INTEGRATION WITH AI/ML AND SYSTEMS BIOLOGY

Particularly for complex diseases such as neurodegenerative disorders, this integration holds unprecedented promise in accelerating the identification of effective, multi-target therapeutics. As single-target approaches continue to yield limited clinical success, a paradigm shift toward systems-level understanding and multi-target intervention is becoming essential. AI&ML provide powerful data-driven tools for identifying candidate molecules with desirable properties, while systems biology enables the modeling of biological complexity at the network level. Together, they constitute a synergistic framework for precision, personalized drug discovery, (Cavalli et al., 2008; Ou-Yang et al., 2012; Sadybekov & Katritch, 2023b; Smith et al., 2018).

The fusion of artificial intelligence AI, ML & systems biology has emerged as a transformative force in drug discovery and development. AI has proven particularly valuable for curation in the context of complex diseases like neurodegenerative disorders, where conventional single-target therapeutic strategies often fall short due to the intricate and multifactorial nature of disease progression. The use of ML algorithm and Systems Biology have revolutionized drug discovery processes, particularly in the context of neurodegenerative disorders and are characterized by multifactorial pathologies, progressive neuronal deterioration, involve numerous interacting genes, proteins, and pathways. Traditional single-target drug discovery approaches often fail to produce meaningful outcomes in such complex diseases. The multi-target drug discovery, driven by computational methods, has become a central strategy for the new drug synthesis. There are some of the complexities associated with the drug synthesis. To address such complexity, algorithm-based predictions and systems-level simulations are being connected to accelerate the discovery of multi-target ligands, elucidate mechanisms of action, and simulate systemic drug responses with higher precision, reduced cost. In this context, AI/ML, systems-level modeling provides complementary strengths. AI/ML offers predictive analytics and pattern recognition, while systems biology helps in mechanistic understanding and simulation of disease pathways, (Carvalho et al., 2017; Cavalli et al., 2008; Smith et al., 2018; S. Q. Yang et al., 2021).

Systems biology complements machine learning by enabling a holistic understanding of biological systems at the molecular, cellular, and organismal levels. The reductionist approaches that focus on isolated pathways or targets, systems biology model complex networks of interactions among genes, proteins, metabolites, and signaling pathways. This system-level perspective is crucial in neurodegenerative research, where disease progression is driven by dynamic crosstalk among multiple molecular components. The goal of systems-level simulation is to predict how perturbations, such as drug interventions propagate through these networks and influence disease outcomes. In a typical procedure for systems biology, the first step is to construct a biological network. This is the beginning of the process. KEGG, which stands for the Kyoto Encyclopedia of Genes and Genomes, Reactome, STRING, and BioGRID are all examples of public datasets that may be used in the process of generating their respective networks. he production of these networks may also be accomplished via the use of experimental data, the curation of literature,

or other sources. In the network, nodes are accountable for representing biological entities like proteins and genes, while edges are accountable for expressing interactions such as activation, inhibition, and binding. Nodes will be liable for representing biological objects. Hubs, which are nodes that are highly connected to one another, bottlenecks, which are key control points, and modules, which are clusters that are functionally coupled to one another are all examples of the types of insights that may be gained from the topologies of these networks. After it has been constructed, the network may be used to mimic the influence that possible drug candidates have on certain disease pathways. This is something that this network may be used for. In order to select therapeutic targets for the goal of multi-target ligand discovery, the discipline of systems biology may be used. To achieve this goal, it is necessary to investigate the ways in which individual proteins influence the behavior of the network as a whole. Through the use of network-based approaches such as randomization with restart, network propagation, and module discovery, it is possible to achieve the task of identifying significant regulators of disease-associated modules. Researchers are able to discover synergistic target combinations that would not be evident from trials that just concentrate on a single target to the extent that they are able to do so via the use of these approaches. In Alzheimer's disease, for instance, treating both BACE1 and tau kinases has the potential to simultaneously reduce the number of amyloid particles and the pathology caused by tau antibodies In comparison to each of the two interventions taken separately, this would result in a more significant therapeutic effect. Systems biology is distinguished by its ability to predict the effect that ligands will have on the operation of the system, which is one of the most important aspects of this field of study. Ordinary differential equations (ODEs), stochastic simulations, or agent-based models that depict dynamic changes over time are used for the aim of modeling drug-induced perturbations. These models are used to describe the effects of changes in the drug. Using these simulations, it is feasible to discover potential compensatory mechanisms, inadvertent repercussions, or long-term adaptations that would be difficult to identify using normal experimental procedures. These are all things that may be discovered for the first time. Although it is feasible that suppressing a neuroinflammatory pathway might initially result in a drop in cytokine levels, it is also plausible that this could ultimately lead to immune suppression. The use of simulations makes it feasible to forecast the outcomes of such situations and to have an impact on the development of solutions that are both more secure and more efficient. In the realm of system-level modeling, the evaluation of route crosstalk is yet another strong tool that is taken into consideration. Many of the systems that are involved in neurodegenerative illnesses are intricately connected to one another. These mechanisms include oxidative stress, mitochondrial failure, autophagy, synaptic plasticity, and protein aggregation. The phenomenon known as crosstalk occurs when one pathway has an effect on another pathway, either directly via components that are shared or indirectly through signaling that occurs farther downstream. Having a thorough knowledge of these interactions is necessary for the goal of developing drugs that target many targets. This is because the change of one pathway may have ramifications on other pathways, therefore it is important to have this information well. With the use of systems biology tools like Cell-Designer, Cytoscape, and Pathway Commons, researchers are able to examine and analyze crosstalk, find common nodes, and forecast the outcomes of multi-pathway therapies. These capabilities are all possible. An example of pathway crosstalk that is crucial to dementia is the connection that takes place between the MAPK pathway and the PI3K-Akt signaling pathway. This interaction is seen in neurodegenerative diseases. Due to the fact that both of these routes are essential to the survival of neurons and the function of synapses, it has

been shown that an imbalance in the regulation of both pathways is associated with a decrease in cognitive capacity. It is feasible that a multi-target medicine that partially activates PI3K-Akt while reducing aberrant MAPK signaling might, in principle, restore balance and increase neuronal resilience. This is something that is possible. Before committing to costly experimental studies, it is possible to validate the notion and simulate these interactions via the use of system-level models. This may be done before an expensive experiment is conducted(Biswas & Chakrabarti, 2020; Ramsay et al., 2018; T. Yang et al., 2020).

By combining AI and ML with biology systems, prediction potential is further increased. Machine learning models that are driven by data have the capacity to recognize correlations and patterns, while mechanistic systems biology models provide causation and interpretability. The combination of the two makes it possible to create hybrid modeling techniques, in which the outputs of machine learning are used to parameterize or restrict dynamic models, while the findings of simulation analysis are utilized to provide features for machine learning. This repeated cycle allows for the development of drug discovery pipelines that are more precise and guided by biological principles. In summing up, the incorporation of machine learning and systems biology into the area of neurodegenerative drug development reflects a paradigm change that is transformational. Machine learning enables high-throughput, data-driven predictions of ligand activity, ADMET properties, and polypharmacological potential, while systems biology provides mechanistic insights into disease pathways and drug effects. Together, they facilitate a comprehensive understanding of drug-disease interactions at both the molecular and systems levels. As data availability continues to expand and computational tools grow more sophisticated, this integrated framework will play an increasingly critical role in identifying and optimizing multi-target ligands capable of addressing the complex nature of neurodegenerative disorders. The future of precision medicine in neurology will undoubtedly rely on this synergistic combination to overcome current therapeutic challenges and pave the way for more effective and personalized treatment strategies(Alvarez-Rodríguez et al., 2019; Choubey et al., 2025; Ellingson et al., 2020; Gelemanović, 2023).

Machine Learning in Ligand Prediction

Machine learning techniques play a pivotal role in predicting the interaction between chemical compounds (ligands) and biological targets. The first step in any ML-based ligand prediction pipeline is feature engineering, where the chemical and structural information of molecules is transformed into numerical representations that algorithms can understand. Machine learning has become a central component of computational drug discovery, particularly in ligand-based drug design and activity prediction. The underlying strength of ML lies in its ability to learn complex, nonlinear relationships between molecular descriptors, biological outcomes, enabling the rapid screening of large chemical libraries and the identification of promising multi-target compounds, (Ballester & Mitchell, 2010; Ellingson et al., 2020; Gelemanović, 2023; Heck et al., 2017).

Feature Engineering and Molecular Representation

One of the first and most crucial steps in ML-based ligand prediction is the conversion of chemical structures into numerical or graphical representations that algorithms can process, a step known as feature engineering. This step significantly influences model performance, inter-

pretability, and generalizability. Features used in ligand prediction include molecular descriptors, structural fingerprints, and graph-based representations(Pang et al., 2012; Zimmermann et al., 2007). These features can be categorized as:

Table 9.

Descriptor Type	Examples	Description
Physicochemical	Molecular weight, logP, TPSA	Encodes general drug-likeness and solubility
Topological	Wiener index, Kier shape index	Describes atom connectivity and molecular shape
Electronic	HOMO-LUMO gap, polarizability	Informs about reactivity and binding potential
Structural fingerprints	ECFP, MACCS, RDKit	Binary vectors representing molecular substructures
Graph representations	Node (atom) and edge (bond) embeddings	Used in GNNs for deep learning-based modeling

Once the features are defined, they are fed into machine learning models for prediction. Various algorithms have been developed and optimized for ligand activity prediction. In recent years, graph-based representations have become increasingly popular, especially for deep learning applications. Graph Neural Networks (GNNs) treat molecules as graphs, use message passing algorithms to learn features that are not explicitly predefined but learned directly from data. These models have outperformed traditional descriptor-based models in many benchmark tasks, including activity prediction and toxicity classification, (Ballester & Mitchell, 2010; Boyles et al., 2020; Ravikumar & Aittokallio, 2018; Zhang et al., 2024).

Common Machine Learning Models

The choice of machine learning model depends on the type of data available, the prediction task (classification vs. regression), and the complexity of the relationships in the dataset.

Table 10.

Model	Description	Use Case
Random Forest (RF)	An ensemble of decision trees trained on random feature subsets, high-dimensional data.	Classification of active/inactive ligands, Bioactivity classification, ADMET prediction
XG-Boost	A gradient boosting technique that improves over weak learners	Multi-target prediction, property regression, Regression, and classification of binding affinities
Support Vector Machines (SVM)	Maximizes decision boundary margin	Classification tasks with small datasets
Artificial Neural Networks (ANNs)	Multi-layered networks that model nonlinear relationships	QSAR regression, multi-label classification
Graph Neural Networks (GNNs)	Learns from molecular graphs without handcrafted features, high accuracy in QSAR tasks	Target binding prediction, de novo drug design, Multitarget ligand prediction, property inference

Among these, Random Forest and XGBoost are especially favored for small-to-medium datasets due to their interpretability and robustness against overfitting. The GNN and other deep

learning models are becoming more prevalent with the advent of big data from high-throughput screening campaigns.

Deep Learning and Multi-Target Drug Discovery

ML models are not only used for predicting ligand-target affinity but also for other tasks such as ADMET profiling, synthetic accessibility, and toxicity estimation. By combining predictive modeling with multi-label classification, ML can identify ligands that act on multiple targets simultaneously, which is essential in neurodegenerative therapy where pathways are deeply interconnected. Deep learning is especially useful for multi-target ligand prediction, which is a concept that is gaining interest in the field of neurodegenerative drug development (Satti et al., 2024; Sharma et al., 2022; Sharma, Gupta, et al., 2021; Sharma, Kumar, et al., 2021; Sharma, Pal, et al., 2024). In this approach, a single molecule is intended to modify numerous targets concurrently. Deep learning models, in particular Graph Neural Networks (GNNs), have shown remarkable performance as a result of their capacity to capture both the spatial and electrical information that molecules contain. Geometric neural networks (GNNs) are capable of learning complicated patterns from raw molecular graphs and do not need explicit feature engineering, (Badria et al., 2025; Boyles et al., 2020; Cichońska et al., 2024; Ji et al., 2021; Liu et al., 2013; Lo et al., 2018; Rodríguez-Pérez & Bajorath, 2021; Zhang et al., 2024). Through the use of iterative message-passing techniques, these networks are able to update atomic representations in accordance with their chemical surroundings.

Advantages and Limitations

Table 11.

Advantages	**Limitations**
High-throughput screening capability	Requires large, high-quality labeled datasets
Can identify complex, non-linear patterns	Interpretability can be limited (black-box nature)
Facilitates multitarget activity prediction	Potential overfitting without proper regularization

Key Techniques

- **Multi-label classification:** Each compound can have multiple active labels corresponding to different targets.
- **Transfer learning:** Models trained on well-annotated targets can be adapted to novel targets with limited data.
- **Generative models (e.g., VAEs, GANs):** Generate novel compounds with optimized multi-target binding profiles.

These approaches are highly useful in designing compounds for Alzheimer's or Parkinson's, where inhibition of both amyloid and tau-related pathways (or dopaminergic and cholinergic systems) is often desired.

Deep Learning and Multi-Target Drug Discovery

Deep learning is especially useful for multi-target ligand prediction, which is a concept that is gaining interest in the field of neurodegenerative drug development. In this approach, a single molecule is intended to modify numerous targets concurrently, (Cichońska et al., 2024; Lo et al., 2018; Shaheen & Melnik, 2025).

Key Techniques

- **Multi-label classification:** Each compound can have multiple active labels corresponding to different targets.
- **Transfer learning:** Models trained on well-annotated targets can be adapted to novel targets with limited data.
- **Generative models (e.g., VAEs, GANs):** Generate novel compounds with optimized multi-target binding profiles.

These approaches are highly useful in designing compounds for Alzheimer's or Parkinson's, where inhibition of both amyloid and tau-related pathways (or dopaminergic and cholinergic systems) is often desired.

Table 12.

Metric	Purpose
Accuracy	Percentage of correctly classified samples
Precision & Recall	Measures of correctness and completeness
F1 Score	Harmonic mean of precision and recall
ROC-AUC	Measures overall classification quality
RMSE/MAE	Error metrics for regression tasks

Systems-Level Simulation of Neurodegenerative Pathways

While machine learning excels at prediction, it often lacks causal interpretability. Systems biology complements this by modeling the mechanistic and dynamic behavior of biological systems. In neurodegenerative diseases, multiple signaling pathways interact over time, creating a network of molecular events. Systems-level simulation models this network to predict how drug interventions affect the overall system (Baloni et al., 2021; Ji et al., 2021). This is particularly important in neurodegenerative diseases, where feedback loops, pathway crosstalk, and multi-organ effects influence treatment outcomes, (Campillo-Sánchez & Gómez-Sanz, 2016; Proctor et al., 2013; Tomaskova et al., 2016; Uleman et al., 2023).

Predicting Systemic Effects of Ligands

Systems biology tools use network-based and dynamic modeling techniques to simulate the propagation of ligand effects across biological pathways. Models can be built using ordinary differential equations (ODEs), Boolean logic, or agent-based systems, depending on the complexity and data availability.

The workflow typically involves:

1. Identifying disease-associated pathways (e.g., KEGG, Reactome).
2. Constructing the interaction network of genes, proteins, and metabolites.
3. Incorporating ligand-target interactions from databases or docking results.
4. Running simulations to observe system-level changes upon perturbation.

Table 13.

Tool	Application
CellDesigner	Pathway diagramming and dynamic simulation
COPASI	Simulation of biochemical networks using ordinary differential equations (ODEs)
Cytoscape	Visualization and analysis of biomolecular interaction networks

For example, targeting the amyloid-beta (Aβ) cascade in Alzheimer's may reduce plaque formation but can also affect downstream oxidative stress and inflammation pathways. Simulating this effect helps in understanding the broader implications of therapeutic intervention.

Pathway Modeling and Biological Networks

Systems biology makes use of a wide range of modeling techniques in order to create an accurate depiction of the intricate interactions that take place inside biological systems that are being studied. KEGG, Reactome, BioGRID, and STRING are some examples of public databases that provide users access to curated data that may be used in the building of these networks. These databases serve as examples of public databases. These are some instances of databases that are available to the public.

Table 14.

Network Type	Nodes	Edges	Purpose
Protein-Protein Interaction (PPI)	Proteins	Physical or functional interactions	Identify hub proteins and druggable clusters
Gene Regulatory Network (GRN)	Genes/TFs	Activation/inhibition relationships	Understand gene expression control
Signaling Pathways	Receptors, kinases, transcription factors	Signal transduction	Analyze drug impact on downstream targets
Metabolic Pathways	Metabolites, enzymes	Biochemical reactions	Study energy and neurotransmitter metabolism

Predicting Systemic Effects of Ligands. Drugs that act on multiple targets can trigger ripple effects across interconnected pathways. Systems-level simulation allows researchers to predict these systemic effects using various mathematical models.

Approaches

- **Ordinary Differential Equations (ODEs):** Simulate time-dependent behavior of pathways (e.g., NF-κB activation).
- **Boolean Networks:** Simplify gene/protein activation states to ON/OFF for logic-based simulation.
- **Agent-Based Models (ABMs):** Simulate interactions between individual cellular agents (e.g., immune cells, neurons).
- **Constraint-based models:** Used in metabolic network simulation (e.g., Flux Balance Analysis).

In dementia, these methods assist in forecasting the impact of interventions on tau phosphorylation, oxidative stress, or neuroinflammation regarding below neuronal survival or synaptic plasticity.

Pathway Crosstalk Analysis and Polypharmacology

Crosstalk refers to the interdependence between biological pathways, where activation or inhibition of one pathway affects another. In neurodegenerative diseases, pathways such as autophagy, apoptosis, mitochondrial dysfunction, and neuroinflammation are highly interconnected. Systems-level analysis can identify key nodes involved in crosstalk, which become strategic targets for multitarget drugs. Consider the following example of crosstalk between pathways in AD:

Table 15.

Pathway Affected	Cross-talking Partner	Mechanistic Interaction
Amyloid-beta pathway	Oxidative stress pathway	Aβ aggregation leads to ROS generation
Tau phosphorylation	Insulin signaling pathway	Tau kinase activation modulated by insulin levels
Neuroinflammation	MAPK signaling pathway	Cytokine production is influenced by the MAPK cascade

By simulating perturbations at shared nodes (e.g., tau kinases, ROS-producing enzymes), researchers can identify optimal points for therapeutic intervention that simultaneously modulate multiple pathological processes. Systems biology allows for the simulation of drug perturbations in these crosstalk scenarios, enabling the identification of therapeutic combinations that exert synergistic effects or avoid adverse interactions.

Table 16.

Pathway 1	Pathway 2	Crosstalk Impact
PI3K/Akt	MAPK	Balances survival vs. apoptosis signals
Nrf2/ARE	NF-κB	Antioxidant and inflammatory response regulation
Wnt	GSK-3β	Affects tau phosphorylation and synaptic plasticity
mTOR	Autophagy	Modulates the clearance of protein aggregates

Case Example: Systems Simulation in Alzheimer's Disease

In Alzheimer's, drugs targeting β-secretase (BACE1) to reduce amyloid-beta levels must also consider downstream effects on tau protein phosphorylation and neuroinflammation. A systems model incorporating: Amyloid cascade, Tau hyperphosphorylation, Microglial activation, and Synaptic dysfunction can simulate how BACE1 inhibition, GSK-3β modulation, and anti-inflammatory interventions interact within the disease network. Such models help design multi-modal drugs or drug combinations with enhanced efficacy and reduced toxicity, (Gelemanović, 2023; Rollo et al., 2023; Shaheen & Melnik, 2025; Zhang et al., 2024).

Integration with AI/ML

The integration of ML and systems biology enables a feedback loop where ML models inform network parameters and network simulation results refine feature selection and target prioritization. For instance, ML can identify novel compounds predicted to inhibit tau kinases, and systems biology can simulate the systemic impact of these inhibitors within the AD pathway network.

This hybrid modeling approach enhances drug discovery in several ways:

- Increases confidence in predicted drug effects
- Reduces off-target risks
- Enables rational design of multi-target ligands

As more multi-omics data (e.g., transcriptomics, proteomics, metabolomics) become available, systems biology models become increasingly accurate, and AI/ML algorithms can incorporate these datasets to enhance prediction accuracy. The integration of AI/ML with systems biology represents a powerful, holistic approach to multi-target drug discovery for neurodegenerative disorders. Machine learning excels in high-throughput, data-driven prediction of ligand properties and activities, while systems biology provides a mechanistic understanding of how these ligands interact within the complex cellular environment. Together, they form a synergistic framework that accelerates the identification, validation, and optimization of multi-target ligands with enhanced therapeutic potential. Computational tools become more sophisticated and data availability improves; this integrated strategy is poised to play a central role in developing the next generation of neurodegenerative therapeutics. AI/ML and systems biology are increasingly being integrated into hybrid modeling frameworks. For instance, the learning algorithm can be used to predict drug-target interactions and generate perturbation data. These predictions are then

fed into dynamic systems biology models to simulate long-term effects. Simulation outputs (e.g., time series of protein expression) can be used to generate new ML features for phenotype prediction, (Kolodkin et al., 2012; Rollo et al., 2023; Shaheen & Melnik, 2025; Uleman et al., 2023).

CHALLENGES AND FUTURE DIRECTIONS

Despite their potential, the integration of AI/ML and systems biology is not without challenges. The data heterogeneity and quality, inconsistent annotations and missing values in biological datasets has a major challenge in the accurate disease detection and diagnosis. Computational complexity on large-scale simulations and deep models is resource intensive. Interpretability in deep learning models often act as black boxes, which may be unsuitable for regulatory approval without transparent validation. The advances in cloud computing, explainable AI (XAI), and better data standards (e.g., FAIR principles) are mitigating these challenges. The emergence of digital twin models, which simulate an individual patient's disease progression and drug response, will rely heavily on AI-driven systems biology. Personalized medicine for neurodegenerative diseases will thus become increasingly feasible, (Campillo-Sánchez & Gómez-Sanz, 2016; Rodríguez-Pérez & Bajorath, 2021; Shaheen & Melnik, 2025; Uleman et al., 2023).

In conclusion the integration of AI/ML and systems biology into the drug discovery pipeline represents a paradigm shift, particularly for complex diseases like neurodegeneration. Machine learning enables the efficient prediction of ligand activity, ADMET properties, and polypharmacological profiles, while systems biology offers mechanistic insights into disease processes and therapeutic interventions at the systems level. Together, they provide a comprehensive, data-driven, and mechanistically informed framework for multi-target drug discovery. This interaction has the potential to not only shorten development timelines and reduce failure rates but also usher in a new era of precision medicine tailored to the intricate networks that underlie neurological diseases, (Kumar & Sharma, 2023; Lankadasu et al., 2024; Satti et al., 2024; Sharma & Kumar, 2022).

EXPERIMENTAL VALIDATION CONSIDERATIONS

While computational methods such as virtual screening, QSAR modeling, and molecular docking play a central role in accelerating the identification of multi-target ligands, these in silico predictions must ultimately be validated through robust experimental methods. The process of experimental validation guarantees that drugs that have been computationally chosen to display true biological activity, specificity, and pharmacokinetic qualities when these attributes are tested under physiological settings. When it comes to medication candidates that are intended to treat complicated neurodegenerative illnesses, the validation procedure often consists of a mix of in vitro biochemical assays, cell-based testing, and in vivo investigations conducted on appropriate animal models. This section provides an overview of the most important approaches and factors to take into account while conducting experimental validation of multi-target ligands, with a special emphasis on neurodegenerative applications. The assessment process is broken down into two phases: in vitro and in vivo.

In Vitro Assays for Multi-Target Validation

When it comes to determining whether or whether computational predictions are relevant to biological processes, in vitro experiments are often the first step. Under controlled laboratory circumstances, these tests are aimed to determine whether or not the drug binds to the molecular targets that are supposed to be targeted and whether or not it affects the activity of those targets. Assays conducted in vitro must evaluate the activity of multi-target medications against various proteins either concurrently or sequentially. This is done to ensure that the treatments are effective without causing any off-target harm.

Enzyme Inhibition Assays

For the purpose of verifying small molecule inhibitors, the enzyme inhibition test is one of the most frequent in vitro techniques. By evaluating metrics such as IC_{50} (half-maximal inhibitory concentration) or Ki (inhibition constant), these tests determine whether or not a substance has the capacity to decrease the activity of a certain enzyme(Campillo-Sánchez & Gómez-Sanz, 2016; Johnson et al., 2021; Kasabov et al., 2011; Kolodkin et al., 2012; Tomaskova et al., 2016). Specific enzyme targets that may be useful in the setting of neurodegenerative illnesses include the following:

- **Acetylcholinesterase (AChE):** Associated with cognitive decline in Alzheimer's disease.
- **Monoamine oxidaseB (MAO-B):** Involved in dopaminergic degradation in Parkinson's disease.
- **β-secretase (BACE1):** Key enzyme in amyloid-beta production.
- **GSK-3β and CDK5:** Kinases involved in tau protein phosphorylation.

The basic principle involves incubating the enzyme with its substrate in the presence or absence of the inhibitor and measuring the reaction product using spectrophotometry, fluorescence, or luminescence. In the enzyme inhibition assay is simple and cost effective, the assay performs the high throughput screening. The quantitative and reproducible in nature. Despite some of the advantages the current system has some limitations also. Limitation like the assay may not reflect the cellular environment and lack information on compound permeability or bioavailability in nature.

Binding Affinity Assays

While inhibition assays indicate functional effects, binding assays directly measure the affinity between a ligand and its target, often expressed as the dissociation constant (Kd). These are essential for confirming that a compound interacts with its predicted target at biologically relevant concentrations.

Table 17.

Technique	Principle	Applications
Surface Plasmon Resonance (SPR)	Measures real-time interaction kinetics using light reflection	High sensitivity, useful for small molecule-protein interactions
Isothermal Titration Calorimetry (ITC)	Measures heat released/absorbed during binding	Provides thermodynamic parameters (ΔG, ΔH, ΔS)
Microscale Thermophoresis (MST)	Detects movement of molecules in temperature gradients	Effective with low sample quantities
Differential Scanning Fluorimetry (DSF)	Detects thermal shift in protein stability upon ligand binding	Simple setup, widely used in screening workflows

Common Techniques Include

These assays are particularly useful when confirming dual or triple binding affinity to different targets. For instance, a dual AChE/MAO-B inhibitor can be validated by performing independent binding assays with both enzymes.

Cell-Based Functional Assays. Cell-based assays provide a more physiologically relevant environment, incorporating cell membrane permeability, metabolic stability, and functional response. These assays measure cellular outcomes such as:

- Neurotransmitter levels
- Reactive oxygen species (ROS) production
- Apoptosis markers
- Phosphorylation of specific proteins
- Intracellular calcium signaling

For example, neuroblastoma (e.g., SH-SY5Y), glioblastoma (e.g., U-87 MG), or microglial cell lines (e.g., BV2) can be used to assess compound activity in neural-relevant cellular contexts. In case of multi-target validation, one can use genetically engineered cell lines overexpressing two or more relevant targets to measure poly-pharmacological efficacy simultaneously. Toxicity and Off-Target Screening, the cytotoxicity assays (e.g., MTT, LDH, or ATP-based assays) are crucial to assess the compound's safety at effective concentrations. Moreover, off-target profiling using panels like CEREP or Eurofins safety screen helps to identify undesirable interactions with unrelated proteins such as hERG (cardiotoxicity marker), cytochrome P450 enzymes (drug metabolism), or GPCRs.

In Vivo Studies and Translational Models

While in vitro assays provide essential information, in vivo models are critical for evaluating the pharmacodynamics, pharmacokinetics, and therapeutic potential of candidate compounds in a whole-organism context. This includes understanding how the drug distributes throughout the body, whether it crosses the blood-brain barrier (BBB), its metabolism and excretion pathways, and how it affects disease phenotypes in animal models(Enciu et al., 2011; Nguyen et al., 2021; Sweeney et al., 2019; Tăuţan et al., 2021).

Blood-Brain Barrier (BBB) Penetration Studies

Crossing the BBB is a non-negotiable requirement for any neurotherapeutic agent. The BBB is a highly selective, semipermeable border formed by endothelial cells, astrocyte end-feet, and pericytes, preventing most drugs from entering the central nervous system (CNS). Computational BBB permeability models can predict CNS penetration, but these must be confirmed with empirical data, (Gupta et al., 2020; Heifetz, 2020; Mohan et al., 2021; Sadybekov & Katritch, 2023a; Sweeney et al., 2018; Tautermann, 2020). Methods to assess BBB penetration:

Table 18.

Method	Description	Use Case
In Situ Brain Perfusion	Measures compound uptake in brain tissue directly through perfused vessels	Accurate and quantifiable BBB transport
CSF Sampling	Measures drug concentration in cerebrospinal fluid	Non-invasive but indirect BBB assessment
LC-MS/MS Analysis	High-resolution quantification in brain homogenates	Standard method for pharmacokinetic studies
Imaging (PET/SPECT)	Uses radiolabeled compounds to visualize BBB penetration	Useful for real-time, spatial distribution

Neurotoxicity and Behavioral Studies. Once BBB permeability is confirmed, the next step is to evaluate neurotoxicity and functional outcomes. In vivo neurotoxicity assays monitor signs such as:

- Locomotor activity
- Seizure thresholds
- Changes in body weight or grooming
- Memory and cognitive function using maze tests (e.g., Morris water maze, Y-maze)

Rodent models are commonly used for neurodegenerative research. For example:

Table 19.

Animal Model	Disease Context	Application
5xFAD or APP/PS1 mice	Alzheimer's disease	Amyloid plaque burden, memory tests, synaptic dysfunction
MPTP-treated mice	Parkinson's disease	Dopaminergic neuron loss, motor deficits
SOD1-G93A mice	Amyotrophic Lateral Sclerosis (ALS)	Motor neuron degeneration, survival analysis
Tau P301L or rTg4510 mice	Frontotemporal dementia / Tauopathy	Neurofibrillary tangle formation, cognitive decline

In these models, administration of multi-targeted ligands can be followed by histological and behavioral analysis to assess both biochemical efficacy and functional recovery.

Translational and Humanized Models

The ultimate goal of in vivo validation is translation to human therapy. Traditional animal models do not always recapitulate the human pathophysiology of neurodegenerative diseases. Therefore, the field is gradually shifting towards translationally relevant models, such as:

- Induced pluripotent stem cells (iPSCs) derived from patient cells, differentiated into neurons or glial cells for patient-specific testing.
- Organoids or brain-on-a-chip systems, which replicate 3D architecture, cell-cell interactions, and even microvasculature.
- Humanized mouse models, genetically modified to express human proteins implicated in disease (e.g., human APP, tau, α-synuclein).

These models allow for more accurate evaluation of compound efficacy, target engagement, and toxicity, reducing the translational gap between preclinical and clinical research.

Pharmacokinetic (PK) and Pharmacodynamic (PD) Studies

In addition to efficacy, understanding the drug's behavior over time within the body is essential. Pharmacokinetic parameters such as:

- Tmax (time to peak concentration)
- Cmax (peak concentration)
- AUC (area under the concentration-time curve)
- t1/2 (elimination half-life)

The PK and PD are measured in plasma and brain tissue to determine optimal dosing schedules, bioavailability, and drug accumulation. In contrast, pharmacodynamic investigations are conducted to assess the molecular and cellular reactions that occur as a result of the administration of medication. A decrease in amyloid or tau pathology, a rise in synaptic markers, or a regulation of neuroinflammation are all things that fall under this category. Within the realm of clinical application, experimental validation acts as a crucial link between computer prediction and clinical application. In vivo investigations give insights into pharmacokinetics, BBB permeability, neurotoxicity, and behavioral effects, while in vitro tests provide approaches that are both quick and regulated for confirming the binding and activity of a target. In the context of the development of multi-target ligands for neurodegenerative illnesses, these validation methodologies need to be broadened such that they incorporate action across many disease pathways and numerous targets. The combination of conventional methods with contemporary models, such as neurons produced from induced pluripotent stem cells (iPSCs) and brain organoids, has the potential to improve translational potential and pave the way for individualized neurotherapeutic approaches. In the end, the combination of in silico design and experimental validation serves as the foundation of a drug development process that is rational, efficient, and successful in the treatment of complicated neurological illnesses, (Budd Haeberlein & Harris, 2015; Carvalho et al., 2017; Hou et al., 2019; Migliore & Coppedè, 2002; Ou-Yang et al., 2012; S. Q. Yang et al., 2021).

CONCLUSION

Alzheimer's disease, Parkinson's disease, Huntington's disease, and amyotrophic lateral sclerosis (ALS) are examples of neurodegenerative illnesses that are characterized by complicated molecular pathways that overlap with one another. These mechanisms include many genetic, proteomic, and cellular components. The progressive character of these ailments, the complex nature of their genesis, and the limited efficacy of traditional single-target treatments continue to make them a hard obstacle for modern medicine to overcome. In this environment, multi-target drug development, which is led by in silico techniques, appears as a transformational way to generating therapies that are more effective and that change illness.

A complete computational drug discovery workflow that has been designed for the identification of multi-target ligands in neurodegenerative situations has been detailed in this chapter. Beginning with the pathophysiological basis, we focused on highlighting important molecular targets, including acetylcholinesterase (AChE), b-acetylcholinesterase (BACE1), monoamine oxidase (MAO-B), tau protein, neurotransmitter receptors (NMDA), and α-synuclein. Amyloidogenesis, tau hyperphosphorylation, oxidative stress, and neuroinflammation are all associated with these proteins, which play a crucial role in the processes that cause illness. The shift away from reductionist, single-target methods and toward more comprehensive polypharmacological paradigms is required because of the interdependent functions that they play.

Approaches known as ligand-based drug design (LBDD) and structure-based drug design (SBDD) are both included in the computational workflow. In order to develop predictive models from pre-existing ligand datasets, LBDD makes use of many mathematical methods, such as QSAR modeling and pharmacophore mapping. With SBDD, on the other hand, molecular docking, virtual screening, and binding site analysis are used in order to examine interactions that occur at the interface between the protein and the ligand. Through the reduction of the chemical space and the prioritization of lead compounds with highly anticipated effectiveness, these strategies greatly speed the early stages of drug development that are now underway. In order to exclude candidates that have poor drug-likeness, inadequate pharmacokinetics, or significant safety risks, the ADMET and toxicity prediction models are integrated at an early stage in the pipeline. The permeability of the blood-brain barrier (BBB), hepatotoxicity, cardiotoxicity, and metabolic stability are some of the parameters that are evaluated with the use of platforms such as SwissADME, pkCSM, and ADMETlab. Because of this, late-stage failure rates are decreased, and clinical translatability is improved, which is particularly important for medications that target the central nervous system (CNS).

In identifying promising multi-target ligands, strategies such as data curation, target fishing, network pharmacology, multi-target QSAR, and parallel docking workflows are employed. The use of databases like ChEMBL, ZINC, and PDB, combined with network-based tools like STRING and DisGeNET, supports target prioritization and compound profiling. Multi-label machine learning algorithms enable activity prediction across multiple proteins simultaneously, while consensus docking strategies enhance the accuracy of binding affinity estimations.

Advancing beyond conventional cheminformatics, the author has explored the integration of artificial intelligence (AI) and systems biology. AI/ML methods including Random Forest, XGBoost, and Graph Neural Networks (GNNs) enable high-throughput predictions and feature learning from complex molecular data. These are particularly useful for identifying novel scaffolds with multitarget capabilities. Systems biology offers a mechanistic perspective, enabling

simulation of drug responses across interconnected pathways, such as amyloid-beta, tau phosphorylation, neuroinflammation, oxidative stress, and synaptic dysfunction. Tools like Cytoscape, CellDesigner, and COPASI support simulation, visualization, and dynamic analysis of pathway crosstalk vital for anticipating systemic effects and minimizing adverse outcomes.

Computational predictions must be substantiated by experimental validation. In vitro assays include enzyme inhibition, binding affinity profiling, and cell-based functional studies confirm activity, specificity, and cytotoxicity. In vivo studies, using animal models and advanced imaging techniques, assess blood-brain barrier permeability, pharmacokinetics, neurotoxicity, and behavioral effects. Translational platforms such as iPSC-derived neurons, brain organoids, and humanized mouse models bridge the gap between preclinical and clinical studies, enhancing the relevance and applicability of multi-target drug candidates.

In sum, this chapter has provided a multidimensional framework for the rational in silico identification and experimental validation of multi-target ligands aimed at treating neurodegenerative disorders. The synergy between cheminformatics, AI/ML, systems biology, and translational pharmacology offers a powerful roadmap for discovering next-generation CNS therapeutics. As data grows in volume and precision, and as computational tools continue to evolve, the future of neurodegenerative drug discovery lies in integrated, predictive, and personalized approaches that address the complexity of these devastating diseases with scientific rigor and translational promise.

REFERENCES

Alvarez-Rodríguez, J. M., Zuñiga, R. M., Pelayo, V. M., & Llorens, J. (2019). Challenges and opportunities in the integration of the Systems Engineering process and the AI/ML model lifecycle. *INCOSE International Symposium*, *29*(1), 560–575. DOI: 10.1002/j.2334-5837.2019.00621.x

Armstrong, R., Richard, P., & Armstrong, A. (2020). What causes neurodegenerative disease? *Folia Neuropathologica*, *58*(2), 93–112. DOI: 10.5114/fn.2020.96707 PMID: 32729289

Badria, F. A., De Filippis, B., El-Magd, M. A., Elbadawi, M. M., Hamdi, A., & Elgazar, A. A. (2025). Editorial: Multi-target drug discovery and design for complex health disorders. *Frontiers in Pharmacology*, *16*, 1633600. DOI: 10.3389/fphar.2025.1633600 PMID: 40584615

Ballester, P. J., & Mitchell, J. B. O. (2010). A machine learning approach to predicting protein–ligand binding affinity with applications to molecular docking. *Bioinformatics (Oxford, England)*, *26*(9), 1169–1175. DOI: 10.1093/bioinformatics/btq112 PMID: 20236947

Baloni, P., Funk, C. C., Readhead, B., & Price, N. D. (2021). Systems modeling of metabolic dysregulation in neurodegenerative diseases. *Current Opinion in Pharmacology*, *60*, 59–65. DOI: 10.1016/j.coph.2021.06.012 PMID: 34352486

Berdigaliyev, N., & Aljofan, M. (2020). An overview of drug discovery and development. *Future Medicinal Chemistry*, *12*(10), 939–947. DOI: 10.4155/fmc-2019-0307 PMID: 32270704

Biswas, N., & Chakrabarti, S. (2020). Artificial Intelligence (AI)-Based Systems Biology Approaches in Multi-Omics Data Analysis of Cancer. *Frontiers in Oncology*, *10*, 588221. DOI: 10.3389/fonc.2020.588221 PMID: 33154949

Boyles, F., Deane, C. M., & Morris, G. M. (2020). Learning from the ligand: Using ligand-based features to improve binding affinity prediction. *Bioinformatics (Oxford, England)*, *36*(3), 758–764. DOI: 10.1093/bioinformatics/btz665 PMID: 31598630

Budd Haeberlein, S. L., & Harris, T. J. R. (2015). Promising Targets for the Treatment of Neurodegenerative Diseases. *Clinical Pharmacology and Therapeutics*, *98*(5), 492–501. DOI: 10.1002/cpt.195 PMID: 26250447

Campillo-Sánchez, P., & Gómez-Sanz, J. (2016). Modelling and Simulation of Alzheimer's Disease Scenarios. *Procedia Computer Science*, *83*, 353–360. DOI: 10.1016/j.procs.2016.04.136

Carvalho, D., Paulino, M., Polticelli, F., Arredondo, F., Williams, R. J., & Abin-Carriquiry, J. A. (2017). Structural evidence of quercetin multi-target bioactivity: A reverse virtual screening strategy. *European Journal of Pharmaceutical Sciences*, *106*, 393–403. DOI: 10.1016/j.ejps.2017.06.028 PMID: 28636950

Cavalli, A., Bolognesi, M. L., Mìnarini, A., Rosini, M., Tumiatti, V., Recanatini, M., & Melchiorre, C. (2008). Multi-target-directed ligands to combat neurodegenerative diseases. *Journal of Medicinal Chemistry*, *51*(3), 347–372. DOI: 10.1021/jm7009364 PMID: 18181565

Choubey, J., Choudhari, J. K., & Sahariah, B. P. (2025). Future directions on systems biology. *Systems Biology and In-Depth Applications for Unlocking Diseases: Principles, Tools, and Application to Disease*, 319–328. DOI: 10.1016/B978-0-443-22326-6.00025-0

Cichońska, A., Ravikumar, B., & Rahman, R. (2024). AI for targeted polypharmacology: The next frontier in drug discovery. *Current Opinion in Structural Biology, 84*, 102771. DOI: 10.1016/j.sbi.2023.102771 PMID: 38215530

Cummings, J. (2017). Disease modification and Neuroprotection in neurodegenerative disorders. *Translational Neurodegeneration, 6*(1), 1–7. DOI: 10.1186/s40035-017-0096-2 PMID: 29021896

Dar, K. B., Bhat, A. H., Amin, S., Reshi, B. A., Zargar, M. A., Masood, A., & Ganie, S. A. (2020). Elucidating Critical Proteinopathic Mechanisms and Potential Drug Targets in Neurodegeneration. *Cellular and Molecular Neurobiology, 40*(3), 313–345. DOI: 10.1007/s10571-019-00741-0 PMID: 31584139

de la Fuente, A. G., Pelucchi, S., Mertens, J., Di Luca, M., Mauceri, D., & Marcello, E. (2023). Novel therapeutic approaches to target neurodegeneration. *British Journal of Pharmacology, 180*(13), 1651–1673. DOI: 10.1111/bph.16078 PMID: 36965025

De Pedro-Cuesta, J., Rábano, A., Martínez-Martín, P., Ruiz-Tovar, M., Alcalde-Cabero, E., Almazán-Isla, J., Avellanal, F., & Calero, M. (2015). Comparative Incidence of Conformational, Neurodegenerative Disorders. *PLoS One, 10*(9), e0137342. DOI: 10.1371/journal.pone.0137342 PMID: 26335347

Ellingson, S. R., Davis, B., & Allen, J. (2020). Machine learning and ligand binding predictions: A review of data, methods, and obstacles. *Biochimica et Biophysica Acta (BBA) -. Biochimica et Biophysica Acta. G, General Subjects, 1864*(6), 129545. DOI: 10.1016/j.bbagen.2020.129545 PMID: 32057823

Enciu, A. M., Nicolescu, M. I., Manole, C. G., Mureşanu, D. F., Popescu, L. M., & Popescu, B. O. (2011). Neuroregeneration in neurodegenerative disorders. *BMC Neurology, 11*(1), 1–7. DOI: 10.1186/1471-2377-11-75 PMID: 21699711

Gelemanović, A. (2023). Using AI/ML to transform molecular biology databases. *4th Belgrade Bioinformatics Conference, 4*(14), 9–9. https://imagine.imgge.bg.ac.rs/handle/123456789/1944

Gupta, P. P., Bastikar, V. A., Bastikar, A., Chhajed, S. S., & Pathade, P. A. (2020). Computational Screening Techniques for Lead Design and Development. *Computer-Aided Drug Design*, 187–222. DOI: 10.1007/978-981-15-6815-2_9

Harrington, J. S., Ryter, S. W., Plataki, M., Price, D. R., & Choi, A. M. K. (2023). MITOCHONDRIA IN HEALTH, DISEASE, AND AGING. *Physiological Reviews, 103*(4), 2349–2422. DOI: 10.1152/physrev.00058.2021 PMID: 37021870

Heck, G. S., Pintro, V. O., Pereira, R. R., de Ávila, M. B., Levin, N. M. B., & de Azevedo, W. F. (2017). Supervised Machine Learning Methods Applied to Predict Ligand- Binding Affinity. *Current Medicinal Chemistry, 24*(23), 2459–2470. DOI: 10.2174/092986732466617062309250 3 PMID: 28641555

Heifetz, A. (Ed.). (2020). *Quantum Mechanics in Drug Discovery. 2114*. DOI: 10.1007/978-1-0716-0282-9

Hou, Y., Dan, X., Babbar, M., Wei, Y., Hasselbalch, S. G., Croteau, D. L., & Bohr, V. A. (2019). Ageing as a risk factor for neurodegenerative disease. *Nature Reviews. Neurology, 15*(10), 565–581. DOI: 10.1038/s41582-019-0244-7 PMID: 31501588

Ji, B., He, X., Zhai, J., Zhang, Y., Man, V. H., & Wang, J. (2021). Machine learning on ligand-residue interaction profiles to significantly improve binding affinity prediction. *Briefings in Bioinformatics, 22*(5), 1–14. DOI: 10.1093/bib/bbab054 PMID: 33758923

Johnson, A. M., Dudek, J. M., Edwards, D. K., Myers, T. A., Joseph, P., Laffin, J. J., & Bruinsma, J. J. (2021). Analytical validation of a novel multi-target blood-based test to detect hepatocellular carcinoma. *Expert Review of Molecular Diagnostics, 21*(11), 1245–1252. DOI: 10.1080/14737159.2021.1981290 PMID: 34581651

Josephs, K. A., Ahlskog, J. E., Parisi, J. E., Boeve, B. F., Crum, B. A., Giannini, C., & Petersen, R. C. (2009). Rapidly progressive neurodegenerative dementias. *Archives of Neurology, 66*(2), 201–207. DOI: 10.1001/archneurol.2008.534 PMID: 19204156

Kasabov, N., Schliebs, R., & Kojima, H. (2011). Probabilistic computational neurogenetic modeling: From cognitive systems to alzheimer's disease. *IEEE Transactions on Autonomous Mental Development, 3*(4), 300–311. DOI: 10.1109/TAMD.2011.2159839

Khanna, I. (2012). Drug discovery in pharmaceutical industry: Productivity challenges and trends. *Drug Discovery Today, 17*(19–20), 1088–1102. DOI: 10.1016/j.drudis.2012.05.007 PMID: 22627006

Kolodkin, A., Simeonidis, E., Balling, R., & Westerhoff, H. V. (2012). Understanding complexity in neurodegenerative diseases: In silico reconstruction of emergence. *Frontiers in Physiology, 3*(JUL), 25275. DOI: 10.3389/fphys.2012.00291 PMID: 22934043

Kovacs, G. G. (2018). Concepts and classification of neurodegenerative diseases. *Handbook of Clinical Neurology, 145*, 301–307. DOI: 10.1016/B978-0-12-802395-2.00021-3 PMID: 28987178

Kumar, R., & Sharma, A. (2023). Computational strategies and tools for protein tertiary structure prediction. *Basic Biotechniques for Bioprocess and Bioentrepreneurship*, 225–242. DOI: 10.1016/B978-0-12-816109-8.00015-5

Lankadasu, N. V. Y., Pesarlanka, D. B., Sharma, A., Sharma, S., & Gochhait, S. (2024). Skin Cancer Classification Using a Convolutional Neural Network: An Exploration into Deep Learning. *2024 ASU International Conference in Emerging Technologies for Sustainability and Intelligent Systems, ICETSIS 2024*, 1047–1052. DOI: 10.1109/ICETSIS61505.2024.10459368

Lavé, T., Parrott, N., Grimm, H. P., Fleury, A., & Reddy, M. (2007). Challenges and opportunities with modelling and simulation in drug discovery and drug development. *Xenobiotica, 37*(10–11), 1295–1310. DOI: 10.1080/00498250701534885 PMID: 17968746

Levy, G. (2007). The relationship of Parkinson disease with aging. *Archives of Neurology, 64*(9), 1242–1246. DOI: 10.1001/archneur.64.9.1242 PMID: 17846263

Liu, X., Zhu, F., & Ma, H., X., Shi, Z., Y. Yang, S., Q. Wei, Y., & Z. Chen, Y. (. (2013). Predicting Targeted Polypharmacology for Drug Repositioning and Multi- Target Drug Discovery. *Current Medicinal Chemistry*, *20*(13), 1646–1661. DOI: 10.2174/0929867311320130005 PMID: 23410165

Lo, Y. C., Rensi, S. E., Torng, W., & Altman, R. B. (2018). Machine learning in chemoinformatics and drug discovery. *Drug Discovery Today*, *23*(8), 1538–1546. DOI: 10.1016/j.drudis.2018.05.010 PMID: 29750902

Migliore, L., & Coppedè, F. (2002). Genetic and environmental factors in cancer and neurodegenerative diseases. *Mutation Research/Reviews in Mutation Research*, *512*(2–3), 135–153. DOI: 10.1016/S1383-5742(02)00046-7 PMID: 12464348

Mohan, A., Banerjee, S., & Sekar, K. (2021). Role of Advanced Computing in the Drug Discovery Process. *Innovations and Implementations of Computer Aided Drug Discovery Strategies in Rational Drug Design*, 59–90. DOI: 10.1007/978-981-15-8936-2_4

. Nguyen, B., Bix, G., & Yao, Y. (2021). Basal lamina changes in neurodegenerative disorders. *Molecular Neurodegeneration 2021 16:1*, *16*(1), 1–25. DOI: 10.1186/s13024-021-00502-y

Ou-Yang, S. S., Lu, J. Y., Kong, X. Q., Liang, Z. J., Luo, C., & Jiang, H. (2012). Computational drug discovery. *Acta Pharmacologica Sinica*, *33*(9), 1131–1140. DOI: 10.1038/aps.2012.109 PMID: 22922346

Pang, M. H., Kim, Y., Jung, K. W., Cho, S., & Lee, D. H. (2012). A series of case studies: Practical methodology for identifying antinociceptive multi-target drugs. *Drug Discovery Today*, *17*(9–10), 425–434. DOI: 10.1016/j.drudis.2012.01.003 PMID: 22269134

Proctor, C. J., Boche, D., Gray, D. A., & Nicoll, J. A. R. (2013). Investigating Interventions in Alzheimer's Disease with Computer Simulation Models. *PLoS One*, *8*(9), e73631. DOI: 10.1371/journal.pone.0073631 PMID: 24098635

Ramsay, R. R., Majekova, M., Medina, M., & Valoti, M. (2016). Key targets for multi-target ligands designed to combat neurodegeneration. *Frontiers in Neuroscience*, *10*(AUG), 207966. DOI: 10.3389/fnins.2016.00375 PMID: 27597816

Ramsay, R. R., Popovic-Nikolic, M. R., Nikolic, K., Uliassi, E., & Bolognesi, M. L. (2018). A perspective on multi-target drug discovery and design for complex diseases. *Clinical and Translational Medicine*, *7*(1), 1–14. DOI: 10.1186/s40169-017-0181-2 PMID: 29340951

Ravikumar, B., & Aittokallio, T. (2018). Improving the efficacy-safety balance of polypharmacology in multi-target drug discovery. *Expert Opinion on Drug Discovery*, *13*(2), 179–192. DOI: 10.1080/17460441.2018.1413089 PMID: 29233023

Rodríguez-Pérez, R., & Bajorath, J. (2021). Evaluation of multi-target deep neural network models for compound potency prediction under increasingly challenging test conditions. *Journal of Computer-Aided Molecular Design*, *35*(3), 285–295. DOI: 10.1007/s10822-021-00376-8 PMID: 33598870

Rollo, J., Crawford, J., & Hardy, J. (2023). A dynamical systems approach for multiscale synthesis of Alzheimer's pathogenesis. *Neuron, 111*(14), 2126–2139. DOI: 10.1016/j.neuron.2023.04.018 PMID: 37172582

Sadybekov, A. V., & Katritch, V. (2023a). Computational approaches streamlining drug discovery. *Nature, 616*(7958), 673–685. DOI: 10.1038/s41586-023-05905-z PMID: 37100941

Sadybekov, A. V., & Katritch, V. (2023b). Computational approaches streamlining drug discovery. *Nature 2023 616:7958, 616*(7958), 673–685. DOI: 10.1038/s41586-023-05905-z

Satti, S. R., Lankadasu, J. S. K., Sharma, A., Sharma, S., & Gochhait, S. (2024). Deep Learning in Medical Image Diagnosis for COVID-19. *2024 ASU International Conference in Emerging Technologies for Sustainability and Intelligent Systems, ICETSIS 2024*, 1858–1865. DOI: 10.1109/ICETSIS61505.2024.10459430

Shaheen, H., & Melnik, R. (2025). Brain Network Dynamics and Multiscale Modeling of Neurodegenerative Disorders: A Review. *IEEE Access : Practical Innovations, Open Solutions*, *13*, 33074–33100. DOI: 10.1109/ACCESS.2025.3542634

Sharma, A., Guleria, V., & Jaiswal, V. (2022). The Future of Blockchain Technology, Recent Advancement and Challenges. *Studies in Big Data*, *105*, 329–349. DOI: 10.1007/978-3-030-95419-2_15

Sharma, A., Gupta, A., & Jaiswal, V. (2021). Solving Image Processing Critical Problems Using Machine Learning. *Studies in Big Data*, *82*, 213–248. DOI: 10.1007/978-981-15-9492-2_11

Sharma, A., Kala, S., Guleria, V., & Jaiswal, V. (2021). IoT-based data management and systems for public healthcare. *Assistive Technology Intervention in Healthcare*, 189–224. https://doi.org/DOI: 10.1201/9781003207856-13/IOT-BASED-DATA-MANAGEMENT-SYSTEMS-PUBLIC-HEALTHCARE-AJAY-SHARMA-SHASHI-KALA-VANDANA-GULERIA-VARUN-JAISWAL

. Sharma, A., Kala, S., Kumar, A., Sharma, S., Gupta, G., & Jaiswal, V. (2024). Deep Learning in Genomics, Personalized Medicine, and Neurodevelopmental Disorders. *Intelligent Data Analytics for Bioinformatics and Biomedical Systems*, 235–264. https://doi.org/DOI: 10.1002/9781394270910.CH10;SUBPAGE:STRING:ABSTRACT;WEBSITE:WEBSITE:PERICLES;CTYPE:STRING:BOOK

Sharma, A., & Kumar, R. (2022). Recent Advancement and Challenges in Deep Learning, Big Data in Bioinformatics. *Studies in Big Data*, *105*, 251–284. DOI: 10.1007/978-3-030-95419-2_12

Sharma, A., Kumar, R., & Jaiswal, V. (2021). Classification of Heart Disease from MRI Images Using Convolutional Neural Network. *Proceedings of IEEE International Conference on Signal Processing,Computing and Control, 2021-October*, 358–363. DOI: 10.1109/ISPCC53510.2021.9609408

Sharma, A., Pal, T., Naithani, U., Gupta, G., & Jaiswal, V. (2024). Emerging Trends of Big Data in Bioinformatics and Challenges. *Intelligent Data Analytics for Bioinformatics and Biomedical Systems*, 265–290. https://doi.org/DOI: 10.1002/9781394270910.CH11;CSUBTYPE:STRING:EDITED

Smith, J. S., Roitberg, A. E., & Isayev, O. (2018). Transforming Computational Drug Discovery with Machine Learning and AI. *ACS Medicinal Chemistry Letters*, *9*(11), 1065–1069. DOI: 10.1021/acsmedchemlett.8b00437 PMID: 30429945

Sweeney, M. D., Sagare, A. P., & Zlokovic, B. V. (2018). Blood-brain barrier breakdown in Alzheimer disease and other neurodegenerative disorders. *Nature Reviews. Neurology*, *14*(3), 133–150. DOI: 10.1038/nrneurol.2017.188 PMID: 29377008

Sweeney, M. D., Zhao, Z., Montagne, A., Nelson, A. R., & Zlokovic, B. V. (2019). Blood-brain barrier: From physiology to disease and back. *Physiological Reviews*, *99*(1), 21–78. DOI: 10.1152/physrev.00050.2017 PMID: 30280653

Tăuţan, A. M., Ionescu, B., & Santarnecchi, E. (2021). Artificial intelligence in neurodegenerative diseases: A review of available tools with a focus on machine learning techniques. *Artificial Intelligence in Medicine*, *117*, 102081. Advance online publication. DOI: 10.1016/j.artmed.2021.102081 PMID: 34127244

Tautermann, C. S. (2020). Current and Future Challenges in Modern Drug Discovery. *Methods in Molecular Biology (Clifton, N.J.)*, *2114*, 1–17. DOI: 10.1007/978-1-0716-0282-9_1 PMID: 32016883

Tomaskova, H., Kuhnova, J., Cimler, R., Dolezal, O., & Kuca, K. (2016). Prediction of population with Alzheimer's disease in the European Union using a system dynamics model. *Neuropsychiatric Disease and Treatment*, *12*, 1589–1598. DOI: 10.2147/NDT.S107969 PMID: 27418826

Uleman, J. F., Melis, R. J. F., Ntanasi, E., Scarmeas, N., Hoekstra, A. G., Quax, R., & Rikkert, M. G. M. O. (2023). Simulating the multicausality of Alzheimer's disease with system dynamics. *Alzheimer's & Dementia*, *19*(6), 2633–2654. DOI: 10.1002/alz.12923 PMID: 36794757

Van Der Schyf, C. J. (2011). The use of multi-target drugs in the treatment of neurodegenerative diseases. *Expert Review of Clinical Pharmacology*, *4*(3), 293–298. DOI: 10.1586/ecp.11.13 PMID: 22114774

Wang, Y., Xing, J., Xu, Y., Zhou, N., Peng, J., Xiong, Z., Liu, X., Luo, X., Luo, C., Chen, K., Zheng, M., & Jiang, H. (2015). In silico ADME/T modelling for rational drug design. *Quarterly Reviews of Biophysics*, *48*(4), 488–515. DOI: 10.1017/S0033583515000190 PMID: 26328949

Wu, Y., Chen, M., & Jiang, J. (2019). Mitochondrial dysfunction in neurodegenerative diseases and drug targets via apoptotic signaling. *Mitochondrion*, *49*, 35–45. DOI: 10.1016/j.mito.2019.07.003 PMID: 31288090

Yang, S. Q., Ye, Q., Ding, J. J., Ming-Zhu, Y., Lu, A. P., Chen, X., Hou, T. J., & Cao, D. S. (2021). Current advances in ligand-based target prediction. *Wiley Interdisciplinary Reviews. Computational Molecular Science*, *11*(3), e1504. DOI: 10.1002/wcms.1504

Yang, T., Sui, X., Yu, B., Shen, Y., & Cong, H. (2020). Recent Advances in the Rational Drug Design Based on Multi-target Ligands. *Current Medicinal Chemistry*, *27*(28), 4720–4740. DOI: 10.2174/0929867327666200102120652 PMID: 31894741

Zádori, D., Klivényi, P., Plangár, I., Toldi, J., & Vécsei, L. (2011). Endogenous neuroprotection in chronic neurodegenerative disorders: With particular regard to the kynurenines. *Journal of Cellular and Molecular Medicine*, *15*(4), 701–717. DOI: 10.1111/j.1582-4934.2010.01237.x PMID: 21155972

Zhang, Y., Li, S., Meng, K., & Sun, S. (2024). Machine Learning for Sequence and Structure-Based Protein-Ligand Interaction Prediction. *Journal of Chemical Information and Modeling*, *64*(5), 1456–1472. DOI: 10.1021/acs.jcim.3c01841 PMID: 38385768

Zimmermann, G. R., Lehár, J., & Keith, C. T. (2007). Multi-target therapeutics: When the whole is greater than the sum of the parts. *Drug Discovery Today*, *12*(1–2), 34–42. DOI: 10.1016/j.drudis.2006.11.008 PMID: 17198971

Chapter 7
Advancements in Predictive Modeling and Neuromodulation for Disorders of Consciousness:
A Synergistic Approach

Fateha Soobia
https://orcid.org/0009-0006-9399-7090
Taylor's University, Malaysia

Mohsin Qadeer
https://orcid.org/0000-0001-7509-6885
Jinnah Medical and Dental College, Pakistan

ABSTRACT

Disorders of Consciousness (DoC), such as Unresponsive Wakefulness Syndrome (UWS) and the Minimally Conscious State (MCS), have an indelible effect on the patients and their families at very high stakes. Growing evidence shows that neuromodulation, especially deep brain stimulation, has the potential to restore consciousness in some DoC patients. There are efforts to propose an ai predictive model for the condition of coma-like patients undergoing treatment via neuromodulation. The research will center on the centromedian-parafascicular complex of the thalamus, especially when hypoxia or trauma affects one side of the brain more than the other. A longitudinal approach using EEG and neuroimaging methods for preprocessing and data segregation is combined with a GCSVM (Glasgow Coma Scale Support Vector Machine) model for continuous follow-up. AI model detects subtle neurological changes ensures early intervention to prevent the development of irreversible musculoskeletal conditions with related complications.

DOI: 10.4018/979-8-3373-4627-4.ch007

INTRODUCTION

Consciousness is a multifaceted and often ambiguous concept that has sparked passionate debates across multiple disciplines. It is widely believed to arise from reciprocal connections between specialized networks of gray matter within the cortical and subcortical regions of the brain. Absence of an encyclopedic approach to consciousness to address the way these might marry with the basic characteristics has rendered its study challenging and complex (Fischer & Edlow, 2024).

Within the clinical formulation of consciousness, two variables emerge: awareness and arousal. They both have their own neural correlates and specifications. Awareness is the content of consciousness, which can be quantified by clinical measures such as command-following, eye tracking, or responses to stimulation localized to pain. This is a reflection of activity in the large fronto-parietal network and associative cortices, (Kazazian *et.al,* 2024). Arousal, on the other hand, is defined as a state of wakefulness and attentiveness that can be measured by responses, especially the opening of the ocular eyelid, associated primarily with structures in the brainstem and hypothalamus. Remarkably, despite the fact that awareness and arousal are necessary for several physiological states, such as sleep, their intrinsic and functional respects vary greatly (Bodien *et.al*, 2024). For example, REM sleep is associated with the continued presence of internal consciousness, while there is a great suppression of wakefulness; in contrast, in cases involving vegetative states and unresponsive wakefulness syndrome, arousal remains intact, and awareness fails. This dissociation sharply pronounces the disparity in functional connectivity at times, thereby intensifying the need for functional neuropathological explorations, (Zamora *et.al*, 2023).

Patients in a state of VS/UWS–their awareness is, for all intents and purposes, zeroed out and are otherwise referred to as unresponsive wakefulness syndrome–provide an important option for a lesion-based approach to understanding the neural correlates of awareness. Unlike comatose patients, these patients may awaken from nonconsciousness and are valuable in the case of knowledge about the functions of awareness of states. They pose significant diagnostic and prognostic challenges in clinical terms, (Weitzel & Bavishi, 2024).

This review attempts to piece together and extract relevant revelations on (un)consciousness from research exploring all conditions from coma, VS/UWS, and minimally conscious states (MCS) to disorders of consciousness (DoC) following brain injury. In this light, we would like to better understand the neuropathological and clinical complexities surrounding consciousness for the pursuit of more precise diagnostics and therapeutic interventions, (Newcombe, 2024).

LITERATURE SEARCH

The author undertook an extensive electronic search to identify studies that are relevant. The search was exhaustive and included databases such as ClinicalTrials.gov, Evidence Based Medicine Reviews, Scopus, EMBASE, MEDLINE, and henceforth into Web of Science. Specific keywords were used for each type of stimulation-taken into consideration in this investigation-to cover transcranial random noise stimulation (RNS), low-field magnetic therapy (MFMS), electroshock treatment, deep brain stimulation (DBS), and vagal nerve stimulation (VNS). Suicidal behaviors or tendencies, self-inflicted injuries or harm, self-mutilation, and completed suicide

were some other keywords we searched for, so as to deepen our understanding of this issue and refine the selection of appropriate data sources (Lejeune *et.al*, 2024).

STUDY SELECTION AND DATA EXTRACTION

In this research, the PRISMA framework is utilized for the process selection systematically to identify and remove inappropriate and duplicate articles-articles which have been thoroughly reviewed as to them of the inclusion criteria or exclusion ones. It should also be mentioned that this research includes studies addressed on suicide and mainly reported primary-qualified outcomes. Studies reporting transition in the rating scale scores from baseline to the last available follow-up were included in this study, (Cronberg *et.al*, 2021). If there was no agreement between the two primary reviewers on the inclusion or exclusion of studies, a third reviewer (C.P.L.) was called for consensus. The included studies were also screened for further references. The eligibility studies included retrospective studies, open-label trials, and randomized controlled trials. The exclusions were reviews, meta-analyses, case studies, case reports, and congress abstracts. This also includes outcome studies that look at suicide incidence, such as suicidal ideation or event occurrence, rating scales measuring suicidal behavior or ideation, or binary classifications indicating presence or absence of suicidal behavior or ideation, (Gosseries & Laureys, 2022).

How Can the Condition of Disorders of Consciousness (DoC) in Coma Patients Be Investigated, and How Can the trauma State of a Coma Patient Be Identified?

Disorders of Consciousness (DoC) encompass conditions arising from neural system injuries that alter levels of arousal or awareness. As defined by Kondziella et al. [16], DoC includes coma, unresponsive wakefulness syndrome (UWS), and minimally conscious state (MCS), which are classified based on the degree of residual consciousness. Coma patients are completely unconscious, showing no response to external stimuli, including painful sensations. Usually, the coma terminates after a few weeks (Hermann et.al, 2021; Morris and Wong, 2022); Huang *et.al,* 2023). A person in a minimally conscious state (MCS) exhibits sporadic yet reproducible signs of consciousness; for instance, the patient may follow simple commands, track objects with his or her eyes, or respond to specific stimuli. The disorder previously known as vegetative state is in contrast to MCS in that it refers to a condition where an individual is unable to assess self-awareness, interaction with others, or awareness of the environment (Burns and Cervantes-Arslanian 2021; Reimann and Niendorf., 2020). Trauma usually is the cause of both MCS and UWS, as indicated by studies in which non-traumatic brain injuries, including ischemic strokes and cerebral hemorrhages, or acute hypoxia–ischemia due to cardiac arrest are also included (Kondziella *et.al*, 202). The prevalence of UWS in the U.S ranges from 56 to 140 cases per million, while MCS is said to be ten times more prevalent than UWS (Thibaut *et.al*, 2019; Bonanno *et.al*, 2022; Chen *et.al*, 2022). This provides diagnoses, specifically for MCS and UWS, using an essential tool such as the Coma Recovery Scale-Revised (CRS-R). CRS-R, developed by Giacino et al. in (Floel 2014; Formica *et.al,* 2021), is a validated tool that assesses neurobehavioral functions and has proven reliability. In terms of treatment, amantadine is the

drug that usually cures severe central thalamic inhibition. However, drug resistance develops in some of the patients with DoC, (Spindler, 2023).

Advancements in emergency medicine have led to higher survival rates following severe brain trauma, increasing the clinical prevalence of DoC (Fan *et.al*, 2022; Posner *et.al*, 2019). Coma is marked by an absence of eye-opening, voluntary behaviors, and spontaneous or stimulus-induced responses (Bonhomme et.al, 2024). This condition may result from bilateral brain damage or abnormalities in the brainstem-reticular system (Fischer *et al*, 2016). Outcomes from coma vary: some patients may progress to UWS/VS, recover consciousness, or experience brain death. The prognosis depends on factors such as the cause of injury and duration. Traumatic injuries typically have better outcomes compared to non-traumatic ones. For instance, permanent damage in non-traumatic cases usually occurs within three months, whereas for traumatic cases, it takes up to 12 months (Schiff, 2018).

Patients in MCS exhibit minimal awareness and occasional self-recognition behaviors. The MCS population is further divided into subgroups based on behavioral intensity:

- MCS-: Displays limited actions like visual tracking or emotional responses.
- MCS+: Shows intentional behaviors such as command-following or rudimentary communication.

Patients may transition from MCS to full consciousness once they demonstrate functional use of objects or reliable communication (Facco and Tressoldi, 2021; Luppi *et.al,* 2023) While MCS patients generally have better recovery prospects than UWS patients, the temporal limits of irreversible MCS remain uncertain. Differential diagnosis of DoC also requires distinguishing between conditions like Locked-In Syndrome (LIS), which is caused by brainstem lesions affecting corticospinal and corticobulbar pathways. LIS patients lose voluntary muscle control but can communicate through eye movements (Jiang *et.al*, 2023). The diagnosis and management of DoC involve significant ethical and medical challenges, including pain management and end-of-life decisions (Xia *et.al,* 2021). Further research is essential to enhance diagnostic precision and treatment outcomes.

What is the Pathogenesis of DoC, and How Can Cerebral Network Activity Be Restored in Coma Patients Using Neuromodulation Techniques?

Comas result from various types of brain injuries, which can occur in isolation or combination. These injuries include diffuse bihemispheric lesions, bilateral rostral paramedian brainstem lesions, unilateral diencephalon and bilateral brainstem involvement, as well as toxic or metabolic encephalopathies. Such conditions disrupt corticothalamic circuits and their connections with the limbic system and basal ganglia, leading to the suppression of synaptic activity in the cerebral cortex, regardless of etiology. This suppression, known as "disfacilitation," reduces neuronal firing rates due to loss or decreased input to neocortical and thalamic neurons. Disfacilitation involves the blockade of excitatory neurotransmission, potassium leakage, and neuronal hyper-

polarization, causing disorganized, slow cortical-thalamic waveforms (Sadeghihassanabadi *et.al,* 2022; Kazazian *et.al,* 2024).

Recovery from coma involves restoring excitatory neurotransmission within corticocortical, thalamocortical, and thalamostriatal connections. The "mesocircuit model" is central to this recovery, focusing on the anterior forebrain mesocircuit, which includes the frontostriatal connections, central thalamic neurons, and the frontoparietal network. Activation of this network supports the graded return of behavioral responsiveness in disorders of consciousness (DoC).

The anterior forebrain mesocircuit is an eventful structure integrating components like the frontal and prefrontal cortices and the striatopallidal feedback loop for modulating thalamic outflow to the cortex and striatum. It thus ends up being highly vulnerable to trauma-induced injury due to its extensive anatomical connections. The frontoparietal network consists of two subnetworks:

1. The Default Mode Network (DMN), anchored in the posterior cingulate, precuneus, and medial prefrontal cortex, is responsible for internal awareness.
2. The Executive Control Network, anchored in the dorsolateral prefrontal and posterior parietal cortices, manages attention and environmental awareness.

During recovery, metabolic activity and functional connectivity increase within the anterior forebrain mesocircuit and the frontoparietal network. Patients transition through states, from coma to vegetative state/unresponsive wakefulness syndrome (VS/UWS), minimally conscious state (MCS), confusional state, and finally full cognitive recovery. Neuromodulation techniques, such as electrical stimulation of the central thalamus, have shown potential in restoring activity in these networks (Edlow *et.al,* 2022; Janson *et.al,* 2022). Tools like the Coma Recovery Scale-Revised (CRS-R) evaluate motor function and cognitive emergence in patients. In cases of covert cognition, functional MRI (fMRI) and EEG assessments can detect cortical processing in non-behavioral patients. Neuromodulation offers promise in enhancing recovery trajectories by reactivating disrupted neural pathways, improving outcomes for individuals with DoC (Redinbaugh *et.al,* 2022).

How is the Mesocircuit Model Implemented to Aid the Recovery of Consciousness in Coma Patients?

Severe brain injuries leading to a comatose state are characterized by a significant reduction in synaptic background activity. This reduction arises either from focal damage in the paramedian mesodiencephalon (encompassing the central thalamus and rostral brainstem tegmentum) or from widespread neuronal death, dysfunction, or disconnection across the neocortex, striatum, and thalamus. Central thalamic neurons play a pivotal role by integrating the loss of input across multiple brain targets, contributing to widespread disfacilitation of neocortical, striatal, and thalamic neurons.

A reduction in the inhibition of medium spiny neurons in the globus pallidus internal (GPi) actively suppresses central thalamic components, such as the central lateral nucleus (CL). Collectively, these processes downregulate anterior forebrain activity, causing behavioral responses to be limited or fluctuate. The mesocircuit model supports recovery by targeting this network. Direct stimulation of the CL via electrical or optogenetic methods activates the frontal cortex and striatum. This process aligns with observed changes in the corticothalamic system's neuronal

firing patterns, reflected in EEG spatiotemporal dynamics. Additionally, individual neurons' capacity to integrate synaptic information improves under the influence of background synaptic input (Tasserie et.al, 2022; Edlow *et al,* 2019).

However, normalizing resting EEG background activity alone may not fully restore cognitive function. Factors like inadequate resource distribution and the inability to maximize the neocortical neurons' dynamic range also contribute significantly to ongoing deficits. The mesocircuit model, as illustrated in Figure 1 (a sagittal image of a human brain specimen), highlights potential pharmaceutical and non-pharmacological intervention targets. Key components include the pedunculotegmental nucleus (PTg) and the thalamic reticular nucleus (Ret), indicated by blue arrows in the figure. These targets underscore the anatomical and functional basis for therapeutic strategies aimed at restoring consciousness (Danilova, 2022).

Figure 1. Thalamic reticular nucleus

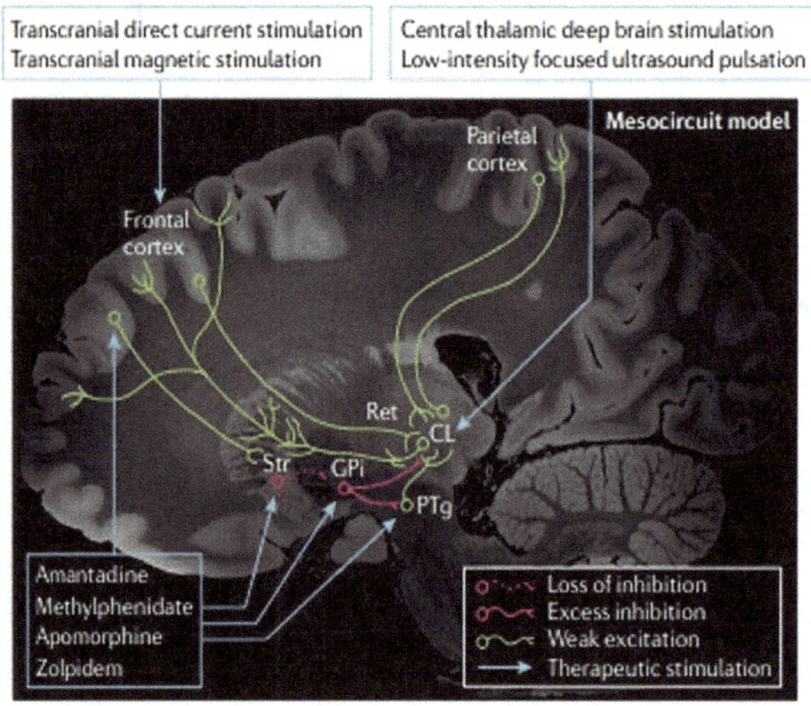

How are Artificial Intelligence Techniques Utilized to Identify the Current Condition of Coma Patients?

Memming Park, during his middle school years, constructed his first artificial neural network at Stony Brook University. His award-winning research, *Personalized Landscape of Unconsciousness*, was driven by his long-standing interest in understanding the brain's functions. Park

credits his conversation with Dr. Charles Mikell at Stony Brook University as a pivotal moment that inspired his research into neurotechnologies and machine learning techniques for analyzing coma patients' brain activity. Mikell had already been using his own data analysis tools to capture signals from the human brain during surgeries, and these brain implants piqued interest as potential therapies for conditions like seizures. "They would notice a specific pattern of brain activity before a seizure occurs and stimulate the brain to stop it," Park explained (Lozano *et.al*, 2019; Chen *et.al,* 2019).

Given the success of these devices for treating neurological conditions and the lack of standard treatment for Coma, Park and Mikell focused on using these brain implants to wake Coma patients. The primary challenge was that each patient's condition is unique, with brain damage and unconsciousness stemming from different causes. According to Park, "Humans are not capable of completing this process; it involves identifying patterns within extremely complex signals." To address this, AI and machine learning play a critical role in Park's research, as they are designed to recognize patterns and extract computational information from brain signals that are interpretable by humans. Beyond silico testing, Park expanded his work to current testing with AI-based algorithms, including studies involving animal research or "mini-brains" (biological cultures), to prepare for human trials. The ultimate goal of Park's work is to demonstrate that these technologies and algorithms can successfully reawaken unconscious patients. A key focus of Park's research is the application of machine learning to model complex systems. Although machine learning is commonly used for predictions, it is also effective in simulating brain activity in response to stimulation. This is particularly important because deep brain stimulation aims to manipulate and enhance the intricate networks of interconnected brain regions. For instance, Krylov et al. used a reinforcement learning model in simulation research to reduce inappropriate synchronous oscillations in degenerating neurons to treat Parkinson's disease. This approach shows promise in tailoring brain stimulation to the unique anatomy of each patient, potentially offering personalized treatments for coma patients (Morais *et.al*, 2023; Craik *et.al*, 2019; Ahmed *et.al,* 2022; Watts *et.al,* 2022).

How Does Deep Brain Stimulation Work to Identify Brain Activity Disorders Using Artificial Intelligence Techniques?

One treatment that modifies brain activity to control symptoms is deep brain stimulation (DBS). The complexity of addressing brain disorders with DBS has led to an investigation into artificial intelligence (AI) methodologies. A branch of AI called "machine learning" utilizes computers to identify patterns in data and has a wide range of applications in the medical field, including clinical decision support, personalized medication, and diagnostic assistance. However, machine learning models often have undetermined decision-making processes. The core of explainable AI (XAI) is to generate interpretable solutions from machine learning models (Bouthour *et.al*, 2019; Pascual-Valdunciel *et.al,* 2022; Krauss *et.al,* 2022).

To enhance a patient's clinical state, DBS involves implanting a device that sends electrical currents into the brain. DBS is generally considered safe and effective for treating a range of neurological and psychiatric conditions. Chronic electrical stimulation changes the cellular and molecular structures of brain circuits responsible for behaviors, though the underlying mechanisms are still being investigated. A key question in DBS research is how to customize neurostimulation to the individual patient. This can be addressed using AI techniques, such as

adjusting stimulation regimens based on machine learning models of brain activity that indicate the stage of sleep. However, there is a distinction between applying machine learning to explain mechanistic properties and to discover functional links. While machine learning can identify patterns of brain activity, it may not reveal the processes behind brain function changes (Brocker *et.al*,2017; Döbrössy *et.al*, 2021)

This study synthesizes current literature and proposes a novel approach—explainable AI—that enables the extraction of knowledge from machine learning models. From a decision-making standpoint, DBS implementation requires optimizing decisions, which AI can assist with. For example, closed-loop DBS systems can use neural activity to identify symptoms and modify stimulation parameters in real-time. These systems might rely on computer models of brain activity to determine how to adjust stimulation and prevent undesirable behaviors, such as tremors, before they occur. This technique of adaptive stimulation changes stimulation parameters based on the difference between intended neural activity and the present neural uproar using a sensor-trigger protocol. One way to go about this is by constructing the pre-trained computer model on stimulation features with the cost function simulating symptoms (Sutton *et.al*, 2020).

An important improvement that AI algorithms very much need in DBS research is the understanding of decision making by a model. One step towards making AI more interpretable in DBS will be the derivation of the reasoning from the decisions made by machine learning algorithms. This way, the understanding of the features that make up the model can be translated for clinicians to share with patients and other colleagues. For instance, PECLIDES is a custom-made clinical decision support system, based on random forests, which diagnoses conditions related to neurology, such as Parkinson's disease, where one of the additional outputs is a list of if-then rules that assist the clinician to understand how the model arrived at its conclusion, in addition to diagnosis. This transparency preserves human oversight, which is beneficial for clinical decision-making. For instance, machine learning algorithms have been used to create models for predicting clinical outcomes after DBS, such as medication dosages and stimulation parameter settings. These models have the potential to show a physician predicted clinical outcomes from different treatment strategies and suggest the best treatment approach to minimize symptoms. However, without explainable AI, the physician may not understand why the model predicted a certain treatment strategy. An explainable approach to AI could extract rules explaining the decision and highlight the key patient factors that influenced the decision (Guidotti *et.al*, 2019).

Figure 2. In two patient groups, the electrodes showed a notable rise in spectral energy after stimulation compared to pre-stimulation. In the R− group, energy increased in the alpha2 and beta1 bands of the F8 electrodes, while the R+ group showed increased energy primarily in the alpha2 and beta1 bands

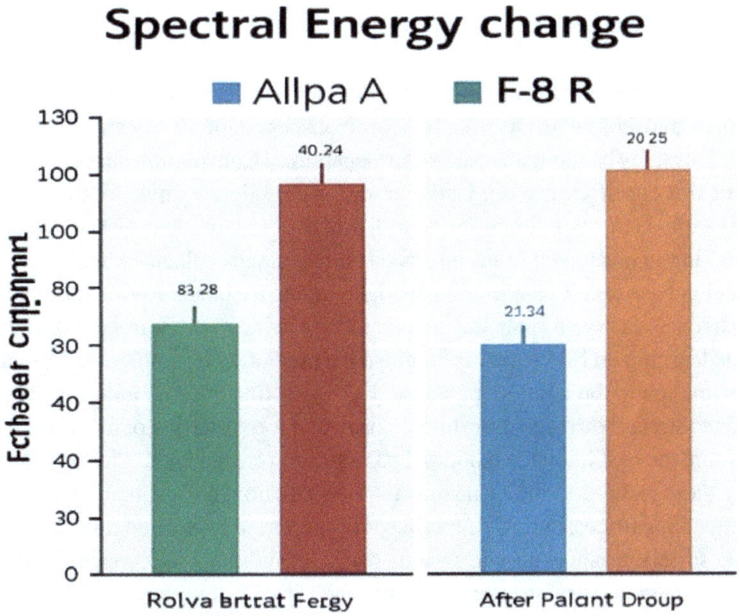

Electroencephalography (EEG) Recording and Processing

In this study, the Nicolet EEG amplifier (Natus Neurology Inc., Middleton, WI, USA) and 32 electrodes from the international standard 10–20 system were used. Before the trial, electrode impedance was kept below 5 kg. A ten-minute EEG recording was taken. Some patients were awake during EEG collection due to the CRS-R arousal stimulation technique applied before the EEG. If the patient closed their eyes for more than a few seconds or exhibited sleep features (such as sleep spindles or K-complex waves), the EEG recording was stopped and the data discarded. The CRS-R awakening technique, including EEG capture, was repeated. No nourishment (parenteral or enteral) was given to patients prior to the 30-minute EEG recording. Offline preprocessing of EEG data was performed using self-programmed scripts and EEGLAB in a MATLAB environment. First, the EEG data were band-pass filtered (0.5–40 Hz) to remove alternating current (AC) noise (50 Hz IF signal), and a notched filter (48–52 Hz) was applied. The data were then re-referred using an average amplitude after reducing the sampling rate to 500 Hz. The EEG signal was divided into five-second epochs. The analysis included complementing bad channels with spherical interpolation and manually removing bad segments. Independent component analysis (ICA) was used to assess the remaining data. These were examined over epochs concerning spectrum, topography, and weights to identify components corresponding to

eye blinks and movements. EEG segments that had a retention rate of 80% or less were deemed to be invalid. In an effort to reduce the volume conduction of EEG signals before the evaluation of their characteristics, current source density (CSD) analysis was performed.

GENERAL DISCUSSION

This paper describes a new, aggressive method for predicting patients who have profound unconsciousness and those with Disorders of Consciousness (DoC) by means of neuromodulation AI modeling. This study has uniquely placed the Generalized Convolution Support Vector Machine (GCSVM) for this specific purpose. Unlike traditional models such as logistic regression and linear regression, which often do not work well when a large number of features are included, prediction making in our model relies on advanced techniques enhancement.

The model is based on 7 whole-brain spatial complexity bands for features and behavioral scale responsiveness factors for labeling to categorize the patient's awareness-threshold. A two-layer machine learning architecture was employed: a prediction evaluation in the outer loop and parameter estimation in the inner loop, whose data separation ensured independence for testing and validation to strengthen result robustness. Through rigorous testing of models and parameters in the inner loop, the best model and optimal parameters were selected. The outer loop was then used to apply these features to independent data for prediction, and evaluation through accuracy metrics, confusion matrices, and AUC metrics was supported by permutation testing with 1000 iterations. These performance measures were critical for judging the proposed model's efficacy.

With respect to model performance, from the analysis, SVM with a linear kernel showed the highest predictive performance compared to Random Forest (RF), Linear Discriminant Analysis (LDA), and K-Nearest Neighbors (KNN). This gave an area under the curve:

Advancements in Non-Invasive Brain Stimulation (NIBS)

The advancement of techniques using Non-Invasive Brain Stimulation (NIBS) has recently shown promise in reflecting their thought therapy on treatment outcomes of patients who are in DoC status. It now includes other modalities like the now-popularized terms TMS (transcranial magnetic stimulation) and tDCS (transcranial direct current stimulation) involving neural activity modulation and providing means for maintaining recovery of neural networks. Based on the neuroplasticity theory anchoring this study, such NIBS could potentially inspire and inhibit many processes related to neural pathways; thus, it may help recovery of consciousness in patients with DoC. Treatment followed by cortical enhancement or inhibition can be performed, based on the frequency and pattern of stimulation, to ameliorate cognitive functions, such as attention and consciousness.

The Role of Arousal Networks in Consciousness Recovery

The connectivity between the frontoparietal network, the anterior forebrain mesocircuit, as well as the ascending arousal system is necessary to explain the possible restoration of consciousness in patients suffering from DoC. In the condition of coma recovery, the lateral thalamic nucleus selectively arouses by concerting action with brainstem arousal nuclei for consciousness. The

research indicates the centrality of such networks for recovery, implying that coactivation of both networks might be pivotal for re-establishing consciousness via consolidation with the ascending arousal network, and they need to continue exploring this idea into specific neural nodes and connections critical to this process.

Limitations of EEG in Restoring Cognitive Function

However, the normalization of resting EEG patterns may suggest a measure of recovery, it does not imply that cognitive restoration is at hand. From the results, it appears that recovery of neocortical neuronal firing patterns-defined through the EEG power spectrum-is critical for interpreting the consciousness level in DoC patients. Indeed, postoperative recovery might not entirely signify cognitive recovery since deficits in resource allocation and inactivation of the full dynamic range of neocortical neurons influence overall function.

AI Systems in Predicting Consciousness Recovery

An interesting instance of prediction of consciousness recovery by AI is reported from the study conducted at the Chinese Academy of Sciences and PLA General Hospital in Beijing. Traumatic brain injury predictive AI system designed for recovery outcome predictability in unconscious patients could show about 90% accuracy. This AI system adopts machine learning algorithms to recognize brain activity patterns, offering new insights into the restoration of consciousness. This study illustrates the increasing use of AI in clinical decision-making for providing prognostic data, influencing interventions among patients with DoC.

Efficacy of HD-tDCS in DOC Treatment

The application of highly-definition transcranial direct current stimulation (HD-tDCS) has been investigated for a period of two weeks in a cohort of 45 patients suffering from disorders of consciousness (DoC) in a study done in China. The positive portion of the results exhibited strong promise for improvements in consciousness recovery through HD-tDCS application with most of the patients improving significantly. It has been done ethically and the evidence of the good outcomes support further credence into NIBS therapies including HD-tDCS for prognostic gain in DoC patients. Therefore, these initial observations serve to fuel the ever-increasing acceptance of NIBS as an effective means of improving recovery of consciousness.

The combination of neuromodulation techniques, such as tDCS, with even more advanced AI models such as GCSVM will, for the first time, be a breakthrough technique in predicting and handling patients with DoC scenarios on profound unconsciousness. Our study now lays a very strong foundation by utilizing whole-brain spatial complexity features along with behavioral responsiveness factors towards improving prognosis in the individual patient. Future research may include looking toward other models and optimizing treatment protocols for the patients. The applications of AI within clinical practice will take great wings in improving our comprehension and management of DoC, promising better recovery and rehabilitation possibilities.

PROPOSED MODEL FOR COMA PATIENT DIAGNOSIS USING NEUROMODULATION AND DEEP BRAIN STIMULATION TECHNIQUES WITH SEGMENTATION OF EEG AND MRI IMAGES

We utilize Support Vector Machine (SVM) and Electroencephalogram (EEG) to monitor brain activity using neuromodulation techniques. Accuracy and quality are paramount in the medical industry; thus, addressing challenges such as unclear MRI images, irrelevant features, or missing boundaries is critical before applying any image segmentation techniques. To overcome these issues, our proposed method integrates SVM with a graph cut segmentation approach, which filters out noise and irrelevant features from images. We also employ k-means clustering algorithms for storing data across multi-classification zones, addressing SVM's limitation in classifying multiple classes independently.

SVM remains a widely used classification method for image recognition. However, it not only minimizes errors but also actively handles issues related to misclassification during multi-class classification, which is managed through SVM applications connected to diverse image types.

Training Sample Selection and Feature Calculation

SVM selects the training sample images, and their feature vectors are computed. The MRI image pixel points undergo feature vector calculation through SVM to facilitate classification.

Classification using Trained SVM

The trained SVM classifies the image points in the target dataset based on sample points previously selected.

SEGMENTATION AND BRAIN SIGNAL IDENTIFICATION

To segment the image and identify brain signals of coma patients, the next step is to enhance the points of interest in the targeted region. This is achieved by reconstructing EEG and MRI images using neuromodulation techniques, assisted by the graph cut algorithm. The GrabCut segmentation technique is employed for this purpose. GrabCut segments EEG images using a graph-cut algorithm, detecting both edges and regions to create energy functions that minimize and produce segments. The process involves constructing a graph where nodes represent pixels, with two additional special nodes ("sink" and "source") that help separate background from foreground regions in the image.

HISTOGRAM CONSTRUCTION AND SEGMENTATION

The histogram of grayscale EEG images, which have an intensity range of 0–255 per pixel, is constructed with 256 bins, each representing the frequency of pixels with similar intensities in the image. By combining information from both foreground and background, histograms are created to help segment EEG images. This segmentation uses the foreground probability to de-

termine node weights, while source-node probabilities guide decisions within the "background" nodes (Figure 3).

Figure 3. Foreground and Background Histogram Models in EEG Image Segmentation. 3(a): Brain MRIs from patients not eligible for DBS implantation using T1 MPRAGE imaging in the axial plane. 3(b): Patients with DoC caused by intracerebral hemorrhage, showing a significant lesion at the brainstem and thalamus. 3(c): MRI scans showing global ischemic cortical, basal ganglia, and brainstem changes due to cardiac arrest, resulting in DoC cases. 4(d): MRI scans identifying septic embolization causing significant lesions.

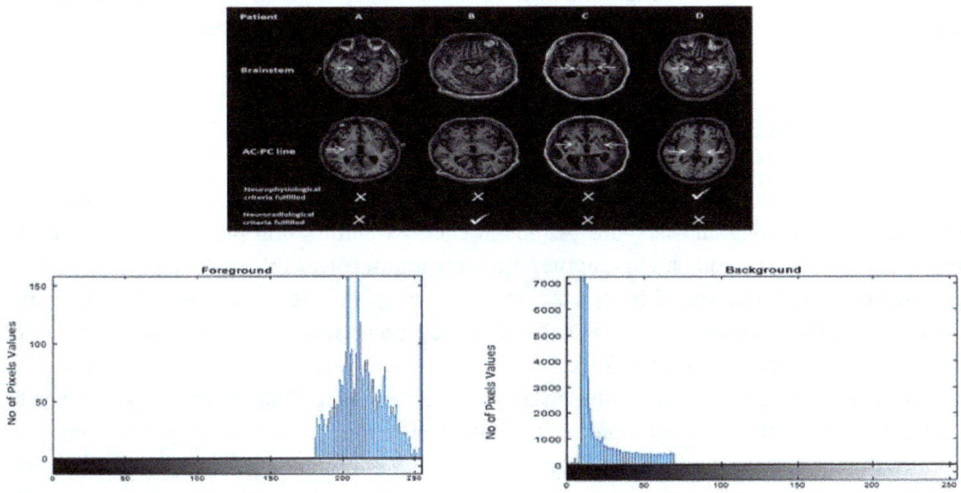

Figure 3 represents the EEG has inherent limitations, including its inability to measure neural activity beneath the brain's surface layers, low signal-to-noise ratios, and the inability to locate drug or neurotransmitter effects. To overcome these challenges and reveal hidden information, we use the foreground and background regions during image labeling with the graph cut algorithm:

Edge Cutting Based on Intensity Difference

The greater the intensity difference between neighboring pixels, the lower the cost, making edge cutting easier. In this manner, edges are cut more efficiently than intensity-coherent regions.

Clue Marking for Pixel Labels

Pixels labeled during the clue-marking stage are never relabeled due to the large constant ensuring high edge weights.

Intensity-based Region Classification

The intensity of an unlabeled pixel determines whether it belongs to the foreground or background based on its position in the histogram. Pixels with high-intensity values are more likely to belong to the background, while low-intensity pixels are associated with the foreground.

The analysis shows that pixels with high intensity values are more likely to appear in the background histogram than in the foreground, resulting in stronger edge weights connecting these pixels to the Sink node. Conversely, low-intensity pixels are more likely to appear in the foreground histogram, resulting in stronger edge weights connecting these pixels to the Source node. Both foreground and background distributions are used to guide the EEG image segmentation process, generating binary labels for foreground and background regions.

SVM AND GRABCUT SEGMENTATION INTEGRATION

The GCSVM method combines the graph cut algorithm with SVM to enhance image resolution during training and labeling. Although energy minimization problems can affect the effectiveness of graph cuts, a min-cut/max-flow algorithm solves this by treating the image as a structured graph. Each pixel is represented as a vertex, and edges link pixels based on similarities with their neighbors. For multi-label images, each label has a unique terminal vertex that assigns pixel probabilities relative to their connection weights. This method allows us to find labelled segmental solutions that maximize the margins of learning algorithms, thereby maximizing classification performance, by cutting at minimum cost. Energy functions were applied to analyze EEG data while maintaining boundary information and improving processing efficiency with. This novel approach meets the segmentation requirements for Coma patients, thus leading to massive improvements on the entire quality of medical image analysis. GCSVM technique uses 2D or 3D features to create hyperplanes that classify various classes of medical images efficiently. Once classified by a binary classifier, appropriate EEG images were further processed to identify their category.

CONCLUSION

The GCSVM technique is a new and novel approach to predicting deep unconsciousness through EEG images classification and neuromodulation-based artificial intelligence. GCSVM, by means of weight matrices and bias for each label, defines hyperplane decision boundaries crucial for effective classification. The improvement in accuracy of the method is a function of improved segmentation and preprocessing techniques employed for EEG-based images. This not only enhances image quality but also gives rise to reduced redundancy and hence energy savings in the segmentation process. The SVM model effectively classifies brain activity in coma patients by accurately calculating the hyperplane distance; thus providing the means for predicting unconscious states in a clinical environment.

ACKNOWLEDGMENTS

This work was supported by the Department of Neurosurgery, Faculty of Surgery, Medicare Cardiac and General Hospital (MCGH)

REFERENCES

Ahmed, I., Jeon, G., & Piccialli, F. (2022). From artificial intelligence to explainable artificial intelligence in Industry 4.0: A survey on what, how, and where. *IEEE Transactions on Industrial Informatics*, *18*(6), 5031–5042. DOI: 10.1109/TII.2022.3146552

Bodien, Y. G., Allanson, J., Cardone, P., Bonhomme, A., Carmona, J., Chatelle, C., Chennu, S., Conte, M., Dehaene, S., Finoia, P., Heinonen, G., Hersh, J. E., Kamau, E., Lawrence, P. K., Lupson, V. C., Meydan, A., Rohaut, B., Sanders, W. R., Sitt, J. D., & Schiff, N. D. (2024). Cognitive motor dissociation in disorders of consciousness. *The New England Journal of Medicine*, *391*(7), 598–608. DOI: 10.1056/NEJMoa2400645 PMID: 39141852

Bonanno, M., De Luca, R., De Nunzio, A. M., Quartarone, A., & Calabro, R. S. (2022). Innovative technologies in the neurorehabilitation of traumatic brain injury: A systematic review. *Brain Sciences*, *12*(12), 1678. DOI: 10.3390/brainsci12121678 PMID: 36552138

Bonhomme, V., Putensen, C., Böttiger, B. W., Stevens, M. F., Marczin, N., Arnal, D., Brotfain, E., Raz, A., Defresne, A., Bogossian, E., Sviri, S., Cardone, P., Mair, A., Robba, C., Dilmen, O. K., Ly, J., Crisan, M. I., De Graaff, J. C., Najafi, N., & Khalifa, C. (2024). Brain health: A concern for anaesthesiologists and intensivists. *European Journal of Anaesthesiology and Intensive Care*, *3*(6), e0063. DOI: 10.1097/EA9.0000000000000063 PMID: 39917635

Bouthour, W., Mégevand, P., Donoghue, J., Lüscher, C., Birbaumer, N., & Krack, P. (2019). Biomarkers for closed-loop deep brain stimulation in Parkinson disease and beyond. *Nature Reviews. Neurology*, *15*(6), 343–352. DOI: 10.1038/s41582-019-0166-4 PMID: 30936569

Brocker, D. T., Swan, B. D., So, R. Q., Turner, D. A., Gross, R. E., & Grill, W. M. (2017). Optimized temporal pattern of brain stimulation designed by computational evolution. *Science Translational Medicine*, *9*(404), eaah3532. DOI: 10.1126/scitranslmed.aah3532 PMID: 28053151

Burns, J. D., & Cervantes-Arslanian, A. M. (Eds.). (2021). *Neurologic Emergencies, An Issue of Neurologic Clinics, E-Book: Neurologic Emergencies, An Issue of Neurologic Clinics, E-Book* (Vol. 39, No. 2). Elsevier Health Sciences.

Chen, J.-M., Chen, Q.-F., Wang, Z.-Y., Chen, Y.-J., Zhang, N.-N., Xu, J.-W., & Ni, J. (2022). Influence of high-frequency repetitive transcranial magnetic stimulation on neurobehavioral and electrophysiology in patients with disorders of consciousness. *Neural Plasticity*, *2022*, 1606542. DOI: 10.1155/2022/7195699 PMID: 36437902

Chen, Y., Gong, C., Hao, H., Guo, Y., Xu, S., Zhang, Y., Yin, G., Cao, X., Yang, A., Meng, F., Ye, J., Liu, H., Zhang, J., Sui, Y., & Li, L. (2019). Automatic sleep stage classification based on subthalamic local field potentials. *IEEE Transactions on Neural Systems and Rehabilitation Engineering*, *27*(1), 118–128. DOI: 10.1109/TNSRE.2018.2890272 PMID: 30605104

Craik, A., He, Y., & Contreras-Vidal, J. L. (2019). Deep learning for electroencephalogram (EEG) classification tasks: A review. *Journal of Neural Engineering*, *16*(3), 031001. DOI: 10.1088/1741-2552/ab0ab5 PMID: 30808014

Cronberg, T., Greer, D. M., Lilja, G., Moulaert, V., Swindell, P., & Rossetti, A. O. (2020). Brain injury after cardiac arrest: From prognostication of comatose patients to rehabilitation. *Lancet Neurology*, *19*(7), 611–622. DOI: 10.1016/S1474-4422(20)30117-4 PMID: 32562686

Danilova, N. N. (2022). Frequency-Selective Generators of Oscillatory Brain Activity as Mapping Structure and Dynamics of Cognitive Processes. In *Russian Cognitive Neuroscience* (pp. 275–296). Brill. DOI: 10.1163/9789004505667_013

Döbrössy, M. D., Ramanathan, C., Ashouri Vajari, D., Tong, Y., Schlaepfer, T., & Coenen, V. A. (2021). Neuromodulation in psychiatric disorders: Experimental and clinical evidence for reward and motivation network deep brain stimulation: Focus on the medial forebrain bundle. *The European Journal of Neuroscience*, *53*(1), 89–113. DOI: 10.1111/ejn.14975 PMID: 32931064

Edlow, B. L., Claassen, J., Schiff, N. D., & Greer, D. M. (2021). Recovery from disorders of consciousness: Mechanisms, prognosis and emerging therapies. *Nature Reviews. Neurology*, *17*(3), 135–156. DOI: 10.1038/s41582-020-00428-x PMID: 33318675

Edlow, B. L., Mareyam, A., Horn, A., Polimeni, J. R., Witzel, T., Tisdall, M. D., Augustinack, J. C., Stockmann, J. P., Diamond, B. R., Stevens, A., Tirrell, L. S., Folkerth, R. D., Wald, L. L., Fischl, B., & van der Kouwe, A. (2019). 7 Tesla MRI of the ex vivo human brain at 100-micron resolution. *Scientific Data*, *6*(1), 244. DOI: 10.1038/s41597-019-0254-8 PMID: 31666530

Facco, E., Fracas, F., & Tressoldi, P. (2021). Moving beyond the concept of altered state of consciousness: The Non-Ordinary Mental Expressions (NOMEs). *Advances in Social Sciences Research Journal*, *8*(3), 615–631. DOI: 10.14738/assrj.83.9935

Fan, J., Zhong, Y., Wang, H., Aierken, N., & He, R. (2022). Repetitive transcranial magnetic stimulation improves consciousness in some patients with disorders of consciousness. *Clinical Rehabilitation*, *36*(7), 916–925. DOI: 10.1177/02692155221089455 PMID: 35322709

Fischer, D., & Edlow, B. L. (2024). Coma prognostication after acute brain injury: A review. *JAMA Neurology*, *81*(4), 405. DOI: 10.1001/jamaneurol.2023.5634 PMID: 38436946

Fischer, D. B., Boes, A. D., Demertzi, A., Evrard, H. C., Laureys, S., Edlow, B. L., Liu, H., Saper, C. B., Pascual-Leone, A., Fox, M. D., & Geerling, J. C. (2016). A human brain network derived from coma-causing brainstem lesions. *Neurology*, *87*(23), 2427–2434. DOI: 10.1212/WNL.0000000000003404 PMID: 27815400

Floel, A. (2014). TDCS-enhanced motor and cognitive function in neurological diseases. *NeuroImage*, *85*, 934–947. DOI: 10.1016/j.neuroimage.2013.05.098 PMID: 23727025

Formica, C., De Salvo, S., Corallo, F., Alagna, A., Logiudice, A. L., Todaro, A., Bramanti, P., & Marino, S. (2021). Role of neurorehabilitative treatment using transcranial magnetic stimulation in disorders of consciousness. *The Journal of International Medical Research*, *49*(2), 0300060520976472. DOI: 10.1177/0300060520976472 PMID: 33535855

Gosseries, O., & Laureys, S. (2022). Severe brain damage: coma and related disorders of consciousness. In *Neuroscience in the 21st Century: From Basic to Clinical* (pp. 3757–3790). Springer International Publishing. DOI: 10.1007/978-3-030-88832-9_95

Guidotti, R., Monreale, A., Ruggieri, S., Turini, F., Giannotti, F., & Pedreschi, D. (2019). A survey of methods for explaining black box models. *ACM Computing Surveys*, *51*(5), 1–42. DOI: 10.1145/3236009

Hermann, B., Sangaré, A., Munoz-Musat, E., Salah, A. B., Perez, P., Valente, M., Faugeras, F., Axelrod, V., Demeret, S., Marois, C., Pyatigorskaya, N., Habert, M.-O., Kas, A., Sitt, J. D., Rohaut, B., & Naccache, L. (2021). Importance, limits and caveats of the use of "disorders of consciousness" to theorize consciousness. *Neuroscience of Consciousness*, *2021*(2), niab048. DOI: 10.1093/nc/niab048 PMID: 35369675

Huang, W., Chen, Q., Liu, J., Liu, L., Tang, J., Zou, M., & Jiang, Q. (2023). Transcranial magnetic stimulation in disorders of consciousness: An update and perspectives. *Aging and Disease*, *14*(4), 1171. PMID: 37163434

Janson, A. P., Baker, J. L., Sani, I., Purpura, K. P., Schiff, N. D., & Butson, C. R. (2021). Selective activation of central thalamic fiber pathway facilitates behavioral performance in healthy non-human primates. *Scientific Reports*, *11*(1), 23054. DOI: 10.1038/s41598-021-02270-7 PMID: 34845232

Jiang, S., Yang, C., Wang, R., & Bao, X. (2023). Resting-state functional connectivity in a non-human primate model of cortical ischemic stroke in area F1. *Magnetic Resonance Imaging*, *104*, 121–128. DOI: 10.1016/j.mri.2023.10.005 PMID: 37844784

Kazazian, K., Edlow, B. L., & Owen, A. M. (2024). Detecting awareness after acute brain injury. *Lancet Neurology*, *23*(8), 836–844. DOI: 10.1016/S1474-4422(24)00209-6 PMID: 39030043

Kazazian, K., Edlow, B. L., & Owen, A. M. (2024). Detecting awareness after acute brain injury. *Lancet Neurology*, *23*(8), 836–844. DOI: 10.1016/S1474-4422(24)00209-6 PMID: 39030043

Kondziella, D., Bender, A., Diserens, K., van Erp, W., Estraneo, A., Formisano, R., Laureys, S., Naccache, L., Ozturk, S., Rohaut, B., Sitt, J. D., Stender, J., Tiainen, M., Rossetti, A. O., Gosseries, O., & Chatelle, C. (2020). European Academy of Neurology guideline on the diagnosis of coma and other disorders of consciousness. *European Journal of Neurology*, *27*(5), 741–756. DOI: 10.1111/ene.14151 PMID: 32090418

Krauss, J. K., Lipsman, N., Aziz, T., Boutet, A., Brown, P., Chang, J. W., Davidson, B., Grill, W. M., Hariz, M. I., Horn, A., Schulder, M., Mammis, A., Tass, P. A., Volkmann, J., & Lozano, A. M. (2021). Technology of deep brain stimulation: Current status and future directions. *Nature Reviews. Neurology*, *17*(2), 75–87. DOI: 10.1038/s41582-020-00426-z PMID: 33244188

Lejeune, N., Fritz, P., Cardone, P., Szymkowicz, E., Vitello, M. M., Martial, C., & Gosseries, O. (2024, April). Exploring the Significance of Cognitive Motor Dissociation on Patient Outcome in Acute Disorders of Consciousness. In *Seminars in Neurology*. Thieme Medical Publishers, Inc. DOI: 10.1055/s-0044-1785507

Lozano, A. M., Lipsman, N., Bergman, H., Brown, P., Chabardes, S., Chang, J. W., Matthews, K., McIntyre, C. C., Schlaepfer, T. E., Schulder, M., Temel, Y., Volkmann, J., & Krauss, J. K. (2019). Deep brain stimulation: Current challenges and future directions. *Nature Reviews. Neurology*, *15*(3), 148–160. DOI: 10.1038/s41582-018-0128-2 PMID: 30683913

Luppi, A. I., Hansen, J. Y., Adapa, R., Carhart-Harris, R. L., Roseman, L., Timmermann, C., Golkowski, D., Ranft, A., Ilg, R., Jordan, D., Bonhomme, V., Vanhaudenhuyse, A., Demertzi, A., Jaquet, O., Bahri, M. A., Alnagger, N. L. N., Cardone, P., Peattie, A. R. D., Manktelow, A. E., & Stamatakis, E. A. (2023). In vivo mapping of pharmacologically induced functional reorganization onto the human brain's neurotransmitter landscape. *Science Advances*, *9*(24), eadf8332. DOI: 10.1126/sciadv.adf8332 PMID: 37315149

Morais, P. L., Rubio-Garrido, P., de Lima, R. M., Córdoba-Claros, A., de Nascimento, E. S.Jr, Cavalcante, J. S., & Clascá, F. (2023). The arousal-related "central thalamus" stimulation site simultaneously innervates multiple high-level frontal and parietal areas. *The Journal of Neuroscience : The Official Journal of the Society for Neuroscience*, *43*(46), 7812–7821. DOI: 10.1523/JNEUROSCI.1216-23.2023 PMID: 37758474

Morris, B., & Wong, J. (2022). A scoping review of treatments for the vegetative and minimally conscious states. *Brain Network and Modulation*, *1*(2), 57–79. DOI: 10.4103/2773-2398.348252

Newcombe, V. (2024). Detection of awareness after brain injury: Time for change. *Lancet Neurology*, *23*(8), 757–759. DOI: 10.1016/S1474-4422(24)00262-X PMID: 39030028

Pascual-Valdunciel, A., Lopo-Martinez, V., Sendra-Arranz, R., Gonzalez-Sanchez, M., Perez-Sanchez, J. R., Grandas, F., Torricelli, D., Moreno, J., Barroso, F. O., Pons, J., & Gutierrez, A. (2022). Prediction of pathological tremor signals using long short-term memory neural networks. *IEEE Journal of Biomedical and Health Informatics*, *26*(12), 5930–5941. Advance online publication. DOI: 10.1109/JBHI.2022.3209316 PMID: 36170410

Posner, J. B., Saper, C. B., Schiff, N. D., & Claassen, J. (2019). *Plum and Posner's Diagnosis and Treatment of Stupor and Coma* (5th ed.). Oxford University Press. DOI: 10.1093/med/9780190208875.001.0001

Redinbaugh, M. J., Afrasiabi, M., Phillips, J. M., Kambi, N. A., Mohanta, S., Raz, A., & Saalmann, Y. B. (2022). Thalamic deep brain stimulation paradigm to reduce consciousness: Cortico-striatal dynamics implicated in mechanisms of consciousness. *PLoS Computational Biology*, *18*(7), e1010294. DOI: 10.1371/journal.pcbi.1010294 PMID: 35816488

Reimann, H. M., & Niendorf, T. (2020). The (un) conscious mouse as a model for human brain functions: Key principles of anesthesia and their impact on translational neuroimaging. *Frontiers in Systems Neuroscience*, *14*, 8. DOI: 10.3389/fnsys.2020.00008 PMID: 32508601

Sadeghihassanabadi, F., Frey, B. M., Backhaus, W., Choe, C. U., Zittel, S., Schön, G., Bönstrup, M., Cheng, B., Thomalla, G., Gerloff, C., & Schulz, R. (2022). Structural cerebellar reserve positively influences outcome after severe stroke. *Brain Communications*, *4*(6), fcac203. DOI: 10.1093/braincomms/fcac203 PMID: 36337341

Schiff, N. D. (2018). Resolving the role of the paramedian thalamus in forebrain arousal mechanisms. *Annals of Neurology*, *84*(6), 812–813. DOI: 10.1002/ana.25378 PMID: 30421449

Spindler, L. (2023). *Where Does it Stem From?-Functional Neuroimaging of Monoaminergic Brainstem Nuclei in Altered States of Consciousness: Translational, Diagnostic and Therapeutic Implications* (Doctoral dissertation).

Sutton, R. T., Pincock, D., Baumgart, D. C., Sadowski, D. C., Fedorak, R. N., & Kroeker, K. I. (2020). An overview of clinical decision support systems: Benefits, risks, and strategies for success. *NPJ Digital Medicine*, *3*(1), 17. DOI: 10.1038/s41746-020-0221-y PMID: 32047862

Tasserie, J., Uhrig, L., Sitt, J. D., Manasova, D., Dupont, M., Dehaene, S., & Jarraya, B. (2022). Deep brain stimulation of the thalamus restores signatures of consciousness in a nonhuman primate model. *Science Advances*, *8*(11), eabl5547. DOI: 10.1126/sciadv.abl5547 PMID: 35302854

Thibaut, A., Schiff, N., Giacino, J., Laureys, S., & Gosseries, O. (2019). Therapeutic interventions in patients with prolonged disorders of consciousness. *Lancet Neurology*, *18*(6), 600–614. DOI: 10.1016/S1474-4422(19)30031-6 PMID: 31003899

Watts, J., Khojandi, A., Shylo, O., & Ramdhani, R. (2020). Machine learning's application in deep brain stimulation for Parkinson's disease: A review. *Brain Sciences*, *11*(8), 809. DOI: 10.3390/brainsci10110809 PMID: 33139614

Weitzel, L., & Bavishi, S. (2024). Disorders of consciousness. *Physical Medicine and Rehabilitation Clinics of North America*, *35*(3), 493–506. DOI: 10.1016/j.pmr.2024.02.003 PMID: 38945646

Xia, C., Zhou, J., Lu, C., Wang, Y., Tang, T., Cai, Y., & Ju, S. (2021). Characterizing diaschisis-related thalamic perfusion and diffusion after middle cerebral artery infarction. *Stroke*, *52*(7), 2319–2327. DOI: 10.1161/STROKEAHA.120.032464 PMID: 33971741

Zamora, E., Chun, K. J., & Zamora, C. (2023). Neuroimaging in Coma, Brain Death, and Related Conditions. *Neurographics*, *13*(3), 190–209. DOI: 10.3174/ng.2200001

Chapter 8
Neurodegeneration Protein Structure: A Promising Catalyst for Drug Targets – Decoding Enzyme Dynamics in Neurodegenerative Pathways

Ashwani Mishra
https://orcid.org/0000-0002-5527-4557
Narsee Monjee Institute of Management Studies, Indore, India

Prashant Tiwari
Dayananda Sagar University, India

Dilpreet Singh
Chandigarh University, India

Sunil Kumar Kadiri
Dayananda Sagar University, India

ABSTRACT

Neurodegenerative diseases affect over 55 million people globally, with 10 million new cases annually. Despite advances in symptom management, curative treatments remain elusive. This chapter explores enzyme-targeted strategies as promising therapeutic avenues, focusing on enzymes involved in oxidative stress, neuroinflammation, protein aggregation, and neurotransmitter metabolism. Integrative modeling techniques like homology modeling, molecular docking, and AlphaFold simulations help visualize enzyme-ligand interactions, aiding rational drug design. Multi-omics data and bioinformatics tools accelerate target validation, highlighting enzymes such as MAO, GSK3β, and ASM for their disease-modifying potential. The chapter advocates a shift from descriptive pathology to precision-targeted interventions, paving the way for next-generation neurodegenerative therapeutics.

DOI: 10.4018/979-8-3373-4627-4.ch008

INTRODUCTION

The loss of neuron is the important and primary feature of neurodegenerative diseases. The two most prevalent and common neurodegenerative illnesses are Parkinson's and Alzheimer's disease. The extremely effective blood–brain barrier nevertheless poses a significant obstacle to the proper management of neurodegeneration, (Davenport 2023) As per the current statistics, around 55 million individuals globally affected with dementia, a severe neurogenerative disease. Out of these affected individuals more than 60% residing in middle-income and low-income nations. Along with it around 10 million new cases reported annually.

Dementia, which is brought on by several kinds of diseases and brain injuries. The most general kind of dementia, which has involvement in 60–70% of cases is Alzheimer's disease. (WHO,2024) It was generally accepted that the primary risk factor for the onset of all neurodegenerative disorders was age, but new research shows that both an individual's genetic composition and environmental circumstances might raise their risk of developing neurodegeneration. According to recent data, over 65 age 5% suffer from Parkinson's. while over 85 up to 30% of the people have Alzheimer's disease. (Shusharina,2023) The two major reason of concerned and sign of neurogenerative disorders are cognitive decline and memory loss brought on by a lack of neural function. Agitation, irritability, and abnormal motor behavior are common signs of neurodegenerative illnesses in various forms of dementia. Alzheimer's along with dementia and Parkinson's disease, in some cases undiagnosed dementia have all been reported to have certain neurogenerative disorder symptoms (Figure 1). Moreover, diverse kinds of dementia were found to exhibit symptoms including disinhibition, apathy, hallucinations, and aberrant hunger, underscoring the range of symptoms throughout behavior and psychological neurodegenerative illnesses. This is now a novel issue in contemporary social and economic life, (Kim, 2020; Derrick, 2015). Neurodegenrative disease has been associated with several factors: (i) accumulation of misfolded amyloidogenic proteins along with tau, another one is α-synuclein, and amyloid-β (Aβ) (ii) dyshomeostasis of metal ions; (iii) deficiency in cholinergic receptors (iv) more reactive oxygen species (ROS)basically responsible for oxidative stress, (Savelieff, 2018; Kalia, 2015; Kayed, 2003).

Figure 1. Major nurodegenerative illness

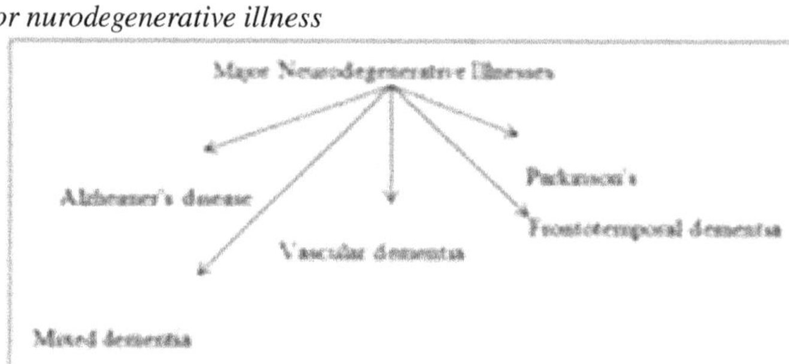

Structural neuroimaging techniques may be used in the diagnosis of NDDs like positron emission tomography (PET). The other effective technique is single-photon emission computed

tomography (SPECT), even computed tomography can be utilized for the same purpose, which are quick new methods. In addition to tomography techniques functional magnetic resonance imaging (fMRI) can be utilized, it is primarily utilized to determine the correlation of numerous physiological processes during NDDs as opposed to direct imaging of neural activities, (Derrick, 2015).

Neurodegenerative disease diagnosis can be made using metabolomics. Alzheimer's disease is indicated by a reduction in the metabolism of fluorodeoxyglucose-PET. Genetic markers connected to established neurodegenerative illnesses can even be used to make the diagnosis. Alzheimer's disease is diagnosed based on a number of characteristics, including presenilin gene mutations, polymorphism, amyloid precursor protein and apolipoprotein E (APOE), (Kayed, 2003).

Therapeutic Strategies

Degenerative diseases currently have no cure, but certain traditional medications like for Alzheimer's cholinesterase inhibitors and levo-dopa for Parkinson's can help relieve symptoms, (Kayed, 2003). Drugs like dopaminergics are utilized to treat movement disorders and Parkinson's disease (Wu, 2006), cognitive disorders can be treated by cholinesterase inhibitors, for the prevention of behavioural and cognitive symptoms in dementia patients' antipsychotic drugs can be used (Tagaris, 2018) and analgesic drugs can treat pain, (Kayed, 2003). Metabolomics can be used to diagnose neurodegenerative diseases. A decrease in fluorodeoxyglucose-PET metabolism is indicative of Alzheimer's disease, (Wilkins, 2018). The diagnosis may even be made using genetic markers linked to known neurodegenerative diseases. Alzheimer's disease can be easily diagnosed based on a number of specific characteristics, including apolipoprotein E (APOE), presenilin gene mutations, amyloid precursor protein, and polymorphism. As an alternative form of therapy, scientists are creating medications that inhibit the progression of illnesses. Examples of these include non-steroidal anti-inflammatory drugs as alternative for the Alzheimer's disease (García, 2018), caffeine A2A receptor antagonists, and CERE-120 for inhibiting the illness and neuroprotection in Parkinson's disease, (Shaw, 2007).

Medicine should be such that, it should only treat the profound symptoms of illnesses but also taking into account all associated symptoms and attempting to enhance the patients' quality of activities of daily living. Enzymes can be targeted in the treatment of disease as nearly every reaction in the human body is catalyzed by enzymes, which are significant protein molecules. Without enzymes, no biological pathway in the human body can function properly, (Desai, 2007).

Enzymatic Targets

Enzymes are incredibly effective biocatalysts that guarantee the smooth operation of every metabolic and biochemical route within the human body. Moreover, enzymes are employed as disease indicators. From a diagnostic perspective, a rise or fall in a particular enzyme level can lead to a medical issue. Enzymes are also important because they play dual role some enzymes are protective and some of them play detrimental role in different neurological diseases. Some enzymes are significantly involved in protective function while some worsen the disease due to aberrations in enzyme expression or protein structure. NADP oxidases are a novel set of pharmacological targets employed in neurodegeneration treatment due to their involvement in producing oxidants and likely regulating microglia activation (Figure 2). The production of hydrogen per-

oxide (H2O2) and superoxide anion (O2•–) is the special role of NOX. Nonetheless, they exhibit contradictory characteristics when considering neuroinflammation, as the NOX mediate production of O2•/H2O2 and/or O2•–/H2O2 based origination of secondary reactive oxygen species ROS which can result in either neuronal oxidative injury or the resolution of inflammation. An essential regulator of ROS generation in the central nervous system is NADPH Oxidase (NOX). In animal models of ALS, NOX inhibition improves survival and slows the course of the disease, (Wilkins, 2018). A NOX inhibitor Apocynin, has been reported to reduce O_2 levels specially in glioblastoma cells of human that express SOD mutant, relieve symptoms, and lengthen treated mice's survival significantly (Stewart, 1997). Nevertheless, these findings could not be repeated in subsequent research, (Marks, 2008). Different NOX inhibitors are Diphenyleneiodonium, GSK2795039, A subset of *N*-substituted phenothiazines, Ebselen, and Celastrol, (Connor, 2006).

Figure 2. Crystal structure 3D of dehydrogenase domain of Cylindrospermum stagnale NADPH-Oxidase 5 (Smallfield, 2017)

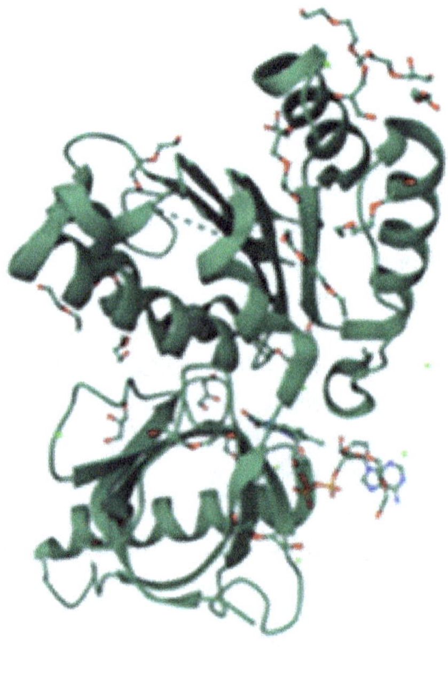

γ-secretase

Loss of neurons and synapses in the brain is one of the causes of neurodegenerative diseases. Senile plaques carry amyloid β-peptide (Aβ) are one of the prominent characteristics of Alzheimer's disease (AD). The proteolytic cleavages of Amyloid precursor protein (APP) through γ-secretase and β-secretase to create Aβ. The hallmark and pathogenic even of Alzheimer's disease

is the polymerization of Aβ into amyloid plaques. γ-secretase has been extensively researched as a possible and promising therapeutic target for the targeting of AD because it causes the final cleavage that liberates Aβ [20]. By binding to presenilin active site, γ-secretase inhibitors prevent γ-secretase cleavage, which lowers the amount of Aβ produced overall. γ-secretase has been extensively studied using γ-secretase inhibitors including L-685, 45835, 115, BrA-1-Bt34, III-31C116, DAPT117, and Merck C57, as well as γ-secretase inhibitors -based chemical probes (Figure 3). A photoaffinity experiment based on γ-secretase inhibitors analysis revealed that less than 14% of PS1 is catalytically active and integrated into active γ-secretase complexes, with the remaining PS1 being part of inactive γ-secretase complexes (Wu,2006). Therefore, it is essential to distinguish enzymatically inactive complexes from active γ-secretase complexes using γ-secretase inhibitors -based chemical probes.

Figure 3. Structure of human gamma-secretase in complex with E2012 and L685458 as 3D CryoEM (Harraz, 2008)

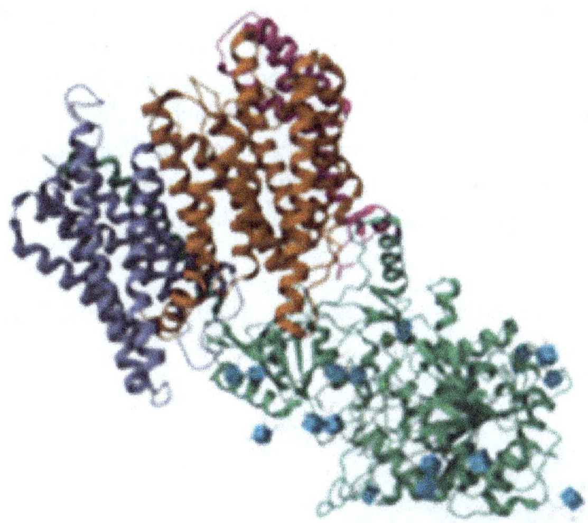

Asparagine endopeptidase (AEP), also known as legumain, is a cysteine protease enzyme that plays a role in protein degradation. AEP is involved in the cleavage of proteins at specific asparagine residues, leading to their fragmentation (Trumbull,2012). In the context of neurodegenerative diseases, including Alzheimer's disease (AD), The processing of amyloid precursor protein (APP) and the production of amyloid beta (Aβ) peptides have been linked to AEP. APP is a transmembrane protein that is cleaved by various proteases to produce Aβ peptides. AEP cleaves APP at specific sites, leading to the generation of Aβ peptides, which can then aggregate to form amyloid plaques, a hallmark pathology of AD, (Silvia, 2017). It is known to cleave Tau, the protein linked with axonal microtubules, and APP, the precursor protein of amyloid, both of them may protect axon regeneration after peripheral nerve injury (PNI). Peripheral nerve injuries contained fragments of APP (APP N585), Tau (Tau N368), and active AEP (Hur, 2022).

However, translating AEP-targeted therapies to clinical trials for AD poses several challenges. One concern is the potential for off-target effects. Furthermore, the blood-brain barrier presents a challenge for delivering AEP-targeted therapies to the brain in sufficient quantities to exert a therapeutic effect. Despite these challenges, AEP remains a promising target for AD therapy, and further research is needed to elucidate its precise role in AD pathogenesis and develop safe and effective AEP-targeted therapies.

ACETYLCHOLINESTERASE (ACHE)

Anti-cholinesterase's, or AChE inhibitors, stop the cholinesterase enzyme from breaking down ACh, increasing the amount and duration of the neurotransmitter effect. Based on how they work, AChE inhibitors can be divided into two classes: irreversible and reversible, (Lai, 2003). Competitive or noncompetitive reversible inhibitors. Reversible Acetylcholinesterase Inhibitors are *Donepezil, Rivastigmine, Galantamine and* Carbamates. *Donepezil* is a reversible, selective AChE inhibitor that attaches to the peripheral anionic site to treat AD symptoms as well as cause-related consequences by delaying the onset of amyloid plaque, (Yang, 2021). *Rivastigmine*is a potent, slowly reversible carbamate inhibitor that binds to the esteratic region of the active site to decrease cholinesterase action. In contrast to donepezil, which blocks AChE specifically (Figure 4). *Galantamine* is an alkaloid that has been extracted from the Galanthus woronowii plant and used to treat mild to moderate AD. It interacts with both the anionic subsite and the aromatic gorge and is a selective, competitive, fast-reversible AChE inhibitor.

Figure 4. Complexed 3D Structure of Torpedo californica acetylcholinesterase with N-piperidinopropyl-galanthamine, (English, 2021)

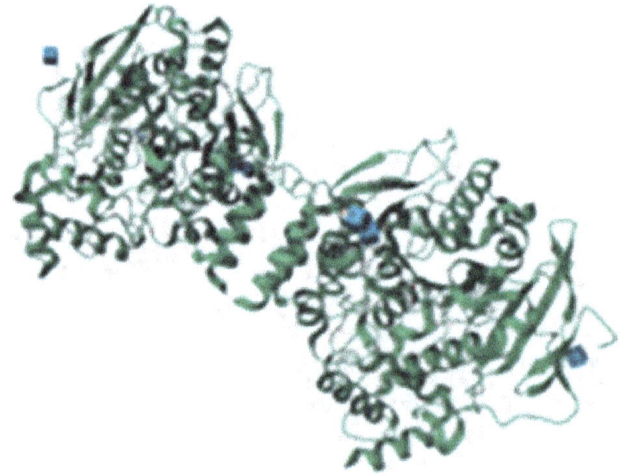

BUTYRYLCHOLINESTERASE (BUCHE)

According to recent research, double acetyl and butyryl cholinesterase inhibitors, often known as butyrylcholinesterase (BuChE) inhibitors, have less adverse effects and a greater ability to treat AD than individual AChE inhibitors (Figure 5) The study of dual target cholinesterase inhibitors has emerged as a new area of interest for anti-AD medications. Acetylcholine levels in the brain decrease as AD progresses due to an increase in cholinesterase activity (Chen,1998). Since cholinergic signaling is crucial for both learning and long-term memory, its disruption has significant ramifications, (Li, 2003; Gleenon, 1999) Because of this pathology, acetylcholine levels are protected by cholinesterase inhibitors, which have been essential in the treatment of Alzheimer's disease. By restoring cholinesterase levels, these inhibitors alleviate symptoms; however, they also increase the amount of time it takes for individuals with the condition to get more intensive care, such as care in a nursing home.

Despite the fact that BChE specific inhibition seems to have prospective benefits for treating AD, doctors are presently unable to take advantage of this distinction because BChE specific medications are not readily available. The FDA has approved four cholinesterase inhibitors—tacrine, rivastigmine, galantamine, and donepezil for the treatment of AD but none of them is BChE specific.

Figure 5. Human butyrylcholinesterase in complex with tacrine (Bartolucci, 2010)

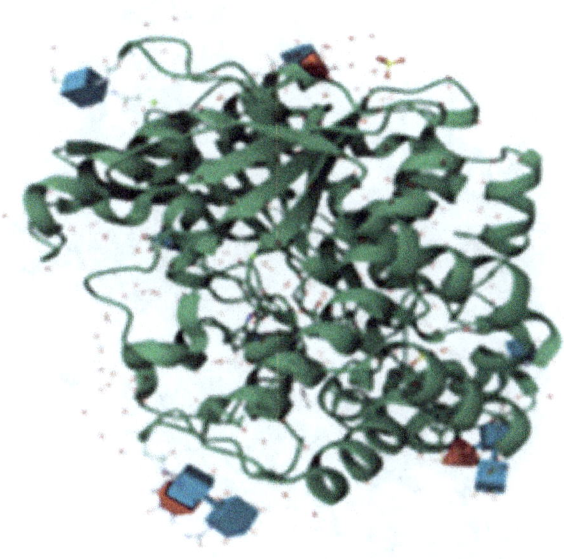

Neprilysin

Neprilysin, also known as neutral endopeptidase (NEP), is an enzyme that has a role in the significant breakdown of various peptides, including amyloid beta (Aβ) peptides (Figure 6). It is a metallopeptidase that is integrally attached to the membrane and has a broad range of substrates and physiological functions, (Kihara, 2004). It is crucial for immunological response, cardiovascular control, fetal development, renal proteolytic processes, and cell proliferation. Amyloid beta peptides are a important feature of Alzheimer's disease, as they accumulate and form plaques in the brain, contributing to neurodegeneration and cognitive decline. Research has shown that neprilysin levels decrease with age, and this drop in levels might be a factor in the build-up of Aβ peptides in the brain, (Woolf, 2006). Therefore, increasing neprilysin activity could potentially enhance the clearance of Aβ peptides and reduce their accumulation, which is a promising approach for the treatment of Alzheimers disease. Several preclinical studies have investigated the use of neprilysin as a specific therapeutic target for Alzheimer's disease. These studies have demonstrated that increasing neprilysin activity through various means, such as gene therapy or pharmacological agents, can lead to the reduction of Aβ peptide levels and amelioration of cognitive deficits in animal models of Alzheimers disease, (Woolf, 1998).

Figure 6. 3D Structure of neprilysin with potent inhibitor

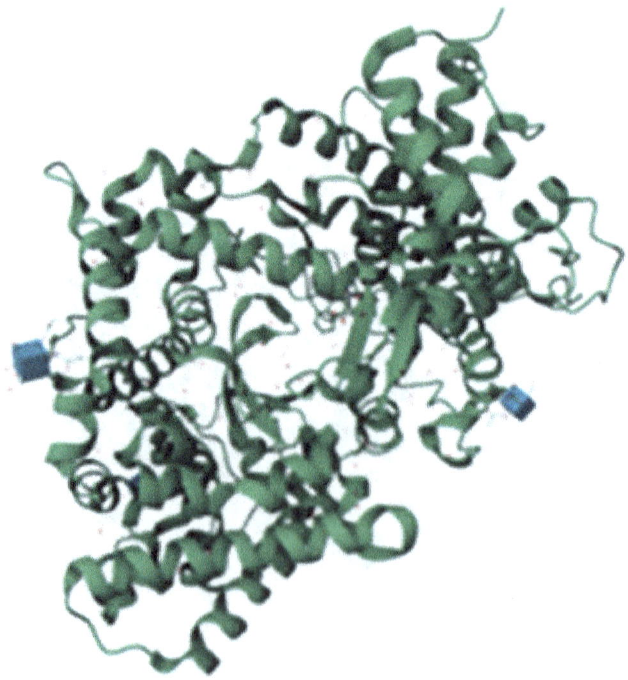

INSULIN-DEGRADING ENZYME (IDE)

IDE stands for insulin-degrading enzyme. It is a zinc metallopeptidase that is majorly used in in the degradation and clearance of different peptides, including insulin and amyloid betapeptides (Figure 7). Because of its involvement in the removal of Aβ peptides, IDE has attracted interest in relation to Alzheimer's disease (AD), (Williams, 2019). The structure of IDE has two relatively equal-sized (~55 kDa) domains that make up IDE are IDE-N and IDE-C.Together, the two parts form a crypt that encloses its substrates and prevents them from leaving or entering, hence the name "crypt forming peptidase." The crypt's volume is roughly 15,700 Å3, and peptides with more than 70 amino acids are not included in it, (Nachon, 2013).

Insulin and Aβ are catabolized by IDE, a metallopeptidase that is zinc-dependent and 113 kDa, (Oefner, 2004; Feygina, 2019). IDE is primarily found in the cytosol. A 28-amino acid loop joins the two IDE domains, IDE-N and IDE-C, that share the same size. Numerous hydrogen bonds between the two domains keep the catalytic site, which is found in IDE-N, closed, (Fang, 2016; Woo, 2009). E111 functions as a base to initiate the hydrolysis of substrates by catalytic water (Nalivaeva, 2020). Aβ peptides are the primary component of amyloid plaques, which are pathological hallmarks of AD. The brain's build-up of Aβ peptides is thought to have an impact in the neurodegeneration and cognitive impairment known as AD. IDE is one of the enzymes responsible for breaking down and clearing Aβ peptides from the brain.

Figure 7. Cryo-EM structure of human insulin degrading enzyme Elife **7s**

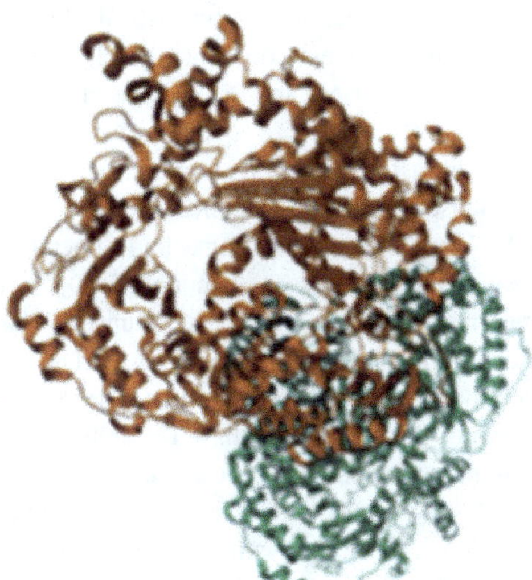

ADAM10

ADAM10, also known as disintegrin and metalloproteinase 10, is a type I transmembrane protein belonging to the ADAM family of proteases. ADAM10 is majorly expressed in different tissues and performs important roles in diverse physiological processes, which includes cell adhesion, proteolysis of cell surface protein and migration, (Tundo, 2017).

After being created in the ER, ADAM10 is transferred to the Golgi where the prodomain is removed to allow for maturation and activation. The developed ADAM10 in the Golgi apparatus is 68 kDa in size, not activated, and still possessing prodomain, (Malito, 2008) ADAM10 has attracted plenty of research in regard to Alzheimer's disease (AD) due to its role in the proteolytic processing for the amyloid precursor protein (APP). Alzheimer's disease characteristic disease, amyloid plaques, develop when amyloid beta (Aβ) peptides, produced by the sequential cleavage of the transmembrane protein APP by proteases, assemble. ADAM10 is one of the proteases involved in the non-amyloidogenic processing of APP. It cleaves APP within the Aβ domain, leading to the release of soluble APPα (sAPPα) and the generation of a smaller, non-toxic fragment. This non-amyloidogenic pathway reduces the production of Aβ peptides, which are neurotoxic and contribute to AD pathology [44] Citrus limon peels (LPE) have an effect on oxidative stress-related enzymes such as superoxide dismutase (SOD), aggregation of Aβ1–40, and key cholinergic and aminergic neurotransmission enzymes such as monoamine oxidases and butyryl cholinesterase. In vitro experiments, Citrus limon peels acts as an enzyme inhibitor on SOD 1/2, MAO-A/B, BuChE, and prevents the aggregation of Aβ1–40 peptides. These findings show that citrus limon peels functions as a multitargeting drug against important Alzheimer's disease and Parkinson's disease components by lowering Aβ-fibril aggregation and inhibiting BuChE, MAOs, and SODs to varying degrees. Consequently, LPE presents a viable option for managing and preventing the symptoms of AD and PD when used in conjunction with pharmaceutical treatments, (Çakir, 2012).

Nicotinamide phosphoribosyltransferase from a structural perspective, NAD+ is made up of an adenosine diphosphate ribose (ADP-ribose) molecule joined to a nicotinamide (NAM) molecule. Intracellular NAD+ levels are essential for cells to operate properly since NAD+ is involved in different types of cellular processes. Although NAD+ levels in cells seem to be rather constant, NAD+ homeostasis is a very dynamic mechanism. A balance between NAD+ production and NAD+ consumption is necessary to maintain NAD+ homeostasis. NAD+ can be oxidized or reduced reversibly during energy metabolism. The variable levels of NAD+ are not caused by this usage. Enzymes that use NAD+ have the ability to alter NAD+ levels, and free NAM and ADP-ribose are the end products of these processes. NAD+ levels are carefully regulated in healthy states, but NAD+ homeostasis can be upset in pathological circumstances, leading to a different issue such as metabolic dysfunction and oxidative stress (Zhang,2018; Endres,2018). Thus, the equilibrium between production and consumption governs NAD+ homeostasis, (Wolfsberg,1995).

NAD+ depletion has been documented in both accelerated and typical aging (Figure 8). A number of diseases that cause rapid aging, including Cockayne syndrome, ataxia telangiectasia, and xeroderma pigmentosum group A, are associated with neurodegeneration. NAD+ reduction has been demonstrated in the brain tissues of mice with AT, XPA, and CS models as well as in C. elegans. Numerous NAD+ augmentation techniques, like therapy with the NAD+ precursors NR or NMN, treatment with a PARP1 inhibitor, or treatment with a SIRT1 activator, enhanced

health and life span in the rapidly aging animal models. These findings are consistent with the significance of NAD+ depletion in neurodegeneration, (Elsworthy, 2022; Arcone, 2023). Additionally, increasing NAD+ boosts bioenergetics and mitochondrial function, which helps in cognitive performance and neuronal survival.

Figure 8. Association of NAD^+ with the ten hallmarks of brain aging

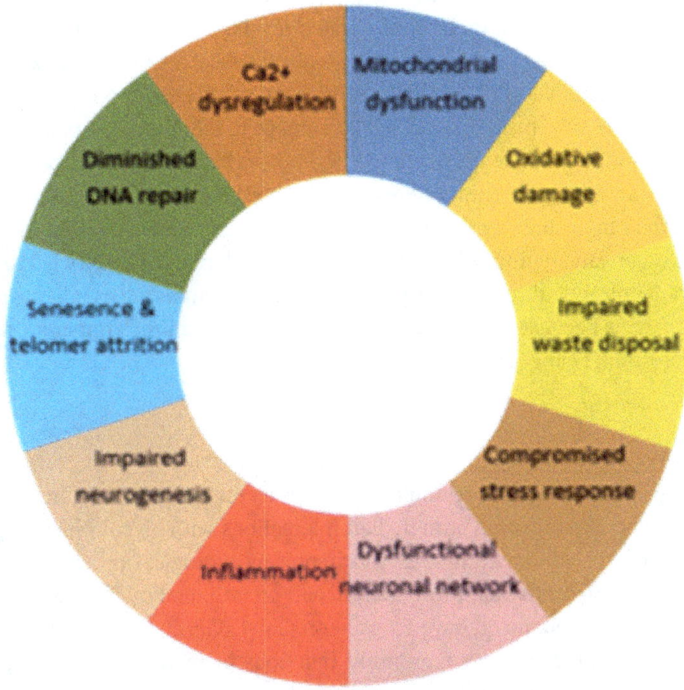

Sestrins were initially discovered to be transcription repressors in yeast, scientists have also discovered that they are present in bacteria and eukaryotes, which includes mammals. The seven members of the family (SIRT1–7) in humans are either deacetylases or mono-ADP ribosyltransferases. Sirtuins are thought to be important for cell metabolism and play a major part in the way that cells respond to a range of stimuli, including oxidative and genotoxic stress. Antioxidant properties have been linked to a number of pathways. The primary process involves peroxiredoxins, which are important enzymes for the safety of antioxidant system. This further degrades living organisms' peroxides. Another vital component alkyl hydroperoxide reductase (AhpD) acts as defense system of bacterial antioxidant, has a redox-active domain that is similar to sestrins. AhpD can catalyze alkyl hydroperoxide reductase C (AhpC) reduction to restore overoxidized bacterial peroxiredoxins, (Rajman, 2018). Preliminary results indicate that pure sestrin2 protein, rather than AhpD, which is a disulfide reductase, ncreases the over-oxidized peroxiredoxin-I ATP-dependent lowering in vitro, revealing that sestrins are none other than cysteine sulfinyl

reductases (Canto,2021). Subsequent research revealed that unlike sulfiredoxin, sestrin2 does not function as a reductase of cysteine sulfinic acid of peroxiredoxins, (Covarrubias,2021).

Sestrins have shown anti-ageing potential, Senescent cells build up in numerous tissues with age, preventing those tissues from functioning properly. Senescent cells strongly influence neighboring cells. Through the secretion of certain cytokines, chemokines, and inflammatory mediators, they alter the microenvironment. One of the reasons for the low-grade inflammation seen in elderly people is this secretory phenotype, which can also promote tumor growth and cause nearby cells to senesce. In addition to their secretory phenotype, senescent cells show a number of other characteristics, including elevated levels of cell cycle inhibitors, granularity, DNA damage, and senescence-associated with β-galactosidase activity. Age-related increases in DNA damage are caused by a decrease in the effectiveness of DNA repair mechanisms. Cellular senescence is believed to be primarily caused by damage to DNA. It is associated with both replicative (Telomeres that are extremely short are thought to be double strand breaks in DNA. and stress-induced (oxidative, genotoxic) senescence. DNA damage is linked to appropriate cellular function, and cells can be adequately protected from its accumulation by effective repair mechanisms. On the other hand, aging-related reductions in DNA repair capacity led to an increase in damage accumulation and, ultimately, cellular senescence. Sirtuins are excellent anti-senescence and anti-aging targets because they are essential for DNA repair, inflammatory regulation, and antioxidant protection, (Fang, 2014).

Galectins

A type of β-galactoside-binding proteins known as lectins, as galactins, are widely expressed practically in all essential organs. Through their interactions with glycolipids and glycoproteins, gals control a range of cellular responses and important biological processes, such as immunological response, differentiation, proliferation, cell growth, and migration. In past few years, some important studies conducted have focused on Gal-1, Gal-3, and Gal-9 gaining particular attention as Gal superfamily. The superfamily functions in regulating neurodegenerative and neuroinflammatory processes have been emphasized.

Numerous studies have connected Gal-1 to neurodegeneration, and Gal-1 expression level differ with different NDs, (Fang, 2016; Budanov, 2009). Compared to healthy control higher levels of Gal-1 observed in neurological disorders patients, (Woo, 2009) Associations between hosts and pathogens, immune system activity, adhesion, tumor suppressor improvement, and signaling are all controlled by the pro-inflammatory cytokine protein Gal-1, (Chen, 2019; Grabowska, 2017). As demonstrated by the expansion of the mouse olfactory bulb neural system, Gal-1 is also essential for the development of sensory neurons during the embryonic stage and neural cord synaptic connections also formed by its help.

It has long been considered that Gal-1, which is a glycan-restricting lectin that is encoded by LGALS1 for human beings, is crucial in regulation of microglia activation, (Li, 2020). Over time, Gal-1 slows neurodegeneration and boosts neuroprotection through promoting M1 microglia deactivation as well as elevating the phenotype of M2 microglia stimulation (Figure 9). Gal-3 levels in brain stalks and spinal cords of ALS patients were found to be substantially greater than those of normal controls, (Bonsack, 2019). Gal-3 has been connected to many different cellular functions, just like fragmentation, apoptosis, immunological response, inflammation, differentiation, and cellular adhesion, (He, 2017; Huflejt, 1993). Research indicates that Gal-3

may have a role in the neurophysiological process of ALS, however ALS patients had around twice as much Gal-3 in their CSF as individuals with other neurological illnesses, like dementia and stroke, (Oefner, 2004). Gal-3 levels in the plasma is further accelerated the ALS progression, suggesting that it might have a neuroprotective impact.

Figure 9. Role of galectins in microglia and astrocyte activation

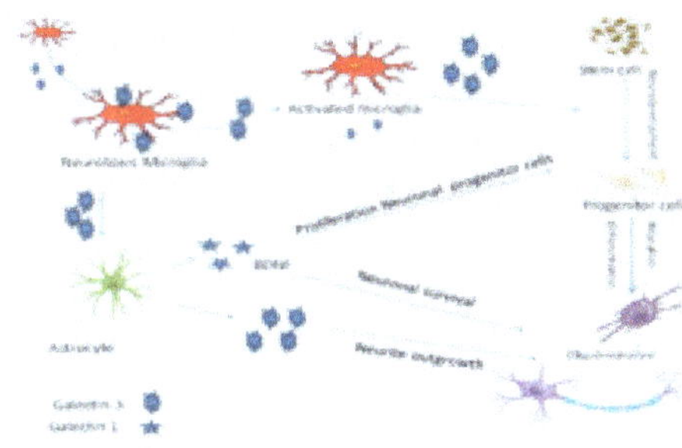

Casein Kinases (CK1, TTBK, CK2)

Protein kinase CK1 is widely expressed It is a member of the constitutively active and second messenger-independent kinases family. Seven isoforms of CK1 (α, β, γ1, γ2, γ3, δ, and ε) and splicing of their alternative variants exist in monomeric form and are encoded by distinct genes (Fulcher,2020). The kinase activity and significantly roles, biochemical characteristics, and subcellular localization of the many CK1 isoforms vary, (Zhang, 1996). The molecular weights of these proteins range from 37 to 51 kDa, with CK1α which is being the smallest and the largest one is CK1γ3(Meggio,1992). Numerous studies have demonstrated the critical function that CK1 plays in NDDs, with a focus on tauopathies like AD. A comparison between AD and healthy brains using a study of distribution of all CK1 isoforms showed that CK1 is present in fibrillar lesions as well as in the matrix consisting of granulovacuolar degeneration bodies, (Ghoshal,1999) Enhanced activity levels of CK1δ (33-fold) and CK1ε (9-fold) have been observed in the brain tissue after post-mortem from Alzheimer patients and Amyotrophic Lateral Sclerosis patients.

CK1α modifies a number of proteins linked to neurological illnesses, including parkin (Mbefo,2015) α-synuclein (Yamamoto, 2005), and β-secretase (Walter, 2001) In a similar vein, it has been found that CK1δ phosphorylates a number of proteins linked to several neurodegenerative disorder in vitro. The tau protein is phosphorylated by CK1δ, which causes it to aggregate and eventually form neurofibrillary tangles, (Baier, 2022) In a similar vein, it has been observed that CK1δ phosphorylates a number of proteins linked to several Neurodegenerative disorders in vitro. The tau protein is phosphorylated by CK1δ, which causes to aggregate and eventually form neurofibrillary tangles, (Li, 2004). Other proteins linked to neurodegenerative disorders, such as TDP43, presenilin-2, β-secretase, LRRK2, parkin, α-synuclein, and tau, have also been exhibited to be phosphorylated in a CK1δ-dependent manner, (De Wit, 2018). Consequently, it has been reported that inhibition of CK1δ/ε has positive impact on Amyotrophic Lateral Sclerosis, Frontotemporal dementia, and Parkinson's disease phenotypes in vivo, (Palomo, 2020).

CONCLUSION

The topic of studying enzyme targets for the prevention of neurodegenerative diseases is active and fast developing. The best targets for treating neurodegenerative disorders include enzymes such as NADP oxidases, γ-secretase, asparagine endopeptidase, acetylcholinesterase (AChE), butyrylcholinesterase (BuChE), neprilysin, insulin-degrading enzyme, ADAM10, citrus limon peel, nicotinamide phosphoribosyl transferase, sestrins, galectins, and casein kinases. Recent advances emphasize the significance of interdisciplinary collaboration, cutting-edge technologies, and translational research efforts in advancing the field towards more effective treatments for these debilitating diseases. They also underscore the vitality of enzymatic modulation as a therapeutic strategy of providing therapeutic benefit.

ACKNOWLEDGEMENT

The authors gratefully acknowledge Dayananda Sagar University for offering the workspace and ongoing support.

AUTHORS' CONTRIBUTION

Prashant Tiwari: Writing – original draft, Investigation, Resources Formal analysis, Ashwani Mishra and Dilpreet Singh: Data curation, Writing – review & editing, Investigation. Sunil Kumar Kadiri: Conceptualization, Supervision Resources, Visualization.

REFERENCES

Arcone, R., D'Errico, A., Nasso, R., Rullo, R., Poli, A., Di Donato, P., & Masullo, M. (2023). Inhibition of enzymes involved in neurodegenerative disorders and Aβ1-40 aggregation by *Citrus limon* peel polyphenol extract. *Molecules*, *28*(17), Article 6332. DOI: 10.3390/molecules28176332

Baier, A., & Szyszka, R. (2022). CK2 and protein kinases of the CK1 superfamily as targets for neurodegenerative disorders. *Frontiers in Molecular Biosciences*, *9*. *Frontiers in Molecular Biosciences*, *916063*, 916063. Advance online publication. DOI: 10.3389/fmolb.2022.916063 PMID: 36275622

Bartolucci, C., Haller, L. A., Jordis, U., Fels, G., & Lamba, D. (2010). Crystal structure of a potent acetylcholinesterase inhibitor. *Journal of Medicinal Chemistry*, *53*(3), 745–751. https://doi.org/DOI: 10.1021/jm901348x

Bonsack, F., & Sukumari-Ramesh, S. (2019). Differential cellular expression of galectin-1 and galectin-3 after intracerebral hemorrhage. *Frontiers in Cellular Neuroscience*, *13*. *Frontiers in Cellular Neuroscience*, *157*, 157. Advance online publication. DOI: 10.3389/fncel.2019.00157 PMID: 31156388

Budanov, A. V., Sablina, A. A., Feinstein, E., Koonin, E. V., & Chumakov, P. M. (2004). Regeneration of peroxiredoxins by p53-regulated sestrins, homologs of bacterial AhpD. *Science*, *304*(5670), 596–600. DOI: 10.1126/science.1095569

Çakir, B., Dağliyan, O., Dağyildiz, E., & others. (2012). Structure based discovery of small molecules to regulate the activity of human insulin degrading enzyme. *PLoS ONE*, *7*(2), Article e31787. DOI: 10.1371/journal.pone.0031787

Canto, C., Menzies, K. J., & Auwerx, J. (2015). NAD+ metabolism and the control of energy homeostasis: A balancing act between mitochondria and the nucleus. *Cell Metabolism*, *22*(1), 31–53. DOI: 10.1016/j.cmet.2015.05.023

Carlos, C. P., Silva, A. A., Gil, C. D., & Oliani, S. M. (2018). Pharmacological treatment with galectin-1 protects against renal ischaemia-reperfusion injury. *Scientific Reports*, *8*(1), Article 9568. DOI: 10.1038/s41598-018-27907-y

Chen, J. M., Dando, P. M., Stevens, R. A., Fortunato, M., & Barrett, A. J. (1998). Cloning and expression of mouse legumain, a lysosomal endopeptidase. *Biochemical Journal*, *335*(Pt 1), 111–117. DOI: 10.1042/bj3350111

Chen, S. D., Yang, J. L., Lin, T. K., & Yang, D. I. (2019). Emerging roles of sestrins in neurodegenerative diseases: Counteracting oxidative stress and beyond. *Journal of Clinical Medicine*, *8*(7), Article 1001. DOI: 10.3390/jcm8071001

Covarrubias, A. J., Perrone, R., Grozio, A., & Verdin, E. (2021). NAD+ metabolism and its roles in cellular processes during ageing. *Nature Reviews Molecular Cell Biology*, *22*(2), 119–141. DOI: 10.1038/s41580-020-00313-x

Davenport, F., Gallacher, J., Kourtzi, Z., Koychev, I., Matthews, P. M., Oxtoby, N. P., Parkes, L. M., Priesemann, V., Rowe, J. B., Smye, S. W., & Zetterberg, H. (2023). Neurodegenerative disease of the brain: A survey of interdisciplinary approaches. *Journal of the Royal Society Interface*, *20*(198), Article 20220406. DOI: 10.1098/rsif.2022.0406

De Wit, T., Baekelandt, V., & Lobbestael, E. (2019). Inhibition of LRRK2 or casein kinase 1 results in LRRK2 protein destabilization. *Molecular Neurobiology*, *56*(7), 5273–5286. https://doi.org/DOI: 10.1007/s12035-018-1449-6

Derrick, J. S., & Lim, M. H. (2015). Tools of the trade: Investigations into design strategies of small molecules to target components in Alzheimer's disease. *ChemBioChem*, *16*(6), 887–898. https://doi.org/DOI: 10.1002/cbic.201402471

Desai, A. K., & Grossberg, G. T. (2005). Diagnosis and treatment of Alzheimer's disease. *Neurology*, *64*(12, Suppl. 3), S34–S39. DOI: 10.1212/WNL.64.12_suppl_3.S34

Elsworthy, R. J., Hill, E. J., Dunleavy, C., & Aldred, S. (2022). The role of ADAM10 in astrocytes: Implications for Alzheimer's disease. *Frontiers in Aging Neuroscience*, *14*. *Frontiers in Aging Neuroscience, 1056507*, 1056507. Advance online publication. DOI: 10.3389/fnagi.2022.1056507 PMID: 36533182

Endres, K., & Deller, R. (2017). Regulation of α-secretase ADAM10 in vitro and in vivo: Genetic, epigenetic, and protein-based mechanisms. *Frontiers in Molecular Neuroscience*, *10*. *Frontiers in Molecular Neuroscience, 56*. Advance online publication. DOI: 10.3389/fnmol.2017.00056 PMID: 28367112

English, A. W., Liu, X., Mistretta, O. C., Ward, P. J., & Ye, K. (2021). Asparagine endopeptidase (δ-secretase), an enzyme implicated in Alzheimer's disease pathology, is an inhibitor of axon regeneration in peripheral nerves. *eNeuro*, *8*(1), Article ENEURO.0155-20.2020. DOI: 10.1523/ENEURO.0155-20.2020

Fang, E. F., Kassahun, H., Croteau, D. L., Scheibye-Knudsen, M., Marosi, K., Lu, H., Shamanna, R. A., Kalyanasundaram, S., Bollineni, R. C., Wilson, M. A., & others. (2016). NAD+ replenishment improves lifespan and healthspan in ataxia telangiectasia models via mitophagy and DNA repair. *Cell Metabolism*, *24*(4), 566–581. DOI: 10.1016/j.cmet.2016.09.004

Fang, E. F., Scheibye-Knudsen, M., Brace, L. E., Kassahun, H., SenGupta, T., Nilsen, H., & Bohr, V. A. (2014). Defective mitophagy in XPA via PARP-1 hyperactivation and NAD+/SIRT1 reduction. *Cell*, *157*(4), 882–896. DOI: 10.1016/j.cell.2014.03.020

Feygina, E. E., Katrukha, A. G., & Semenov, A. G. (2019). Neutral endopeptidase (neprilysin) in therapy and diagnostics: Yin and yang. *Biochemistry (Moscow)*, *84*(11), 1346–1358. https://doi.org/DOI: 10.1134/S0006297919110083

Fulcher, L. J., & Sapkota, G. P. (2020). Functions and regulation of the serine/threonine protein kinase CK1 family: Moving beyond promiscuity. *Biochemical Journal*, *477*(23), 4603–4621. DOI: 10.1042/BCJ20200506

García, J. C., & Bustos, R. H. (2018). The genetic diagnosis of neurodegenerative diseases and therapeutic perspectives. *Brain Sciences*, *8*(12), Article 222. DOI: 10.3390/brainsci8120222

Ghoshal, N., Smiley, J. F., DeMaggio, A. J., Hoekstra, M. F., Cochran, E. J., Binder, L. I., & others. (1999). A new molecular link between the fibrillar and granulovacuolar lesions of Alzheimer's disease. *American Journal of Pathology*, *155*(4), 1163–1172. https://doi.org/DOI: 10.1016/S0002-9440(10)65219-8

Grabowska, W., Sikora, E., & Bielak-Zmijewska, A. (2017). Sirtuins, a promising target in slowing down the ageing process. *Biogerontology*, *18*(4), 447–476. DOI: 10.1007/s10522-017-9685-9

Harraz, M. M., Marden, J. J., Zhou, W., Zhang, Y., Williams, A., Sharov, V. S., Nelson, K., Luo, M., Paulson, H., Schöneich, C., & others. (2008). SOD1 mutations disrupt redox-sensitive Rac regulation of NADPH oxidase in a familial ALS model. *Journal of Clinical Investigation*, *118*(2), 659–670. DOI: 10.1172/JCI34060

He, X. W., Li, W. L., Li, C., Liu, P., Shen, Y. G., Zhu, M., & Jin, X. P. (2017). Serum levels of galectin-1, galectin-3, and galectin-9 are associated with large artery atherosclerotic stroke. *Scientific Reports*, *7*(1), Article 40994. DOI: 10.1038/srep40994

Huflejt, M. E., Turck, C. W., Lindstedt, R., Barondes, S. H., & Leffler, H. (1993). L-29, a soluble lactose-binding lectin, is phosphorylated on serine 6 and serine 12 in vivo and by casein kinase I. *Journal of Biological Chemistry*, *268*(35), 26712–26718. https://doi.org/DOI: 10.1016/S0021-9258(19)74360-4

Hur, J. Y. (2022). γ-Secretase in Alzheimer's disease. *Experimental & Molecular Medicine*, *54*(4), 433–446. DOI: 10.1038/s12276-022-00754-8

Kalia, L. V., & Lang, A. E. (2015). Parkinson's disease. *The Lancet*, *386*(9996), 896–912. DOI: 10.1016/S0140-6736(14)61393-3

Kayed, R., Head, E., Thompson, J. L., & others. (2003). Common structure of soluble amyloid oligomers implies common mechanism of pathogenesis. *Science*, *300*(5618), 486–489. DOI: 10.1126/science.1079469

Kihara, T., & Shimohama, S. (2004). Alzheimer's disease and acetylcholine receptors. *Acta Neurobiologiae Experimentalis*, *64*(1), 99–105.

Kim, N., & Lee, H. J. (2020). Target enzymes considered for the treatment of Alzheimer's disease and Parkinson's disease. *BioMed Research International*, *2020*. *BioMed Research International, 2010728*(1), 2010728. Advance online publication. DOI: 10.1155/2020/2010728 PMID: 33224974

Lai, M. T., & others. (2003). Presenilin-1 and presenilin-2 exhibit distinct yet overlapping gamma-secretase activities. *Journal of Biological Chemistry*, *278*(25), 22475–22481. DOI: 10.1074/jbc.M300974200

Li, D. N., Matthews, S. P., Antoniou, A. N., Mazzeo, D., & Watts, C. (2003). Multistep autoactivation of asparaginyl endopeptidase in vitro and in vivo. *Journal of Biological Chemistry*, *278*(40), 38980–38990. https://doi.org/DOI: 10.1074/jbc.M305383200

Li, G., Yin, H., & Kurent, J. (2004). Casein kinase 1 delta phosphorylates tau and disrupts its binding to microtubules. *Journal of Biological Chemistry*, *279*(16), 15938–15945. https://doi.org/DOI: 10.1074/jbc.M314101200

Li, Y., Chen, N., Wu, C., Lu, Y., Gao, G., Duan, C., Yang, H., & Lu, L. (2020). Galectin-1 attenuates neurodegeneration in Parkinson's disease model by modulating microglial MAPK/IκB/NFκB axis through its carbohydrate-recognition domain. *Brain, Behavior, and Immunity*, *83*, 214–225. DOI: 10.1016/j.bbi.2019.10.015

Malito, E., Hulse, R. E., & Tang, W. J. (2008). Amyloid β-degrading cryptidases: Insulin degrading enzyme, presequence peptidase, and neprilysin. *Cellular and Molecular Life Sciences*, *65*(17), 2574–2585. DOI: 10.1007/s00018-008-8112-4

Marks, W. J., Jr., Ostrem, J. L., Verhagen, L., & others. (2008). Safety and tolerability of intraputaminal delivery of CERE-120 (adeno-associated virus serotype 2–neurturin) to patients with idiopathic Parkinson's disease: An open-label, phase I trial. *The Lancet Neurology*, *7*(5), 400–408. DOI: 10.1016/S1474-4422(08)70065-6

Mbefo, M. K., Fares, M.-B., Paleologou, K., Oueslati, A., Yin, G., Tenreiro, S., & others. (2015). Parkinson disease mutant E46K enhances α-synuclein phosphorylation in mammalian cell lines, in yeast, and in vivo. *Journal of Biological Chemistry*, *290*(15), 9412–9427. DOI: 10.1074/jbc.M114.610774

Mc Gleenon, B. M., Dynan, K. B., & Passmore, A. P. (1999). Acetylcholinesterase inhibitors in Alzheimer's disease. *British Journal of Clinical Pharmacology*, *48*(4), 471–480. DOI: 10.1046/j.1365-2125.1999.00026.x

Meggio, F., Perich, J. W., Marin, O., & Pinna, L. A. (1992). The comparative efficiencies of the Ser(P)-, Thr(P)-, and Tyr(P)-residues as specificity determinants for casein kinase-1. *Biochemical and Biophysical Research Communications*, *182*(3), 1460–1465. https://doi.org/DOI: 10.1016/0006-291X(92)91864-9

Mizuno, Y. (2014). Recent research progress in and future perspective on treatment of Parkinson's disease. *Integrative Medicine International*, *1*(2), 67–79. DOI: 10.1159/000365070

Nachon, F., Carletti, E., Ronco, C., Trovaslet, M., Nicolet, Y., Jean, L., & Renard, P. (2013). Crystal structures of human cholinesterases in complex with huprine W and tacrine: Elements of specificity for anti-Alzheimer's drugs targeting acetyl- and butyryl-cholinesterase. *Biochemical Journal*, *453*(3), 393–399. DOI: 10.1042/BJ20130013

Nalivaeva, N. N., Zhuravin, I. A., & Turner, A. J. (2020). Neprilysin expression and functions in development, ageing and disease. *Mechanisms of Ageing and Development*, *192*. *Mechanisms of Ageing and Development, 111363*, 111363. Advance online publication. DOI: 10.1016/j.mad.2020.111363 PMID: 32987038

O'Connor, C. C., Wen, L. M., Rissel, C. E., & Shaw, M. (2006). Sexual behaviour and risk in Vietnamese men living in metropolitan Sydney. *Sexually Transmitted Infections*, *82*(1), 47–51. https://doi.org/DOI: 10.1136/sti.2005.016188

Oefner, C., Roques, B. P., Fournie-Zaluski, M. C., & Dale, G. E. (2004). Structural analysis of neprilysin with various specific and potent inhibitors. *Acta Crystallographica Section D: Biological Crystallography*, *60*(Pt 2), 392–396. https://doi.org/DOI: 10.1107/S0907444903028407

Palomo, V., Nozal, V., Rojas-Prats, E., Gil, C., & Martinez, A. (2021). Protein kinase inhibitors for amyotrophic lateral sclerosis therapy. *British Journal of Pharmacology*, *178*(6), 1316–1335. DOI: 10.1111/bph.15221

Rajman, L., Chwalek, K., & Sinclair, D. A. (2018). Therapeutic potential of NAD-boosting molecules: The in vivo evidence. *Cell Metabolism*, *27*(3), 529–547. DOI: 10.1016/j.cmet.2018.02.011

Reiner, R. E., Kraulhacker, B., Simeon, V., & Skinjaric-Spoiler, M. (1975). Mechanisms of inhibition in vitro of mammalian acetylcholinesterase and cholinesterase in solutions of 0,0-dimethyl 2,2,2-trichloro-1-hydroxyethyl phosphate (trichorphon). *Biochemical Pharmacology*, *24*(7), 717–722. https://doi.org/DOI: 10.1016/0006-2952(75)90243-8

Savelieff, M. G., Nam, G., Kang, J., Lee, H. J., Lee, M., & Lim, M. H. (2019). Development of multifunctional molecules as potential therapeutic candidates for Alzheimer's disease, Parkinson's disease, and amyotrophic lateral sclerosis in the last decade. *Chemical Reviews*, *119*(2), 1221–1322. DOI: 10.1021/acs.chemrev.8b00138

Shaw, L. M., Korecka, M., Clark, C. M., Lee, V. M.-Y., & Trojanowski, J. Q. (2007). Biomarkers of neurodegeneration for diagnosis and monitoring therapeutics. *Nature Reviews Drug Discovery*, *6*(4), 295–303. DOI: 10.1038/nrd2176

Shusharina, N., Yukhnenko, D., Botman, S., Sapunov, V., Savinov, V., Kamyshov, G., Sayapin, D., & Voznyuk, I. (2023). Modern methods of diagnostics and treatment of neurodegenerative diseases and depression. *Diagnostics*, *13*(3), Article 573. DOI: 10.3390/diagnostics13030573

Smallfield, S., & Heckenlaible, C. (2017). Effectiveness of occupational therapy interventions to enhance occupational performance for adults with Alzheimer's disease and related major neurocognitive disorders: A systematic review. *American Journal of Occupational Therapy*, *71*(5), 7105180010p1–7105180010p9. DOI: 10.5014/ajot.2017.024752

Sorce, S., Stocker, R., Seredenina, T., Holmdahl, R., Aguzzi, A., Chio, A., Depaulis, A., Heitz, F., Olofsson, P., Olsson, T., Duveau, V., Sanoudou, D., Skosgater, S., Vlahou, A., Wasquel, D., Krause, K.-H., & Jaquet, V. (2017). NADPH oxidases as drug targets and biomarkers in neurodegenerative diseases: What is the evidence? *Free Radical Biology and Medicine*, *112*, 387–396. DOI: 10.1016/j.freeradbiomed.2017.08.006

Stewart, W. F., Kawas, C., Corrada, M., & Metter, E. J. (1997). Risk of Alzheimer's disease and duration of NSAID use. *Neurology*, *48*(3), 626–632. DOI: 10.1212/WNL.48.3.626

Sundblad, V., Quintar, A. A., Morosi, L. G., Niveloni, S. I., Cabanne, A., Smecuol, E., Mauriño, E., Mariño, K. V., Bai, J. C., Maldonado, C. A., & Rabinovich, G. A. (2018). Galectins in intestinal inflammation: Galectin-1 expression delineates response to treatment in celiac disease patients. *Frontiers in Immunology*, *9*. *Frontiers in Immunology*, *379*, 379. Advance online publication. DOI: 10.3389/fimmu.2018.00379 PMID: 29545799

Tagaris, A., Kollias, D., Stafylopatis, A., Tagaris, G., & Kollias, S. (2018). Machine learning for neurodegenerative disorder diagnosis—Survey of practices and launch of benchmark dataset. *International Journal of Artificial Intelligence Tools*, *27*(3), Article 1850011. https://doi.org/DOI: 10.1142/S0218213018500110

Trumbull, K. A., McAllister, D., Gandelman, M. M., Fung, W. Y., Lew, T., Brennan, L., Lopez, N., Morré, J., Kalyanaraman, B., & Beckman, J. S. (2012). Diapocynin and apocynin administration fails to significantly extend survival in G93A SOD1 ALS mice. *Neurobiology of Disease*, *45*(1), 137–144. DOI: 10.1016/j.nbd.2011.08.003

Tundo, G. R., di Muzio, E., Ciaccio, C., & others. (2016). Multiple allosteric sites are involved in the modulation of insulin-degrading enzyme activity by somatostatin. *The FEBS Journal*, *283*(20), 3755–3770. DOI: 10.1111/febs.13841

Tundo, G. R., Sbardella, D., Ciaccio, C., & others. (2017). Multiple functions of insulin-degrading enzyme: A metabolic crosslight? *Critical Reviews in Biochemistry and Molecular Biology*, *52*(5), 554–582. DOI: 10.1080/10409238.2017.1337707

Walter, J., Fluhrer, R., Hartung, B., Willem, M., Kaether, C., Capell, A., & others. (2001). Phosphorylation regulates intracellular trafficking of β-secretase. *Journal of Biological Chemistry*, *276*(18), 14634–14641. DOI: 10.1074/jbc.M011116200

Wilkins, J. M., & Trushina, E. (2018). Application of metabolomics in Alzheimer's disease. *Frontiers in Neurology*, *8*. *Frontiers in Neurology*, *719*, 719. Advance online publication. DOI: 10.3389/fneur.2017.00719 PMID: 29375465

Williams, A., Zhou, S., & Zhan, C. G. (2019). Discovery of potent and selective butyrylcholinesterase inhibitors through the use of pharmacophore-based screening. *Bioorganic & Medicinal Chemistry Letters*, *29*(24), Article 126754. DOI: 10.1016/j.bmcl.2019.126754

Woo, H. A., Bae, S. H., Park, S., & Rhee, S. G. (2009). Sestrin 2 is not a reductase for cysteine sulfinic acid of peroxiredoxins. *Antioxidants & Redox Signaling*, *11*(4), 739–745. https://doi.org/DOI: 10.1089/ars.2008.2238

Woolf, N. T. (1998). A structural basis for memory storage in mammals. *Progress in Neurobiology*, *55*(1), 59–77. https://doi.org/DOI: 10.1016/S0301-0082(98)00002-9

Woolf, N. T. (2006). Acetylcholine, cognition, and consciousness. *Journal of Molecular Neuroscience*, *30*(1–2), 219–222. DOI: 10.1385/JMN:30:1:219

World Health Organization. (2024, May 3). *Dementia*. https://www.who.int/news-room/fact-sheets/detail/dementia

Wu, D. C., Ré, D. B., Nagai, M., Ischiropoulos, H., & Przedborski, S. (2006). The inflammatory NADPH oxidase enzyme modulates motor neuron degeneration in amyotrophic lateral sclerosis mice. *Proceedings of the National Academy of Sciences*, *103*(32), 12132–12137. DOI: 10.1073/pnas.0603670103

Wu, Y., Le, W., & Jankovic, J. (2011). Preclinical biomarkers of Parkinson disease. *Archives of Neurology*, *68*(1), 22–30. DOI: 10.1001/archneurol.2010.321

Yamamoto, A., Friedlein, A., Imai, Y., Takahashi, R., Kahle, P. J., & Haass, C. (2005). Parkin phosphorylation and modulation of its E3 ubiquitin ligase activity. *Journal of Biological Chemistry*, *280*(5), 3390–3399. DOI: 10.1074/jbc.M407724200

Yang, G., Zhou, R., Guo, X., Yan, C., Lei, J., & Shi, Y. (2021). Structural basis of γ-secretase inhibition and modulation by small molecule drugs. *Cell*, *184*(3), 521–533.e14. DOI: 10.1016/j.cell.2020.11.049

Zhang, J., Gross, S. D., Schroeder, M. D., & Anderson, R. A. (1996). Casein kinase I α and αL: Alternative splicing-generated kinases exhibit different catalytic properties. *Biochemistry*, *35*(51), 16319–16327. https://doi.org/DOI: 10.1021/bi962019u

Zhang, Z., Liang, W. G., Bailey, L. J., Tan, Y. Z., Wei, H., Wang, A., Farcasanu, M., Woods, V. A., McCord, L. A., Lee, D., Shang, W., Deprez-Poulain, R., Deprez, B., Liu, D. R., Koide, A., Koide, S., Kossiakoff, A. A., Li, S., Carragher, B., Potter, C. S., & Tang, W. J. (2018). Ensemble cryoEM elucidates the mechanism of insulin capture and degradation by human insulin degrading enzyme. *eLife*, *7*, Article e36666. DOI: 10.7554/eLife.36666

Chapter 9
Current Advancement of Enzymatic Targets for the Mitigation of Neurodegenerative Disorders:
Neuroinflammatory Mediators as Biomarkers for Diagnosis, Prognosis, and Treatment of AD

Sonal Dubey
https://orcid.org/0000-0003-3073-1173
College of Pharmaceutical Sciences, Dayananda Sagar University, India

Nahid Abbas
https://orcid.org/0000-0002-2877-760X
Akshaya Institute of Pharmacy, Rajiv Gandhi University of Health Science, India

ABSTRACT

Neurodegenerative disorders such as Parkinson's disease (PD), Alzheimer's disease (AD), and multiple sclerosis (MS) are characterized by the abnormal accumulation of misfolded proteins within the central nervous system (CNS). These pathological protein aggregates—including β-amyloid in AD, mutant huntingtin in Huntington's disease (HD), ubiquitinated proteins in amyotrophic lateral sclerosis (ALS), and tau in MS—are central to disease progression. The development of novel therapeutic and diagnostic agents aimed at early detection, improved efficacy, and reduced side effects is critical. This chapter reviews recent advancements in enzymatic targets that offer promising avenues for mitigating neurodegenerative disorders by addressing their underlying molecular mechanisms.

DOI: 10.4018/979-8-3373-4627-4.ch009

INTRODUCTION

Neuro-regeneration is the phenomena of formation of new neurons, dendrons, dendrites and glia, (Adolfsson et al., 1979). It is the development and correction of damaged nerves over a period of time. The CNS is damaged due to death of the cell, demyelination, failure to regenerate axone and genetic factors. All these disorders are collectively classified under neurodegenerative disorders. They cause the brain and neurons to malfunction, (Aisen, Vellas, & Hampel, 2013). Particularly slow decline in sensory, motor, and cognitive function, or possibly complete loss, (Allard et al., 1990; Alzheimer's Association, 2012; Armulik et al., 2010; Bäckman & Farde, 2001; Barbanti et al., 2000).

Various neurodegenerative disorders have different forms; it is often characterized by different physiological and morphological changes in the brain. AD is due to β-amyloid deposition in the brain; HD is caused by misfolded Huntington protein aggregation. Ubiquitinated proteins aggregation is observed in amyotrophic lateral sclerosis. Tau and β-amyloid accumulation are found in MS plaques. Whereas α-synuclein is found in PD. In accidental brain injuries Tau neurofibrillary tangles are indicated. Occurrence of misfolded proteins is another evidence of the progression of the disease, (Barnum, 1977; Bell et al., 2012; Bhujbal & Hah, 2023; Blennow, de Leon, & Zetterbeg, 2006; Blokhuis et al., 2013; Bonner & Peskind, 2002; Bratkowski et al., 2022).

The degeneration of neurons occurs when there is abnormal deposition of the above-mentioned proteins. The amyloid αβ plaques and fibrils, tau plaques, Lewy bodies-having misfolded α-synuclein (α-syn), Neurofilament light protein (Nfl) which is formed due to degeneration of myelinated axons. Post-synaptic degeneration results in the deposition of neurogranin, while pre-synaptic vesicle 2A (SV2A) and glial acidic fibrillary protein (GFAP), monocyte chemoattractant protein-1 (MCP-1), and triggering receptor expressed on myeloid cells 2 (TREM2) exhibit aberrant expression in disease conditions. Figure 1 depicts the various neuron degeneration sites, (Burdakov, 2020; Chen et al., 2021; Cotman, Monaghan, & Ganong, 1988; Danbolt, 2001; Danysz et al., 2000).

These diseases have a substantial impact on different brain regions, resulting in unique phenotypes, similar to the progressive loss of cognitive and motor sensory-motor abilities, (Danysz et al., 2000). However, their cellular etiology is comparable. Therefore, it's critical to comprehend and identify treatment strategies for a variety of neurodegenerative diseases that share symptoms. The most common of them are multiple sclerosis (MS), Parkinson's disease (PD), Alzheimer's disease (AD), and Huntington's disease (HD). As per WHO 2024 reports, around one billion people in the world are affected by neurological disorders. Table 1 summarizes some of the drugs which are under clinical trials / treatment for some neurodegenerative disorders.

Figure 1. Neuron degeneration sites

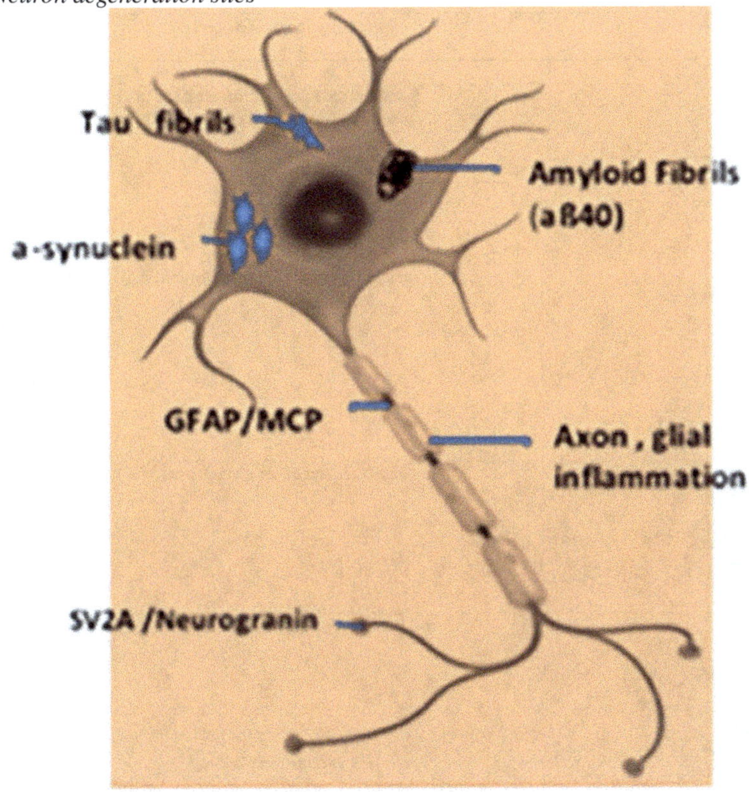

Table 1. Drug candidates in the clinical phase trial for the treatment of neurodegenerative disorders

Drug Candidate	Enzymatic Target	Clinical Trial Phase/ Treatment
SMALL MOLECULES:		
(GSM)776890 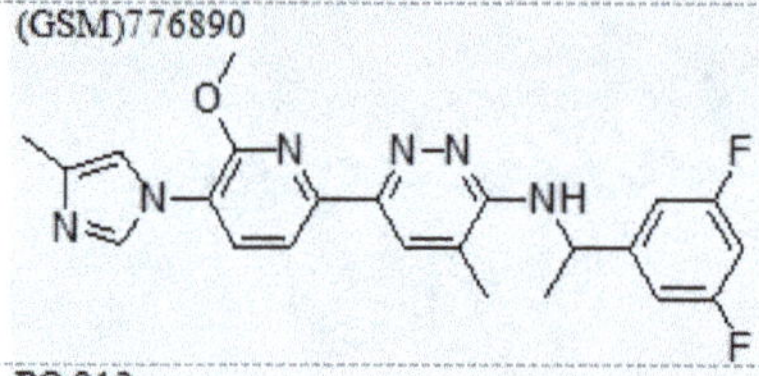	γ-secretase, allosteric modulator of amyloid precursor protein (APP)	Phase I To treat Alzheimer's
PQ912 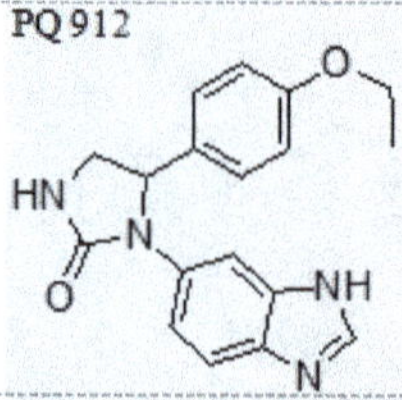	glutaminyl cyclase (QC) inhibitor	Phase II To treat Inflammation in neurons
CT1812 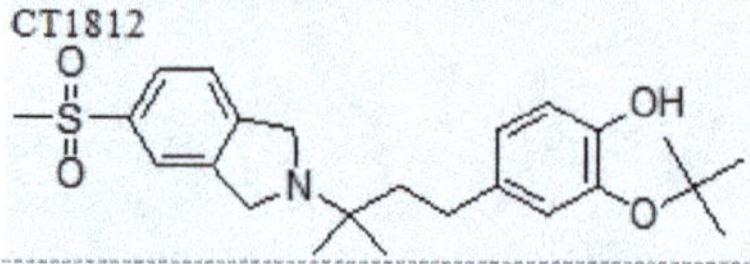	sigma2 receptor antagonist	Phase II To treat Alzheimer's
ALZ-801 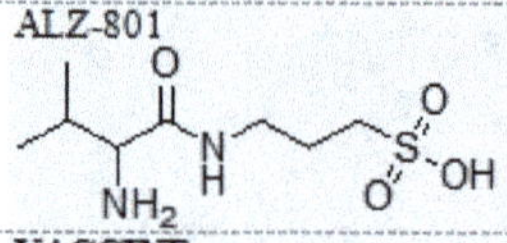	Inhibits Aß oligomer formation	Phase III To treat Alzheimer's
VACCINE:		
AV-1959D,	it targets amyloid-β	Phase I To treat Alzheimer's it's a vaccine
BAN2401,	anti-amyloid-ß antibody	Phase III To treat Alzheimer's

There is currently no fully effective treatment for neurodegenerative illnesses, particularly if they are advanced in nature. Nonetheless, it has become important to treat the physiological and cognitive deficiencies of these illnesses through the development of therapeutic techniques, (David & Tayebi, 2014). In this chapter, current advancement of various enzymatic targets for the mitigation of neurodegenerative disorders have been discussed.

TARGETS INVOLVED IN TREATMENT

JNK3 (c-Jun N-Terminal Kinase 3)

JNKs are members of the mitogen-activated protein kinase, or MAPK, family, which is a type of serine-threonine protein kinases activated by stress, (Duffy, Rapport, & Graf, 1980). From cell division to cell death, they are in charge. While JNK3 is expressed in the heart, testis, smooth muscle, and CNS, JNK1 and JNK2 are present in every bodily tissue. It has been discovered

to play a unique part in cerebral ischemia, Parkinson's disease, Alzheimer's disease, and other CNS related illnesses.

In these disease conditions the JNK3 level increases in the CSF, leading to cognitive decline, synaptic dysfunction and spine loss. Thus, it serves as a biomarker for the detection of these disorders. Thus, JNK3 holds a good potential for the treatment of neurodegenerative disorders. Covalent inhibitors have been discovered which bind to cysteine154 a critical residue present in the JNK3's binding site by crossing the blood–brain barrier (BBB). Three pan-JNK inhibitors SP600125, AS-602801, and Tanzisertib have been recognized as neuro-regenerators, (Gage & Temple, 2013; Gill et al., 2009).

Figure 2.

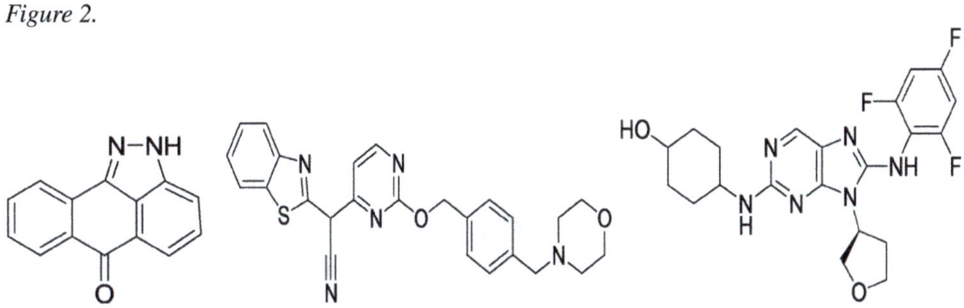

SP600125 AS-602801 Tanzisertib

NLRP3 Inhibitors

The NLRP3 inflammasome is the main cause for innate immune-mediated inflammation, it leads to different type neurodegenerative diseases. Clinically proven NLRP3 inflammasome inhibitors are not available. Yun *et al.* discovered RRx-001, an anticancer molecule undergoing phase III clinical trials. This strong NLRP3 inhibitor attaches to NLRP3's cysteine409 via its bromoacetyl group, preventing the NLRP3-NEK7 interaction, which is a precursor for inflammation. MCC950 is an NLRP3 inflammasome inhibitor, (Goetz, 2011).

Figure 3.

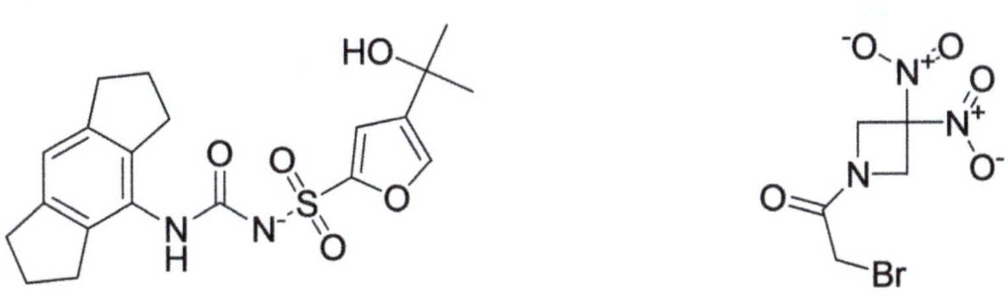

MCC950 RRx-001

NAD (Nicotinamide Adenine Dinucleotide) Hydrolase SARM1 Inhibitors

Nicotinamide adenine dinucleotide hydrolase sterile alpha toll/interleukin receptor motif containing-1 (SARM1) is an enzyme that catalyzes the hydrolysis of NAD+ to form nicotinamide and a mixture of adenosine diphosphate ribose (ADPR) and cADPR. SARM1 is a central metabolic sensor and executioner of axon degeneration, a pathological event that occurs early in many neurological diseases. SARM1 inhibitors could be a therapeutic target for neurodegenerative disorders, peripheral neuropathies, and traumatic brain injuries. Bratkowski *et al.* (2022) revealed fascinating neuroprotective treatments for arresting the degenerative progression. DSRM-3716 is a small molecule which brings SARM-I inhibition, (Hatters, 2008).

Figure 4.

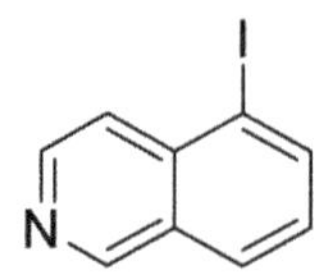

DSRM-3716

Inhibitors of Phosphoinositide 3-Kinase (PI3K), Protein Kinase B (AKT), and mTOR (Mammalian Target of Rapamycin)

The phosphoinositide 3-kinase (PI3K)/protein kinase B (AKT)/mammalian target of rapamycin (mTOR) pathway has been identified as a potentially effective target for the treatment of neurodegenerative disorders in recent studies. As ATP-competitive inhibitors, allosteric inhibitors, covalent inhibitors, and proteolysis-targeting chimeras for the PI3K/AKT/mTOR pathway, Huang et al. documented their significance in the most recent development to significantly lower neurotoxicity. PI3K inhibitors are currently being developed, some of the good inhibition is being shown by NVP-BKM120, BAY80-6946, PX866, XL147, and GDC-0941. An intriguing Akt inhibitor is MK-2206. While AZD2014, MLN0128, and OSI-027 are effective mTOR inhibitors based on clinical trials. For the inhibition of PI3K/mTOR, dual target inhibitors such as PI-103 and NVP-BEZ235 are utilized. The search for a multi target inhibitor is this field is still on, (Huang et al., 2022).

Figure 5.

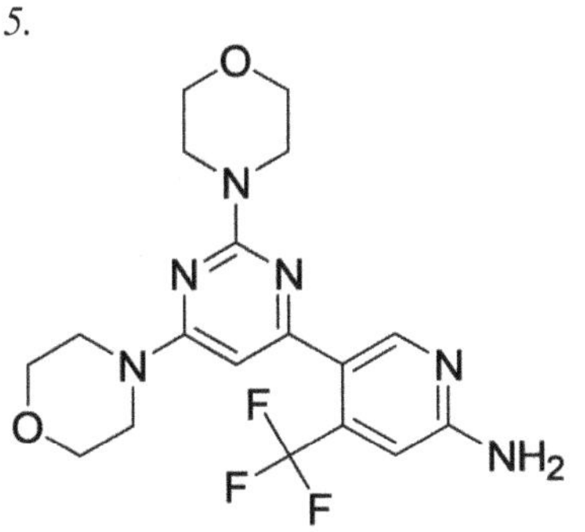

NVP-BKM120

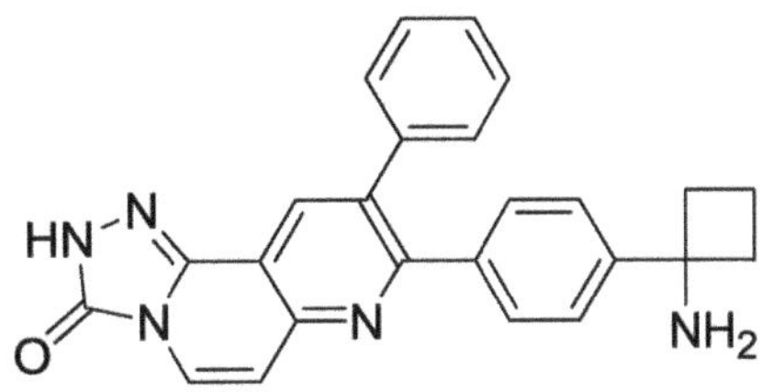

MK-2206

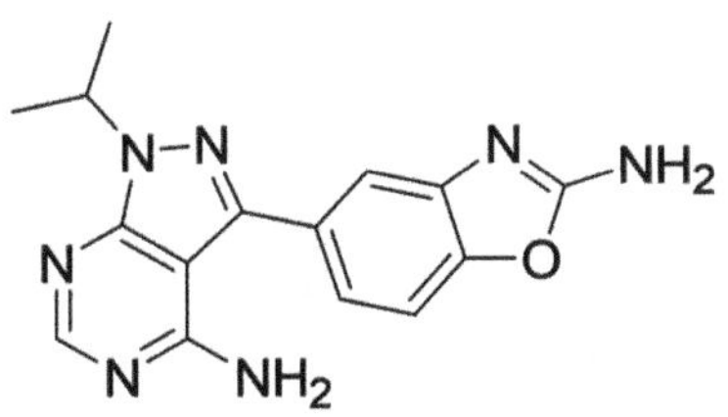

MLN0128

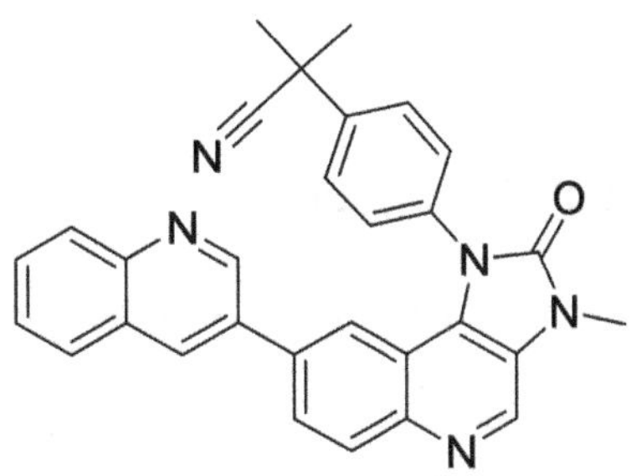

NVP-BEZ235

Cholinesterase Inhibitors

In advance neurodegenerative disease condition, the death of brain cells is observed. With loss of synaptic condition of neurons, exhibiting worst cognitive symptoms. Impairing memory and thinking abilities of patients. Cholinesterase inhibitors are the best medications to treat conditions related to memory, judgment, thinking, and communication. They act by prevention of acetylcholine breakdown. A neurotransmitter for learning and memory. Rivastigmine is used in the Parkinsons disease; Donezipil and Galantamine are used to treat Alzheimer's disease, (Hussain et al., 2018; Inglis, 2002; Jun et al., 2023; Jun et al., 2023; Kang et al., 1987; Kinney, 2018).

Figure 6.

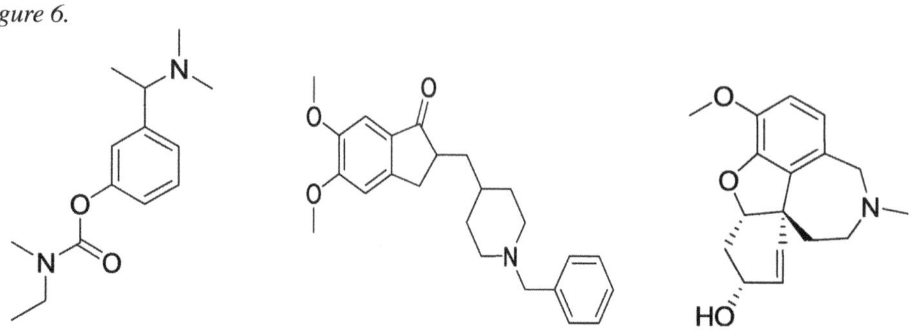

Rivastigmine Donezipil Galantamine

Glutamate Regulators

At synapses and neuronal survival, excitatory glutamatergic neurotransmission working through the N-methyl-d-aspartate receptor (NMDAR) is essential. However, NMDAR activity results in excitotoxicity and encourages cell death, which leads to neurodegeneration, (Krasemann et al., 2017; Lucke-Wold et al., 2014). Glutamate regulators are drugs given to improve reasoning, thinking, improving concentration and motor activities. They work by regulating the activity of glutamate. Ionic channels are formed by the assembly of 18 genes that make up the glutamate receptor, which transmit excitatory synaptic signals from the central nervous system to other cells via an agonist binding site. Numerous functions in the brain, spinal cord, retina, and peripheral nervous system are regulated by these receptors. As a result, these receptors are essential in many neurological disorders. The brain uses this chemical messenger to process information. The drug memantine is NMDA blocker which is used to treat advanced Alzheimer's disease, (Malberg et al., 2000; Masters et al., 1985).

Figure 7.

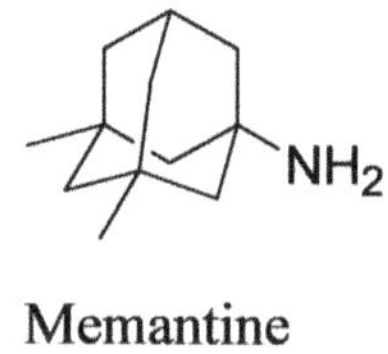

Memantine

Orexin Receptor Antagonist

Two neuropeptides generated by orexin neurons in the lateral hypothalamus make up orexins. G protein-coupled orexin type 1 and type 2 receptors OX1Rs and OX2Rs, respectively are bind

and are activated by orexins. They control hunger, reward, emotion, motivation, sleep-wake cycles, and reward systems. Dementia and Stress-induced anxiety behaviors were reversed by orexinergic blockade in the hippocampus, which revealed that the hippocampal orexins were promising therapeutic targets to minimize stress-induced impairments in AD patients. Suvorexant is the drug used for treating insomnia in Alzheimer patients, (Mayanji et al., 2015; Mayne et al., 2020; McGeer et al., 1988; McGeer, Itagaki, & McGeer, 1988; McGeer et al., 1987; Mehta, Adem, & Sabbagh, 2012).

Figure 8.

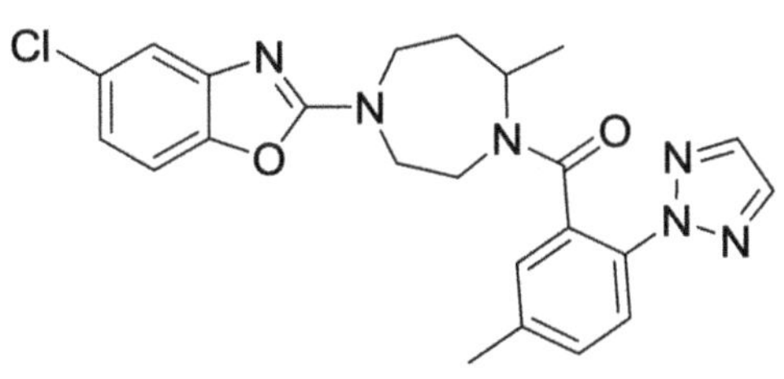

Suvorexant

Amyloid Target by Inhibiting β- Secretase

Mostly found in the brain's grey matter, amyloid plaques, also referred to as neuritic plaques, amyloid beta plaques, or senile plaques, are extracellular deposits of the amyloid beta (Aβ) protein. Amyloid plaques are seen on astrocytes and microglia. Alzheimer's disease is associated with an increase in plaques and neurofibrillary tangles.

The plaque size is 400-450 square micrometers (μm^2) to less than 200 μm^2. Plaques form when Aβ misfolds with the help of β- secretase and γ- secretase, which further aggregates into oligomers and longer polymers to form fibrils, (Montagne et al., 2020; Mukherjee & Grimster, 2018).

Treatment strategies against amyloid focus on beta-amyloid at various phases of plaque development. An intravenous (IV) anti-amyloid antibody infusion molecule audatenumab is under clinical trials. A genetic risk factor known as ApoE ε4 gene carriers may put some individuals at higher risk of developing ARIAs (amyloid-related imaging abnormalities). Another drug in market for eliminating beta-amyloid from the brain is lecanemab. Lecanemab-irmb (Leqembi) is a monoclonal antibody that reduces amyloid beta plaques in the brain. It binds to amyloid beta (Aβ) peptide, the main component of amyloid plaques, and removes soluble toxic Aβ aggregates. This can potentially slow disease progression and affect disease pathology. It addressed Alzheimer's patients' declining cognitive and functional abilities, (Parkinson, 2002; Prober, 2018).

Dopamine and Serotonin Chemical Pathway Targets

The limbic system and cortex contain dopamine receptors, which regulate mood and emotional stability. Memory in AD is correlated with hippocampal D2R. Dopamine increases cortical excitability through D2-like receptors and increases cortical acetylcholine release through D1-like

receptors. Nonetheless, AD patients have lower dopamine levels. The administration of L-dopa improves the cognitive function of AD patients by modulating cholinergic cortical excitability. Elderly patients with psychosis related to dementia are treated with antipsychotic medications that interfere with the brain's serotonin and dopamine chemical pathways. Brexpiprazole- a novel D2 dopamine and serotonin 1A partial agonist called serotonin-dopamine activity modulator (SDAM) is used to treat agitation brought on by Alzheimer's disease-related dementia, (Rogers et al., 1988; Rubinsztein, 2006; Safieh, Korczyn, & Michaelson, 2019; Soya & Sakurai, 2020; Summers et al., 2020).

Figure 9.

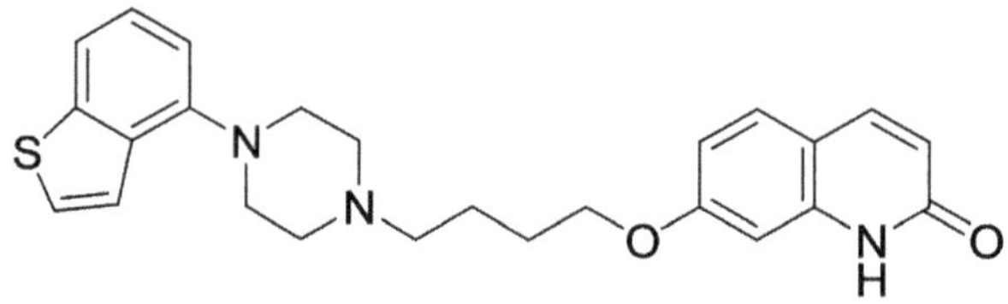

Brexpiprazole

APOE-TREM2 Pathway Targets

In various neurodegenerative diseases, including AD, APOE can bind with the intracellular domain of TREM2 and cause microglia to change from a homeostatic to a neurodegenerative phenotype. A proinflammatory signaling pathway is the APOE-TREM2 pathway. In addition to microglia and astrocytes, APOE control pericyte activation. By controlling pericyte activation and apoptosis for BBB integrity, APOE also influences BBB function. The transgenic mice that expressed human APOE4 showed uncontrolled expression of proinflammatory cyclophilin A (CypA) in pericytes. This, in turn, triggered the activation of NF-kB and matrix metalloproteinase 9 (MMP9), ultimately leading to the breakdown of the blood-brain barrier. Even in the absence of tau or Aβ pathology, APOE4 causes cognitive decline, most likely via the CypA-MMP9 pathway. Consequently, AD progresses due to APOE4-mediated inflammation, and it was discovered that APOE4 carriers respond better to NSAIDs treatment. Ketorolac, Diflunisal, aspirin are the common NSAID's used for treating neuroinflammation, (Triantafylidis et al., 2018; Vadakkan, 2016; Willie et al., 2001; Woolley et al., 2011).

Figure 10.

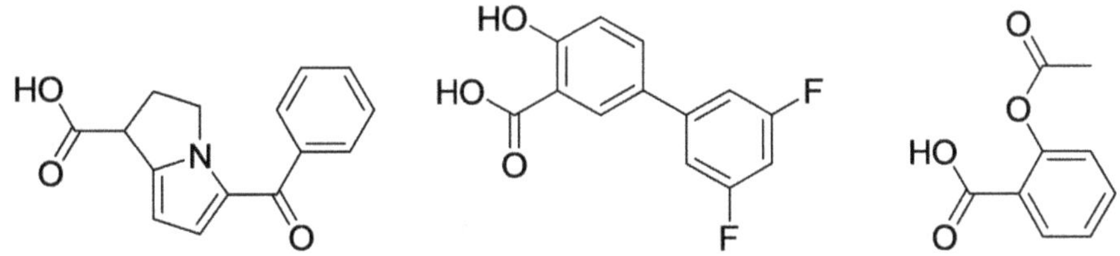

Ketorolac Diflunisal Aspirin

CONCLUSION

The current advancements in targeting enzymatic pathways offer promising therapeutic avenues for mitigating neurodegenerative disorders, which continue to be a significant challenge in medical science. The strategic intervention in specific biochemical pathways holds potential not just for symptom management but also for altering the course of diseases like Alzheimer's, Parkinson's, Huntington's, and multiple sclerosis. JNK3 Inhibition- Targeting JNK3, a kinase implicated in stress responses and synaptic dysfunction, could prevent cognitive decline and neuronal loss. Inhibitors like SP600125, AS-602801, and Tanzisertib demonstrate the capacity to cross the blood-brain barrier and offer neuroregenerative benefits. NLRP3 Inhibition- The NLRP3 inflammasome is a critical player in neuroinflammation, a common feature of neurodegenerative diseases. Inhibitors such as MCC950 and the anticancer agent RRx-001 have shown promise in blocking inflammation pathways, potentially slowing disease progression. SARM1 Inhibition-By inhibiting NAD hydrolase SARM1, researchers aim to protect axonal integrity and prevent neurodegeneration. Compounds like DSRM-3716 represent a new class of neuroprotective agents that intercept NAD hydrolysis, critical for maintaining neuronal health. PI3K/AKT/mTOR Pathway-This signalling pathway is crucial for cell survival and metabolism. Inhibitors targeting different components of this pathway, such as NVP-BKM120 and MK-2206, are in various stages of clinical trials, showing potential to reduce neurotoxicity and promote cell survival. Cholinesterase Inhibition-Drugs like Donepezil, Galantamine, and Rivastigmine enhance cholinergic transmission by preventing acetylcholine breakdown, thereby improving cognitive functions and slowing symptom progression in Alzheimer's and other dementias. Glutamate Regulation-Overactivity of glutamate receptors leads to excitotoxicity and neuronal death. Regulators like Memantine help mitigate these effects, improving cognitive and motor functions in patients with severe Alzheimer's disease. Orexin Receptor Antagonism-Orexin receptors, involved in regulating the sleep-wake cycle and emotional responses, are targeted by drugs like Suvorexant to treat insomnia and stress-induced impairments in Alzheimer's patients. Amyloid Beta-Secretase Inhibition-Targeting the formation and accumulation of amyloid plaques, with drugs like Aducanumab and Lecanemab, represents a critical strategy in treating Alzheimer's by directly addressing one of its core pathological features. Dopamine and Serotonin Pathway Targets-Managing dopamine and serotonin pathways can alleviate symptoms of dementia-related

psychosis and agitation. Brexpiprazole, for instance, helps stabilize mood and cognitive function in affected individuals. APOE-TREM2 Pathway Targets-The APOE-TREM2 pathway's role in neuroinflammation and blood-brain barrier integrity is a promising target. Anti-inflammatory drugs like Ketorolac and aspirin show potential in reducing APOE4-mediated cognitive decline.

The convergence of these targeted therapeutic strategies highlights a multifaceted approach to tackling neurodegenerative diseases. While no definitive cure has been discovered, these advancements offer significant hope. They represent a move towards more personalized and precise treatments, capable of addressing the underlying mechanisms of these disorders rather than merely alleviating symptoms. Ongoing research and clinical trials remain essential, as they will further elucidate these pathways and lead to the development of more effective treatments, ultimately improving the quality of life for millions affected by neurodegenerative conditions.

REFERENCES

Adolfsson, R., Gottfries, C. G., Roos, B. E., & Winblad, B. (1979). Changes in the brain catecholamines in patients with dementia of Alzheimer type. *British Journal of Psychiatry*, *135*(3), 216–223. DOI: 10.1192/bjp.135.3.216

Aisen, P. S., Vellas, B., & Hampel, H. (2013). Moving towards early clinical trials for amyloid-targeted therapy in Alzheimer's disease. *Nature Reviews Drug Discovery*, *12*(4), 324–324. DOI: 10.1038/nrd3842

Allard, P., Alafuzoff, I., Carlsson, A., Eriksson, K., Ericson, E., & others. (1990). Loss of dopamine uptake sites labeled with [3H]GBR-12935 in Alzheimer's disease. *European Neurology*, *30*(4), 181–185. DOI: 10.1159/000117339

Alzheimer's Association. (2012). 2012 Alzheimer's disease facts and figures. *Alzheimer's & Dementia*, *8*(2), 131–168. DOI: 10.1016/j.jalz.2012.02.001

Armulik, A., Genové, G., Mäe, M., Nisancioglu, M. H., Wallgard, E., Niaudet, C., He, L., Norlin, J., Lindblom, P., Strittmatter, K., Johansson, B. R., & Betsholtz, C. (2010). Pericytes regulate the blood-brain barrier. *Nature*, *468*(7323), 557–561. DOI: 10.1038/nature09522

Bäckman, L., & Farde, L. (2001). Dopamine and cognitive functioning: Brain imaging findings in Huntington's disease and normal aging. *Scandinavian Journal of Psychology*, *42*(3), 287–296. DOI: 10.1111/1467-9450.00238

Barbanti, P., Fabbrini, G., Ricci, A., Bruno, G., Cerbo, R., & others. (2000). Reduced density of dopamine D2-like receptors on peripheral blood lymphocytes in Alzheimer's disease. *Mechanisms of Ageing and Development*, *120*(1–3), 65–75. DOI: 10.1016/S0047-6374(00)00183-4

Barnum, D. W. (1977). Spectrophotometric determination of catechol, epinephrine, dopa, dopamine, and other aromatic vic-diols. *Analytica Chimica Acta*, *89*(1), 157–166. DOI: 10.1016/S0003-2670(01)83081-6

Bell, R. D., Winkler, E. A., Singh, I., Sagare, A. P., Deane, R., Wu, Z., Holtzman, D. M., Betsholtz, C., Armulik, A., Sallstrom, J., Berk, B. C., & Zlokovic, B. V. (2012). Apolipoprotein E controls cerebrovascular integrity via cyclophilin A. *Nature*, *485*(7399), 512–516. DOI: 10.1038/nature11087

Bhujbal, S. P., & Hah, J.-M. (2023). An intriguing purview on the design of macrocyclic inhibitors for unexplored protein kinases through their binding site comparison. *Pharmaceuticals*, *16*(7), Article 1009. DOI: 10.3390/ph16071009

Blennow, K., de Leon, M. J., & Zetterberg, H. (2006). Alzheimer's disease. *The Lancet*, *368*(9533), 387–403. DOI: 10.1016/S0140-6736(06)69113-7

Blokhuis, A. M., Groen, E. J., Koppers, M., van den Berg, L. H., & Pasterkamp, R. J. (2013). Protein aggregation in amyotrophic lateral sclerosis. *Acta Neuropathologica*, *125*(6), 777–794. DOI: 10.1007/s00401-013-1125-6

Bonner, L. T., & Peskind, E. R. (2002). Pharmacologic treatments of dementia. *Medical Clinics of North America*, *86*(3), 657–674. DOI: 10.1016/S0025-7125(02)00007-X

Bratkowski, M., Burdett, T. C., Danao, J., Wang, X., Mathur, P., Gu, W., Beckstead, J. A., Talreja, S., Yang, Y.-S., Danko, G., & others. (2022). Uncompetitive adduct-forming SARM1 inhibitors are neuroprotective in preclinical models of nerve injury and disease. *Neuron*, *110*(22), 3711–3726.e16. DOI: 10.1016/j.neuron.2022.08.017

Burdakov, D. (2020). How orexin signals bias action: Hypothalamic and accumbal circuits. *Brain Research*, *1731*. *Brain Research, 145943*, 145943. Advance online publication. DOI: 10.1016/j.brainres.2018.09.011 PMID: 30205111

Chen, Y., He, H., Lin, B., Chen, Y., Deng, X., Jiang, W., & Zhou, R. (2021). RRx-001 ameliorates inflammatory diseases by acting as a potent covalent NLRP3 inhibitor. *Cellular & Molecular Immunology*, *18*(6), 1425–1436. https://doi.org/DOI: 10.1038/s41423-021-00648-4

Cotman, C. W., Monaghan, D. T., & Ganong, A. H. (1988). Excitatory amino acid neurotransmission: NMDA receptors and Hebb-type synaptic plasticity. *Annual Review of Neuroscience*, *11*, 61–80. DOI: 10.1146/annurev.ne.11.030188.000425

Danbolt, N. C. (2001). Glutamate uptake. *Progress in Neurobiology*, *65*(1), 1–105. DOI: 10.1016/S0301-0082(00)00067-8

Danysz, W., & Parsons, C. G. (2003). The NMDA receptor antagonist memantine as a symptomatological and neuroprotective treatment for Alzheimer's disease: Preclinical evidence. *International Journal of Geriatric Psychiatry*, *18*(S1), S23–S32. DOI: 10.1002/gps.938

Danysz, W., Parsons, C. G., Möbius, H. J., Stöffler, A., & Quack, G. (2000). Neuroprotective and symptomatological action of memantine relevant for Alzheimer's disease—A unified glutamatergic hypothesis on the mechanism of action. *Neurotoxicity Research*, *2*(2–3), 85–97. DOI: 10.1007/BF03033787

David, M. A., & Tayebi, M. J. (2014). Detection of protein aggregates in brain and cerebrospinal fluid derived from multiple sclerosis patients. *Frontiers in Neurology*, *5*. *Frontiers in Neurology, 251*. Advance online publication. DOI: 10.3389/fneur.2014.00251 PMID: 25520699

Duffy, P. E., Rapport, M., & Graf, L. (1980). Glial fibrillary acidic protein and Alzheimer-type senile dementia. *Neurology*, *30*(7), 778–782. DOI: 10.1212/WNL.30.7.778

Gage, F. H., & Temple, S. (2013). Neural stem cells: Generating and regenerating the brain. *Neuron*, *80*(3), 588–601. DOI: 10.1016/j.neuron.2013.10.037

Gill, S. S., Anderson, G. M., Fischer, H. D., Bell, C. M., Li, P., Normand, S. L., & Rochon, P. A. (2009). Syncope and its consequences in patients with dementia receiving cholinesterase inhibitors: A population-based cohort study. *Archives of Internal Medicine*, *169*(9), 867–873. DOI: 10.1001/archinternmed.2009.43

Goetz, C. G. (2011). The history of Parkinson's disease: Early clinical descriptions and neurological therapies. *Cold Spring Harbor Perspectives in Medicine*, *1*(1), Article a008862. DOI: 10.1101/cshperspect.a008862

Hatters, D. M. (2008). Protein misfolding inside cells: The case of huntingtin and Huntington's disease. *IUBMB Life*, *60*(11), 724–728. DOI: 10.1002/iub.111

Huang, J., Chen, L., Wu, J., Ai, D., Zhang, J.-Q., Chen, T.-G., & Wang, L. (2022). Targeting the PI3K/AKT/mTOR signaling pathway in the treatment of human diseases: Current status, trends, and solutions. *Journal of Medicinal Chemistry*, *65*(23), 16033–16061. https://doi.org/DOI: 10.1021/acs.jmedchem.2c01237

. Hussain, R., Zubair, H., Pursell, S., & Shahab, M. (2018). Neurodegenerative diseases: Regenerative mechanisms and novel therapeutic approaches. *Brain Sciences*, *8*(9), Article 177. DOI: 10.3390/brainsci8090177

Inglis, F. (2002). The tolerability and safety of cholinesterase inhibitors in the treatment of dementia. *. *International Journal of Clinical Practice. Supplement*, (127), 45–63. PMID: 12139367

Jun, J., Moon, H., Yang, S., Lee, J., Baek, J., Kim, H., Cho, H., Hwang, K., Ahn, S., Kim, Y. J., & others. (2023). Carbamate JNK3 inhibitors show promise as effective treatments for Alzheimer's disease: In vivo studies on mouse models. *Journal of Medicinal Chemistry*, *66*(9), 6372–6390. DOI: 10.1021/acs.jmedchem.3c00173

Jun, J., Yang, S., Lee, J., Moon, H., Kim, J., Jung, H., Im, D., Oh, Y., Jang, M., & Cho, H. J. (2023). Discovery of novel imidazole chemotypes as isoform-selective JNK3 inhibitors for the treatment of Alzheimer's disease. *European Journal of Medicinal Chemistry*, *245*(Pt 1), Article 114894. DOI: 10.1016/j.ejmech.2022.114894

Kang, J., Lemaire, H. G., Unterbeck, A., Salbaum, J. M., Masters, C. L., Grzeschik, K. H., & others. (1987). The precursor of Alzheimer's disease amyloid A4 protein resembles a cell-surface receptor. *Nature*, *325*(6106), 733–736. DOI: 10.1038/325733a0

Kinney, J. W. (2018). Inflammation as a central mechanism in Alzheimer's disease. *Alzheimer's & Dementia: Translational Research & Clinical Interventions*, *4*, 575–590. DOI: 10.1016/j.trci.2018.06.014

Krasemann, S., Madore, C., Cialic, R., Baufeld, C., Calcagno, N., El Fatimy, R., Beckers, L., & others. (2017). The TREM2-APOE pathway drives the transcriptional phenotype of dysfunctional microglia in neurodegenerative diseases. *Immunity*, *47*(3), 566–581.e9. DOI: 10.1016/j.immuni.2017.08.008

Lucke-Wold, B. P., Turner, R. C., Logsdon, A. F., Bailes, J. E., Huber, J. D., & Rosen, C. L. (2014). Linking traumatic brain injury to chronic traumatic encephalopathy: Identification of potential mechanisms leading to neurofibrillary tangle development. *Journal of Neurotrauma*, *31*(13), 1129–1138. DOI: 10.1089/neu.2013.3303

Malberg, J. E., Eisch, A. J., Nestler, E. J., & Duman, R. S. (2000). Chronic antidepressant treatment increases neurogenesis in adult rat hippocampus. *Journal of Neuroscience*, *20*(24), 9104–9110. DOI: 10.1523/JNEUROSCI.20-24-09104.2000

Masters, C. L., Simms, G., Weinman, N. A., Multhaup, G., McDonald, B. L., & Beyreuther, K. (1985). Amyloid plaque core protein in Alzheimer disease and Down syndrome. *Proceedings of the National Academy of Sciences*, *82*(12), 4245–4249. DOI: 10.1073/pnas.82.12.4245

Mavanji, V., Perez-Leighton, C. E., Kotz, C. M., Billington, C. J., Parthasarathy, S., Sinton, C. M., & others. (2015). Promotion of wakefulness and energy expenditure by orexin-A in the ventrolateral preoptic area. *Sleep*, *38*(9), 1361–1370. DOI: 10.5665/sleep.4970

Mayne, K., White, J. A., McMurran, C. E., Rivera, F. J., & de la Fuente, A. G. (2020). Aging and neurodegenerative disease: Is the adaptive immune system a friend or foe? *Frontiers in Aging Neuroscience*, *12*. *Frontiers in Aging Neuroscience, 572090*, 572090. Advance online publication. DOI: 10.3389/fnagi.2020.572090 PMID: 33173502

McGeer, P. L., Itagaki, S., Boyes, B. E., & McGeer, E. G. (1988). Reactive microglia are positive for HLA-DR in the substantia nigra of Parkinson's and Alzheimer's disease brains. *Neurology*, *38*(8), 1285–1291. DOI: 10.1212/WNL.38.8.1285

McGeer, P. L., Itagaki, S., McGeer, E. G. (1988). Expression of the histocompatibility glycoprotein HLA-DR in neurological disease. *Acta Neuropathologica*, *76*(6), 550–557. DOI: 10.1007/BF00689592

McGeer, P. L., Itagaki, S., Tago, H., & McGeer, E. G. (1987). Reactive microglia in patients with senile dementia of the Alzheimer type are positive for the histocompatibility glycoprotein HLA-DR. *Neuroscience Letters*, *79*(1–2), 195–200. DOI: 10.1016/0304-3940(87)90696-3

Mehta, M., Adem, A., & Sabbagh, M. (2012). New acetylcholinesterase inhibitors for Alzheimer's disease. *International Journal of Alzheimer's Disease*, *2012*. *International Journal of Alzheimer's Disease, 728983*, 1–8. Advance online publication. DOI: 10.1155/2012/728983 PMID: 22216416

Montagne, A., Nation, D. A., Sagare, A. P., Barisano, G., Sweeney, M. D., Chakhoyan, A., Pachicano, M., Joe, E., Nelson, A. R., D'Orazio, L. M., Buennagel, D. P., Harrington, M. G., Benzinger, T. L. S., Fagan, A. M., Ringman, J. M., Schneider, L. S., Morris, J. C., Reiman, E. M., Caselli, R. J., Chui, H. C., Tcw, J., Chen, Y., Pa, J., Conti, P. S., Law, M., Toga, A. W., & Zlokovic, B. V. (2020). APOE4 leads to blood-brain barrier dysfunction predicting cognitive decline. *Nature*, *581*(7806), 71–76. DOI: 10.1038/s41586-020-2247-3

Mukherjee, H., & Grimster, N. P. (2018). Beyond cysteine: Recent developments in the area of targeted covalent inhibition. *Current Opinion in Chemical Biology*, *44*, 30–38. DOI: 10.1016/j.cbpa.2018.05.011

Parkinson, J. (2002). An essay on the shaking palsy. *Journal of Neuropsychiatry and Clinical Neurosciences*, *14*(2), 223–236. (Original work published 1817). DOI: 10.1176/jnp.14.2.223

Prober, D. A. (2018). Discovery of hypocretin/orexin ushers in a new era of sleep research. *Trends in Neurosciences*, *41*(2), 70–72. DOI: 10.1016/j.tins.2017.11.006

Rogers, J., Luber-Narod, J., Styren, S. D., & Civin, W. H. (1988). Expression of immune system-associated antigens by cells of the human central nervous system: Relationship to the pathology of Alzheimer's disease. *Neurobiology of Aging*, *9*(4), 339–349. DOI: 10.1016/S0197-4580(88)80079-4

Rubinsztein, D. C. (2006). The roles of intracellular protein-degradation pathways in neurodegeneration. *Nature*, *443*(7113), 780–786. DOI: 10.1038/nature05291

Safieh, M., Korczyn, A. D., & Michaelson, D. M. (2019). ApoE4: An emerging therapeutic target for Alzheimer's disease. *BMC Medicine*, *17*(1), Article 64. DOI: 10.1186/s12916-019-1299-4

Soya, S., & Sakurai, T. (2020). Orexin as a modulator of fear-related behavior: Hypothalamic control of noradrenaline circuit. *Brain Research*, *1731*. *Brain Research, 146037*, 146037. Advance online publication. DOI: 10.1016/j.brainres.2018.11.032 PMID: 30481504

Summers, C. H., Yaeger, J. D. W., Staton, C. D., Arendt, D. H., & Summers, T. R. (2020). Orexin/hypocretin receptor modulation of anxiolytic and antidepressive responses during social stress and decision-making: Potential for therapy. *Brain Research*, *1731*. *Brain Research, 146085*, 146085. Advance online publication. DOI: 10.1016/j.brainres.2018.12.036 PMID: 30590027

Triantafylidis, L. K., Clemons, J. S., Peron, E. P., Roefaro, J., & Zimmerman, K. M. (2018). Brain over bladder: A systematic review of dual cholinesterase inhibitor and urinary anticholinergic use. *Drugs & Aging*, *35*(1), 27–41. DOI: 10.1007/s40266-017-0500-8

Vadakkan, K. I. (2016). Neurodegenerative disorders share common features of "loss of function" states of a proposed mechanism of nervous system functions. *BioMedicine*, *83*(2), 412–430. https://doi.org/DOI: 10.1016/j.biomed.2016.07.006

Willie, J. T., Chemelli, R. M., Sinton, C. M., & Yanagisawa, M. (2001). To eat or to sleep? Orexin in the regulation of feeding and wakefulness. *Annual Review of Neuroscience*, *24*, 429–458. DOI: 10.1146/annurev.neuro.24.1.429

Woolley, J. D., Khan, B. K., Murthy, N. K., Miller, B. L., & Rankin, K. P. (2011). The diagnostic challenge of psychiatric symptoms in neurodegenerative disease: Rates of and risk factors for prior psychiatric diagnosis in patients with early neurodegenerative disease. *Journal of Clinical Psychiatry*, *72*(2), 126–133. DOI: 10.4088/JCP.10m06382oli

Chapter 10

Tyrosine Kinase as the Therapeutic Target for Neurodegenerative Diseases

Nandita Mandal
Sanaka Educational Trust's Group of Institutions, India

Avijit Bej
https://orcid.org/0009-0006-8419-3007
Mahadeva Lal Schroff College of Pharmacy, Aurangabad, India

Anwesha Das
https://orcid.org/0000-0002-0182-9422
Sanaka Educational Trust's Group of Institutions, India

Arijit Nandi
https://orcid.org/0000-0003-0437-7879
Sanaka Educational Trust's Group of Institutions, India

ABSTRACT

Treatment based on the inhibition of tyrosine kinases can provide relief to patients with severe neurodegenerative phenomena, for example, Alzheimer's disease, multiple sclerosis, Parkinson's disease, and amyotrophic lateral sclerosis. All these conditions involve ongoing neuronal disruptions and neuro-degeneration, sharing several common traits: the build-up of abnormal protein aggregates, oxidative stress, mitochondrial dysfunction, DNA damage, neurotrophin irregularities, and persistent neuro-inflammation. Pathways participating in neurodegenerative diseases' progression and development, accompanied by the expression of biomarkers, are dependent on the activities of proteins called tyrosine kinases and phosphatases.

DOI: 10.4018/979-8-3373-4627-4.ch010

INTRODUCTION

Today, neurodegenerative disorders represent a significant health challenge. Recent studies have shown that aging is associated with a growing susceptibility to various neurodegenerative conditions, including Huntington's disease (HD), Parkinson's disease (PD), frontotemporal dementia (FTD), amyotrophic lateral sclerosis (ALS), and Alzheimer's disease (AD) (Gitler et al., 2017). Even though these conditions are grouped into neurodegenerative diseases (NDDs), the pathophysiology behind them is distinctly different: some of them impair memory, while others impact cognition, motion, speech, or breathing. This fact partly explains the limited success in finding a pharmacological cure for these diseases (Spagnuolo et al., 2018). One of the modern and trending strategies in finding a cure for these pathophysiologies is the exertion of combined therapies that target multiple pathophysiology aspects. However, further understanding of these therapies and their pathophysiologies is needed to evolve with advanced and successful treatment (Ahmed et al., 2020). Molecular, pathological, genetic, and biochemical studies over the past century have established that proteins with altered physical-chemical properties are aggressively deposited in the human brain in NDDs. It should be noted that these proteins are not only accumulated in neurons but also in glial cells. This kind of participation of proteins in the pathogenesis of NDDs has led to the emergence of the concept of" conformational diseases" (Kovacs et al., 2010). In substance, the theory is that the architectural conformation of the regular protein is changed in such a way that its activity is altered or toxic deposition accumulates within or beyond the cells. Mutations in genes liable for encoding those proteins are responsible for hereditarily controlled diseases. The new classification of previously known diseases, based on molecular, pathological, genetic, and biochemical research, introduced fresh possibilities for the development of biomarkers and the creation of new treatment approaches (Kovacs, 2014). Kinases represent a group of enzymes tasked with facilitating the phosphate group transfer from a high energy (typically ATP)-containing donor molecule to a substrate molecule (Guo et al., 2019). They are classified according to the substrate they phosphorylate, resulting in two primary divisions: metabolic kinases and protein kinases (Backus et al., 2019). Within the protein kinase category, there are three subtypes: serine/threonine-specific kinases, tyrosine-specific kinases, and kinases of mixed specificity (Bhujbal & Hah, 2023; H. Cheng et al., 2016). Tyrosine kinases bring about the modulation of intracellular signaling pathways, which crucially take place in the case of neurodegenerative disorders. A planar irregularity in the phosphorylation of the tyrosine residues of the signaling molecules of the intracellular parts, the activity of which is controlled by protein tyrosine phosphatases (PTPs) and protein tyrosine kinases (PTKs), has been related to the neurodegenerative disorder development like AD, PD etc. (Shu et al., 2023). These anomalous phosphorylation events are the cause of processes like neuroinflammation and the accumulation of pathological proteins such as tau and β-amyloid plaques that are NDDs typical features (Mahato & Sidorova, 2020). Research studies have shown tyrosine kinase inhibitors (TKIs) as potential neuro-therapeutic options to manage the progression of degenerative diseases, which are mostly related to neurological disorders. TKIs and activators are promising therapeutic agents for treating neurodegenerative disorders, with numerous compounds currently undergoing clinical trials to evaluate their efficacy and safety. Secondly, it was found that PTPs can be considered suitable targets for drug design in recent studies (Das et al., 2023; Ricke et al., 2020). Research work done on this subject has demonstrated that the administration of hybrid molecules that can inhibit protein tyrosine phosphatase 1B (PTP1B) can help reverse hippocampal neuron loss

and cognitive impairment in AD (Kanno et al., 2016). These inhibitors target protein tyrosine phosphorylation-related signaling pathways, which is a promising way to develop new and innovative treatments for these horrible diseases (Mehdi et al., 2016; Upadhyay et al., 2024). The tyrosine receptor kinase RET (Rearranged during transfection) has likewise shown that it is a determinant of NDDs. RET is involved in multiple wide-spread vital cellular processes that allow for the maintenance and supply of the nervous system. Disturbances of RET signaling can cause severe diseases, for example, neurodegenerative disorders. Understanding RET's structure, communication pathways, and role in normal and diseased states gives clinicians the basis to develop drugs for neurodegenerative disorders and those related to them (Chattaraj, Khanal, et al., 2023; Mahato & Sidorova, 2020).

NEURODEGENERATIVE MECHANISMS

Neurodegeneration is a systematic process that involves cells and molecules in the degradation of neurons for NDDs. This suggests that various disorders share common pathophysiological mechanisms, indicating the possibility of targeting these shared pathways for therapeutic interventions. (Gan et al., 2018). Important mechanisms include ubiquitin-proteasome system malfunction and defective protein aggregation and misfolding mechanisms, mitochondrial dysfunction, oxidative stress, DNA harm, and neuroinflammatory responses (Figure 1).(Auti et al., 2022; Koziorowski et al., 2021). AD is marked by the degeneration of synapses and neurons and the formation of cell-damaging Aβ oligomers. This results in deficits at the synapse, alterations in glutamate receptors, mitochondrial dysfunction, and signaling events in the realm of synapse plasticity and neurogenesis (Crews & Masliah, 2010). Similar pathophysiological signatures include selective neuronal death; depositions of non-fibrillar proteins and fibrillary alpha-synuclein tangles; and degeneration of dopaminergic neurons, although there are different clinical manifestations between Parkinsonian dementias and PD (Brunelli et al., 2020; Chattaraj, Nandi, et al., 2023).

Neurodegenerative conditions involving tyrosine kinase activity encompass AD, ALS, multiple sclerosis (MS), and PD. These conditions are defined by abnormal protein phosphorylation regulated by PTKs and PTPs, leading to pathological events such as neuroinflammation and the buildup of misfolded proteins, including β-amyloid and tau, within the central nervous system (CNS) (Shu et al., 2023). Furthermore, other neurodegenerative ailments like FTD and Lewy body dementia (LBD) are similarly linked to tyrosine kinase irregularities and are being addressed in clinical trials utilizing TKIs (Hebron & Moussa, 2015).

Figure 1. Overall mechanisms of neurodegenerative disorders

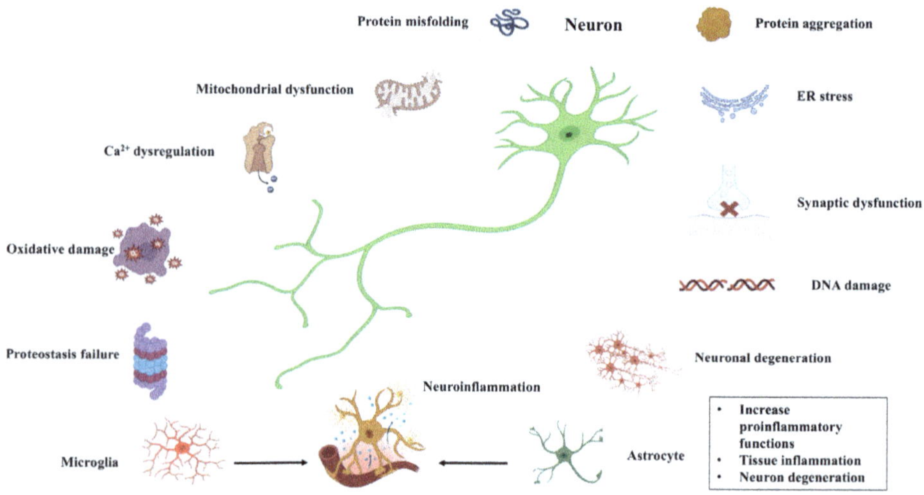

Protein Aggregation and Misfolded Proteins

Misfolded proteins and protein aggregation are the main causes of the development of neurodegenerative disorders such as HD, AD, and PD (Table 1). In these illnesses, certain proteins undergo misfolding, transforming into harmful forms that induce cellular toxicity and advance the disease process (Nandi, Das, Lin, et al., 2023; Sweeney et al., 2017). The emergence of misfolded protein aggregates characterizes neurodegenerative proteinopathies, resulting in cellular harm and toxicity. Neurodegenerative disorders are often associated with the misfolded protein accumulation within the brain. These accumulations can be located either inside or outside cells and are linked to altered biochemical processes, often resulting in the loss of neurons (Chattaraj et al., 2022; Hardy & Allsop, 1991). For instance, in AD, histopathological features include extracellular beta-amyloid deposits forming amyloid plaques and intracellular tau fibrils (Grundke-Iqbal et al., 1986). In PD, misfolded alpha-synuclein clusters form intracellular Lewy bodies, while HD presents intracellular aggregates of mutated huntingtin protein in brain and Creutzfeldt-Jakob disease (CJD)caused by infectious misfolded prion protein. These deposits mainly comprise the fibrils of protein and have traditionally been viewed as the primary drivers of cellular dysfunctions that result in the pathologies observed in these NDDs (Cremades et al., 2012; Nandi, Mandal, et al., 2024). These aberrant proteins can interact with mitochondria, disturbing their function and affecting neuronal energy levels, crucial for proper neuronal communication (Ludtmann & Abramov, 2016). The buildup of pathological proteins and impaired mitochondria sets off a harmful cycle, intensifying the progression of neurodegeneration (Jishi & Qi, 2022).

Table 1. Misfolded proteins responsible for NDDs

Disorders Related to Protein Misfolding	Aggregated Protein
ALS	Superoxide dismutase 1 (SOD1)
Huntington's disease	mutant huntingtin (mHTT)
AD	Aβ peptide, Tau
Multiple tauopathies	Tau protein
Parkinson disease	α-Synuclein
Spongiform encephalopathies	Prion proteins

(Sweeney et al., 2017)

Oxidative Stress and Mitochondrial Dysfunction

Dysfunction in mitochondria and oxidative stress are intricately linked to neurodegenerative disorders, notably PD. Mitochondrial dysfunction and atypical protein aggregation significantly contribute to the decline of dopaminergic neurons in PD (Xie et al., 2010). Research indicates that mutations in Parkinson's-related genes such as PINK1 and parkin influence the regulation of mitochondrial quality control mechanisms, whereas the accumulation of alpha-synuclein aggregates represents a significant pathological aspect in individuals with PD. The interplay between misfolded proteins and mitochondria can result in mitochondrial impairment, oxidative stress, and the death of neuronal cells, thus playing a role in the progression of neurodegeneration (Hashimoto et al., 2003). Oxidative stress, resulting from an imbalance between the generation of reactive oxygen species (ROS) and the body's antioxidant defenses, can lead to the mutations of mitochondrial DNA, disrupt the mitochondrial respiratory chain, alter membrane integrity, and disturb the balance of calcium ions, as well as the mitochondrial defense mechanisms. These alterations are linked to the initiation of neurodegenerative disorders, exacerbating dysfunction of neurons and initiating neurodegeneration (Guo et al., 2019).

Numerous studies have indicated that oxidative stress is significantly involved in the development of AD. In this condition, mitochondrial dysfunction and the abnormal accumulation of transition metals can lead to an overproduction of ROS and the aggregation of abnormal amyloid beta or tau proteins, which exacerbate the disease. Additionally, vascular and metabolic impairments, alongside mitochondrial issues, are now acknowledged as contributing factors to Alzheimer's. Vascular impairments reduce cerebral blood flow, while mitochondrial dysfunction disrupts calcium ion regulation and heightens the production of free radicals/ROS, both of which are associated with neuroinflammation (Buchholz et al., 2007; Nandi, Auti, et al., 2024; Wojda et al., 2008). Elevated levels of ROS prompt pro-inflammatory genes' activation, resulting in the cytokine release like TNF-α, IL-6, and IL-1 along with chemokines, which in turn trigger neuroinflammation. On the contrary, inflammatory reactions stimulate microglia and astrocytes to generate substantial quantities of ROS. This indicates a dual association wherein neuroinflammation can both instigate and be a consequence of chronic oxidative stress (Calabrese et al., 2018). This interplay between neuroinflammation and oxidative stress contributes to the production of beta-amyloid. The accumulation of beta amyloid peptide within brain initiates the formation of neurofibrillary tangles and inflammatory reactions leading to cell death and dementia (Kamat et al., 2016).

DNA Damage and Neuro-Inflammation

DNA damage and neuroinflammation in NDDs are interconnected processes that contribute to the pathogenesis of conditions like PD, AD, and ALS. Studies highlight that DNA damage, coupled with factors like irregular protein processing, oxidative stress, and impaired mitochondrial function, are common underlying mechanisms in these conditions (Welch & Tsai, 2022). Neuroinflammation, marked by microglial and astrocytal activation, is pivotal in these disorders, with research suggesting that inflammation may precede protein aggregation and contribute to the progression of neurodegeneration. Damage to DNA during processes like replication and transcription can trigger inflammation in microglial cells, which then interact with astrocytes and neurons, ultimately fostering neuro-degeneration (Nandi, Nigar, et al., 2023; Wang et al., 2023). DNA damage can occur through various means, such as the addition or disruption of bases, errors during replication, or breaks in either single or both strands. Significant types of DNA damage include single-strand and double-strand breaks, which involve the rupture of phosphodiester bonds in one or both strands. While single-strand breaks are more prevalent, double-strand breaks are particularly harmful, posing a greater risk of genetic instability and consequently being more detrimental. Additionally, single-strand breaks have the potential to convert into more severe double-strand breaks (Chatterjee & C, 2010). Various research shows that DNA damage prompts an inflammatory response in neuronal cells associated with NDDs comprising microglia, astrocytes, and neurons. The accumulation of DNA damage, especially in neurons, due to their high energy demands and long lifespan, can lead to dysfunctional repair processes, ultimately contributing to the inhibition of tyrosine kinases has become an attractive strategy to eradicate NDDs and neuroinflammation. The connection between DNA damage and neuroinflammation highlights the intricate relationship between these processes in the pathogenesis of NDDs (Konopka & Atkin, 2022; Nandi, Das, Dey, et al., 2023).

KINASE ENZYME AND THEIR TYPES

A kinase is an enzyme responsible for transferring a phosphate group from ATP (Adenosine triphosphate) to a specific substrate molecule, frequently a protein, through a process called phosphorylation. This alteration can either activate or deactivate the protein of interest. Kinases usually contain a conserved catalytic domain capable of binding both ATP and the protein substrate (H. C. Cheng et al., 2011). The phosphate group is subsequently covalently linked to particular amino acid residues, usually serine, threonine, or tyrosine, on the substrate. This phosphorylation occurrence can modify the function, cellular positioning, or associations with other proteins of the target protein (Ardito et al., 2017).

Various Types of Kinase Enzymes

i. Serine/Threonine Kinases (STPKs): These enzymes phosphorylate serine and threonine residues in target proteins, influencing cellular processes such as cell growth, proliferation, and programmed cell death (apoptosis). Examples include protein kinase A (PKA) and cyclin-dependent kinases (CDKs) (Rajpurohit et al., 2022).

ii. Tyrosine Kinases: This group of kinases phosphorylates tyrosine residues within target proteins, serving essential functions in cellular communication, proliferation, and survival. Instances include the epidermal growth factor receptor (EGFR) and the insulin receptor (Perona, 2006).
iii. Dual Specificity Protein Kinases (DSPKs): These kinases have the capability to phosphorylate serine, threonine, and tyrosine residues. An instance of such a kinase is MEK (MAPKK), which plays a role in the MAP kinase cascade (Caunt & Keyse, 2013).
iv. Histidine-Specific Protein Kinases: These kinases, structurally distinct, are primarily found in prokaryotes as components of two-component signal transduction mechanisms. They phosphorylate histidine residues and are involved in signaling processes (Wolanin et al., 2002).
v. Aspartic Acid/Glutamic Acid-Specific Protein Kinases: These kinases act on aspartic acid and glutamic acid residues in proteins, contributing to various cellular pathways (Ammerpohl & Kalthoff, 2007).

Each type of kinase enzyme has a specific function in cellular signaling, regulation, and metabolic pathways, underscoring their importance in maintaining proper cellular function and their potential as targets for therapeutic intervention.

TARGETING TYROSINE KINASE AS A TREATMENT STRATEGY

Targeting tyrosine kinase has become a promising approach for treating neurodegenerative disorders, for example, AD. Tyrosine kinases are pivotal in developing these conditions, rendering them appealing focal points for pharmaceutical research and development. Tyrosine kinase inhibition has surfaced as a hopeful method for treating NDDs (Fowler et al., 2019). It has been discovered that the use of inhibitors of Abelson (Abl) tyrosine kinase along with Discoidin Domain Receptors (DDRs) and Src kinases can be a means of treating neurodegenerative conditions. Several inhibitors of multi-kinases such as LCB-03-0110, Bosutinib, and Nilotinib have been established to reduce the neurotoxic proteins such as tau, amyloid beta, and alpha-synuclein whether the amount of these proteins are high in the brain or specific to Abl (Motaln & Rogelj, 2023). Moreover, these multi-kinase inhibitors can target multiple tyrosine kinases including Abl, DDRs, and Src and this is advantageous in the treatment of NDDs (Bhujbal & Hah, 2023). Its ability to lower toxic protein levels and protect neurons further supports the idea that tyrosine kinases should be therapeutic targets for neurodegeneration. Such an approach will facilitate the development of therapeutics capable of modulating critical signaling events in the neuro-degeneration process, providing a glimmer of hope for the restoration of these devastating conditions (Motaln & Rogelj, 2023).

Roles Played by Tyrosine Kinase in the Cases of Neurodegenerative Pathways

Tyrosine kinases, especially receptor tyrosine kinases (RTKs), play a critical role in numerous cellular functions like growth, movement, specialization, and metabolism. Their improper functioning can result in neuro-degeneration (Du & Lovly, 2018). Abnormalities in the phosphorylation

of tyrosine of internal signaling molecules by PTKs and PTPs are linked to neurodegenerative ailments such as AD, PD, ALS, and MS (Shu et al., 2023). These anomalies contribute to processes like neuro-inflammation and the accumulation of misfolded proteins like tau and amyloid beta plaques, those are the characteristics of these diseases (Mehdi et al., 2016). Targeting tyrosine kinases with inhibitors has displayed potential in regulating these crucial pathological mechanisms in NDDS, presenting promising avenues for therapeutic intervention in these intricate conditions (Ferguson & Gray, 2018). The non-receptor tyrosine kinase c-Abl plays a significant role in neurodegeneration (Figure 2). It is essential for normal brain development, but its abnormal expression or activation contributes to pathological processes (Motaln & Rogelj, 2023). c-Abl exerts its influence by phosphorylating cytoskeletal proteins, regulating interactions at cell-cell and cell-matrix junctions, and initiating inflammatory responses (Benn & Dawson, 2020). One critical pathway involves the c-Abl activation, and its target, p73. In models of PD, there is an increase in the levels of phosphorylation of both c-Abl and p73, which triggers the induction of the pro-apoptotic isoform of p73, TAp73. When drugs like Imatinib inhibit c-Abl, it prevents the phosphorylation of p73, thereby averting the upregulation of TAp73 and protecting dopaminergic neurons from apoptosis (Marín et al., 2022).

The aberrant phosphorylation of tyrosine residues on intracellular signaling molecules, under the control of both PTPs and PTKs, significantly contributes to the pathological mechanisms involved in neuro-inflammation and the aggregation of misfolded proteins seen in neurodegenerative disorders. Inhibiting tyrosine kinases can induce autophagy, which facilitates the clearance of toxic proteins and enhances the survival of post-mitotic neurons (Hebron & Moussa, 2015; Mou et al., 2021; Shu et al., 2023).

Additional tyrosine kinases such as ZAK and arginase 2 represent promising targets for drug intervention, as their inhibition could enhance the removal of toxic proteins associated with neurodegenerative disorders. TKIs can stimulate autophagy, facilitating the clearance of misfolded proteins without triggering neuronal apoptosis. Furthermore, TKIs might influence myeloid cells to generate growth factors that support neuronal viability (Hebron & Moussa, 2015). Fyn, a type of non-receptor tyrosine kinase within the Src family, has been associated with numerous processes like myelination, the transmission of signals between neurons, and the development of certain neurodegenerative conditions. These conditions include demyelination, the abnormal buildup of proteins, neuro-inflammation, and impairment in cognitive function (Guglietti et al., 2021). Kinases such as CSF1R contribute to regulate the proliferation of microglia, which increases neurodegenerative disorders. The DLK-JNK pathway is a well-known controller of neuronal degeneration post-injury and has been linked to pathways involved in PD and AD (Benn & Dawson, 2020). Overall, tyrosine kinases are crucial regulators of numerous pathological processes in neurodegeneration. Targeting specific kinases like c-Abl, ZAK, and CSF1R could offer therapeutic advantages by decreasing neuro-inflammation, eliminating harmful proteins, and supporting neuronal survival (Motaln & Rogelj, 2023). However, further investigation is necessary to create kinase inhibitors that can penetrate the brain effectively and selectively for clinical use in neurodegenerative disorders (Hebron & Moussa, 2015).

Figure 2. The contribution of c-Abl tyrosine kinase in brain along with its pathologies

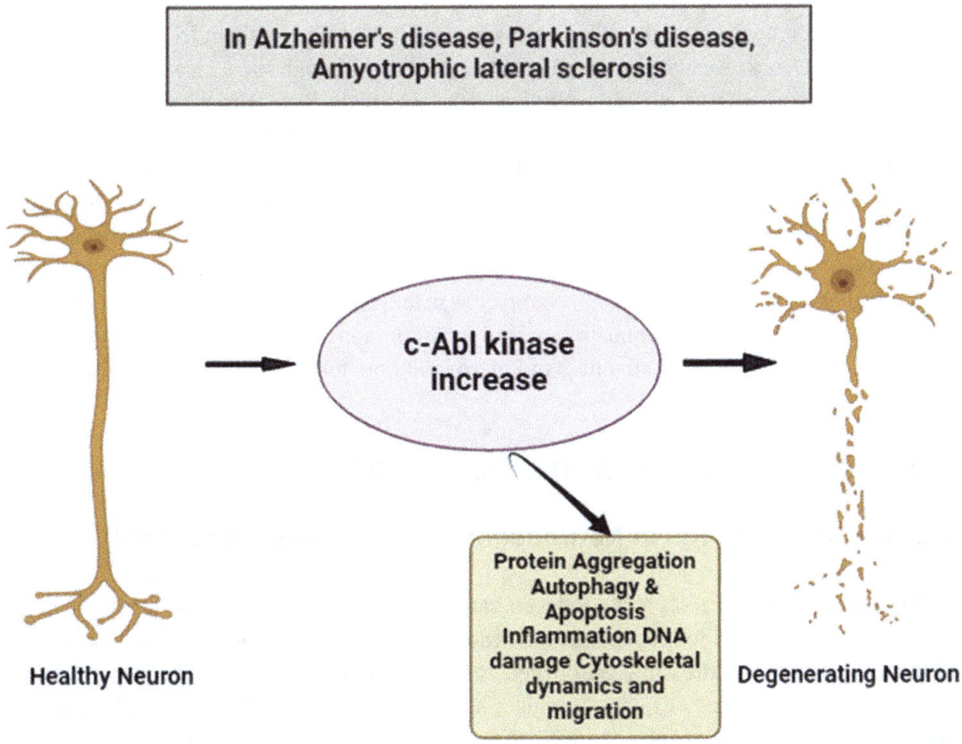

Strategies for Tyrosine Kinase Inhibition

Recently, inhibiting tyrosine kinase was found a potential solution to deal with neurodegenerative disorders like AD (Fagiani et al., 2020). A lot of trials have been conducted on the ability of TKIs that are used to treat cancer, as well as other forms of dementia like AD, to be considered as disease-modifying treatments (Bhujbal & Hah, 2023). This strategy is established on tyrosine kinases being the most important regulators of the intracellular pathways that control cell metabolism and replication. The pathways mentioned, in the context of cancer and neurodegenerative disease, are damaged causing abnormal cells that demand treatment. Through the prevention of malignant kinase, TKIs work to curb neurodegenerative disease development (Fagiani et al., 2020). This preclinical research using animal models not only showed promise but also some encouraging results. As an instance, the tyrosine kinase inhibitor ibrutinib notably reduces amyloidβ plaques, hyperphosphorylation of tau, and neuro-inflammation in 5xFAD mice which model the early stage of Alzheimer that is usually observed among the patients (Kim et al., 2022). Yet, all TKIs do not show therapeutic advantageous effects; some of them rather contribute to the manifestation of pathology in this mouse model. This shows the need for optimizing drug dosage, administration mode, and timing when transferring TKIs for the therapy of neurodegenerative disorders (Lee et al., 2023). Covalent kinase inhibitors, which are

covalently bound to the target enzyme, represent a new approach that can, potentially, translate to improved potency and selectivity, as compared to conventional reversible inhibitors (Sutanto et al., 2020). Obtaining the isoform-selective covalent inhibitors, among them JNK3 kinase, which is mapped to AD, is a research goal now (Lee et al., 2023). Although some kinase inhibitors have shown great in vitro activity, all of the clinical trials investigating such drugs for AD have failed. Possibly, AD's multifactorial and complex nature which could involve simultaneous targeting of multiple kinases through combinational therapy is the reason for this type of therapy failure (Fagiani et al., 2020). Next, the serious toxicity of kinase inhibitors along with other side effects is another problem that has to be overcome (Caldemeyer et al., 2016). However, despite that, TKIs seem to have great potential in the ailment of neurodegenerative disorders, but there are still several obstacles that need to be overcome to use these inhibitors in practice. Improvements in drug design, titration and administration, and incorporation of combination therapy may help to improve the therapeutic effectiveness of kinase inhibitors for these diseases(Cui, 2014).

CLINICAL APPLICATIONS AND CHALLENGES

Current Status of TKIs in Neurodegenerative Disease Treatment

The current status of TKIs in neurodegenerative disease treatment is a rapidly evolving field with significant potential for therapeutic applications. Research has centered on the contribution of kinase inhibitors in addressing neurodegenerative conditions like AD, PD, and ALS (Bhujbal & Hah, 2023). Studies have explored covalent kinase inhibitors, including c-Abl inhibitors like Imatinib, Nilotinib, and others, to target key pathways involved in neuro-degeneration. These inhibitors have demonstrated efficacy in mitigating amyloid-β plaque formation, reducing hyperphosphorylation of tau, alleviating neuro-inflammation, and enhancing cognitive function in animal models (Brahmachari et al., 2017).

In AD, research stated that TKIs have the potential to regulate autophagy, protein degradation, and neuronal continuation, which progress the disease. Inhibiting tyrosine kinases such as c-Abl and Fyn has demonstrated neuro-protective effects, possibly by diminishing the buildup of harmful proteins and enhancing cellular. Also the use of anti-cancer drugs, like nilotinib has been explored for their potential in repurposing for non-oncological indications like AD (Table 2) (Lee et al., 2023).

In PD, inhibiting c-Abl kinase activity has been associated with halting neuro-degeneration, and medications used for cancer treatment have displayed positive effects in animal models of PD. Extensive research has investigated the connection between c-Abl and α-synuclein, a protein involved in PD pathology, revealing that inhibiting c-Abl can mitigate neuro-degeneration induced by α-synuclein (Lindholm et al., 2016).

In ALS, tyrosine kinases' role in the disease's progression has been investigated, and inhibitors like masitinib have been found to modulate neuro-inflammation and slow disease progression in preclinical models. The efficacy of masitinib in treating ALS has been demonstrated by its ability to prolong the survival of SOD1 G93A rats, a commonly used model for inherited ALS (Lonskaya et al., 2013).

Table 2. Cancer kinase inhibitors in AD in clinical trials

Drugs / Substances	Phase	Mode of action	Therapeutic purpose
Nilotinib (AMN107)	Phase II active, not enlisting	TKI of Bcr-Abl	Reduce the phosphorylation levels of tau and amyloid proteins
Tideglusib (NP031112)	Phase I and II have done	Inhibitor of GSK-3 by selectively targeting sites other than ATP-binding sites	Reduced amyloid buildup, hyperphosphorylation of tau proteins, and neuronal loss
Saracatinib (AZD0530)	Phase II (completed)	TKI of Src	Effect on the cerebral glucose metabolic rate
Neflamapimod	Phase II (completed)	Inhibitor of p38 MAPKα, an enzyme responsible for the transduction of signal	Reduces the plaques of amyloid
DNL747	Phase I active, not enlisting	Inhibitor of receptor-interacting protein kinase 1 (RIPK1)	Reduce levels of cytokines and other inflammatory factors
Masitinib (AB1010)	Phase III active, not enlisting	TKI that targets c-Kit, platelet-derived growth factor receptors, and to a lesser extent, Lyn, Fyn, and the FAK pathway	Impacts on mast cells, and the regulation of inflammatory processes

(Fagiani et al., 2020)

Challenges and Limitations in Targeting Tyrosine Kinase for Therapy

Developing TKIs for the ailment of NDDs presents several challenges. Although protein kinases show promise as potential therapeutic targets for neurodegenerative therapy, there are challenges and limitations in effectively addressing them. While these kinases hold potential as targets for conditions like AD, the development of therapies focusing on kinases for CNS disorders faces obstacles (Hussain et al., 2018).

i. Cytochrome P450-mediated metabolism: Cytochrome P450-dependent metabolism may cause rapid elimination of TKIs, which can compromise their effectiveness. Therefore, enhancing their pharmacokinetic characteristics is crucial (Fagiani et al., 2020).
ii. The potential toxicity and unintended impacts of TKIs, including issues like cardiovascular, gastrointestinal, and hematologic complications, require thorough management and monitoring (Jabbour et al., 2011).
iii. Overcoming the obstacle of blood-brain barrier penetration poses a significant challenge, as many TKIs struggles to enter the central nervous system. It is crucial to develop inhibitors specifically designed to penetrate the CNS effectively (Mehdi et al., 2016).
iv. Concentrating exclusively on a single tyrosine kinase may not yield the desired results due to the complex nature of diseases like AD. Therefore, employing combination therapies or inhibitors targeting multiple factors could be essential (Maramai et al., 2020).
v. The delay in CNS drug discovery, in contrast to other disease domains such as cancer, has resulted in fewer TKIs being developed and evaluated for neurodegenerative uses. Further research in this field is imperative (Benn & Dawson, 2020)
vi. Translational Gap: The complexity of human NDDs may not be fully mirrored by animal models, which presents difficulties in accurately predicting the effectiveness of TKIs in clinical trials(Tello et al., 2022).

POTENTIAL SIDE EFFECTS OF TKIS IN NDDS

TKIs, initially developed for the ailment of cancer, are now being explored as potential treatments for neurodegenerative disorders like PD and AD (Benn & Dawson, 2020). While preclinical studies show promise as they manipulate autophagy and facilitate the degradation of harmful proteins, TKIs also pose significant risks of adverse effects (Bhullar et al., 2018).

The most commonly observed cardiovascular complications associated with TKIs include hypertension, atrial fibrillation, diminished cardiac function, heart failure, and sudden death. Neurological impairment, such as an increased occurrence of cerebral infarction (stroke), is noted among chronic myeloid leukemia patients subjected to prolonged courses of higher doses of nilotinib (Sunder et al., 2023). Gastrointestinal issues such as diarrhea are frequent, followed by the symptoms like fatigue, fluid retention, muscle cramps (Brümmendorf et al., 2015).

Skin-related adverse effects such as rashes are commonly observed (Druker et al., 2006).

Potential interactions with other drugs, supplements, and certain food items may either diminish the efficacy of TKIs or result in unsafe elevations of TKI concentrations in the bloodstream. Patients often report cognitive difficulties and depressive symptoms that may not be fully recognized by healthcare providers (Hyland et al., 2023; Schoenbeck et al., 2020). Further investigation is needed to gain deeper insights into the mechanisms underlying the adverse effects and to devise efficacious strategies for their management.

POTENTIAL BENEFITS OF USING TKIS IN COMBINATION WITH OTHER TREATMENTS FOR NEURODEGENERATIVE PATHWAYS

The potential advantages of employing TKIs alongside other therapies for neurodegenerative pathways include:

i. **Enhanced Treatment Effectiveness:** By combining TKIs with other treatments, there's a possibility of achieving better therapeutic results as it targets various mechanisms and pathways implicated in neurodegenerative conditions (Lee et al., 2023)
ii. **Diminished Adverse Effects:** Through the precise targeting of specific kinases and pathways, the amalgamation of TKIs with other therapies might reduce the side effects associated with singular treatment approaches, thereby improving the overall safety and tolerability of the regimen (Fagiani et al., 2020).
iii. **Expanded Targeted Therapy:** Integrating TKIs with other treatments could broaden the scope of targeted therapy by addressing multiple kinases and pathways linked to NDDs, potentially enhancing the efficacy of disease modification strategies (Bhujbal & Hah, 2023).
iv. **Enhanced Patient Outcomes:** Combining TKIs with other treatments holds the promise of better patient outcomes by tackling various aspects of NDDs, including neuro-inflammation, oxidative stress, and the dysfunction of proteasomes (Fagiani et al., 2020; Lee et al., 2023).
v. **Advanced Insight into Disease Mechanisms:** The combination of TKIs with other therapies can offer valuable insights into the fundamental pathophysiology of NDDs, paving the path for the creation of more effective therapeutic approaches (Bhujbal & Hah, 2023).

FUTURE PERSPECTIVES

Tyrosine kinases have become an auspicious focal point for addressing neurodegenerative conditions in the future. DYRKs have been found to play a key role in various neuronal cellular functions implicated in neurodegeneration like DNA repair, cell survival, and synaptic plasticity. Moreover, the protein kinases related to DYRKs have significant potential in investigating treatments for NDDs like AD (Bellantoni & Wagner, 2021). These advances have further highlighted the need to understand the role of tyrosine kinases as strategic targets in the ailment of NDDs. Future research should endeavor to focus more on the discovery of newer tyrosine kinase targets that are closely associated with neurodegeneration. Intensive screening and use of state-of-the-art bioinformatics tools will ensure fast observation of such new targets. Therefore, the next step should be generating better therapeutic approaches that address the fundamental mechanisms by which abnormal tyrosine phosphorylation causes neuro-degeneration (Ferguson & Gray, 2018). TKIs can be combined with anti-inflammatory and neuro-protective drugs to yield increased efficacy. Continued advancements in research and collaborative efforts across disciplines offer promising prospects for tyrosine kinase-targeted therapies, with the potential to significantly enhance outcomes for individuals affected by severe neurodegenerative disorders (Dunkel et al., 2012).

CONCLUSION

NDDs have a variety of brain disorders with a concept of multilevel and multifactorial processes in the brain. This state is marked by the progressive decline in cognitive, mnemonic, and motor abilities. On the other hand, even though there have been considerable achievements in understanding the mechanisms and pathogenesis of NDDs, drug development efforts still do not lead to any effective treatments, stressing the pressing need for new clinical approaches. Recent studies reveal the influence of abnormal protein tyrosine phosphorylation of many proteins on the occurrence of these diseases. Many PTPs and PTKs have been observed to be dysregulated in the brain during neurological disorders, and the treatment of these enzymes with particular inhibitors or activators has shown to have therapeutic potential for NDDs. PTK inhibitors are currently being explored in some clinical trials. Nevertheless, there is still a lot about the roles of the numerous PTK and PTP members in the neurodegenerative disease development that are unknown. The chapter addresses the current state of research on protein tyrosine phosphorylation in NDDs, intending to provide the theoretical foundation and directions for future studies.

ACKNOWLEDGEMENT

All the authors are thankful to the Principal and Head of the Department of Pharmacy, Sanaka Educational Trusts Group of Institutions, Durgapur, West Bengal, 713212, for their encouragement of this work.

REFERENCES

Ahmed, T., Zulfiqar, A., Arguelles, S., Rasekhian, M., Nabavi, S. F., Silva, A. S., & Nabavi, S. M. (2020). Map kinase signaling as therapeutic target for neurodegeneration. *Pharmacological Research, 160*, 105090. DOI: 10.1016/j.phrs.2020.105090

Ammerpohl, O., & Kalthoff, H. (2007). The role of protein kinases in pancreatic carcinogenesis. *Clinica Chimica Acta, 381*(1), 56–62. DOI: 10.1016/j.cca.2007.02.024

Ardito, F., Giuliani, M., Perrone, D., Troiano, G., & Lo Muzio, L. (2017). The crucial role of protein phosphorylation in cell signalingand its use as targeted therapy [Review]. *International Journal of Molecular Medicine, 40*(2), 271–280. DOI: 10.3892/ijmm.2017.3036

Auti, P. S., Nandi, A., Kumari, V., & Paul, A. T. (2022). Design, synthesis, biological evaluation and molecular modelling studies of oxoacetamide warhead containing indole-quinazolinone based novel hybrid analogues as potential pancreatic lipase inhibitors. *New Journal of Chemistry, 46*(24), 11648–11661. DOI: 10.1039/D2NJ01210C

Backus, K. M., Cao, J., & Maddox, S. M. (2019). Opportunities and challenges for the development of covalent chemical immunomodulators. *Bioorganic & Medicinal Chemistry, 27*(15), 3421–3439. DOI: 10.1016/j.bmc.2019.05.050

Bellantoni, A. J., & Wagner, L. M. (2021). Pursuing precision: Receptor tyrosine kinase inhibitors for treatment of pediatric solid tumors. *Cancers (Basel), 13*(14), 1–22. DOI: 10.3390/cancers13143531

Benn, C. L., & Dawson, L. A. (2020). Clinically Precedented Protein Kinases: Rationale for Their Use in Neurodegenerative Disease. *Frontiers in Aging Neuroscience, 12*(September), 1–29. DOI: 10.3389/fnagi.2020.00242

Bhujbal, S. P., & Hah, J. M. (2023). An Innovative Approach to Address Neurodaegenerative Diseases through Kinase-Targeted Therapies: Potential for Designing Covalent Inhibitors. *Pharmaceuticals (Basel, Switzerland), 16*(9), 1295–1308. DOI: 10.3390/ph16091295

Bhullar, K. S., Lagarón, N. O., McGowan, E. M., Parmar, I., Jha, A., Hubbard, B. P., & Rupasinghe, H. P. V. (2018). Kinase-targeted cancer therapies: Progress, challenges and future directions. *Molecular Cancer, 17*(1), 1–20. DOI: 10.1186/s12943-018-0804-2

Brahmachari, S., Karuppagounder, S. S., Ge, P., Lee, S., Dawson, V. L., Dawson, T. M., & Ko, H. S. (2017). C-Abl and Parkinson's Disease: Mechanisms and Therapeutic Potential. *Journal of Parkinson's Disease, 7*(4), 589–601. DOI: 10.3233/JPD-171191

Brümmendorf, T. H., Cortes, J. E., de Souza, C. A., Guilhot, F., Duvillié, L., Pavlov, D., Gogat, K., Countouriotis, A. M., & Gambacorti-Passerini, C. (2015). Bosutinib versus imatinib in newly diagnosed chronic-phase chronic myeloid leukaemia: Results from the 24-month follow-up of the BELA trial. *British Journal of Haematology, 168*(1), 69–81. DOI: 10.1111/bjh.13108

Brunelli, F., Valente, E. M., & Arena, G. (2020). Mechanisms of neurodegeneration in Parkinson's disease: Keep neurons in the PINK1. *Mechanisms of Ageing and Development, 189*(May), 111277–111284. DOI: 10.1016/j.mad.2020.111277

Buchholz, J. N., Behringer, E. J., Pottorf, W. J., Pearce, W. J., & Vanterpool, C. K. (2007). Age-dependent changes in Ca2+ homeostasis in peripheral neurones: Implications for changes in function. *Aging Cell, 6*(3), 285–296. DOI: 10.1111/j.1474-9726.2007.00298.x

Calabrese, V., Santoro, A., Monti, D., Crupi, R., Di Paola, R., Latteri, S., Cuzzocrea, S., Zappia, M., Giordano, J., Calabrese, E. J., & Franceschi, C. (2018). Aging and Parkinson's Disease: Inflammaging, neuroinflammation and biological remodeling as key factors in pathogenesis. *Free Radical Biology and Medicine, 115*(October 2017), 80–91. DOI: 10.1016/j.freeradbiomed.2017.10.379

Caldemeyer, L., Dugan, M., Edwards, J., & Akard, L. (2016). Long-Term Side Effects of Tyrosine Kinase Inhibitors in Chronic Myeloid Leukemia. *Current Hematologic Malignancy Reports, 11*(2), 71–79. DOI: 10.1007/s11899-016-0309-2

Caunt, C. J., & Keyse, S. M. (2013). Dual-specificity MAP kinase phosphatases (MKPs) Shaping the outcome of MAP kinase signalling. *The FEBS Journal, 280*(2), 489–504. DOI: 10.1111/j.1742-4658.2012.08716.x

Chattaraj, B., Khanal, P., Nandi, A., Das, A., Sharma, A., Mitra, S., & Dey, Y. N. (2023). Network pharmacology and molecular modelling study of Enhydra fluctuans for the prediction of the molecular mechanisms involved in the amelioration of nephrolithiasis. *Journal of Biomolecular Structure & Dynamics, 0*(0), 1–11. DOI: 10.1080/07391102.2023.2189476

Chattaraj, B., Nandi, A., Anwesha, D., Sharma, A., Kumar, D., Dey, N. Y., & Rajagopal, M. (2022). In vitro antilithiatic activity of Enhydra fluctuans Lour. on calcium oxalate crystallisation and the elucidation of the possible mechanism involved therein through in silico studies. *Frontiers in Pharmacology, 13*, 1–29.

Chattaraj, B., Nandi, A., Das, A., Baidya, A., Mahata, S., Chowdhury, A., Mitra, S., Roy, S., Chakraborty, S., & Dey, Y. N. (2023). Enhydra fluctuans Lour. aqueous extract inhibited the growth of calcium phosphate crystals: An in vitro study. *Food Chemistry Advances, 2*(August 2022), 100287. DOI: 10.1016/j.focha.2023.100287

Chatterjee, N., & C, W. G. (2010). Mechanisms of DNADamage, Repair, and Mutagenesis. *Environmental and Molecular Mutagenesis, 405*(April), 391–405. DOI: 10.1002/em

Cheng, H., Nair, S. K., & Murray, B. W. (2016). Recent progress on third generation covalent EGFR inhibitors. *Bioorganic & Medicinal Chemistry Letters, 26*(8), 1861–1868. DOI: 10.1016/j.bmcl.2016.02.067

Cheng, H. C., Qi, R. Z., Paudel, H., & Zhu, H. J. (2011). Regulation and function of protein kinases and phosphatases. *Enzyme Research, 2011*(1), 7–9. DOI: 10.4061/2011/794089

Cremades, N., Cohen, S. I. A., Deas, E., Abramov, A. Y., Chen, A. Y., Orte, A., Sandal, M., Clarke, R. W., Dunne, P., Aprile, F. A., Bertoncini, C. W., Wood, N. W., Knowles, T. P. J., Dobson, C. M., & Klenerman, D. (2012). Direct observation of the interconversion of normal and toxic forms of α-synuclein. *Cell, 149*(5), 1048–1059. DOI: 10.1016/j.cell.2012.03.037

Crews, L., & Masliah, E. (2010). Molecular mechanisms of neurodegeneration in Alzheimer's disease. *Human Molecular Genetics*, *19*(1), 12–20. DOI: 10.1093/hmg/ddq160

Cui, J. J. (2014). A new challenging and promising era of tyrosine kinase inhibitors. *ACS Medicinal Chemistry Letters*, *5*(4), 272–274. DOI: 10.1021/ml500091p

Das, A., Nandi, A., Kumari, V., & Alvala, M. (2023). FBDD & De Novo Drug Design. In *Applied Computer-Aided Drug Design: Models and Methods* (pp. 159–201). BENTHAM SCIENCE PUBLISHERS. DOI: 10.2174/9789815179934123010008

Druker, B. J., Guilhot, F., O'Brien, S. G., Gathmann, I., Kantarjian, H., Gattermann, N., Deininger, M. W. N., Silver, R. T., Goldman, J. M., Stone, R. M., Cervantes, F., Hochhaus, A., Powell, B. L., Gabrilove, J. L., Rousselot, P., Reiffers, J., Cornelissen, J. J., Hughes, T., Agis, H., & Larson, R. A. (2006). Five-Year Follow-up of Patients Receiving Imatinib for Chronic Myeloid Leukemia. *The New England Journal of Medicine*, *355*(23), 2408–2417. DOI: 10.1056/NEJMoa062867

Du, Z., & Lovly, C. M. (2018). Mechanisms of receptor tyrosine kinase activation in cancer. *Molecular Cancer*, *17*(1), 1–13. DOI: 10.1186/s12943-018-0782-4

Dunkel, P., Chai, C. L., Sperlágh, B., Huleatt, P. B., & Mátyus, P. (2012). Clinical utility of neuroprotective agents in neurodegenerative diseases: Current status of drug development for Alzheimer's, Parkinson's and Huntington's diseases, and amyotrophic lateral sclerosis. *Expert Opinion on Investigational Drugs*, *21*(9), 1267–1308. DOI: 10.1517/13543784.2012.703178

Fagiani, F., Lanni, C., Racchi, M., & Govoni, S. (2020). Targeting dementias through cancer kinases inhibition. *Alzheimer's & Dementia: Translational Research & Clinical Interventions*, *6*(May), 1–10. DOI: 10.1002/trc2.12044

Ferguson, F. M., & Gray, N. S. (2018). Kinase inhibitors : The road ahead. *Nature Reviews. Drug Discovery*, *17*(5), 353–376. DOI: 10.1038/nrd.2018.21

Fowler, A. J., Hebron, M., Missner, A. A., Wang, R., Gao, X., Kurd-Misto, B. T., Liu, X., & Moussa, C. E. H. (2019). Multikinase Abl/DDR/Src Inhibition Produces Optimal Effects for Tyrosine Kinase Inhibition in Neurodegeneration. *Drugs in R&D.*, *19*(2), 149–166. DOI: 10.1007/s40268-019-0266-z

Gan, L., Cookson, M. R., Petrucelli, L., & La Spada, A. R. (2018). Converging pathways in neurodegeneration, from genetics to mechanisms. *Nature Neuroscience*, *21*(10), 1300–1309. DOI: 10.1038/s41593-018-0237-7

Gitler, A. D., Dhillon, P., & Shorter, J. (2017). Neurodegenerative disease: Models, mechanisms, and a new hope. *Disease Models & Mechanisms*, *10*(5), 499–502. DOI: 10.1242/dmm.030205

Grundke-Iqbal, I., Iqbal, K., Tung, Y. C., Quinlan, M., Wisniewski, H. M., & Binder, L. I. (1986). Abnormal phosphorylation of the microtubule-associated protein τ (tau) in Alzheimer cytoskeletal pathology. *Proceedings of the National Academy of Sciences of the United States of America*, *83*(13), 44913–44917. DOI: 10.1073/pnas.83.13.4913

Guglietti, B., Sivasankar, S., Mustafa, S., Corrigan, F., & Collins, L. E. (2021). Fyn Kinase Activity and Its Role in Neurodegenerative Disease Pathology : A Potential Universal Target? *Molecular Neurobiology*, *58*(11), 5986–6005. DOI: 10.1007/s12035-021-02518-3

Guo, Y., Liu, Y., Hu, N., Yu, D., Zhou, C., Shi, G., Zhang, B., Wei, M., Liu, J., Luo, L., Tang, Z., Song, H., Guo, Y., Liu, X., Su, D., Zhang, S., Song, X., Zhou, X., Hong, Y., & Wang, Z. (2019). Discovery of Zanubrutinib (BGB-3111), a Novel, Potent, and Selective Covalent Inhibitor of Bruton's Tyrosine Kinase. *Journal of Medicinal Chemistry*, *62*(17), 7923–7940. DOI: 10.1021/acs.jmedchem.9b00687

Hardy, J., & Allsop, D. (1991). Amyloid deposition as the central event in the aetiology of Alzheimer's disease. *Trends in Pharmacological Sciences*, *12*, 383–388. DOI: 10.1016/0165-6147(91)90609-V

Hashimoto, M., Rockenstein, E., Crews, L., & Masliah, E. (2003). Role of Protein Aggregation in Mitochondrial Dysfunction and Neurodegeneration in Alzheimer's and Parkinson's Diseases. In *NeuroMolecular Medicine* (Vol. 4, Issues 1–2, pp. 21–35). DOI: 10.1385/NMM:4:1-2:21

Hebron, M., & Moussa, C. E. H. (2015). Two sides of the same coin: Tyrosine kinase inhibition in cancer and neurodegeneration. *Neural Regeneration Research*, *10*(11), 1767–1769. DOI: 10.4103/1673-5374.165320

Hussain, R., Zubair, H., Pursell, S., & Shahab, M. (2018). Neurodegenerative diseases: Regenerative mechanisms and novel therapeutic approaches. *Brain Sciences*, *8*(9), 1–37. DOI: 10.3390/brainsci8090177

Hyland, K. A., Eisel, S. L., Hoogland, A. I., Root, J. C., Bowles, K., James, B., Nelson, A. M., Booth-Jones, M., Jacobsen, P. B., Ahles, T. A., Jim, H. S. L., & Gonzalez, B. D. (2023). Cognition in patients treated with targeted therapy for chronic myeloid leukemia: A controlled comparison. *Leukemia & Lymphoma*, *64*(2), 415–423. DOI: 10.1080/10428194.2022.2148208

Jabbour, E., Deininger, M., & Hochhaus, A. (2011). Management of adverse events associated with tyrosine kinase inhibitors in the treatment of chronic myeloid leukemia. *Leukemia*, *25*(2), 201–210. DOI: 10.1038/leu.2010.215

Jishi, A., & Qi, X. (2022). Altered Mitochondrial Protein Homeostasis and Proteinopathies. *Frontiers in Molecular Neuroscience*, *15*(April), 1–16. DOI: 10.3389/fnmol.2022.867935

Kamat, P. K., Kalani, A., Rai, S., Swarnkar, S., Tota, S., Nath, C., & Tyagi, N. (2016). Mechanism of Oxidative Stress and Synapse Dysfunction in the Pathogenesis of Alzheimer's Disease: Understanding the Therapeutics Strategies. *Molecular Neurobiology*, *53*(1), 648–661. DOI: 10.1007/s12035-014-9053-6

Kanno, T., Tsuchiya, A., Tanaka, A., & Nishizaki, T. (2016). Combination of PKCε Activation and PTP1B Inhibition Effectively Suppresses Aβ-Induced GSK-3β Activation and Tau Phosphorylation. *Molecular Neurobiology*, *53*(7), 4787–4797. DOI: 10.1007/s12035-015-9405-x

Kim, J., Lee, H., Park, J. H., Cha, B. Y., & Hoe, H. S. (2022). Nilotinib modulates LPS - induced cognitive impairment and neuroinflammatory responses by regulating P38 / STAT3 signaling. *Journal of Neuroinflammation*, *19*(187), 1–28. DOI: 10.1186/s12974-022-02549-0

Konopka, A., & Atkin, J. D. (2022). DNA Damage, Defective DNA Repair, and Neurodegeneration in Amyotrophic Lateral Sclerosis. *Frontiers in Aging Neuroscience*, *14*(April), 1–15. DOI: 10.3389/fnagi.2022.786420

Kovacs, G. G. (2014). Current Concepts of Neurodegenerative Diseases. *Neurology*, *1*(July), 78–86. DOI: 10.33590/emjneurol/10314777

Kovacs, G. G., Botond, G., & Budka, H. (2010). Protein coding of neurodegenerative dementias: The neuropathological basis of biomarker diagnostics. *Acta Neuropathologica*, *119*(4), 389–408. DOI: 10.1007/s00401-010-0658-1

Koziorowski, D., Figura, M., Milanowski, Ł. M., Szlufik, S., Alster, P., Madetko, N., & Friedman, A. (2021). Mechanisms of neurodegeneration in various forms of parkinsonism—Similarities and differences. *Cells*, *10*(3), 1–29. DOI: 10.3390/cells10030656

Lee, H., Hwang, J.-W., Park, J.-H., Jeong, Y. J., Jang, J.-Y., & Hoe, H.-S. (2023). Profiling tyrosine kinase inhibitors as AD therapeutics in a mouse model of AD. *Molecular Brain*, *16*(63), 1–5. DOI: 10.1186/s13041-023-01051-9

Lindholm, D., Pham, D. D., Cascone, A., Eriksson, O., Wennerberg, K., & Saarma, M. (2016). C-Abl inhibitors enable insights into the pathophysiology and neuroprotection in Parkinson's disease. *Frontiers in Aging Neuroscience*, *8*, 6–11. DOI: 10.3389/fnagi.2016.00254

Lonskaya, I., Hebron, M. L., Desforges, N. M., Franjie, A., & Moussa, C. E. H. (2013). Tyrosine kinase inhibition increases functional parkin-Beclin-1 interaction and enhances amyloid clearance and cognitive performance. *EMBO Molecular Medicine*, *5*(8), 1247–1262. DOI: 10.1002/emmm.201302771

Ludtmann, M. H. R., & Abramov, A. Y. (2016). *Protein Misfolding and Aggregation: Implications for Mitochondrial Dysfunction and Neurodegeneration Marthe* (2nd ed.). Mitochondrial Dysfunction in Neurodegenerative Disorders., DOI: 10.1007/978-3-319-28637-2

Mahato, A. K., & Sidorova, Y. A. (2020). Ret receptor tyrosine kinase: Role in neurodegeneration, obesity, and cancer. *International Journal of Molecular Sciences*, *21*(19), 1–21. DOI: 10.3390/ijms21197108

Maramai, S., Benchekroun, M., Gabr, M. T., & Yahiaoui, S. (2020). Multitarget Therapeutic Strategies for Alzheimer's Disease: Review on Emerging Target Combinations. *BioMed Research International*, *2020*(1), 1–27. DOI: 10.1155/2020/5120230

Marín, T., Valls, C., Jerez, C., Elgueta, D., Vidal, L., Alvarez, A. R., & Cancino, G. I. (2022). The c-Abl / p73 pathway induces neurodegeneration in a Parkinson ' s disease model. *IBRO Neuroscience Reports, 13*(January), 378–387. DOI: 10.1016/j.ibneur.2022.10.006

Mehdi, S. J., Barger, S. W., Paule, M. G., Ali, S. F., & Imam, S. Z. (2016). Tyrosine Kinase Inhibitors and Neurodegenerative Disorders. *Inflammation, Aging, and Oxidative Stress, Oxidative Stress in Applied Basic Research and Clinical Practice*, 81–91. DOI: 10.1007/978-3-319-33486-8_5

Motaln, H., & Rogelj, B. (2023). The Role of c-Abl Tyrosine Kinase in Brain and Its Pathologies. *Cells, 12*(16), 1–23. DOI: 10.3390/cells12162041

Mou, L., Tian, X., Zhou, B., Zhan, Y., Chen, J., Lu, Y., Deng, J., Deng, Y., Wu, Z., Li, Q., Song, Y., Zhang, H., Chen, J., Tian, K., Ni, Y., & Pu, Z. (2021). Improving Outcomes of Tyrosine Kinase Inhibitors in Hepatocellular Carcinoma: New Data and Ongoing Trials. *Frontiers in Oncology, 11*(October), 1–11. DOI: 10.3389/fonc.2021.752725

Nandi, A., Auti, P. S., Jagtap, U. A., & Paul, A. T. (2024). Investigating the role of indole and quinazolinone-based hybrid analogues with ketoamide fragment and alkyl extension for potential PL inhibition. *Journal of Molecular Structure, 1301*, 137337. DOI: 10.1016/j.molstruc.2023.137337

Nandi, A., Das, A., Dey, Y. N., & Roy, K. K. (2023). The Abundant Phytocannabinoids in Rheumatoid Arthritis: Therapeutic Targets and Molecular Processes Identified Using Integrated Bioinformatics and Network Pharmacology. *Life (Basel, Switzerland), 13*(3), 1–19. DOI: 10.3390/life13030700

Nandi, A., Das, A., Lin, W.-Y., & Chakraborty, P. (2023). Antiviral Drugs - in Past and Current Pandemics. In *Current Trends in the Identification and Development of Antimicrobial Agents* (pp. 167–194). BENTHAM SCIENCE PUBLISHERS., DOI: 10.2174/9789815080056123020009

Nandi, A., Mandal, N., Das, A., & Dey, Y. N. (2024). Approaches Based on Network Pharmacology and Molecular Docking to Predict the Molecular Mechanism of Plumbago zeylanica ' s Anti-Inflammatory Action. *Journal of Biological Regulators and Homeostatic Agents, 38*(3), 2055–2067.

Nandi, A., Nigar, T., Das, A., & Dey, Y. N. (2023). Network pharmacology analysis of Plumbago zeylanica to identify the therapeutic targets and molecular mechanisms involved in ameliorating hemorrhoids. *Journal of Biomolecular Structure & Dynamics, 0*(0), 1–15. DOI: 10.1080/07391102.2023.2280681

Perona, R. (2006). Cell signalling: Growth factors and tyrosine kinase receptors. *Clinical & Translational Oncology, 8*(2), 77–82. DOI: 10.1007/s12094-006-0162-1

Rajpurohit, Y. S., Kumar, D., & Misra, H. S. (2022). Research in Microbiology Involvement of serine / threonine protein kinases in DNA damage response and cell division in bacteria. *Research in Microbiology, 173*(1-2), 103883–103893. DOI: 10.1016/j.resmic.2021.103883

Ricke, K. M., Cruz, S. A., Qin, Z., Farrokhi, K., Sharmin, F., Zhang, L., Zasloff, M. A., Stewart, A. F. R., & Chen, H. H. (2020). Neuronal protein tyrosine phosphatase 1B hastens amyloid β-associated Alzheimer's disease in mice. *The Journal of Neuroscience : The Official Journal of the Society for Neuroscience, 40*(7), 1581–1593. DOI: 10.1523/JNEUROSCI.2120-19.2019

Schoenbeck, K. L., Tummala, S., Goyal, N. G., Smith, C. C., & Shah, N. P. (2020). Cognitive Dysfunction Associated with Tyrosine Kinase Inhibitors in Patients with CML in Chronic Phase. *Blood*, *136*(1, Supplement 1), 2–3. DOI: 10.1182/blood-2020-142997

Shu, L., Du, C., & Zuo, Y. (2023). Abnormal phosphorylation of protein tyrosine in neurodegenerative diseases. *Journal of Neuropathology and Experimental Neurology*, *82*(10), 826–835. DOI: 10.1093/jnen/nlad066

Spagnuolo, C., Moccia, S., & Russo, G. L. (2018). Anti-inflammatory effects of flavonoids in neurodegenerative disorders. *European Journal of Medicinal Chemistry*, *153*, 105–115. DOI: 10.1016/j.ejmech.2017.09.001

Sunder, S. S., Sharma, U. C., & Pokharel, S. (2023). Adverse effects of tyrosine kinase inhibitors in cancer therapy : pathophysiology, mechanisms and clinical management. In *Signal Transduction and Targeted Therapy* (Vol. 8, Issue 1, p. 262). Springer US. DOI: 10.1038/s41392-023-01469-6

Sutanto, F., Konstantinidou, M., & Dömling, A. (2020). Covalent inhibitors: A rational approach to drug discovery. *RSC Medicinal Chemistry*, *11*(8), 876–884. DOI: 10.1039/D0MD00154F

Sweeney, P., Park, H., Baumann, M., Dunlop, J., Frydman, J., Kopito, R., McCampbell, A., Leblanc, G., Venkateswaran, A., Nurmi, A., & Hodgson, R. (2017). Protein misfolding in neurodegenerative diseases: Implications and strategies. *Translational Neurodegeneration*, *6*(1), 1–13. DOI: 10.1186/s40035-017-0077-5

Tello, J. A., Williams, H. E., Eppler, R. M., Steinhilb, M. L., & Khanna, M. (2022). Animal Models of Neurodegenerative Disease: Recent Advances in Fly Highlight Innovative Approaches to Drug Discovery. *Frontiers in Molecular Neuroscience*, *15*(April), 1–21. DOI: 10.3389/fnmol.2022.883358

Upadhyay, D. B., Mokariya, J. A., Patel, P. J., Patel, S. G., Das, A., Nandi, A., Nogales, J., More, N., Kumar, A., Rajani, D. P., Narayan, M., Kumar, J., Banerjee, S., Sahoo, S. K., & Patel, H. M. (2024). Indole clubbed 2,4-thiazolidinedione linked 1,2,3-triazole as a potent antimalarial and antibacterial agent against drug-resistant strain and molecular modeling studies. *Archiv Der Pharmazie, December 2023*, 1–20. DOI: 10.1002/ardp.202300673

Wang, Z. X., Li, Y. L., Pu, J. L., & Zhang, B. R. (2023). DNA Damage-Mediated Neurotoxicity in Parkinson's Disease. *International Journal of Molecular Sciences*, *24*(7), 1–21. DOI: 10.3390/ijms24076313

Welch, G., & Tsai, L.-H. (2022). Mechanisms of DNA damage-mediated neurotoxicity in neurodegenerative disease. *EMBO Reports*, *23*(6), 1–16. DOI: 10.15252/embr.202154217

Wojda, U., Salinska, E., & Kuznicki, J. (2008). Calcium ions in neuronal degeneration. *IUBMB Life*, *60*(9), 575–590. DOI: 10.1002/iub.91

Wolanin, P. M., Thomason, P. A., & Stock, J. B. (2002). Protein family review Histidine protein kinases : Key signal transducers outside the animal kingdom. *Genome Biology*, *3*(10), 1–8. DOI: 10.1186/gb-2002-3-10-reviews3013

Xie, W., Wan, O. W., & Chung, K. K. K. (2010). New insights into the role of mitochondrial dysfunction and protein aggregation in Parkinson's disease. *Biochimica et Biophysica Acta. Molecular Basis of Disease*, *1802*(11), 935–941. DOI: 10.1016/j.bbadis.2010.07.014

Chapter 11
Recent Development on Anti-Amyloid Monoclonal Antibodies to Mitigate CNS Disorders

Rupam Hazra
https://orcid.org/0009-0003-0332-2128
Global Institute of Management and Technology, India

Parag Chatterjee
https://orcid.org/0000-0003-1243-9582
Global Institute of Management and Technology, India

Soumen Ghosh
https://orcid.org/0009-0008-3778-6090
Global Institute of Management and Technology, India

ABSTRACT

Neurodegenerative diseases like Alzheimer's, Parkinson's, ALS, and Huntington's are rising globally due to aging populations and longer life expectancy. Marked by progressive neuronal loss, these disorders share common features such as protein misfolding, mitochondrial dysfunction, oxidative stress, and chronic neuroinflammation. Current diagnostics often detect disease at late stages, and available treatments mainly alleviate symptoms without altering progression. However, advances in molecular biology, biotechnology, and imaging are enabling earlier detection and targeted interventions. Promising innovations include anti-amyloid antibodies, enzyme therapy, gene editing, and precision diagnostics. This chapter reviews key mechanisms, diagnostic challenges, and emerging therapies, highlighting the need for interdisciplinary research and policy support to translate scientific progress into effective clinical care.

DOI: 10.4018/979-8-3373-4627-4.ch011

INTRODUCTION TO NEURODEGENERATIVE DISORDERS

Neurodegenerative diseases represent one of the most urgent and complex challenges in modern medicine. As global populations age and life expectancies increase, the prevalence of conditions such as Alzheimer's disease, Parkinson's disease, amyotrophic lateral sclerosis (ALS), and Huntington's disease continues to rise sharply. These disorders are characterized by the progressive loss of neuronal structure and function, leading to devastating impairments in cognition, mobility, and overall quality of life. Most current therapies provide only symptomatic relief and fail to halt or reverse disease progression. A major reason for this therapeutic stagnation is the intricate interplay of molecular mechanisms underlying neurodegeneration—including protein misfolding, mitochondrial dysfunction, oxidative stress, and chronic neuroinflammation. These interrelated processes form a vicious cycle that accelerates neuronal injury and poses significant barriers to treatment. However, recent scientific advances are beginning to reshape the therapeutic landscape. Innovations in monoclonal antibody therapies, gene editing technologies, enzyme modulation, and precision diagnostics offer new hope for early intervention and disease modification. Concurrently, improved biomarker development and neuroimaging techniques are enabling earlier diagnosis and more personalized treatment strategies. This chapter explores the epidemiology, pathophysiology, and societal impact of neurodegenerative disorders. It critically examines the limitations of current diagnostic and treatment approaches, delves into the molecular mechanisms driving disease, and highlights promising developments in therapeutic innovation. The discussion also underscores the importance of collaborative research, translational science, and supportive policy frameworks in accelerating progress toward effective, accessible, and durable solutions.

Epidemiology and Societal Impact

Epidemiology plays a crucial role in understanding the distribution, causes, and control of diseases within populations. By identifying patterns and risk factors associated with disease spread, epidemiologists help shape public health policies and interventions. The societal impact of such findings extends beyond healthcare, influencing economic stability, education, and community well-being. Epidemiology enables effective monitoring of disease outbreaks, both infectious and non-communicable. Early detection through surveillance systems helps authorities implement timely preventive measures, such as vaccination campaigns or quarantine protocols, thereby minimizing transmission and fatalities. The effectiveness of these transformative agents will encourage the creation of additional anti-amyloid MABs, various other anti-amyloid treatments, therapies for different targets of AD biology, and innovative strategies for treating a range of neurodegenerative diseases, (Cummings, 2023).

Healthcare Resource Allocation

Data-driven insights from epidemiological studies guide governments and healthcare systems in resource planning. This includes optimizing hospital infrastructure, staffing, and the distribution of medications or vaccines to areas with the greatest need, enhancing overall public health response.

Social and Economic Consequences

Widespread diseases can disrupt education, employment, and economic productivity. Epidemiological research highlights vulnerable populations and informs strategies to mitigate long-term impacts—such as mental health support, social aid programs, and economic relief packages—ensuring a more resilient society.

Common Pathological Feature

Neurodegenerative disorders, though clinically distinct, share several fundamental pathological features that drive disease progression. One of the most prominent is the accumulation of misfolded proteins, such as amyloid-beta and tau in Alzheimer's disease, alpha-synuclein in Parkinson's, and mutant huntingtin in Huntington's disease. These aggregated proteins form toxic intracellular or extracellular deposits that impair cellular function and communication. Progressive neuronal loss is another hallmark, leading to the deterioration of cognitive and motor functions over time. In addition, synaptic dysfunction, mitochondrial damage, and chronic neuroinflammation further exacerbate neuronal injury and contribute to disease symptoms. Additionally, the possible molecular targets emerging from these mechanisms have been examined, along with innovative promising strategies like nanoparticle therapy, neural stem cell transplantation, vaccines, and CRISPR-Cas9 genome editing methods, (Sighencea, 2024).

Protein Aggregation

Protein aggregation is a hallmark of many neurodegenerative diseases, where specific proteins misfold and accumulate abnormally in the brain. Misfolded proteins such as amyloid-beta, tau, and alpha-synuclein form toxic oligomers and fibrils that interfere with neuronal function and connectivity. These aggregates disrupt cellular homeostasis by impairing synaptic signalling, mitochondrial activity, and protein clearance pathways.

Progressive Neuronal Loss

Progressive neuronal loss refers to the gradual degeneration and death of neurons over time, a core feature of most neurodegenerative disorders. As neurons die, the brain's ability to transmit signals deteriorates, leading to cognitive deficits, memory loss, and impaired motor function. This process is often region-specific—affecting the hippocampus in Alzheimer's, the substantia nigra in Parkinson's, or motor neurons in ALS. The brain's limited regenerative capacity makes the damage largely irreversible.

Current Limitations in Diagnosis and Treatment

Despite growing research efforts, neurodegenerative disorders remain notoriously difficult to diagnose and treat effectively. Most diagnoses occur at late stages, once significant neuronal loss has already taken place, limiting the potential for therapeutic intervention. Current diagnostic methods rely heavily on clinical symptoms, which often overlap across disorders and can be subtle or misleading in early stages. Biomarkers and advanced imaging are emerging tools, but

they are not yet widely accessible or standardized. Treatment options are largely symptomatic, addressing cognitive or motor impairments without altering the disease's underlying course.

Late Diagnosis

Late diagnosis is a major hurdle in the management of neurodegenerative diseases, as symptoms often emerge only after significant neuronal damage has occurred. Early-stage pathology can remain clinically silent for years, making detection difficult without advanced biomarkers or imaging techniques. By the time cognitive or motor symptoms manifest, therapeutic interventions may be less effective. This delay also reduces the window of opportunity for enrolling patients in early-phase clinical trials.

Limited Disease-Modifying Therapies

Despite intense research, few therapies have demonstrated the ability to halt or reverse neuronal degeneration. Complex disease mechanisms, including genetic variability and multifactorial pathophysiology, make drug development highly challenging. Recently approved therapies, like certain monoclonal antibodies for Alzheimer's, show promise but still offer limited benefit. Continued innovation and targeted research are needed to develop truly disease-modifying options.

MOLECULAR MECHANISMS UNDERLYING NEURODEGENERATION

Neurodegeneration arises from a complex interplay of molecular mechanisms that disrupt normal neuronal function and survival. One of the central features is protein misfolding and aggregation, where proteins like amyloid-beta, tau, alpha-synuclein, and huntingtin adopt toxic conformations and accumulate in the brain, impairing cellular processes. Mitochondrial dysfunction is another key contributor, leading to energy deficits, oxidative stress, and increased vulnerability to cell death. Additionally, chronic neuroinflammation, driven by activated microglia and astrocytes, creates a toxic environment that further damages neurons and synapses. These mechanisms often overlap and amplify one another, forming a vicious cycle that accelerates disease progression.

Protein Misfolding and Aggregation

Normally, proteins fold into specific three-dimensional structures to function correctly, but under pathological conditions, misfolded proteins can accumulate, form aggregates, and interfere with essential cellular processes. Misfolded proteins are central to the pathology of many neurodegenerative diseases, with each disorder linked to a specific type of protein dysfunction. For example, amyloid-beta and tau aggregates are associated with Alzheimer's disease, alpha-synuclein with Parkinson's, and huntingtin protein with Huntington's disease. These proteins lose their normal conformation and form toxic oligomers and fibrils that accumulate in neurons and surrounding tissues.

Various production and storage conditions have been identified as capable of inducing aggregation of polyclonal and monoclonal antibody (mAb) therapies such as low pH, freezing, light exposure, lyophilisation and increased ionic strength(Sheehan,2025).

Cellular Toxicity and Mechanisms of Damage

Misfolded proteins cause cellular toxicity through multiple mechanisms, including oxidative stress, mitochondrial dysfunction, impaired synaptic signalling, and calcium imbalance. These toxic aggregates interfere with the normal functioning of organelles and disrupt critical cellular pathways, ultimately triggering apoptosis or necrosis. Neurons, being highly specialized and energy-demanding, are particularly vulnerable to such disturbances. Inflammatory responses by activated glial cells further exacerbate the damage. Over time, cumulative toxicity contributes to widespread neuronal degeneration and loss of brain function.

Propagation and Therapeutic Targeting

Recent research suggests that misfolded proteins can propagate from cell to cell in a prion-like manner, spreading pathology across brain regions. This transmission may occur through exosomes, synaptic contacts, or other intercellular routes, contributing to disease progression. Targeting this propagation process is an emerging therapeutic strategy aimed at halting or slowing disease spread. Approaches include antibodies that neutralize extracellular aggregates, small molecules that stabilize native protein conformation, and inhibitors of uptake pathways. Effective targeting of this mechanism holds promise for modifying the course of multiple neurodegenerative diseases.

Mitochondrial Dysfunction and Oxidative Stress

In neurodegenerative diseases, mitochondrial dysfunction and the resulting oxidative stress are key contributors to neuronal damage and disease progression. Mitochondria are the primary energy-producing organelles in neurons, generating ATP through oxidative phosphorylation. In neurodegenerative diseases, mitochondrial enzymes and respiratory chain complexes become dysfunctional, reducing ATP output. This energy deficit compromises critical neuronal functions such as synaptic transmission, ion balance, and axonal transport. Future therapies must aim at addressing various factors of oxidative stress, especially mitochondrial impairment, to improve clinical results and delay neurodegeneration in Alzheimer's disease patients(Alkhalifa,2025).

Increased Production of Reactive Oxygen Species (ROS)

Damaged mitochondria often leak electrons during respiration, leading to the excessive production of reactive oxygen species (ROS). Elevated ROS levels cause oxidative damage to lipids, proteins, and nucleic acids, disrupting cellular integrity. In neurons, oxidative stress impairs membrane function, disturbs signalling pathways, and can activate apoptotic cascades. ROS also exacerbate the misfolding and aggregation of disease-related proteins such as amyloid-beta and alpha-synuclein. Antioxidant defense may be overwhelmed in disease states, further amplifying cellular injury.

Disrupted Mitochondrial Dynamics and Quality Control

Healthy mitochondrial function depends on a balance between fission (division) and fusion (joining), as well as efficient mitophagy—the removal of damaged mitochondria. In neurode-

generative conditions, this dynamic balance is disrupted, leading to fragmented or excessively fused mitochondria that cannot meet cellular demands. Impaired mitophagy allows dysfunctional mitochondria to accumulate, increasing oxidative stress and bioenergetic failure. Key regulatory proteins such as PINK1 and Parkin, often mutated in familial Parkinson's disease, are involved in these processes. Targeting mitochondrial dynamics and enhancing quality control mechanisms are promising therapeutic avenues.

Neuroinflammation and Immune Dysregulation

Neuroinflammation and immune system dysregulation play a critical role in the progression of neurodegenerative diseases. While inflammation is a natural protective response to injury or infection, chronic and uncontrolled neuroinflammation can exacerbate neuronal damage. Glial cells—primarily microglia and astrocytes—are key players in the brain's immune defense system and become activated in response to injury or pathogenic proteins.

Human intravenous immunoglobulin (hIVIG) is used for the treatment of primary immunodeficiency disorders linked to deficient humoral immunity(Puli,2012). In neurodegenerative diseases, this activation becomes chronic and exaggerated, leading to a persistent inflammatory state. Activated microglia release pro-inflammatory mediators such as TNF-α, IL-1β, and nitric oxide, which can damage neurons. Astrocytes, which normally support neurons, may also adopt a reactive phenotype that contributes to toxicity and impairs synaptic function. While initially protective, sustained glial activation exacerbates neuronal dysfunction and accelerates disease progression.

Dysregulated Cytokine Signalling and Immune Responses

Neurodegenerative diseases are associated with an imbalance between pro-inflammatory and anti-inflammatory cytokines, resulting in chronic immune activation. Elevated levels of cytokines like IL-6, IL-1β, and interferon-gamma disrupt homeostasis and promote neuronal injury. In some cases, peripheral immune cells may also infiltrate the CNS, amplifying inflammation. Dysregulated signalling through pathways such as NF-κB and JAK/STAT perpetuates glial activation and impairs the resolution of inflammation. This maladaptive immune response contributes to a toxic environment that hinders repair and regeneration.

Contribution to Disease Progression and Therapeutic Targeting

Chronic neuroinflammation is not just a consequence but a driver of neurodegeneration, amplifying protein aggregation, oxidative stress, and neuronal death. Approaches include microglial inhibitors, cytokine blockers, and small molecules that shift glial cells toward a neuroprotective phenotype. Anti-inflammatory drugs like NSAIDs have shown mixed results, but more targeted immunomodulators are under investigation. Effective control of neuroinflammation could slow disease progression and improve long-term outcomes.

RECENT DEVELOPMENTS IN ANTI-AMYLOID MONOCLONAL ANTIBODIES TO MITIGATE CNS DISORDERS

Recent developments in anti-amyloid monoclonal antibodies (mAbs) have marked a significant advance in the treatment of central nervous system (CNS) disorders, particularly Alzheimer's disease. These biologics are designed to selectively target and clear amyloid-beta plaques, a key pathological hallmark implicated in neuronal toxicity and cognitive decline. Recent clinical trials have demonstrated that certain mAbs, such as aducanumab and lecanemab, can reduce amyloid burden in the brain, slow cognitive deterioration, and potentially modify disease progression. The presence of amyloid plaques and tau tangles triggers the recruitment of microglia, activating these cells and initiating a localized inflammatory response that contributes to neurotoxicity(Skoczeń, 2025).

Advances in antibody engineering have improved their specificity, blood-brain barrier penetration, and safety profiles, though challenges remain in optimizing dosing, minimizing adverse effects like amyloid-related imaging abnormalities (ARIA), and identifying patient populations most likely to benefit.

Mechanism of Amyloid-Beta Clearance by mAbs

Monoclonal antibodies (mAbs) target amyloid-beta (Aβ) peptides, which aggregate abnormally in the brain and are a hallmark of Alzheimer's disease and other central nervous system (CNS) disorders. These antibodies recognize and bind specifically to Aβ species—either monomers, oligomers, or fibrils—facilitating their removal through immune-mediated mechanisms. One major route involves engaging microglia, the brain's resident immune cells, which are activated to phagocytose and degrade the Aβ-antibody complexes. Additionally, mAbs can promote Aβ clearance through peripheral "sink" effects, altering the concentration gradient and encouraging efflux of Aβ from the brain. This targeted immunotherapy aims to reduce plaque burden, preserve neuronal function, and slow cognitive decline in affected individuals.

Amyloid-β (Aβ) has been extensively associated with the development of AD. Multiple mechanisms have been suggested for Aβ clearance, involving receptor-mediated transport of Aβ across the blood-brain barrier and enzyme-mediated degradation of Aβ(Wang,2006).

Fc-Mediated Microglial Activation

Monoclonal antibodies bind to Aβ aggregates and present their Fc region to microglial Fcγ receptors, stimulating phagocytosis. This immune activation promotes the engulfment and degradation of Aβ deposits within the brain. However, overactivation of microglia can also lead to neuroinflammation, which must be carefully regulated. Next-generation mAbs are being engineered to fine-tune Fc-effector functions and minimize adverse effects. This balance is crucial for achieving effective clearance while maintaining safety in long-term treatment.

Disruption of Aβ Aggregates

Some monoclonal antibodies act directly on Aβ fibrils or oligomers, destabilizing their structure. By breaking down these aggregates, mAbs can reduce neurotoxic species that impair

synaptic function. This disassembly may also make Aβ more susceptible to natural clearance pathways. This specificity improves therapeutic efficacy while limiting off-target effects.

Clinical Trial Landscape: Aducanumab, Lecanemab, Donanemab

Anti-amyloid monoclonal antibodies have entered clinical use after years of research, with Aducanumab, Lecanemab, and Donanemab emerging as major therapeutic candidates targeting Alzheimer's disease. These antibodies aim to reduce amyloid-beta burden in the brain and potentially slow cognitive decline. Each has undergone rigorous clinical trials, with varying results in terms of efficacy, safety, and regulatory approval. While the overall goal remains consistent—modifying disease progression rather than just managing symptoms—their clinical performance has influenced scientific, medical, and regulatory perspectives. The causes of AD are intricate, shaped by genetic elements like mutations in the amyloid precursor protein (APP) and presenilin genes, with the apolipoprotein E (APOE-e4) allele representing a major risk factor for late-onset AD(Rahman, 2024).

Aducanumab

Developed by Biogen, Aducanumab was the first anti-amyloid mAb to receive FDA accelerated approval in 2021. It targets aggregated amyloid-beta and demonstrated plaque reduction in early-stage Alzheimer's patients. However, its clinical trials (EMERGE and ENGAGE) produced mixed results—only one showed a statistically significant slowing of cognitive decline. Safety concerns, particularly Amyloid-Related Imaging Abnormalities (ARIA), led to further scrutiny and limited clinical uptake. Despite the controversy, it marked a turning point by validating amyloid as a therapeutic target.

Lecanemab

Lecanemab, jointly developed by Eisai and Biogen, gained FDA traditional approval in 2023 following promising Phase 3 trial results. It selectively binds to soluble protofibrils—an especially toxic form of amyloid-beta—showing a significant slowing of cognitive decline in early Alzheimer's patients. The CLARITY-AD trial demonstrated not only plaque reduction but also measurable clinical benefit with a relatively manageable ARIA incidence. Its faster onset of action and better safety profile compared to Aducanumab have made it a preferred candidate in many settings. It represents a more targeted and refined approach in amyloid therapy.

Donanemab

In the TRAILBLAZER-ALZ trial, Donanemab showed strong plaque clearance and moderate cognitive benefits, especially in patients with low tax burden. One of its notable features is the possibility of limited dosing—patients who achieve significant plaque reduction may discontinue treatment, offering a cost-effective model. However, it also showed ARIA risks, particularly in patients carrying the APOE4 gene variant. Ongoing studies are evaluating its long-term effects and comparing it directly with other anti-amyloid therapies.

ADVANCES IN DIAGNOSTIC STRATEGIES

Advances in diagnostic strategies for neurodegenerative disorders have significantly improved early detection, disease monitoring, and patient stratification, which are crucial for effective intervention. Novel biomarkers—detected through cerebrospinal fluid analysis, blood tests, and advanced neuroimaging techniques—allow for the identification of pathological changes such as amyloid-beta accumulation, tau pathology, and neuroinflammation before clinical symptoms manifest. Positron emission tomography (PET) scans and magnetic resonance imaging (MRI) now provide high-resolution insights into brain structure and function, enabling more precise disease staging. Additionally, developments in genetic testing and machine learning algorithms have enhanced the prediction of disease risk and progression by integrating diverse biological data. Despite significant advancements in healthcare services and a rise in life expectancy, there has been a dramatic surge in the occurrence of central nervous system (CNS) disorders such as brain tumors, neurodegenerative diseases (including Alzheimer's, Parkinson's, amyotrophic lateral sclerosis, and Huntington's), ischemic stroke, and epilepsy, which have severely affected quality of life and greatly escalated economic and social burdens(Zhang,2021). These innovations collectively support personalized medicine approaches, guiding treatment decisions and improving clinical trial design, ultimately fostering more effective therapies for Alzheimer's, Parkinson's, ALS, and related disorders.

Biomarker Discovery in CSF and Blood

Biomarker discovery in cerebrospinal fluid (CSF) and blood is revolutionizing the diagnosis and monitoring of central nervous system (CNS) disorders, particularly neurodegenerative diseases like Alzheimer's. Traditionally, diagnosis relied on clinical symptoms and neuroimaging, but these methods are often invasive, costly, or only conclusive in advanced stages. Pathological situations associated with alteration of the blood– brain barrier, local inflammatory response or an infectious situation in fact lead to an increase of CSF protein content(Roche,2008).

By contrast, fluid biomarkers offer a minimally invasive, scalable approach to detect pathological changes even before clinical symptoms appear. Recent advances have led to the identification of key molecular signatures—such as amyloid-beta, tau proteins, and neurofilament light chain (NFL)—that reflect disease processes like amyloid aggregation, neuroinflammation, and axonal damage. These biomarkers not only support early diagnosis but also help evaluate treatment response, guide patient selection, and track disease progression in clinical trials and practice.

Amyloid-Beta and Tau Levels in CSF

Changes in amyloid-beta (Aβ42) and phosphorylated tau (p-tau) levels in CSF are among the most validated biomarkers for Alzheimer's disease. Decreased Aβ42 and elevated p-tau levels reflect amyloid plaque formation and tau tangle pathology, respectively. These biomarkers have been incorporated into research diagnostic frameworks and correlate strongly with PET imaging results. Their high sensitivity and specificity allow clinicians to distinguish Alzheimer's from other forms of dementia. However, the invasive nature of lumbar punctures limits their routine clinical use.

Blood-Based Biomarkers (Plasma Aβ, p-tau, NFL)

Recent advancements have made it possible to detect Aβ42/40 ratios, p-tau isoforms (e.g., p-tau181, p-tau217), and NFL in blood samples. These plasma biomarkers are less invasive and more accessible than CSF measures, enabling broader screening and monitoring. Studies show strong concordance between blood and CSF levels, making them promising tools for early diagnosis and disease tracking. NFL, in particular, is a general marker of neurodegeneration and can be elevated in multiple CNS disorders. Ongoing trials are working to standardize these measures for routine clinical use.

Imaging Techniques: PET, MRI, and Novel Tracers

Advanced imaging techniques play a pivotal role in diagnosing, tracking, and understanding central nervous system (CNS) disorders, especially neurodegenerative diseases like Alzheimer's. Positron Emission Tomography (PET) and Magnetic Resonance Imaging (MRI) are the primary modalities used to visualize structural, functional, and molecular changes in the brain. PET imaging allows for the in vivo detection of pathological proteins such as amyloid-beta and tau using specialized radiotracers, while MRI provides high-resolution anatomical detail and can assess brain atrophy, white matter changes, and functional connectivity. The ability to fuse images from two or more modalities is always interesting, but to acquire them simultaneously or within a narrow window of a few seconds or minutes is exciting as it opens the potential of utilizing the various functional parameters into a single study(Afaq,2013). These imaging tools support early diagnosis, patient stratification, and treatment monitoring, and they are increasingly integrated into clinical trials and routine practice. The development of novel tracers and hybrid imaging technologies continues to enhance sensitivity, specificity, and the ability to detect disease at preclinical stages.

PET Imaging for Amyloid and Tau Pathology

PET imaging uses radiolabelled tracers like [^{11}C]PiB, [^{18}F]florbetapir, and [^{18}F]flortaucipir to visualize amyloid plaques and tau tangles in the brain. These scans provide direct evidence of pathological protein deposition, allowing clinicians to confirm diagnoses such as Alzheimer's disease with high specificity. Amyloid PET is widely used in clinical trials to screen participants and track treatment effects of anti-amyloid therapies. Tau PET is emerging as a powerful tool for staging disease progression and correlating pathology with cognitive decline.

MRI for Structural and Functional Changes

MRI offers detailed visualization of brain anatomy and function without ionizing radiation. Structural MRI can detect cortical thinning, hippocampal atrophy, and ventricular enlargement, all of which are indicative of neurodegeneration. Advanced techniques such as diffusion tensor imaging (DTI) assess white matter integrity, while functional MRI (fMRI) monitors brain activity and connectivity patterns. MRI is also useful for detecting ARIA (Amyloid-Related Imaging Abnormalities), a key side effect of monoclonal antibody therapies. Its versatility makes it a cornerstone in both diagnosis and safety monitoring.Top of FormBottom of Form

Early Diagnosis and Predictive Modelling Using AI

Artificial Intelligence (AI) is transforming the landscape of early diagnosis and predictive modelling in central nervous system (CNS) disorders, particularly neurodegenerative diseases such as Alzheimer's and Parkinson's. By analysing vast and complex datasets—including medical imaging, genetic information, fluid biomarkers, and electronic health records—AI algorithms can detect subtle patterns and correlations that may escape human observation. Machine learning and deep learning models are being trained to identify early biomarkers, predict disease progression, and stratify patients based on risk profiles. Artificial intelligence (AI) is defined as the technology that uses computer knowledge to represent intelligent behaviour with nominal human involvement, and machine learning (ML) is considered as a subset of AI techniques(Battineni,2020). These tools enable faster, more accurate diagnoses and help clinicians intervene before significant neuronal damage occurs, potentially slowing or altering disease trajectories. Moreover, AI-driven predictive models are increasingly integrated into clinical trial design, helping select suitable candidates, optimize endpoints, and reduce trial failures.

AI in Multimodal Data Integration

AI models can integrate data from diverse sources—such as MRI scans, PET imaging, CSF biomarkers, and cognitive assessments—to generate a comprehensive diagnostic profile. This multimodal fusion enhances diagnostic accuracy by capturing different aspects of disease pathology. Deep learning networks can uncover nonlinear relationships and latent features that traditional statistical methods might miss. By harmonizing imaging and biological data, AI systems can offer individualized assessments and disease staging. This personalized approach improves clinical decision-making and supports more precise treatment plans. The integration of multiomics data with detailed phenotypic insights from electronic health records marks a paradigm shift in biomedical research, offering unparalleled holistic views into health and disease pathways(Nam,2024).

Early Detection from Imaging and Speech Patterns

AI is capable of analysing subtle brain changes in imaging data, such as cortical thinning or microstructural damage, before symptoms manifest. In addition, natural language processing (NLP) tools are being developed to evaluate speech and language for signs of cognitive decline. These models can detect anomalies in vocabulary, fluency, and syntax that often precede clinical symptoms. Early detection from such non-invasive inputs could enable widespread screening and long-term monitoring. This opens up possibilities for accessible, AI-driven diagnostic tools in both clinical and home settings.

ENZYME THERAPY IN NEURODEGENERATIVE DISEASES

Neurodegenerative diseases (NDDs) are a group of debilitating, devastating disorders characterized by the progressive degeneration of nerve cells, which present a significant challenge to public health and medical research(Kumar,2024). This strategy involves the use of enzyme

replacement, enhancement, or inhibition to restore normal cellular processes disrupted by pathological mechanisms such as protein aggregation, lysosomal dysfunction, and impaired metabolism. For example, lysosomal enzyme replacement therapies aim to clear toxic protein aggregates and improve cellular waste degradation, which is crucial in diseases like Parkinson's and Alzheimer's. Advances in gene-editing technologies, such as CRISPR/Cas9, have further expanded the potential of enzyme therapy by enabling precise delivery and sustained expression of therapeutic enzymes within the central nervous system. Additionally, small-molecule enzyme modulators are being developed to regulate enzymatic activity involved in neuroinflammation and oxidative stress.

Lysosomal Enzymes and Their Role in Neuronal Health

Lysosomal enzymes play a vital role in maintaining neuronal health by facilitating the breakdown and recycling of cellular waste, damaged organelles, and misfolded proteins within lysosomes—the cell's primary degradative compartments. In neurons, which are long-lived and highly sensitive to photostatic stress, efficient lysosomal function is essential for clearing neurotoxic substances and maintaining cellular homeostasis. Lysosomes are membrane-bound organelles that are responsible for degrading and recycling macromolecules. Lysosomal dysfunction occurs in enzymatic and non-enzymatic deficiencies, which result in abnormal accumulation of materials(Ashtari,2016). Deficiencies or dysfunctions in lysosomal enzymes can lead to the accumulation of undegraded substrates, contributing to the pathogenesis of several neurodegenerative diseases such as Parkinson's, Alzheimer's, and various lysosomal storage disorders (LSDs). These enzymes also participate in autophagy, a critical process where cells digest their own components to survive under stress and maintain energy balance.

Deficiencies Linked to Neurodegenerative Diseases

Mutations affecting lysosomal enzymes, such as glucocerebrosidase (GCase), are strongly linked to increased risk for Parkinson's disease. Reduced GCase activity leads to the buildup of alpha-synuclein, a protein that forms toxic aggregates in neurons. Similarly, enzyme deficiencies in Niemann-Pick, Tay-Sachs, or Batten disease result in toxic accumulation of lipids or proteins in neural tissues. These dysfunctions trigger inflammation, mitochondrial impairment, and neuronal death. Understanding the genetic and biochemical basis of these enzyme deficiencies is key to developing targeted therapies.

Role in Autophagy and Protein Clearance

Lysosomal enzymes are crucial for the final step of autophagy, where autophagosomes fuse with lysosomes to degrade their contents. Impaired enzymatic activity disrupts this process, leading to the accumulation of damaged proteins and organelles that can impair synaptic function. In Alzheimer's disease, for example, lysosomal dysfunction contributes to the buildup of amyloid-beta and tau proteins. Enhancing autophagic flux through upregulation of lysosomal enzymes has shown neuroprotective effects in experimental models. Thus, these enzymes serve as a central hub linking protein homeostasis with neuronal viability.

Enzyme Replacement Therapy: Mechanisms and Delivery Challenges

Enzyme Replacement Therapy (ERT) is a therapeutic approach designed to restore deficient or non-functional lysosomal enzymes in patients with lysosomal storage disorders (LSDs) and certain neurodegenerative diseases. The core mechanism involves administering recombinant forms of the missing or dysfunctional enzymes, which are taken up by cells via specific receptors (e.g., mannose-6-phosphate receptors) and delivered to lysosomes where they perform their degradative functions. The administration of a molecule leads to multiple interactions that might cause a rapid loss of function or degradation of the enzyme, (De La Fuente, 2021). ERT has shown success in treating several systemic LSDs like Gaucher, Fabry, and Pompe diseases by reducing substrate accumulation and improving organ function. However, its application in central nervous system (CNS) disorders presents unique challenges due to the complexity of neuronal delivery. Overcoming these barriers is crucial to translating the success of ERT from peripheral tissues to the brain.

Blood–Brain Barrier (BBB) Penetration

This physiological barrier protects the brain from harmful substances but also blocks therapeutic macromolecules like recombinant enzymes. As a result, intravenously administered ERT has limited efficacy in treating neurological symptoms of LSDs. Researchers are exploring strategies such as receptor-mediated transcytosis, focused ultrasound, and nanocarrier systems to enhance BBB permeability. Direct intrathecal or intracerebroventricular injections are also being used, though they are invasive and not ideal for long-term treatment.

Immunogenicity and Immune Response

Repeated administration of exogenous enzymes can trigger immune responses, leading to the production of neutralizing antibodies. These antibodies can reduce the therapeutic efficacy of ERT and cause infusion-related reactions or systemic inflammation. The risk is higher in patients with complete enzyme deficiency, as their immune systems recognize the therapeutic enzyme as foreign. Immunosuppressive regimens or enzyme modifications (e.g., PEGylation) are being explored to reduce immunogenicity. Long-term management requires balancing therapeutic benefit with immune safety.

Small-Molecule Enzyme Modulators

Small-molecule enzyme modulators are an emerging class of therapeutics aimed at enhancing the function, stability, or trafficking of lysosomal enzymes, offering a non-invasive alternative to enzyme replacement therapy (ERT), especially in treating central nervous system (CNS) disorders. Unlike large biologic drugs, small molecules can often cross the blood–brain barrier (BBB), making them especially promising for neurodegenerative conditions linked to lysosomal dysfunction. These modulators work through various mechanisms, including acting as pharmacological chaperones that stabilize misfolded enzymes, activators that enhance enzymatic activity, or inhibitors that reduce the buildup of toxic substrates by altering metabolic pathways.

Pharmacological Chaperones

Pharmacological chaperones are small molecules that bind to misfolded lysosomal enzymes, stabilizing them and facilitating their proper folding and transport to the lysosome. These are especially useful in diseases caused by missense mutations, where the enzyme is produced but degraded due to improper folding. Once in the lysosome, the enzyme can function more effectively, reducing substrate accumulation. This approach allows for mutation-specific, personalized treatment.

Enzyme Activators

By binding to active or allosteric sites, they increase enzymatic activity without altering protein structure or expression. This can be particularly useful in cases where residual enzyme activity is present but insufficient for normal function. In Parkinson's research, small-molecule activators of GCase are being developed to restore lysosomal clearance of alpha-synuclein aggregates. These compounds may offer disease-modifying effects without the complexities of protein-based therapies.

GENE EDITING AND ENZYME DELIVERY TECHNOLOGIES

Gene editing and enzyme delivery technologies have revolutionized the potential treatment landscape for neurodegenerative diseases by enabling precise correction of genetic mutations and targeted restoration of enzyme function within affected neurons. Techniques such as CRISPR/Cas9 and base editors allow for the specific modification of disease-causing genes, offering the possibility of correcting mutations responsible for disorders like Huntington's disease and certain familial forms of Alzheimer's and Parkinson's diseases. Concurrently, advanced delivery systems—including viral vectors like adeno-associated viruses (AAVs), lipid nanoparticles, and novel biomaterials—are being developed to transport therapeutic enzymes or gene-editing components across the blood-brain barrier and into neural cells efficiently. These technologies facilitate sustained enzyme production and enhanced clearance of toxic protein aggregates or metabolic byproducts. One of the significant obstacles to their implementation is the secure and effective intracellular delivery of genome-editing biomacromolecules, such as nucleases and nucleic acids, (Yin, 2017). Despite challenges such as immune responses, off-target effects, and delivery efficiency, ongoing innovations continue to improve safety and specificity, positioning gene editing and enzyme delivery at the forefront of personalized, disease-modifying therapies for neurodegenerative disorders.

CRISPR/Cas9 and Base Editing in Neurological Contexts

CRISPR/Cas9 and base editing have opened new avenues in treating genetic neurological disorders by enabling precise gene corrections at the DNA level. These tools offer the potential to repair disease-causing mutations, silence toxic genes, or enhance protective ones directly in brain cells. Base editing, a more refined variant of CRISPR, enables single-nucleotide changes without causing DNA double-strand breaks, thus improving safety. Causative alterations can be

detected by modelling disease-related changes in gene expression through CRISPRi/CRISPRa techniques(Kampmann,2020). Together, they provide a platform for potentially curative interventions in diseases that were once considered untreatable.

Correction of Monogenic Mutations

Many neurological diseases like Huntington's disease, Tay-Sachs, and Rett syndrome are caused by single-gene mutations. CRISPR/Cas9 can target and correct these mutations at their source, restoring normal gene function. In preclinical models, such editing has halted or reversed disease symptoms. The success of such interventions depends on precise delivery and timing. These strategies are especially promising for early-onset, progressive disorders where early correction may prevent irreversible damage.

Base Editing for Improved Safety

Base editors can convert one nucleotide into another (e.g., A→G or C→T) without cutting the DNA strand, reducing the risk of off-target damage. This makes base editing particularly useful in the sensitive environment of the CNS. It allows precise mutation correction with minimal disruption to the genome. This has been successfully demonstrated in preclinical studies of spinal muscular atrophy and certain lysosomal storage diseases. Base editing could enable safer, long-term therapeutic applications in the brain.

Viral and Non-Viral Vectors for Enzyme Delivery

Gene and enzyme therapies rely on delivery vehicles—vectors—to transport therapeutic agents into target cells, especially in the brain. Both viral and non-viral systems are under active development for neurological applications, including lysosomal storage disorders and other neurodegenerative conditions. Gene therapy is defined as the procedure used to treat or improve the health condition of the patient by modifying the patient's cells genetically, (Ramamoorth, 2015). Choosing the appropriate delivery platform is essential for achieving successful outcomes in CNS-targeted therapies.

Adeno-Associated Virus (AAV) Vectors

AAVs are the most commonly used viral vectors for CNS gene therapy due to their high transduction efficiency and relatively low immunogenicity. Certain serotypes like AAV9 can cross the BBB and reach neurons and glial cells. They have been used in clinical trials for spinal muscular atrophy (SMA) and Batten disease, showing promising therapeutic outcomes. However, repeated administration can be challenging due to immune responses. Additionally, AAVs have a limited cargo capacity (~4.7 kb), restricting the size of genes or editing tools they can deliver.

Non-Viral Vectors: Nanoparticles and Liposomes

Non-viral vectors, including lipid nanoparticles (LNPs) and polymer-based systems, offer safer, more flexible alternatives for delivering enzymes or genetic material. These platforms can

be engineered for BBB penetration and targeted delivery to specific brain regions. They avoid some of the immune risks associated with viral vectors and can be administered repeatedly. However, their transfection efficiency is typically lower than that of viral systems. Innovations in surface modifications and encapsulation techniques are helping improve their performance for CNS applications.

Precision Medicine and Patient-Specific Approaches

In neurology, where many diseases are genetically or pathologically heterogeneous, this approach is particularly valuable. By integrating genomic data, fluid biomarkers, and AI-based analytics, clinicians can make more informed decisions about diagnosis, prognosis, and treatment. Precision medicine aims to optimize outcomes while minimizing side effects by ensuring that the right patient gets the right treatment at the right time.

Genomic Profiling for Targeted Therapy

This information is used to guide personalized treatments, such as mutation-specific pharmacological chaperones or CRISPR edits. For example, patients with certain mutations in the GBA gene (linked to Parkinson's) may benefit from therapies that enhance glucocerebrosidase function. Genomic profiling also informs clinical trial selection and treatment eligibility. As sequencing becomes more affordable, its use in routine clinical care is expected to grow.

Use of Biomarkers for Personalized Monitoring

Fluid and imaging biomarkers provide real-time insight into disease activity and treatment response. Measuring amyloid-beta, tau, or neurofilament light chain (NfL) levels in blood or CSF helps stratify patients and track disease progression. These biomarkers can be used to tailor treatment duration, intensity, or drug combinations. AI tools are increasingly being used to interpret multi-modal biomarker data. Personalized biomarker tracking enhances safety and efficacy across diverse patient populations.

TRANSLATING LAB DISCOVERIES INTO CLINICAL THERAPIES

Translating laboratory discoveries into effective clinical therapies for neurodegenerative disorders involves bridging the gap between basic research and patient care through rigorous preclinical and clinical development processes. Advances in understanding molecular mechanisms—such as protein misfolding, mitochondrial dysfunction, and neuroinflammation—have identified numerous therapeutic targets, but successful translation requires overcoming challenges like ensuring drug delivery across the blood-brain barrier, optimizing dosing regimens, and managing adverse effects. Robust animal models and in vitro systems are essential for validating candidate therapies, while biomarker-driven clinical trials enable better patient selection and monitoring of treatment efficacy. Collaborative efforts among academic researchers, pharmaceutical companies, regulatory agencies, and patient advocacy groups accelerate the pipeline from bench to bedside.

Development of anti-oestrogens, angiogenesis inhibitors, imatinib and trastuzumab might be taken as examples of successful translational research, (Simon, 2008).

Despite setbacks in past trials, recent approvals of disease-modifying treatments underscore the progress made and highlight the importance of integrating multidisciplinary approaches to develop safe, effective, and accessible therapies for conditions such as Alzheimer's, Parkinson's, and ALS.

Preclinical Models and Drug Screening Platforms

Preclinical models are essential for understanding disease mechanisms and evaluating the safety and efficacy of therapeutic candidates before human trials. In the context of CNS and lysosomal disorders, these models replicate pathological hallmarks, such as protein aggregation, enzyme deficiencies, or neurodegeneration. High-throughput drug screening platforms built on these models allow rapid testing of small molecules, biologics, and gene therapies. Modern approaches incorporate patient-derived cells, 3D organoids, and CRISPR-modified models to better mimic human physiology. These platforms improve predictive accuracy and help prioritize drug candidates for clinical development.

Animal Models of CNS Disorders

Transgenic mice and other animal models (like zebrafish and non-human primates) are commonly used to mimic the genetic and pathological features of human CNS diseases. They allow researchers to observe disease progression and evaluate the impact of interventions in a living organism. For example, GBA1-mutant mice are used in Parkinson's studies, while tauopathy models help screen Alzheimer's drugs. While informative, species differences can limit translational accuracy.

Patient-Derived iPSC Models

Induced pluripotent stem cells (iPSCs) generated from patients' somatic cells can be differentiated into neurons or glial cells, offering personalized disease models. These cells retain the genetic mutations of the donor, allowing researchers to test therapies in a disease-relevant context. iPSC models are particularly useful for rare or genetically heterogeneous disorders. They enable precise phenotyping, drug testing, and even gene-editing experiments in vitro. This approach is a cornerstone of precision drug screening and toxicity prediction.

From Bench to Bedside: Regulatory and Ethical Hurdles

Translating promising research into clinical therapies involves navigating complex regulatory and ethical landscapes. For CNS-targeted interventions—especially gene editing, enzyme therapies, and biologics—the stakes are high due to the irreversible nature of brain damage and the vulnerability of patients. Regulatory approval requires extensive preclinical safety and efficacy data, often demanding years of rigorous testing. Navigating these challenges is essential to ensure both scientific integrity and patient protection.

Regulatory Approval Pathways

Therapies targeting neurological diseases must comply with strict regulatory standards set by agencies like the FDA, EMA, or CDSCO. These include Investigational New Drug (IND) applications, clinical trial authorizations, and extensive toxicology studies. Regulatory bodies also demand clear evidence of therapeutic benefit, often through biomarker and imaging endpoints. For orphan diseases, fast-track or breakthrough designations may be available, but these still require robust data. Ensuring compliance early in the research process can prevent costly delays later.

Ethical Concerns in Gene and Enzyme Therapies

Advanced therapies like CRISPR or viral vector-based enzyme replacement raise complex ethical questions. These include concerns about long-term effects, germline editing (in the case of early interventions), and the right to withdraw from trials. Special attention is needed when involving pediatric or cognitively impaired populations. Transparency, informed consent, and ongoing oversight by ethics committees are critical. Public trust in biotechnology depends on maintaining high ethical standards throughout development.

Case Studies of Successful Translation

Several groundbreaking therapies in the neurodegenerative and lysosomal disease space have successfully transitioned from research labs to clinical application. These case studies highlight not only scientific innovation but also strategic handling of regulatory, ethical, and logistical challenges. They serve as models for future translational efforts by demonstrating how early-stage discoveries can evolve into life-changing therapies. Factors like patient advocacy, biomarker validation, and interdisciplinary collaboration played a vital role in these successes.

Spinraza for Spinal Muscular Atrophy (SMA)

Spinraza (nusinersen) was the first FDA-approved therapy for SMA and emerged from decades of genetic and antisense oligonucleotide (ASO) research. It modulates SMN2 gene splicing to increase functional SMN protein levels. Its development involved close coordination between academia, biotech, and patient advocacy groups. Clinical trials showed significant improvements in motor function and survival. The case underscores the importance of targeted molecular understanding and robust patient community engagement.

Zolgensma: Gene Therapy Milestone

It overcame major technical challenges, such as BBB crossing and vector design, to achieve widespread CNS delivery. Regulatory success was enabled by compelling early data and designation as a breakthrough therapy. Though its high cost raised ethical concerns about accessibility, it set a precedent for future gene therapies.

THERAPEUTIC STRATEGIES BEYOND ENZYME THERAPY

Therapeutic strategies beyond enzyme therapy are expanding the arsenal against neurodegenerative diseases by targeting various pathological mechanisms to complement or provide alternatives to enzyme-based approaches. These include small-molecule drugs designed to inhibit protein aggregation, modulate neurotransmitter systems, and reduce oxidative stress. Immunotherapies, such as monoclonal antibodies and vaccines, aim to clear toxic protein deposits like amyloid-beta and alpha-synuclein or to modulate immune responses. Gene therapies targeting genetic mutations or enhancing neuroprotective factors offer personalized treatment options. Additionally, lifestyle interventions, including diet, exercise, and cognitive training, are recognized for their potential to slow disease progression and improve quality of life. Emerging modalities such as stem cell therapy and neuroprotective peptides hold promise for neuronal regeneration and repair.

Neuroprotective Agents and Anti-inflammatory Compounds

Neuroprotective agents and anti-inflammatory compounds play a crucial role in preventing or slowing neuronal damage in various central nervous system (CNS) disorders. These agents aim to counteract oxidative stress, excitotoxicity, mitochondrial dysfunction, and chronic inflammation—key pathological processes that contribute to neurodegeneration. While many neuroprotective compounds target cellular pathways to preserve neuron viability, anti-inflammatory drugs focus on modulating the immune response to reduce neuroinflammation, which is increasingly recognized as a driver of disease progression. Together, these agents form an important therapeutic category, either as standalone treatments or as adjuncts to disease-specific therapies.

Mechanisms of Neuroprotection

Neuroprotective agents act through multiple mechanisms, including antioxidant activity to neutralize reactive oxygen species (ROS), calcium channel modulation to prevent excitotoxicity, and enhancement of mitochondrial function to improve cellular energy metabolism. Examples include compounds like edaravone, which scavenges free radicals, and memantine, an NMDA receptor antagonist that reduces excitotoxic damage. By preserving cellular integrity, these agents help maintain synaptic function and delay neuronal loss.

Targeting Neuroinflammation

Chronic neuroinflammation mediated by activated microglia and astrocytes contributes to neuronal injury in many neurodegenerative diseases. Anti-inflammatory compounds, including non-steroidal anti-inflammatory drugs (NSAIDs), corticosteroids, and novel microglial modulators, aim to suppress harmful inflammatory signalling pathways. Balancing immune suppression without impairing essential brain immune functions remains a challenge. Current research focuses on selective modulation of inflammation to achieve neuroprotection without systemic side effects.

Stem Cell and Exosome-Based Therapies

Stem cell and exosome-based therapies represent innovative approaches to repair and regenerate damaged neural tissue in CNS disorders. Additionally, they secrete bioactive factors that promote neuroprotection, angiogenesis, and immune modulation.

Types and Sources of Stem Cells

ESCs have high pluripotency but pose ethical concerns and risk of tumorigenesis. iPSCs circumvent ethical issues and can be patient-specific, reducing immune rejection risks.

Therapeutic Potential of Exosomes

Exosomes derived from stem cells carry a cargo of proteins, microRNAs, and signalling molecules that can modulate inflammation, promote angiogenesis, and stimulate endogenous repair mechanisms. Clinical studies are investigating exosome therapy for neurodegenerative diseases, traumatic brain injury, and stroke. Their scalability and stability make them promising candidates for off-the-shelf therapeutics.

Combination Therapies: Synergistic Effects and Personalization

Combination therapies harness the synergistic effects of multiple treatment modalities to enhance efficacy, reduce side effects, and address the multifactorial nature of neurological disorders. By targeting different disease mechanisms simultaneously—such as protein aggregation, inflammation, and neuronal loss—combination approaches aim to produce more robust and durable clinical benefits. Personalized medicine principles are increasingly integrated into combination therapy design, tailoring treatments based on patient genetics, biomarkers, and disease stage.

Rationale for Combination Approaches

Neurological disorders often involve multiple pathogenic pathways, including protein misfolding, neuroinflammation, oxidative stress, and synaptic dysfunction. Single-agent therapies may fail to address this complexity, leading to limited clinical benefits. Combining neuroprotective agents, anti-inflammatory drugs, enzyme replacement, and gene therapies can target these diverse mechanisms concurrently. Preclinical studies show that such combinations can enhance neuronal survival and functional recovery.

Examples of Successful Combinations

In clinical practice and trials, combinations such as cholinesterase inhibitors with memantine are used in Alzheimer's disease to improve cognition and function. Trials are underway combining anti-amyloid monoclonal antibodies with anti-inflammatory agents to address both protein pathology and inflammation. Gene therapies are paired with small-molecule drugs to enhance efficacy or reduce immune reactions. These combinations have demonstrated additive or synergistic effects compared to monotherapies.

COLLABORATIVE RESEARCH AND POLICY IMPLICATIONS

Collaborative research and informed policy play pivotal roles in advancing the understanding and treatment of neurodegenerative disorders. Given the complexity of these diseases, multidisciplinary collaboration among neuroscientists, clinicians, biotechnologists, and data scientists accelerates innovation by integrating diverse expertise and resources. Large-scale consortia and data-sharing initiatives enhance reproducibility and enable the identification of novel biomarkers and therapeutic targets. Meanwhile, policymakers influence research funding, regulatory pathways, and healthcare infrastructure, shaping the pace at which new treatments reach patients. Effective policies that support early diagnosis, equitable access to therapies, and patient-centered care are essential for maximizing public health impact. Furthermore, fostering global partnerships and public-private collaborations can drive investment in cutting-edge technologies and ensure that advances benefit diverse populations.

The Role of International Consortia and Open Science

International consortia and open science initiatives are critical drivers of progress in neurodegenerative disease research by fostering collaboration, data sharing, and standardization across borders. These collaborative efforts bring together multidisciplinary expertise and large patient cohorts to accelerate discovery and therapy development. Open science principles ensure transparency, reproducibility, and accessibility of research data and tools, which collectively reduce duplication of efforts and enhance innovation. By pooling resources and knowledge, consortia help tackle complex neurological diseases more effectively than isolated efforts.

Collaborative Research Networks

International consortia such as the Alzheimer's Disease Neuroimaging Initiative (ADNI) and the Global Parkinson's Genetics Program (GP2) coordinate multi-site studies and share standardized data sets. These networks enable large-scale genomic, biomarker, and clinical data analyses that improve disease understanding and patient stratification. By uniting academic institutions, industry, and patient organizations, consortia accelerate translation from bench to bedside. They also facilitate harmonized protocols and outcome measures for clinical trials, improving comparability across studies.

Open Data and Tool Sharing

Open science initiatives promote the free exchange of datasets, analytical tools, and software platforms through repositories and public databases. Examples include the AMP-AD Knowledge Portal and the Human Brain Project. This transparency allows researchers worldwide to validate findings, reanalyse data, and generate novel hypotheses without repeating costly experiments. Open-source tools for image analysis, biomarker quantification, and AI modelling empower scientists regardless of institutional resources. The open science model fosters inclusivity, collaboration, and rapid knowledge dissemination.

Funding, Policy Making, and Healthcare Integration

Sustainable funding, effective policy frameworks, and integration of new therapies into healthcare systems are pivotal to translating neurodegenerative research into real-world benefits. Adequate investment supports the costly, long-term research required for developing innovative treatments, while policy decisions influence regulatory approval, reimbursement, and equitable access. Integrating novel therapies into clinical practice demands coordination among healthcare providers, payers, and patients. Policies that incentivize innovation, ensure safety, and promote health equity are crucial for maximizing therapeutic impact.

Public and Private Funding Mechanisms

Neurodegenerative disease research is supported by a combination of government grants, philanthropic organizations, and private sector investment. Agencies like the NIH and EU Horizon programs provide foundational funding for basic and translational science. Ensuring continuous funding flow is vital given the high failure rates and extended timelines typical of CNS drug development.

Regulatory and Policy Frameworks

Clear regulatory guidelines facilitate the approval of innovative therapies while safeguarding patient safety. Policies addressing orphan diseases, accelerated approval pathways, and adaptive trial designs encourage innovation. Policymakers face challenges balancing innovation incentives with healthcare budget constraints. Collaborative dialogue among regulators, industry, and patient groups helps shape pragmatic policies that benefit all stakeholders.

Ethical Considerations in Neurodegenerative Therapy Development

Ethical considerations are central to neurodegenerative therapy development, given the vulnerability of patient populations, complexity of interventions, and potential long-term impacts. Ethical frameworks guide responsible research conduct, informed consent, data privacy, and equitable treatment access. Addressing these issues transparently builds public trust and supports sustainable innovation. Emerging technologies such as gene editing and biomarker-based stratification introduce new ethical challenges that must be proactively managed.

Informed Consent and Patient Autonomy

Patients with neurodegenerative disorders often experience cognitive decline, complicating informed consent for experimental therapies. Ensuring that patients or their legal representatives understand potential risks and benefits is essential. Ongoing consent processes and clear communication help respect patient autonomy. In cases of advanced disease, surrogate decision-making and ethical oversight become critical. Ethical research design prioritizes patient welfare while advancing scientific knowledge.

Data Privacy and Genetic Information

Therapies increasingly rely on genetic and biomarker data, raising concerns about confidentiality, data ownership, and potential discrimination. Robust safeguards and transparent policies are necessary to protect patient information. Ethical frameworks must balance data sharing for research advancement with individual privacy rights. International harmonization of data protection regulations facilitates cross-border research while respecting ethical norms.

CONCLUSIONS

Neurodegenerative diseases represent one of the most complex and pressing challenges in modern healthcare, driven by aging demographics and limited treatment options. These disorders, despite their clinical differences, share core molecular mechanisms—including protein misfolding, mitochondrial dysfunction, oxidative stress, and chronic neuroinflammation—that progressively impair neuronal function and survival. As discussed in this chapter, current diagnostic approaches often detect disease only after significant neuronal damage has occurred, and available treatments primarily aim to manage symptoms rather than halt or reverse progression. However, the landscape is beginning to change. Advances in monoclonal antibody therapies, enzyme replacement, gene editing, and precision diagnostics are paving the way for earlier interventions and more personalized, disease-modifying therapies. This chapter emphasizes the importance of integrating molecular insights with technological innovations, translational research, and supportive policy frameworks. Through promoting cross-disciplinary teamwork and emphasizing early diagnosis and specific therapies, the scientific and medical fields are advancing towards changing the treatment landscape for individuals with Alzheimer's, Parkinson's, ALS, Huntington's disease, and various neurodegenerative conditions. Continued progress will depend on sustained investment, global cooperation, and a commitment to bridging the gap between laboratory discovery and clinical application.

REFERENCES

Afaq, A., Syed, R., & Bomanji, J. (2013). PET/MRI: A new technology in the field of molecular imaging. *British Medical Bulletin, 108*(1), 159–171. DOI: 10.1093/bmb/ldt032

Alkhalifa, A. E., Alkhalifa, O., Durdanovic, I., Ibrahim, D. R., & Maragkou, S. (2025). Oxidative Stress and Mitochondrial Dysfunction in Alzheimer's Disease: Insights into Pathophysiology and Treatment. *Journal of Dementia and Alzheimer's Disease*, *2*(2), 17. DOI: 10.3390/jdad2020017

Ashtari, N., Jiao, X., Rahimi-Balaei, M., Amiri, S. E., Mehr, S., Yeganeh, B., & Marzban, H. (2016). Lysosomal acid phosphatase biosynthesis and dysfunction: A mini review focused on lysosomal enzyme dysfunction in brain. *Current Molecular Medicine*, *16*(5), 439–446. DOI: 10 .2174/1566524016666160429115834

Battineni, G., Sagaro, G. G., Chinatalapudi, N., & Amenta, F. (2020). Applications of machine learning predictive models in the chronic disease diagnosis. *Journal of Personalized Medicine*, *10*(2), 21. DOI: 10.3390/jpm10020021

Cummings, J. (2023). Anti-amyloid monoclonal antibodies are transformative treatments that redefine Alzheimer's disease therapeutics. *Drugs*, *83*(7), 569–576. DOI: 10.1007/s40265-023-01858-9

De La Fuente, M., Lombardero, L., Gómez-González, A., Solari, C., Angulo-Barturen, I., Acera, A., Vecino, E., Astigarraga, E., & Barreda-Gómez, G. (2021). Enzyme therapy: Current challenges and future perspectives. *International Journal of Molecular Sciences*, *22*(17), 9181. DOI: 10.3390/ijms22179181

Kampmann, M. (2020). CRISPR-based functional genomics for neurological disease. *Nature Reviews. Neurology*, *16*(9), 465–480. DOI: 10.1038/s41582-020-0373-z

Kumar, S., Saha, S., Singh, T., Tripathi, R. B., Singh, K., Dwivedi, V., Singh, S., & Chandra, D. (2024). Focusing on Enzyme Suppression in Neurodegenerative Disorders: Promising Approaches for Therapeutic Measures. *Emirates Medical Journal*, *5*(1), e02506882311325. DOI: 10.2174/0102506882311325240815105251

Nam, Y., Kim, J., Jung, S. H., Woerner, J., Suh, E. H., Lee, D. G., Shivakumar, M., Lee, M. E., & Kim, D. (2024). Harnessing artificial intelligence in multimodal omics data integration: Paving the path for the next frontier in precision medicine. *Annual Review of Biomedical Data Science*, *7*(1), 7. DOI: 10.1146/annurev-biodatasci-102523-103801

Puli, L., Pomeshchik, Y., Olas, K., Malm, T., Koistinaho, J., & Tanila, H. (2012). Effects of human intravenous immunoglobulin on amyloid pathology and neuroinflammation in a mouse model of Alzheimer's disease. *Journal of Neuroinflammation*, *9*(1), 1–19. DOI: 10.1186/1742-2094-9-105

Rahman, A., Banu, Z., Rani, R., & Mehdiya, R. (2024). Unravelling Alzheimer's disease: Insights into pathophysiology, etiology, diagnostic approaches, and the promise of aducanumab, lecanemab, and donanemab. *Journal of Phytonanotechnology and Pharmaceutical Sciences*, *4*(3), 1–10. DOI: 10.54085/jpps.2024.4.3.1

Ramamoorth, M., & Narvekar, A. (2015). Non viral vectors in gene therapy-an overview. *Journal of Clinical and Diagnostic Research : JCDR*, *9*(1), GE01. DOI: 10.7860/JCDR/2015/10443.5394

Roche, S., Gabelle, A., & Lehmann, S. (2008). Clinical proteomics of the cerebrospinal fluid: Towards the discovery of new biomarkers. *Proteomics. Clinical Applications*, *2*(3), 428–436. DOI: 10.1002/prca.200780040

Sheehan, K., Jeon, H., Corr, S. C., Hayes, J. M., & Mok, K. H. (2025). Antibody aggregation: A problem within the biopharmaceutical industry and its role in AL amyloidosis disease. *The Protein Journal*, *44*(1), 1–20. DOI: 10.1007/s10930-024-10237-6

Sighencea, M. G., Popescu, R. ., & Trifu, S. C. (2024). From Fundamentals to Innovation in Alzheimer's Disease: Molecular Findings and Revolutionary Therapies. *International Journal of Molecular Sciences*, *25*(22), 12311. DOI: 10.3390/ijms252212311

Simon, R. (2008). Lost in translation: Problems and pitfalls in translating laboratory observations to clinical utility. *European Journal of Cancer (Oxford, England)*, *44*(18), 2707–2713. DOI: 10.1016/j.ejca.2008.09.009

Skoczeń, A., Rutecka, N., Kaczmarek, B., Kuśnierz-Gibała, A., Kruk, A., Kulesza, M., Wawrzynów, W., Miłoś, M., Dorosz, A., & Jakubowska, M. M. (2025). Advancements in Alzheimer's Disease Therapy: The Role of Anti-Amyloid Monoclonal Antibodies-A Literature Review. *Journal of Education, Health and Sport*, *79*, 58362–58362. DOI: 10.12775/JEHS.2025.79.58362

Wang, Y. J., Zhou, H. D., & Zhou, X. F. (2006). Clearance of amyloid-beta in Alzheimer's disease: Progress, problems and perspectives. *Drug Discovery Today*, *11*(19-20), 931–938. DOI: 10.1016/j.drudis.2006.08.004

Yin, H., Kauffman, K. J., & Anderson, D. G. (2017). Delivery technologies for genome editing. *Nature Reviews. Drug Discovery*, *16*(6), 387–399. DOI: 10.1038/nrd.2016.280

Zhang, X., Zhou, J., Gu, Z., Zhang, H., Gong, Q., & Luo, K. (2021). Advances in nanomedicines for diagnosis of central nervous system disorders. *Biomaterials*, *269*, 120492. DOI: 10.1016/j.biomaterials.2020.120492

Chapter 12
Regulatory Challenges in the Development and Approval of Drugs Focusing on Enzyme Pathways in Neurodegenerative Diseases

Popat Mohite
https://orcid.org/0000-0002-4536-4444
AETs St. John Institute of Pharmacy and Research, Palghar, India

Deepak Bharti
St. John Institute of Pharmacy and Research, India

Vaishnavi Gohri
AETs St. John Institute of Pharmacy and Research, Palghar, India

ABSTRACT

Neurodegenerative diseases presents the pathways as promising therapeutic targets,such as protein aggregation, mitochondrial dysfunction, and lysosomal degradation. Enzymes like β-secretase in Alzheimer's disease and glucocerebrosidase in Parkinson's exemplify this therapeutic potential.Emerging therapeutic modalitiessuch as gene therapy and enzyme replacement therapypose additional regulatory scrutiny due to novel delivery mechanisms and long-term safety concerns.Ethical considerations, including informed consent in cognitively impaired patients and equitable trial access, further complicate the regulatory landscape. Ensuring compliance with GMP/GCP is critical but resource-intensive.enzyme pathways offer promising avenues for treating neurodegenerative diseases, overcoming regulatory, ethical, and clinical challenges will require coordinated efforts among researchers, regulators, clinicians, and industry stakeholders.

DOI: 10.4018/979-8-3373-4627-4.ch012

INTRODUCTION

The primary regulatory issues that come up during the development and approval of medications that target enzyme pathways in neurodegenerative illnesses are intended to be identified and clarified by this topic. By addressing these issues, scientists, pharmaceutical companies, and government organizations can more adeptly manage the drug development process for these complicated illnesses and promote the creation of more potent treatments that enhance patient results, (Agarwal, 2019). Proteins called enzymes are responsible for catalyzing several biochemical reactions in the body, such as those involving the production, breakdown, and signaling of neurotransmitters. The etiology of multiple neurodegenerative illnesses, such as Alzheimer's, Parkinson's, Huntington's, and amyotrophic lateral sclerosis (ALS), has been linked to the dysregulation of enzyme pathways, (Ajitkumar & De Jesus, 2024).

Enzyme pathways implicated in the synthesis and elimination of beta-amyloid, a protein that builds up in Alzheimer's disease patients' brains, have been thoroughly investigated. The enzyme beta-secretase and gamma-secretase cleave the amyloid precursor protein (APP) to produce beta-amyloid. One of the main goals of Alzheimer's disease medication development has been the inhibition of these enzymes. Neprilysin and insulin-degrading enzyme (IDE), two enzymes implicated in the clearance of beta-amyloid, have been the focus of therapeutic research efforts, (Amjad et al., 2021)

Enzyme pathways related to the production, metabolism, and release of dopamine a neurotransmitter that is reduced in Parkinson's disease brain have been investigated in the illness. Tyrosine hydroxylase and aromatic L-amino acid decarboxylase (AADC) are two enzymes that catalyze the conversion of tyrosine to L-DOPA and L-DOPA to dopamine, respectively and are involved in the manufacture of dopamine. Drug research efforts have also focused on enzymes that are involved in the metabolism of dopamine, such as catechol-O-methyltransferase (COMT) and monoamine oxidase A (MAO-A), (Arnau, Yaver, & Hjort, 2020).

Enzyme pathways involved in glutamate metabolism have been linked to the pathophysiology of Huntington's disease, a hereditary neurological illness. High quantities of glutamate, an excitatory neurotransmitter, damage neurons. Glutamate dehydrogenase and glutamine synthetase are two examples of the enzymes involved in the breakdown of glutamate that have been investigated as possible targets for medication development, (Bakker et al., 2022; Bali & Miller, 2013). Enzyme pathways that produce and eliminate superoxide radicals, or reactive oxygen species (ROS), which are harmful to neurons, have been researched about acute lung injury (ALS). Xanthine oxidase, nicotinamide adenine dinucleotide phosphate (NADPH) oxidase, and cytochrome c oxidase are among the enzymes that produce superoxide radicals. Superoxide dismutase (SOD), which changes superoxide into hydrogen peroxide, and catalase, which changes hydrogen peroxide into water and oxygen, are two enzymes that help remove superoxide radicals from the body, (Bhave & Menon, 2017). The pathophysiology of neurodegenerative illnesses has been linked to the deregulation of several enzyme pathways. Knowing how particular enzymes function in the pathophysiology of diseases can help identify possible therapeutic targets for these conditions, (Bhaduri & Kipgen, 2018). The pharmaceutical community considers enzymes to be the most appealing targets for drug development. Understanding the responses of enzymes requires accurate characterization, which can only be accomplished through a variety of analytical techniques. Among the essential methods are purification, kinetics, protein stabilization, determining the ideal pH, temperature, and ionic strength, substrate/product binding, ligand/inhibitor/protein interactions, three-dimensional

structure, and conformational changes. The characterization of enzymes has significantly benefited from in silico analysis in recent years, with molecular docking and dynamics being two of the main techniques, (Bloem, Okun, & Klein, 2021).

Because of their critical role in drug development, enzymes are desirable research subjects for the pharmaceutical industry and are significant as follows:

1. Enzymes are remarkably efficient. They are essential components of biological systems because they can precisely perform complicated biochemical processes, (Bloem, Okun, & Klein, 2021)
2. Drugs intended to target a specific enzyme can only alter the desired pathway or reaction because enzymes are frequently very selective in their substrate identification and catalytic activity. This may result in treatments that are more focused, efficient and have fewer adverse effects, (Bortolato, Chen, & Shih, 2008).
3. Because enzymes are highly effective catalysts, even slight variations in their activity can have a big impact on the entire biochemical reaction or pathway. Because of this, enzymes are particularly appealing as therapeutic targets for diseases for which small changes in enzyme activity may be sufficient to provide positive effects, (Breijyeh & Karaman, 2020).
4. Enzymes are accessible for drug targeting because they are frequently found on the surface of cells or in biofluids. Furthermore, a great deal of enzymes have distinct active sites or conformational changes that lend themselves to structure-based drug design, (Bhaduri & Kipgen, 2018).
5. Enzymes are involved in a variety of biological processes and metabolic pathways, focusing on a particular enzyme may be therapeutically beneficial for a wide range of illnesses and ailments.
6. Since several enzymes in the body carry out comparable tasks, a dysregulated enzyme or pathway may be compensated for by another. Targeting several of the enzymes involved in a certain pathway can offer a strong therapeutic strategy that is less prone to side effects or resistance, (Cavalli et al., 2008).
7. It's essential to comprehend how enzymes react; researchers use a variety of techniques to characterize enzymes:
8. Separating and purification of complicated mixes' enzymes.
    - Analyzing substrate binding and reaction rates.
    - Protein Stabilization: Maintaining the stability of enzymes.
    - In Silico Analysis: Making use of computer methods such as dynamics and molecular docking
9. Developing new inhibitors is made possible by focusing on enzymes. Reasonable medication design is aided by research into conformational changes and enzyme processes, (Chaturvedi et al., 2016).

Enzymes are essential targets that propel advances in medication research and healing discoveries. Developing drugs that target enzymes offers several benefits for creating potent treatments. Because enzymes regulate and catalyze the body's biochemical events, altering their activity can have a profound impact on cellular signaling networks, metabolic pathways, and general physiology, (Bloem, Okun, & Klein, 2021). Using enzymes as a target for drugs can be a potent and adaptable strategy for creating medicines that effectively treat a variety of illnesses and ailments.

By understanding the biochemical processes and enzyme regulatory networks that underlie disease pathology, researchers can find specific enzymes and pathways to target, design medications with high specificity and potency, and optimize therapy techniques for maximal efficacy and safety, (Chen et al., 2013). Understanding the regulatory obstacles to the development and approval of medications that target enzyme pathways in neurodegenerative diseases would help researchers better appreciate the intricacies involved in creating medications for complicated illnesses with multifaceted pathologies. In the context of complicated disease biology, developing medications that target certain enzyme pathways presents particular difficulties, such as the lack of validated biomarkers and a strict regulatory framework for drug approval, (Chen, Xu, & Chen, 2021). In this book chapter, the regulatory aspects with respect to target specific enzymes in neurodegenerative disorders like Parkinson's, Alzheimer's, Huntington's and amyotrophic lateral sclerosis are discussed. The manufacturing obstacles are also highlighted.

NEURODEGENERATIVE DISEASES

A class of illnesses known as neurodegenerative disorders gradually impair the composition and functionality of neurons in the brain or peripheral nervous system. Deterioration of cognitive and motor abilities, along with related symptoms such as tremors, altered behaviour, memory loss, and poor motor coordination, characterize these illnesses. Alzheimer's disease, Parkinson's disease, Huntington's disease, and amyotrophic lateral sclerosis (ALS) are a few examples of neurodegenerative illnesses, (Cheng et al., 2015). Numerous variables, including genetic abnormalities, environmental influences, and altered cellular processes, can cause neurodegenerative diseases. Ageing is frequently linked to an increased risk of developing these conditions, and as the population ages, it is anticipated that the frequency of neurodegenerative disorders will rise, (Colović et al., 2013).

Alzheimer's Disease

It is a long-term neurodegenerative condition that damages brain structure and function, gradually impairing behaviour, thought processes, and memory. The buildup of tau protein tangles and beta-amyloid plaques in the brain, which impair regular cellular functions and cause brain cell death, are the main symptoms of the illness, (Davenport et al., 2023). Alzheimer's patients have a wide range of symptoms, such as altered personality, disorientation, memory loss, poor decision-making, trouble speaking, and trouble finishing routine chores. The majority of those affected by this crippling illness are older folks, and the chance of getting Alzheimer's disease rises with age, (de la Fuente et al., 2021). Alzheimer's disease currently has no known cure; instead, available treatments concentrate on symptom management. Current research is examining the fundamental processes of the illness and creating novel therapies that can slow down or stop its progression, (Dicks, 2022; Dorsey et al., 2018).

Parkinson's Disease

It is a neurodegenerative disease that worsens over time, affecting the nervous system and impairing motor abilities. Dopamine levels decline, and motor coordination is compromised as

a result of the condition, which is brought on by the slow death of dopamine-producing neurons in the brain. Bradykinesia, or sluggish movement, rigidity, tremors, and postural instability, are the main signs and symptoms of Parkinson's disease, (Falkowska et al., 2015; Frampton, 2020). Parkinson's disease is more common in those over 60, and the disease's risk grows with advancing age. But younger folks can also experience it. Although the precise aetiology of Parkinson's disease is still unknown, scientists think that a mix of environmental and hereditary variables may play a role in the disease's development, (Franco et al., 2023). Parkinson's disease does not currently have a recognized cure, although several alternatives for treatment can aid with symptom management. Deep brain stimulation, speech therapy, physical therapy, and medicine are some of these treatments. Scientists are still trying to figure out the fundamental causes of Parkinson's disease and find novel ways to stop or even reverse the illness's course, (Frak et al., 2022). Overall, millions of individuals worldwide suffer from the crippling effects of Parkinson's disease. In the upcoming years, there will likely be a rise in the number of people with Parkinson's disease due to the ageing population. Effective therapies and management techniques are, therefore, desperately needed to enhance the quality of life for those who have Parkinson's disease and their families, (Gribkoff & Kaczmarek, 2017).

Huntington's Disease

It is a rare genetic disorder that primarily affects the nervous system, leading to the progressive and irreversible loss of cognitive, behavioural, and motor functions. The disease is caused by a defect in the Huntingtin (HTT) gene, which leads to the production of an abnormal version of the Huntingtin protein. As a result, the protein accumulates in the brain, leading to the death of neurons in specific areas of the brain, (Bali & Miller, 2013). Huntington's disease is an inherited condition, and individuals with one copy of the defective gene from one parent are at risk of developing the disorder. The symptoms of Huntington's disease typically appear between the ages of 30 and 50, and they include involuntary movements, cognitive decline, mood disturbances, and difficulties with speech and swallowing, (Halioua-Haubold et al., 2017). Currently, there is no cure for Huntington's disease, and the available treatments focus on managing symptoms. The management of symptoms includes medication to control involuntary movements, speech therapy, physical therapy, and psychological counselling to support individuals and their families, (Hennigan & Lynch, 2022). Researchers are investigating new treatments that could slow or reverse the progression of Huntington's disease and improve the quality of life for affected individuals. These treatments include the development of gene therapy, stem cell therapy, and approaches that target the abnormal proteins that accumulate in the brain, (Holdgate, Meek, & Grimley, 2018). Overall, Huntington's disease is a complex condition that affects individuals and their families profoundly. Researchers continue to work towards understanding the underlying mechanisms of the disease and developing new therapeutic interventions to improve the lives of individuals living with Huntington's disease, (Halioua-Haubold et al., 2017).

Amyotrophic Lateral Sclerosis

It is a progressive neurological disorder that impacts the neurons in the brain and spinal cord. This condition leads to the degeneration of muscle tissue, thereby affecting the control of voluntary muscles. It's commonly referred to as Lou Gehrig's disease, named after a famous baseball player

who was diagnosed with the condition. ALS impacts various functions of the body, including speech, swallowing, and breathing. There are no known cures for ALS, and treatment primarily focuses on managing symptoms and improving quality of life. Regulate voluntary muscular movements. Neurons in ALS undergo a gradual process of deterioration and degeneration, which ultimately leads to their death. This process primarily affects the motor neurons, which are responsible for controlling voluntary muscle movements, (Huang et al., 2021). Most instances of ALS have no known etiology. However, a tiny percentage are inherited and result from genetic abnormalities. Muscle weakness, especially in the arms and legs, is usually the first symptom of the condition and gets worse with time. Individuals can have trouble breathing, swallowing, and speaking as the illness worsens, (Hur, 2022). There is no known cure for ALS, and current therapies focus on managing symptoms and enhancing the quality of life for those affected. In the later stages of the disease, these therapies can include respiratory assistance, physical therapy to strengthen muscles, and medications to control muscle spasms, (Jankovic, 2008). Despite continuous research efforts, the underlying causes of ALS are still largely unknown. Nevertheless, ongoing studies have revealed potential targets for pharmacological intervention and gene therapy that may alleviate or halt disease progression. These breakthroughs provide hope for the development of more effective ALS treatment strategies and a potential cure in the future. Researchers are continually exploring the biological mechanisms, genetic factors, and environmental risk factors associated with the disease to enhance our understanding of the disease's pathology and design targeted therapeutics, (Jimenez-Sanchez et al., 2017). ALS is a problematic and crippling illness that has a significant impact on patients and their families. There is optimism that in the future, new medications and treatments for people with ALS will be created as more research is being conducted, (Kaur et al., 2021).

Role of Enzyme Dysregulation in Disease Progression

Enzyme dysregulation is a condition when the body's regular biological processes are disrupted due to either an overactive or underactive state of enzymes. The body needs enzymes, which are essential proteins, to catalyze chemical reactions that enable metabolism and other processes. Diseases and malfunction can result from dysregulated enzymes, (Bhaduri & Kipgen, 2018). Numerous variables, such as genetic abnormalities, environmental exposure, and lifestyle choices, can lead to enzyme dysregulation. For instance, an enzyme's gene may occasionally mutate, changing the protein's structure and producing either overactive or underactive enzymes. Numerous illnesses, such as cancer, neurological diseases, and metabolic disorders, have been linked to enzyme dysregulation. For example, several enzymes involved in DNA repair and cell development can become dysregulated, causing unchecked growth and DNA damage that encourages the growth of malignancies. Similar to this, misfolded proteins can build up in the brain as a result of dysregulated enzymes that process and degrade proteins in neurodegenerative illnesses including Parkinson's and Alzheimer's. Then, these protein clumps have the potential to harm neurons and accelerate the onset and course of neurodegenerative, (Khan et al., 2020).

Additionally, dysregulated enzymes involved in nutrition metabolism can lead to an imbalance in metabolic pathways and the buildup of toxic metabolites, which can result in metabolic illnesses like diabetes and heart disease. Studies have demonstrated that a deeper comprehension of the processes underlying enzyme dysregulation in a range of diseases might result in the creation of innovative medications and treatments that specifically target these enzymes and

enhance consequences for those who are impacted. Furthermore, more effective methods of preventing enzyme dysregulation may eventually result in a decline in the prevalence of these related illnesses, (Khan et al., 2022).

Examples of the Diseases Linked to Enzyme Dysregulation

1. A large number of diseases, including cancer, metabolic disorders, cardiovascular diseases, neurodegenerative diseases, and genetic disorders, are significantly influenced by enzyme dysregulation in their early stages, (Kiaei, 2013).
2. The buildup of hazardous misfolded proteins in the brain that result in neuronal damage can be caused by enzyme dysregulation in neurodegenerative illnesses like Alzheimer's, Parkinson's, and Huntington's, (Kim, 2023).
3. Dysregulated enzymes in cancer can cause cancer cells to grow and increase uncontrollably, (Kouli, Torsney, & Kuan, 2018).
4. Enzyme dysregulation, which results in an imbalance of metabolic pathways, an accumulation of toxic metabolites, and insulin resistance, can cause metabolic illnesses such as diabetes and metabolic syndrome, (Koumadorakis, Krokidis, & Dimitrakopoulos, 2023).
5. Enzyme dysregulation can play a role in the development of cardiovascular illnesses such as atherosclerosis, hypertension, and heart failure by impacting blood clotting, blood vessel constriction, and cholesterol metabolism, (Kumar et al., 2024).
6. Gene mutations that result in enzyme shortages produce genetic illnesses, including phenylketonuria, Tay-Sachs disease, and Gaucher disease, (Lamptey et al., 2022).
7. Understanding the fundamental mechanisms of enzyme dysregulation in diverse disease conditions can aid researchers in the development of novel therapies and treatments that target these enzymes and enhance the quality of life for afflicted patients, (Lamptey et al., 2022)

ENZYME PATHWAY AS THERAPEUTIC TARGETS

The Role That Enzyme Pathways Play in Neurodegenerative Illnesses

Enzyme pathways are vital for the brain system's normal functioning, but they can also contribute to the development and progression of neurodegenerative diseases. Enzymes release reactive oxygen species (ROS) that can damage neurons and facilitate neurotransmitter breakdown. Enzyme dysfunction and metabolic waste buildup result in inflammation, reduced cellular function, and neuronal death, contributing to neurodegenerative disorders' onset and advancement, (Bhaduri & Kipgen, 2018). Targeting enzyme pathways has become a promising approach for developing neurodegenerative disease therapies that can improve cognitive and motor function. Enzyme activity modification or reducing metabolic waste buildup through drugs can halt or slow disease progression. Several target enzymes for neurodegenerative diseases include acetylcholinesterase, L-DOPA decarboxylase, and superoxide dismutase, (Li et al., 2021). Numerous medications targeting enzyme pathways have been created and authorized to address neurodegenerative illnesses; here are a few instances:

1. **Acetylcholinesterase (AChE) inhibitors:** Acetylcholine is a neurotransmitter involved in memory and learning that is broken down by the enzyme AChE. Acetylcholine insufficiency is one of the factors contributing to cognitive deterioration in Alzheimer's disease, (Martin, Al Khleifat, & Al-Chalabi, 2017).
2. **L-DOPA decarboxylase inhibitors:** Dopamine, a neurotransmitter important in motor function, is derived from L-DOPA. Dopamine insufficiency is a factor in Parkinson's disease, contributing to motor symptoms such as stiffness and tremors. L-DOPA therapy raises dopamine levels in the brain, yet adverse effects such as nausea and dyskinesia are possible. Carbidopa and benserazide are examples of L-DOPA decarboxylase inhibitors that are used to improve the effectiveness of therapy, (McKeith et al., 2017).
3. **Monoamine oxidase (MAO) inhibitors:** The enzyme MAO breaks down dopamine and other neurotransmitters. MAO inhibitors, such as selegiline and rasagiline, are used to treat Parkinson's disease by raising dopamine levels in the brain and enhancing motor function, (Mead et al., 2023).
4. **Catechol-O-methyltransferase (COMT) inhibitors:** The enzyme COMT breaks down dopamine and other neurotransmitters. COMT inhibitors, such as entacapone and tolcapone, are used to treat Parkinson's disease by improving the efficacy of L-DOPA therapy and lowering its adverse effects, (Mejzini et al., 2019).
5. **Gamma-secretase inhibitors:** Beta-amyloid is a protein that builds up in the brains of Alzheimer's disease patients and is produced by the cleavage of amyloid precursor protein (APP) by the enzyme gamma-secretase. The development of gamma-secretase inhibitors, such as semagacestat, aims to decrease the synthesis of beta-amyloid and decelerate the advancement of Alzheimer's disease. Nevertheless, these medications have shown a great deal of negative effects and poor effectiveness, which has caused clinical trials to stop using them, (Mentz et al., 2016).
6. Aducanumab is a monoclonal antibody medication that specifically targets beta-amyloid, a substance that builds up in the brains of individuals suffering from Alzheimer's disease. It is the first disease-modifying medication for Alzheimer's disease, having received FDA approval in 2021, (Miners et al., 2009).
7. Levodopa/carbidopa intestinal gel (LCIG): This treatment entails the continuous administration of carbidopa and levodopa via a small intestine-inserted tube and pump. Carbidopa is a peripheral decarboxylase inhibitor that stops levodopa from being converted to dopamine outside of the brain. Levodopa is a precursor to dopamine. When oral drugs are no longer adequate for treating advanced Parkinson's disease patients, LCIG is utilized to restore motor function, (Morant, Jagalski, & Vestergaard, 2019).
8. Inebilizumab: It is a monoclonal antibody medication that specifically targets CD19, a protein expressed on the surface of B cells, which are immunological cells. The FDA authorized inbebilizumab in 2020 to treat neuromyelitis optica spectrum disorder (NMOSD), an autoimmune condition that causes damage to the spinal cord and optic nerve. Although the exact enzyme mechanism causing NMOSD is unknown, B cells are believed to be involved in the illness process, (Palanisamy et al., 2023).

Importance of Enzyme Pathways on the Nervous System

Enzyme pathways are extremely important for the nervous system because they control several biochemical processes necessary for normal brain function. The body uses enzymes, proteins that catalyze chemical reactions, to produce and break down neurotransmitters, which are signalling chemicals that let neurons communicate with one another, (Bhaduri & Kipgen, 2018).

1. **Maintenance of neurotransmitter levels:** The manufacture and degradation of neurotransmitters, including acetylcholine, dopamine, and serotonin, are greatly aided by enzymes, (Pathak et al., 2022). Because neurotransmitters are necessary for healthy brain development, imbalances in their amounts can cause deviant behaviour and cognitive decline. Neurotransmitter levels are directly influenced by enzyme pathways, and variations in the activity of these pathways can affect the balance of neurotransmitters inside the brain, (Pereira et al., 2023).
2. **Control of metabolic processes:** The brain's many metabolic activities are regulated by enzyme pathways. They affect the concentrations of chemicals necessary for healthy brain activity, such as fatty acids, glucose, and others. Because they manage the availability of substrates and cofactors, enzyme pathways can govern metabolic processes, (Phuna et al., 2022).
3. **Preservation of neuronal integrity:** The structural integrity of neurons can be preserved by enzyme pathways. Superoxide dismutase is one enzyme that can stop oxidative damage to neurons, which can cause neurodegenerative disorders. Additional enzymes play a role in preserving cellular structural integrity and mending damage to DNA, (Rao & Bredesen, 2004). The preservation of neuronal integrity is essential in preventing neurodegenerative disorders such as Parkinson's and Alzheimer's diseases. Amantadine, an antiviral medication, has been shown to exert its neuroprotective effects by inhibiting the activity of the N-methyl-D-aspartate (NMDA) receptor. For example, a study carried out by Chen et al. (2020) found that amantadine treatment can reduce cell apoptosis and amyloid-β accumulation in a rat model of Alzheimer's disease. Another study by Liu et al. (2020) demonstrated that chronic amantadine administration can alleviate motor symptoms in patients with Parkinson's disease by increasing dopamine release and protecting dopaminergic neurons. Thus, these studies suggest that amantadine's ability to preserve neuronal integrity may improve symptoms and slow the progression of neurodegenerative diseases. However, more research is necessary to fully understand the mechanisms of the drug's effects on these disorders and develop effective therapeutic strategies.
4. **Control of neuroinflammatory processes:** The brain's inflammatory processes are regulated by enzyme pathways. While responding to wounds and infections requires the production of inflammatory responses, persistent inflammation can cause tissue damage and neuronal death. The inflammatory response in the brain can be modulated by enzyme pathways, which also control the generation of pro-inflammatory cytokines and chemokines, (Reeve, Simcox, & Turnbull, 2014). Enzyme pathways are necessary for the nervous system because they control essential functions like inflammation, metabolic processes, neuronal integrity, and the synthesis and breakdown of neurotransmitters. Understanding the brain's enzyme pathways can develop treatments for neurological conditions and enhance brain function, (Reiner, Dragatsis, & Dietrich, 2011).

What Role Do Enzymatic Pathways Play in the Emergence of Neurodegenerative Illnesses?

Enzyme pathways are essential for keeping the nervous system operating as it should. Enzyme malfunction, however, occasionally enzyme pathways have been connected to neurodegenerative disorders in the beginning and progression of these illnesses in the following ways, (Bhaduri & Kipgen, 2018):

1. **Buildup of metabolic waste products:** The brain uses enzymes for several different metabolic functions. Metabolic waste products, such as beta-amyloid in Alzheimer's disease and alpha-synuclein in Parkinson's disease, can build up when enzymes malfunction. These waste products can build up and cause inflammation and oxidative damage, which can accelerate the onset and course of neurodegenerative illnesses, (Robinson, 2015).
2. **Decreased neurotransmitter function:** Enzymes mediate the synthesis and degradation of neurotransmitters. In neurodegenerative illnesses, abnormal enzyme levels can cause imbalances in neurotransmitter levels, which can exacerbate motor and cognitive impairment. For instance, Alzheimer's disease-related cognitive impairment has been connected to deregulation of the enzyme acetylcholinesterase, (Schneider et al., 2014).
3. **Elevated oxidative stress:** These are metabolic byproducts of enzymes that can be detrimental to neurons at high concentrations. The accumulation of ROS leads to oxidative stress, which contributes to the damage and death of neurons. This damage can expedite the onset and progression of various neurodegenerative diseases. Therefore, strategies that aim to reduce oxidative stress could mitigate some of the damage in these diseases, potentially resulting in a delay in progression and improved patient outcomes. Experimental methods for reducing ROS levels include using scavenging antioxidants, chelators, and enzyme inhibitors, which have demonstrated promising results in animal studies, (Shenoy, 2016).
4. **Impaired mitochondrial function**: Enzymes are critical for maintaining mitochondrial activity in neurons. When enzyme dysfunction occurs, it creates deficiencies in mitochondrial activity that lead to compromised ATP synthesis and increased levels of oxidative stress. Elevated oxidative stress contributes to dementia's onset by exacerbating neuronal damage and death. Therefore, therapies that focus on preserving mitochondrial function and reducing oxidative stress may help slow down the progression of dementia. Researchers are currently investigating several strategies, including antioxidants, dietary interventions, and drug therapies, to improve mitochondrial function and reduce oxidative stress, (Sies & Jones, 2020).

Neurodegenerative diseases are believed to arise from enzyme pathways that lead to the accumulation of metabolic waste products, compromised mitochondrial activity, increased oxidative stress, and reduced neurotransmitter function. To develop effective therapeutics for these diseases, a better understanding of enzyme function in these disorders is essential. Targeting specific enzymes has shown promise in the treatment of neurodegenerative disorders. In these diseases, the progressive loss of function and neuronal death in particular brain regions leads to a decline in motor and cognitive abilities. It is considered a hallmark of the disorders. Researchers are continuously studying different enzyme targets in the hopes of identifying novel therapeutic

approaches to slow down disease progression, improve quality of life, and provide better treatment options for patients with neurodegenerative illnesses, (Stansley & Yamamoto, 2015).

The neurodegenerative processes that arise in these disorders may be prevented or postponed with the aid of enzyme targeting.

REGULATORY LANDSCAPE IN DRUG DEVELOPMENT

Globally, neurodegenerative illnesses, including Parkinson's, Alzheimer's, and Huntington's, pose a serious threat to public health. The progressive loss of function and neuronal death in particular brain regions, which results in a deterioration in motor and cognitive function, are the hallmarks of these disorders. Enzyme pathways have emerged as exciting targets because of their crucial role in neurodegenerative processes, even though many different therapeutic targets have been suggested to treat these disorders, (Li et al., 2021; Stem Cells for Huntington's Disease (SC4HD), 2021). Regulators face several obstacles in the development and approval of medications that target the enzyme pathways involved in neurodegenerative disorders. The intricacy of the enzyme pathways implicated in these illnesses is one difficulty. The development of medicines that successfully target these pathways is hampered by the malfunctioning of many enzymes and their interactions. Furthermore, several enzymes are engaged in both sick and healthy activities, which may result in unexpected adverse effects from medications that target these enzymes. The absence of reliable biomarkers for neurodegenerative illnesses is another difficulty. Since they offer an objective gauge of the course of a disease and the effectiveness of a treatment, biomarkers are crucial instruments in the drug development process. However, most neurodegenerative illnesses currently lack validated biomarkers, making it difficult to prove the safety and effectiveness of medications that target specific enzyme pathways. This editorial provides a brief summary of the past, present, and future of neurodegenerative disorders in study and treatment, (Stoker & Barker, 2020).

Neurodegenerative diseases share multiple pathologies and pathways, including the loss of neurons in specific regions like the cortical and hippocampal regions in Alzheimer's disease, the striatal regions in Parkinson's disease, the medium spiny neurons in cortical and striatal areas of Huntington's disease, and the motor neurons in the spinal cord and motor cortex in ALS. The standard molecular theme of neurodegenerative diseases involves various mechanisms like protein misfolding, aggregation, and inclusion body formation (such as Amyloid plaque, fibrillary tangles, Lewy bodies, and polyglutamine aggregates), as well as oxidative stress, neuroinflammation, and mitochondrial dysfunction, (Stone & Darlington, 2013). Regulatory issues are further compounded by the lengthy development schedules and high costs associated with developing medicines for neurodegenerative illnesses, (Li et al., 2021).

Together, dementias are responsible for the most significant societal and economic burden of all diseases in developed countries; in the U.K., 850,000 people have dementia, at an annual cost of more than £26 billion. By 2040, this is expected to have doubled. The "Dementia Moonshot" and the 2021 Life Sciences Vision identify the scope and urgency of the issue as a national government priority. Notwithstanding this dedication to enhancing our comprehension and management of neurodegenerative disorders of the brain, public funding for this kind of research is scarce, and neurodegenerative illnesses continue to pose a significant obstacle to medical progress. The business sector has spent billions of pounds on clinical trials of potential dementia treatments over the

past 20 years, yet it is still challenging to show clinically meaningful disease change. One recent medication, Lecanemab, has shown some benefits. Although the FDA approved Aducanumab, it was rejected by the European Medicines Agency, (Strafella et al., 2018).

Despite these challenges, several drugs that target the enzyme pathways linked to neurodegenerative diseases have been discovered and approved. For instance, Parkinson's illness is treated with drugs that target the enzyme L-DOPA decarboxylase, and Alzheimer's disease is treated with drugs that target the enzyme acetylcholinesterase. However, the financial and time resources required to produce these drugs highlight the significance of having a comprehensive regulatory framework in place that will facilitate the development and approval of drugs that target the enzyme pathways implicated in neurodegenerative diseases, (Sweeney et al., 2017; Szatmári et al., 2024).

Regulatory Measures in the Field of Neurodegenerative Research

1. **Multi-disease Area Workshop**: The U.S. Food and Drug Administration (FDA) and the Critical Path Institute (C-Path) arranged the Neuroscience Annual Workshop in October 2022. Participants in this session included representatives from patient communities, academic institutions, government agencies, and regulatory authorities, in addition to the drug development sector, (Tahami Monfared et al., 2022). The five chronic progressive disorders that were especially covered at the workshop were Huntington's disease, Duchenne muscular dystrophy, Alzheimer's disease, Parkinson's disease, and hereditary ataxias, (Tahami Monfared et al., 2022). The workshop's discussions focused on developing tools and treatments for neurological illnesses in the future. The aim was to find common lessons and offer suggestions that would spur the development of new treatments and medication development tools, (Li et al., 2021). Difficulties in Neurological Drug Development: Approval of drugs for neurological illnesses presents particular challenges. These difficulties include the requirement for patient-focused objectives, the inconsistent nature of disease trajectories, and the absence of trustworthy biomarkers to monitor the beginning and progression of the disease. The prevalence of neurological disorders around the world has raised awareness of the need for novel therapeutic techniques and drug development instruments, (Teleanu et al., 2022).
    1. **FDA Human Gene Therapy Guidance:** The FDA offers suggestions to sponsors creating human gene therapy (G.T.) products for patients with neurodegenerative disorders, both adults and children, (Virolainen et al., 2023).
    2. **Rare Neurodegenerative Diseases Action Plan:** A plan of action to tackle the obstacles in the development of drugs for uncommon neurodegenerative disorders, such as ALS, has been made public by the FDA. The proposal calls for new policy measures, program improvements, and regulatory science activities, (Li et al., 2021).
    3. **Terminology and Product Labels:** For the treatment of neurodegenerative illnesses, regulatory guidelines and product labels for disease-modifying medications approved by the FDA and the EMA have been evaluated. This analysis promotes uniform language use and transparent discussion of therapy modalities, (Wang et al., 2020).
    4. **Progress and Cooperation:** Notwithstanding the difficulties, efforts to develop drugs for neurodegenerative illnesses are making headway. To spur innovation and enhance patient outcomes, stakeholders, including researchers, businesses, patients, and regula-

tory agencies, must work together, (Wareham et al., 2022). The regulatory environment is changing, placing a strong emphasis on patient-focused medication research and providing hope for successful therapies in fields that have traditionally lacked adequate options, (Wu et al., 2023).

Regulatory Guidelines Landscape in Drug Development for Neurodegenerative Diseases

1. While regional regulations differ, they all adhere to the same basic principles to guarantee that drug development programs satisfy ethical and scientific criteria, (Wu et al., 2024).
2. The FDA offers guidelines, such as early interaction with the agency and particular research designs and endpoints, for drug development programs for neurodegenerative illnesses in the United States, (Szatmári et al., 2024).
3. The EMA offers similar guidelines in Europe, emphasizing the significance of dependable outcome measures, proof of the drug's impact on the disease's pathophysiology, and comprehensive safety and efficacy testing.
4. The PMDA offers standards that highlight ethical and scientific rigour in clinical studies that assess medication efficacy and disease progression in Japan. These regulatory criteria encompass several general principles, such as meticulous planning and execution of clinical studies, appropriate biomarker and outcome protocols, as well as thorough testing for effectiveness and safety, (Yiannopoulou & Papageorgiou, 2013).
5. Before a drug is licensed for human use, businesses are required to submit extensive data on its safety and efficacy and report adverse events.
6. Given that neurodegenerative disorders have a substantial influence on both the afflicted individuals and society at large, regulatory bodies are crucial in ensuring that medications for these conditions are safe, effective, and of the highest caliber, (Li et al., 2021). Regulatory milestones achieved in public-private partnerships for nervous system disorders are presented in the table number 1.

Table 1. Regulatory milestones achieved in public-private partnerships for nervous system disorders

Alzheimer's disease: regulatory successes			
2011	**EMA**	**Qualification**	**Qualification opinion of low hippocampal volume (atrophy) by MRI for use in clinical trials for regulatory purpose—in pre-dementia stage of Alzheimer's disease**
2013	FDA	Fit for purpose	Disease model of mild to moderate AD
2013	EMA	Qualification	Disease model of mild to moderate AD
2015	FDA	FDA Biomarker Survey	Recommendation of Alzheimer's biomarkers Neurogranin and Tau PET (*collaboration with Kaj Blennow, Mike Weiner on behalf of CAMD*) in response to: "Biomarker Survey—Identifying Potential Biomarkers for Qualification and Describing Contexts of Use to Address Areas Important to Drug Development"
2015	FDA	Letter of support	Cerebral spinal fluid (CSF) analytes Aβ1-42, t-tau, and p-tau as exploratory prognostic biomarkers for enrichment in AD trials
2015	FDA	Letter of support	Low baseline hippocampal volume as an exploratory prognostic biomarker for enrichment in AD trials

continued on following page

Table 1. Continued

Alzheimer's disease: regulatory successes			
2011	**EMA**	**Qualification**	**Qualification opinion of low hippocampal volume (atrophy) by MRI for use in clinical trials for regulatory purpose—in pre-dementia stage of Alzheimer's disease**
2018	EMA	Letter of support	Model-based clinical trial enrichment tool for clinical trials in amnestic mild cognitive impairment
Parkinson's disease: regulatory successes			
2015	FDA	Letter of support	Exploratory prognostic biomarkers for enrichment in early-stage Parkinson's disease clinical trials; molecular neuroimaging biomarker: dopamine trransporter
2016	EMA	Letter of support	Molecular imaging of the dopamine transporter biomarker as an enrichment biomarker for clinical trials for early Parkinson's disease
2018	EMA	Qualification opinion	Molecular neuroimaging of the dopamine transporter as biomarker to identify patients with early manifest Parkinsonism in Parkinson's disease
2019	FDA	Critical path innovation meeting	Digital drug development tools for early Parkinson's disease clinical trials
2019	EMA	Innovative task force	Digital drug development tools for early Parkinson's disease clinical trials
2022	EMA	Letter of support	Model-based clinical trial simulation platform to optimize design of efficacy evaluation studies in Parkinson's disease

(adapted from Tahami Monfared et al. (2022) under CCBY 4.0)

Role Regulatory Agencies Play in the Safety and Efficacy of Drugs Developed for Neurodegenerative Diseases

The quality of life and pain caused by these diseases can be greatly enhanced in the elderly; thus, it is imperative that any medication developed is safe and does not worsen patients' conditions. To guarantee that all data generated by clinical trials withstand scientific scrutiny and that ethical factors have been taken into account, regulatory bodies place strict requirements on scientific rigour and ethical considerations while developing medications for certain disorders, (Yiannopoulou & Papageorgiou, 2013). Regulatory bodies also ensure that medications created to treat neurodegenerative illnesses effectively prevent or delay the advancement of the illness. It is imperative to ensure that patients receive optimal treatment and that medications are appropriately vetted to yield significant benefits, (Yiannopoulou & Papageorgiou, 2020). Additionally, regulatory bodies assist in ensuring adherence to established safety standards and guidelines, and they are crucial in guaranteeing that pharmaceutical research for neurodegenerative illnesses proceeds in a way that is both morally and scientifically sound. One of the most significant issues for public health now is neurodegenerative illnesses. Regulatory bodies play a crucial role in making sure that medications created to treat these illnesses are thoroughly tested and adhere to strict safety and effectiveness requirements. When approving a medicine for broad use, they carefully review safety and efficacy data. Regulatory bodies examine every facet of medication creation to ensure that it provides patients with clear and significant benefits. In the end, regulatory bodies are essential to guarantee that patients get the greatest care available, (Yiannopoulou & Papageorgiou, 2020)

Navigation of the Regulatory Processes for Enzyme-Targeted Therapy for Drug Developers.

Regulatory bodies have strict guidelines for approval, and the procedure can be expensive and time-consuming. Here are a few things to keep in mind when negotiating enzyme-targeted treatment regulatory procedures, (Younus, 2018). First and foremost, regulatory bodies need thorough evidence to bolster the therapy's efficacy and safety. Since enzyme-targeted treatments frequently have intricate mechanisms of action, their creators must provide proof of their efficacy as well as the target enzymes' specificity and bioactivity. Clinical trials have strict guidelines for patient selection, randomization, and the use of placebo controls. As a result, the procedure can be drawn out and quite demanding. It may be expensive and time-consuming to comply with these regulations, (Yuan et al., 2021).

Second, developing medicines that target specific enzymes presents difficulties. To produce these medicines, living organisms must be used, and specific manufacturing procedures that consider product stability and contamination risk must be followed. Production issues may impact the finished drug's consistency and quality, which may impact regulatory approval, (Younus, 2018). Thirdly, developers must adhere to strict quality standards set by regulatory bodies, which presents difficulties for enzyme-targeted treatments. Regulatory bodies are required to guarantee that the product is of superior quality, that the manufacturing process is suitable, and that the product is replicable. Additionally, enzyme-targeted medicines need to be stable and have a long shelf life. Finally, because enzyme-targeted medicines are distinctive, regulatory bodies must first approve them based on specific knowledge and skills. acceptance. Regulatory bodies guarantee that the treatment complies with strict requirements and that pharmaceutical companies have closely collaborated with industry and academic partners to offer guidance on the creation of scientific concepts that form the foundation of targeted therapies for enzymes. Navigating the regulatory procedures for enzyme-targeted therapy can be difficult. Pharmaceutical companies are subject to stringent regulatory requirements that include, among other things, detailed clinical trial designs, sophisticated manufacturing procedures, precise quality standards, and specialist knowledge and experience. Drug developers can effectively navigate the regulatory process and aid in the research and development of medicines that can significantly improve the lives of patients with diseases targeted by enzymes by preparing ahead of time and utilizing their specific knowledge and skills.

Challenges Faced by Manufacturers During Producing Enzyme-Targeted Therapies

1. **Manufacturing challenges:** To produce enzyme-targeted medicines, living organisms like yeast, bacteria, or mammalian cells must be used. Because these medicines are complicated, specialized manufacturing procedures need to be devised to produce them. During the manufacturing process, contamination is a significant worry that might impact the drug's final quality.
2. **Problems with quality control:** Strict guidelines must be followed in the production of enzyme-targeted medicines. To meet regulatory criteria, the finished product's purity, stability, and reproducibility must be guaranteed. It can be difficult to guarantee uniform quality in each batch, especially when manufacturing large-scale batches of these medicines, and quality control problems can occur, (Li et al., 2021).

3. **Stability:** Because enzyme-targeted medicines are complicated, they may be unstable and have a limited shelf life. Stability is a major difficulty during manufacture, and storage conditions need to be carefully managed.
4. **Cost:** Because enzyme-targeted therapies require specific manufacturing techniques, their production costs may be costly. Some patients may find the healthcare system less cheap as a result of these costs being passed on to them.
5. **Regulatory approval:** Drug authorities must assess enzyme-targeted treatment goods before approving them. To meet regulatory bodies' quality and safety requirements, producers must provide a substantial amount of data, which might take a long time throughout the approval process.

Regulatory Challenges

Regulatory challenges in the development and approval of drugs targeting enzyme pathways in neurodegenerative diseases present a multifaceted landscape influenced by scientific, ethical, and bureaucratic factors. Neurodegenerative diseases, including Alzheimer's, Parkinson's, and Huntington's diseases, among others, are characterized by the progressive degeneration of neurons, often involving complex biochemical pathways, including those governed by enzymes. Here, we'll explore some of the key regulatory challenges faced in this arena:

1. **Complexity of Enzyme Pathways**: Enzyme pathways involved in neurodegenerative diseases are intricate and interconnected. Targeting a single enzyme within such pathways may have unforeseen consequences on other cellular processes. Regulatory agencies, such as the FDA (Food and Drug Administration) in the United States or the EMA (European Medicines Agency) in Europe, require a comprehensive understanding of these pathways and the potential off-target effects of drug candidates.
2. **Biomarker Validation**: Developing reliable biomarkers for neurodegenerative diseases is crucial for assessing drug efficacy and patient stratification. However, identifying and validating biomarkers that accurately reflect disease progression and response to treatment remains a challenge. Regulatory bodies demand robust evidence of biomarker validity and reliability before considering them for drug development and approval.
3. **Clinical Trial Design**: Designing clinical trials for drugs targeting enzyme pathways in neurodegenerative diseases requires careful consideration of numerous factors, including patient selection, outcome measures, and trial duration. Regulatory agencies often require extensive clinical data demonstrating both safety and efficacy, which can be particularly challenging in diseases with long latency periods and heterogeneous symptomatology.
4. **Disease Modification vs. Symptomatic Relief**: Distinguishing between disease-modifying therapies and those providing symptomatic relief is crucial for regulatory approval. While symptomatic treatments may alleviate patient suffering, disease-modifying therapies aim to halt or reverse the underlying pathology. Demonstrating disease modification requires long-term clinical studies and may encounter regulatory scepticism due to the inherent uncertainties in predicting long-term outcomes.
5. **Ethical Considerations**: Neurodegenerative diseases often affect vulnerable populations, such as the elderly or those with cognitive impairments. Ensuring patient autonomy, informed consent, and protection from undue influence or coercion presents ethical challenges

throughout the drug development and approval process. Regulatory agencies scrutinize study protocols to safeguard patient welfare and uphold moral standards.

6. **Regulatory Harmonization**: Discrepancies in regulatory requirements between different jurisdictions can impede the global development and approval of drugs targeting enzyme pathways in neurodegenerative diseases. Achieving regulatory harmonization through initiatives such as the International Council for Harmonisation (ICH) facilitates smoother drug development and accelerates access to innovative treatments worldwide.

CONCLUSION

The complex regulatory hurdles involved in creating pharmaceutical treatments for neurodegenerative diseases underscore the importance of gaining a thorough comprehension of enzyme pathways. By tackling these intricacies, those involved can set the stage for groundbreaking and reliable therapeutic options. Joint endeavours and technological progress will be crucial in surmounting regulatory obstacles and driving forward the creation of impactful treatments for neurodegenerative disorders.

AUTHORS CONTRUBUTION

Vaishnavi Gohri Writing original draft; Data curation, Data curation: Deepak Bharati: Software; Formal analysis, Drawn Figure, Popat Mohite: Conceptualization, Writing – review & editing.

ACKNOWLEDGEMENT

The resources required to effectively conduct this work were provided by AETs St. John Institute of Pharmacy and Research, Manor Road Palghar (E), Maharashtra-401 404, India, for which the authors are grateful.

REFERENCES

Agarwal, P. K. (2019). A biophysical perspective on enzyme catalysis. *Biochemistry*, *58*(6), 438–449. DOI: 10.1021/acs.biochem.8b01004

Ajitkumar, A., & De Jesus, O. (2024). Huntington disease. In *StatPearls*. StatPearls Publishing. https://www.ncbi.nlm.nih.gov/books/NBK559198/

Amjad, S., Nisar, S., Bhat, A. A., Shah, A. R., Frenneaux, M. P., Fakhro, K., Haris, M., Reddy, R., Patay, Z., Baur, J., & Bagga, P. (2021). Role of NAD+ in regulating cellular and metabolic signaling pathways. *Molecular Metabolism*, *49*. *Molecular Metabolism, 101195*, 101195. Advance online publication. DOI: 10.1016/j.molmet.2021.101195 PMID: 33609766

Arnau, J., Yaver, D., & Hjort, C. M. (2020). Strategies and challenges for the development of industrial enzymes using fungal cell factories. In Nevalainen, H. (Ed.), *Grand challenges in fungal biotechnology** (pp. 179–210). Springer International Publishing., DOI: 10.1007/978-3-030-29541-7_7

Bakker, E., Hendrikse, N. M., Ehmann, F., Van der Meer, D. S., Llinares Garcia, J., Vetter, T., & others. (2022). Biomarker qualification at the European Medicines Agency: A review of biomarker qualification procedures from 2008 to 2020. *Clinical Pharmacology & Therapeutics*, *112*(1), 69–80. DOI: 10.1002/cpt.2556

Bali, T., & Miller, T. M. (2013). Management of amyotrophic lateral sclerosis. *Missouri Medicine*, *110*(5), 417–421.

Bhaduri, S., & Kipgen, T. (2018). 'New drugs' approvals in India: An institutional perspective. *Science, Technology and Society*, *23*(3), 444–462. https://doi.org/DOI: 10.1177/0971721818762878

Bhave, A., & Menon, S. (2017). Regulatory environment for clinical research: Recent past and expected future. *Perspectives in Clinical Research*, *8*(1), 11–16. DOI: 10.4103/2229-3485.198551

Bloem, B. R., Okun, M. S., & Klein, C. (2021). Parkinson's disease. *The Lancet*, *397*(10291), 2284–2303. DOI: 10.1016/S0140-6736(21)00218-X

Bortolato, M., Chen, K., & Shih, J. C. (2008). Monoamine oxidase inactivation: From pathophysiology to therapeutics. *Advanced Drug Delivery Reviews*, *60*(13–14), 1527–1533. DOI: 10.1016/j.addr.2008.06.002

Breijyeh, Z., & Karaman, R. (2020). Comprehensive review on Alzheimer's disease: Causes and treatment. *Molecules*, *25*(24), Article 5789. DOI: 10.3390/molecules25245789

Cavalli, A., Bolognesi, M. L., Minarini, A., Rosini, M., Tumiatti, V., Recanatini, M., & others. (2008). Multi-target-directed ligands to combat neurodegenerative diseases. *Journal of Medicinal Chemistry*, *51*(3), 347–372. DOI: 10.1021/jm7009364

Chaturvedi, S., Singh, A. K., Keshari, A. K., Maity, S., Sarkar, S., & Saha, S. (2016). Human metabolic enzymes deficiency: A genetic mutation based approach. *Scientifica*, *2016*. *Scientifica, 9828672*, 1–14. Advance online publication. DOI: 10.1155/2016/9828672 PMID: 27051561

Chen, S., Sayana, P., Zhang, X., & Le, W. (2013). Genetics of amyotrophic lateral sclerosis: An update. *Molecular Neurodegeneration*, *8*. *Molecular Neurodegeneration, 28*(1), 28. Advance online publication. DOI: 10.1186/1750-1326-8-28 PMID: 23941283

Chen, Y., Xu, J., & Chen, Y. (2021). Regulation of neurotransmitters by the gut microbiota and effects on cognition in neurological disorders. *Nutrients*, *13*(6), Article 2099. DOI: 10.3390/nu13062099

Cheng, C. J., Tietjen, G. T., Saucier-Sawyer, J. K., & Saltzman, W. M. (2015). A holistic approach to targeting disease with polymeric nanoparticles. *Nature Reviews Drug Discovery*, *14*(4), 239–247. DOI: 10.1038/nrd4503

Colović, M. B., Krstić, D. Z., Lazarević-Pašti, T. D., Bondžić, A. M., & Vasić, V. M. (2013). Acetylcholinesterase inhibitors: Pharmacology and toxicology. *Current Neuropharmacology*, *11*(3), 315–335. DOI: 10.2174/1570159X11311030006

Davenport, F., Gallacher, J., Kourtzi, Z., Koychev, I., Matthews, P. M., Oxtoby, N. P., & others. (2023). Neurodegenerative disease of the brain: A survey of interdisciplinary approaches. *Journal of the Royal Society Interface*, *20*(198), Article 20220406. DOI: 10.1098/rsif.2022.0406

de la Fuente, M., Lombardero, L., Gómez-González, A., Solari, C., Angulo-Barturen, I., Acera, A., & others. (2021). Enzyme therapy: Current challenges and future perspectives. *International Journal of Molecular Sciences*, *22*(17), Article 9181. DOI: 10.3390/ijms22179181

Dicks, L. M. T. (2022). Gut bacteria and neurotransmitters. *Microorganisms*, *10*(9), Article 1838. DOI: 10.3390/microorganisms10091838

Dorsey, E. R., Elbaz, A., Nichols, E., Abbasi, N., Abd-Allah, F., Abdelalim, A., & others. (2018). Global, regional, and national burden of Parkinson's disease, 1990–2016: A systematic analysis for the Global Burden of Disease Study 2016. *The Lancet Neurology*, *17*(11), 939–953. DOI: 10.1016/S1474-4422(18)30295-3

Falkowska, A., Gutowska, I., Goschorska, M., Nowacki, P., Chlubek, D., & Baranowska-Bosiacka, I. (2015). Energy metabolism of the brain, including the cooperation between astrocytes and neurons, especially in the context of glycogen metabolism. *International Journal of Molecular Sciences*, *16*(11), 25959–25981. DOI: 10.3390/ijms161125939

Frąk, W., Wojtasińska, A., Lisińska, W., Młynarska, E., Franczyk, B., & Rysz, J. (2022). Pathophysiology of cardiovascular diseases: New insights into molecular mechanisms of atherosclerosis, arterial hypertension, and coronary artery disease. *Biomedicines*, *10*(8), Article 1938. DOI: 10.3390/biomedicines10081938

Frampton, J. E. (2020). Inebilizumab: First approval. *Drugs*, *80*(12), 1259–1264. https://doi.org/DOI: 10.1007/s40265-020-01370-7

Franco, P., Jain, R., Rosenkrands-Lange, E., Hey, C., & Koban, M. U. (2023). Regulatory pathways supporting expedited drug development and approval in ICH member countries. *Therapeutic Innovation & Regulatory Science*, *57*(3), 484–514. https://doi.org/DOI: 10.1007/s43441-022-00493-5

Gribkoff, V. K., & Kaczmarek, L. K. (2017). The need for new approaches in CNS drug discovery: Why drugs have failed, and what can be done to improve outcomes. *Neuropharmacology*, *120*, 11–19. DOI: 10.1016/j.neuropharm.2016.03.021

Halioua-Haubold, C. L., Peyer, J. G., Smith, J. A., Arshad, Z., Scholz, M., Brindley, D. A., & others. (2017). Regulatory considerations for gene therapy products in the US, EU, and Japan. *Yale Journal of Biology and Medicine*, *90*(4), 683–693.

Hennigan, J. N., & Lynch, M. D. (2022). The past, present, and future of enzyme-based therapies. *Drug Discovery Today*, *27*(1), 117–133. DOI: 10.1016/j.drudis.2021.09.003

Holdgate, G. A., Meek, T. D., & Grimley, R. L. (2018). Mechanistic enzymology in drug discovery: A fresh perspective. *Nature Reviews Drug Discovery*, *17*(2), 115–132. DOI: 10.1038/nrd.2017.219

Huang, J., Xu, Q., Liu, Z., Jain, N., Tyagi, M., Wei, D.-Q., & others. (2021). Controlling the substrate specificity of an enzyme through structural flexibility by varying the salt-bridge density. *Molecules*, *26*(18), Article 5693. DOI: 10.3390/molecules26185693

Hur, J. Y. (2022). γ-Secretase in Alzheimer's disease. *Experimental & Molecular Medicine*, *54*(4), 433–446. DOI: 10.1038/s12276-022-00754-8

Jankovic, J. (2008). Parkinson's disease: Clinical features and diagnosis. *Journal of Neurology, Neurosurgery & Psychiatry*, *79*(4), 368–376. DOI: 10.1136/jnnp.2007.131045

Jimenez-Sanchez, M., Licitra, F., Underwood, B. R., & Rubinsztein, D. C. (2017). Huntington's disease: Mechanisms of pathogenesis and therapeutic strategies. *Cold Spring Harbor Perspectives in Medicine*, *7*(7), Article a024240. DOI: 10.1101/cshperspect.a024240

Kaur, J., Fahmy, L. M., Davoodi-Bojd, E., Zhang, L., Ding, G., Hu, J., Zhang, Z., Chopp, M., & Jiang, Q. (2021). Waste clearance in the brain. *Frontiers in Neuroanatomy*, *15*. *Frontiers in Neuroanatomy, 665803*, 665803. Advance online publication. DOI: 10.3389/fnana.2021.665803 PMID: 34305538

Khan, M. A., Zubair, H., Anand, S., Srivastava, S. K., Singh, S., & Singh, A. P. (2020). Dysregulation of metabolic enzymes in tumor and stromal cells: Role in oncogenesis and therapeutic opportunities. *Cancer Letters*, *473*, 176–185. DOI: 10.1016/j.canlet.2019.12.003

Khan, T., Waseem, R., Zehra, Z., Aiman, A., Bhardwaj, P., Ansari, J., & others. (2022). Mitochondrial dysfunction: Pathophysiology and mitochondria-targeted drug delivery approaches. *Pharmaceutics*, *14*(12), Article 2657. DOI: 10.3390/pharmaceutics14122657

Kiaei, M. (2013). New hopes and challenges for treatment of neurodegenerative disorders: Great opportunities for young neuroscientists. *Basic and Clinical Neuroscience*, *4*(1), 3–4.

Kim, S.-K. (2023). Enzymes as targets for drug development II. *International Journal of Molecular Sciences*, *24*(4), Article 4130. DOI: 10.3390/ijms24044130

Kouli, A., Torsney, K. M., & Kuan, W.-L. (2018). Parkinson's disease: Etiology, neuropathology, and pathogenesis. In *Parkinson's disease: Pathogenesis and clinical aspects* (pp. 3–26). Exon Publications., DOI: 10.15586/codonpublications.parkinsonsdisease.2018.ch1

Koumadorakis, D. E., Krokidis, M. G., & Dimitrakopoulos, G. N. (2023). A consensus gene regulatory network for neurodegenerative diseases using single-cell RNA-seq data. *Advances in Experimental Medicine and Biology*, *1423*, 215–224. DOI: 10.1007/978-3-031-31978-5_18

Kumar, A., Sidhu, J., Goyal, A., & Tsao, J. W. (2024). Alzheimer disease. In *StatPearls*. StatPearls Publishing. https://www.ncbi.nlm.nih.gov/books/NBK499922/

Lamptey, R. N. L., Chaulagain, B., Trivedi, R., Gothwal, A., Layek, B., & Singh, J. (2022). A review of the common neurodegenerative disorders: Current therapeutic approaches and the potential role of nanotherapeutics. *International Journal of Molecular Sciences*, *23*(3), Article 1851. DOI: 10.3390/ijms23031851

Li, Z., Zhang, Z., Ren, Y., Wang, Y., Fang, J., Yue, H., & others. (2021). Aging and age-related diseases: From mechanisms to therapeutic strategies. *Biogerontology*, *22*(2), 165–187. https://doi.org/DOI: 10.1007/s10522-021-09917-z

Martin, S., Al Khleifat, A., & Al-Chalabi, A. (2017). What causes amyotrophic lateral sclerosis? *F1000Research*, *6*, Article 371. DOI: 10.12688/f1000research.10476.1

McKeith, I. G., Boeve, B. F., Dickson, D. W., Halliday, G., Taylor, J.-P., Weintraub, D., & others. (2017). Diagnosis and management of dementia with Lewy bodies: Fourth consensus report of the DLB Consortium. *Neurology*, *89*(1), 88–100. DOI: 10.1212/WNL.0000000000004058

Mead, R. J., Shan, N., Reiser, H. J., Marshall, F., & Shaw, P. J. (2023). Amyotrophic lateral sclerosis: A neurodegenerative disorder poised for successful therapeutic translation. *Nature Reviews Drug Discovery*, *22*(3), 185–212. DOI: 10.1038/s41573-022-00612-2

Mejzini, R., Flynn, L. L., Pitout, I. L., Fletcher, S., Wilton, S. D., & Akkari, P. A. (2019). ALS genetics, mechanisms, and therapeutics: Where are we now? *Frontiers in Neuroscience*, *13*. *Frontiers in Neuroscience, 1310*, 1310. Advance online publication. DOI: 10.3389/fnins.2019.01310 PMID: 31866818

Mentz, R. J., Hernandez, A. F., Berdan, L. G., Rorick, T., O'Brien, E. C., Ibarra, J. C., & others. (2016). Good clinical practice guidance and pragmatic clinical trials: Balancing the best of both worlds. *Circulation*, *133*(9), 872–880. DOI: 10.1161/CIRCULATIONAHA.115.019902

Miners, J. S., Baig, S., Tayler, H., Kehoe, P. G., & Love, S. (2009). Neprilysin and insulin-degrading enzyme levels are increased in Alzheimer disease in relation to disease severity. *Journal of Neuropathology & Experimental Neurology*, *68*(8), 902–914. DOI: 10.1097/NEN.0b013e3181afe475

Morant, A. V., Jagalski, V., & Vestergaard, H. T. (2019). Labeling of disease-modifying therapies for neurodegenerative disorders. *Frontiers in Medicine*, *6*. *Frontiers in Medicine, 223*, 223. Advance online publication. DOI: 10.3389/fmed.2019.00223 PMID: 31681780

Palanisamy, C. P., Pei, J., Alugoju, P., Anthikapalli, N. V. A., Jayaraman, S., Veeraraghavan, V. P., & others. (2023). New strategies of neurodegenerative disease treatment with extracellular vesicles (EVs) derived from mesenchymal stem cells (MSCs). *Theranostics*, *13*(12), 4138–4165. https://doi.org/DOI: 10.7150/thno.82629

Pathak, N., Vimal, S. K., Tandon, I., Agrawal, L., Hongyi, C., & Bhattacharyya, S. (2022). Neurodegenerative disorders of Alzheimer, Parkinsonism, amyotrophic lateral sclerosis and multiple sclerosis: An early diagnostic approach for precision treatment. *Metabolic Brain Disease*, *37*(1), 67–104. https://doi.org/DOI: 10.1007/s11011-021-00840-8

Pereira, J. B., Kumar, A., Hall, S., Palmqvist, S., Stomrud, E., Bali, D., & others. (2023). DOPA decarboxylase is an emerging biomarker for Parkinsonian disorders including preclinical Lewy body disease. *Nature Aging*, *3*(10), 1201–1209. DOI: 10.1038/s43587-023-00478-y

Phuna, Z. X., Panda, B. P., Shivashekaregowda, N. K. H., & Madhavan, P. (2022). Recent development in nanocrystal based drug delivery for neurodegenerative diseases: Scope, challenges, current and future prospects. *Journal of Drug Delivery Science and Technology*, *68*. *Journal of Drug Delivery Science and Technology, 102921*, 102921. Advance online publication. DOI: 10.1016/j.jddst.2021.102921

Rao, R. V., & Bredesen, D. E. (2004). Misfolded proteins, endoplasmic reticulum stress and neurodegeneration. *Current Opinion in Cell Biology*, *16*(6), 653–662. DOI: 10.1016/j.ceb.2004.09.012

Reeve, A., Simcox, E., & Turnbull, D. (2014). Ageing and Parkinson's disease: Why is advancing age the biggest risk factor? *Ageing Research Reviews*, *14*, 19–30. DOI: 10.1016/j.arr.2014.01.004

Reiner, A., Dragatsis, I., & Dietrich, P. (2011). Genetics and neuropathology of Huntington's disease. *International Review of Neurobiology*, *98*, 325–372. DOI: 10.1016/B978-0-12-381328-2.00014-6

Robinson, P. K. (2015). Enzymes: Principles and biotechnological applications. *Essays in Biochemistry*, *59*, 1–41. DOI: 10.1042/bse0590001

. Schneider, L. S., Mangialasche, F., Andreasen, N., Feldman, H., Giacobini, E., Jones, R., & others. (2014). Clinical trials and late-stage drug development for Alzheimer's disease: An appraisal from 1984 to 2014. *Journal of Internal Medicine*, *275*(3), 251–283. DOI: 10.1111/joim.12191

Shenoy, P. (2016). Multi-regional clinical trials and global drug development. *Perspectives in Clinical Research*, *7*(2), 62–67. DOI: 10.4103/2229-3485.179430

Sies, H., & Jones, D. P. (2020). Reactive oxygen species (ROS) as pleiotropic physiological signalling agents. *Nature Reviews Molecular Cell Biology*, *21*(7), 363–383. DOI: 10.1038/s41580-020-0230-3

Stansley, B. J., & Yamamoto, B. K. (2015). L-Dopa and brain serotonin system dysfunction. *Toxics*, *3*(1), 75–88. DOI: 10.3390/toxics3010075

Stem Cells for Huntington's Disease (SC4HD). (2021). An international consortium to facilitate stem cell-based therapy for Huntington's disease. *Journal of Huntington's Disease*, *10*(2), 221–226. DOI: 10.3233/JHD-210474

Stoker, T. B., & Barker, R. A. (2020). Recent developments in the treatment of Parkinson's disease. *F1000Research*, *9*, Article 620. DOI: 10.12688/f1000research.25634.1

Stone, T. W., & Darlington, L. G. (2013). The kynurenine pathway as a therapeutic target in cognitive and neurodegenerative disorders. *British Journal of Pharmacology*, *169*(6), 1211–1227. DOI: 10.1111/bph.12182

Strafella, C., Caputo, V., Galota, M. R., Zampatti, S., Marella, G., Mauriello, S., Cascella, R., & Giardina, E. (2018). Application of precision medicine in neurodegenerative diseases. *Frontiers in Neurology*, *9*. *Frontiers in Neurology*, *701*, 701. Advance online publication. DOI: 10.3389/fneur.2018.00701 PMID: 30190701

Sweeney, P., Park, H., Baumann, M., Dunlop, J., Frydman, J., Kopito, R., McCampbell, A., Leblanc, G., Venkateswaran, A., Nurmi, A., & Hodgson, R. (2017). Protein misfolding in neurodegenerative diseases: Implications and strategies. *Translational Neurodegeneration*, *6*. *Translational Neurodegeneration*, *6*(1), 6. Advance online publication. DOI: 10.1186/s40035-017-0077-5 PMID: 28293421

Szatmári, S., Szász, J. A., Orbán-Kis, K., Bataga, S., Ciorba, M., Nagy, E., & others. (2024). Starting with 24-h levodopa carbidopa intestinal gel at initiation in a large cohort of advanced Parkinson's disease patients. *Scientific Reports*, *14*(1), Article 3676. https://doi.org/DOI: 10.1038/s41598-024-54123-4

Tahami Monfared, A. A., Tafazzoli, A., Ye, W., Chavan, A., & Zhang, Q. (2022). Long-term health outcomes of lecanemab in patients with early Alzheimer's disease using simulation modeling. *Neurology and Therapy*, *11*(2), 863–880. DOI: 10.1007/s40120-022-00350-y

Teleanu, R. I., Niculescu, A.-G., Roza, E., Vladâcenco, O., Grumezescu, A. M., & Teleanu, D. M. (2022). Neurotransmitters—Key factors in neurological and neurodegenerative disorders of the central nervous system. *International Journal of Molecular Sciences*, *23*(11), Article 5954. DOI: 10.3390/ijms23115954

Virolainen, S. J., VonHandorf, A., Viel, K., Weirauch, M. T., & Kottyan, L. C. (2023). Gene–environment interactions and their impact on human health. *Genes & Immunity*, *24*(1), 1–11. DOI: 10.1038/s41435-022-00192-6

Wang, J., Hu, W. W., Jiang, Z., & Feng, M. J. (2020). Advances in treatment of neurodegenerative diseases: Perspectives for combination of stem cells with neurotrophic factors. *World Journal of Stem Cells*, *12*(5), 323–338. DOI: 10.4252/wjsc.v12.i5.323

Wareham, L. K., Liddelow, S. A., Temple, S., Benowitz, L. I., Di Polo, A., Wellington, C., & others. (2022). Solving neurodegeneration: Common mechanisms and strategies for new treatments. *Molecular Neurodegeneration*, *17*(1), Article 23. DOI: 10.1186/s13024-022-00524-0

Wu, X., Xu, M., Geng, M., Chen, S., Little, P. J., Xu, S., & others. (2023). Targeting protein modifications in metabolic diseases: Molecular mechanisms and targeted therapies. *Signal Transduction and Targeted Therapy*, *8*(1), Article 220. DOI: 10.1038/s41392-023-01439-y

Wu, Y. C., Bogale, T. A., Koistinaho, J., Pizzi, M., Rolova, T., & Bellucci, A. (2024). The contribution of β-amyloid, tau and α-synuclein to blood–brain barrier damage in neurodegenerative disorders. *Acta Neuropathologica*, *147*(1), Article 39. https://doi.org/DOI: 10.1007/s00401-023-02667-8

Yiannopoulou, K. G., & Papageorgiou, S. G. (2013). Current and future treatments for Alzheimer's disease. *Therapeutic Advances in Neurological Disorders*, *6*(1), 19–33. DOI: 10.1177/1756285612461679

Yiannopoulou, K. G., & Papageorgiou, S. G. (2020). Current and future treatments in Alzheimer disease: An update. *Journal of Central Nervous System Disease*, *12*. *Journal of Central Nervous System Disease, 1179573520907397.* Advance online publication. DOI: 10.1177/1179573520907397 PMID: 32165850

Younus, H. (2018). Therapeutic potentials of superoxide dismutase. *International Journal of Health Sciences*, *12*(3), 88–93.

Yuan, M. M., Peng, X., Zeng, T. Y., Wu, M. L., Chen, Y., Zhang, K., & others. (2021). The illness experience for people with amyotrophic lateral sclerosis: A qualitative study. *Journal of Clinical Nursing*, *30*(9–10), 1455–1463. DOI: 10.1111/jocn.15694

Chapter 13
Exploring the Role of Phytomedicines in Neurodegenerative Disorders

V. Keerthi
Vels Institute of Science, Technology, and Advanced Studies, India

P. Jayashree
https://orcid.org/0009-0008-6957-9256
Vels Institute of Science, Technology, and Advanced Studies, India

S. S. Meenambiga
https://orcid.org/0000-0002-5445-525X
Vels Institute of Science, Technology, and Advanced Studies, India

P. Prakash
Sathyabama Institute of Science and Technology, India

P. Vivek
Vels Institute of Science, Technology, and Advanced Studies, India

S. Ivo Romauld
https://orcid.org/0000-0003-0610-0646
Vels Institute of Science, Technology, and Advanced Studies, India

ABSTRACT

In today's world, neurological disorders, which encompass a variety of neurodegenerative, neuropsychiatric, and neurodevelopmental issues, are the leading causes of disability and mortality. One of the main causes of genesis of several brain disorders and the neuronal damage is oxidative stress, which is generated by an excess of reactive oxygen species (ROS). The aim of this study is to present an unbiased assessment of the evidence in favor of using phytomedicines to treat brain disorders. There is a captivating case for multidisciplinary teamwork among neuroscientists, pharmacologists, clinicians, and practitioners of traditional medicine, especially growing interest in plant medicine to improve the potential of phytomedicines in neurology. Phytomedicines offer a potential new frontier in the treatment of brain disorders with their multifaceted therapeutic approach based on natural sources.

DOI: 10.4018/979-8-3373-4627-4.ch013

INTRODUCTION

Neurodegenerative diseases (NDs) is one of the largest healthcare issues globally which impact millions and put a huge economic and social burden on the healthcare system. Such diseases, such as multiple sclerosis (MS), Parkinson's disease (PD), amyotrophic lateral sclerosis (ALS), Huntington's disease (HD), and Alzheimer's disease (AD), are all defined by progressive neuronal degeneration and the resulting cognitive and motor impairments, (Kakoti et al., 2022). Prevalence of these diseases is growing at an alarming pace as the world population is aging rapidly. As per the World Health Organization (WHO), more than 55 million individuals suffered from dementia in 2022, and by the year 2050, that number is projected to double (Misrani A et al., 2021). Between 60 and 70 percent of the cases of dementia are due to Alzheimer's disease alone. Equally, about 10 million people across the globe live with Parkinson's disease, whose rate of incidence has more than doubled over the last 25 years. Such dramatic figures highlight the need for the development of sound preventative and therapeutic interventions, (Kumar et al., 2025).

Phytochemicals, also referred to as phytonutrients, are a structurally diverse group of secondary metabolites that plants synthesize using complex biochemical pathways. These compounds possess significant bioactive properties, including antioxidant, anti-inflammatory, antibacterial, anticancer, and neuroprotective actions, but they are not essential for human survival like vital micronutrients. Extensive structural and functional diversity is exhibited by their diversity, encompassing polyphenols, flavonoids, carotenoids, alkaloids, terpenoids, glucosinolates, and saponins, (Hossain et al., 2025).

One of the most ubiquitous and studied groups is polyphenols, consisting of lignans, flavonoids, phenolic acids, and stilbenes. The C6-C3-C6 flavonoid structural motif containing flavanols (quercetin, kaempferol), flavones, isoflavones, and anthocyanins is particularly significant since it impacts antioxidant activity and interfaces with cellular signalling pathways, (Chagas et al., 2022). Anthocyanins are rich in berries, purple cabbage, and maize, which have also been noted to exhibit cardioprotective and anti-inflammatory actions beyond their role in visual pigmentation, (Kumar et al., 2023).

Carotenoids like lutein, lycopene, and β-carotene are isoprenoid pigments with a function in regulation of oxidative stress and photoprotection. They have preventive action against cardiovascular and chronic eye diseases and are vitamin A precursors. Compounds like artemisinin, menthol, and saponins are examples of terpenes and terpenoids that are structurally biosynthesized from five-carbon units of isoprene and have antimalarial, antibacterial, and lipid-lowering activity (Thakur M et al., 2020).

Alkaloids are nitrogen-containing compounds mostly found in medicinal plants with well-established pharmacological properties in both conventional and alternative medicine. Examples of these include morphine, caffeine, and berberine, (Aggarwal et al., 2025). Glucosinolates, which are found in plants of the Brassicaceae family, break down into physiologically active isothiocyanates, which are strong chemo preventive agents that activate detoxifying enzymes and modify epigenetics, (Connolly et al., 2021). In this review paper, we are going to discuss about pathophysiology, etiologic and role of herbs in the neurogenerative disorder.

PATHOPHYSIOLOGY OF NEURODEGENERATIVE DISORDERS

The central nervous system promptly responds to injury and infection as a component of a robust immune system. In pathological circumstances, macrophages and other peripheral immune cells have the ability to penetrate the blood–brain barrier (BBB). The discovery and clarification of a robust network for interaction between the immune system and the central nervous system is one of the most significant recent advancements in medicine. The somatodendritic and axonal compartments are two functionally and physically separate regions in neurones, which make them highly polarised cells. Axons and dendrites are typically formed by a single long neurone. Neural circuits are highly specialised and very dependent on spatiotemporally controlled cargo movement for correct operation because to the high degree of morphological and functional polarisation. Transport of cargo along axons is facilitated by a process called axonal transport (AT), which relies on microtubules (MT). Motor proteins, adaptors, cargos, and MTs make up the AT machinery. MTs, intermediate filaments, and actin filaments make up the cytoskeleton, which is where AT takes place. Motor proteins, such as kinesin and dynein, transport cargo along longitudinally aligned MTs that run down the axon. The adaptors help bind and localise the payloads to the motor proteins by acting as linkers. Maintaining the structural and biochemical heterogeneity that characterises axonal subdomains is mediated by AT, which also controls the delivery of organelles bound by membranes from the cell body to synaptic compartments, removes and degrades old materials, and mediates the turnover of non-synaptic membranes and metabolic and cytoskeletal elements. Therefore, AT can be considered a key cellular activity that underlies the establishment and upkeep of neural architecture and connection across neurones' lifetimes. The somato-dendritic and axonal compartments are two functionally and physically separate regions in neurones, which make them highly polarised cells. Axons and dendrites are typically formed by a single long neurone. Neural circuits are highly specialised and very dependent on spatiotemporally controlled cargo movement for correct operation because to the high degree of morphological and functional polarisation. Transport of cargo along axons is facilitated by a process called axonal transport (AT), which relies on microtubules (MT). Motor proteins, adaptors, cargos, and MTs make up the AT machinery. MTs, intermediate filaments, and actin filaments make up the cytoskeleton, which is where AT takes place. Motor proteins, such as kinesin and dynein, transport cargo along longitudinally aligned MTs that run down the axon. The adaptors help bind and localise the payloads to the motor proteins by acting as linkers. Maintaining the structural and biochemical heterogeneity that characterises axonal subdomains is mediated by AT, which also controls the delivery of organelles bound by membranes from the cell body to synaptic compartments, removes and degrades old materials, and mediates the turnover of non-synaptic membranes and metabolic and cytoskeletal elements. Therefore, AT can be considered a key cellular activity that underlies the establishment and upkeep of neural architecture and connection across neurones' lifetimes. Reactive oxygen species can be beneficial in preventing the development of infections; however, they can also exacerbate neurological ailments. An overabundance of reactive oxygen species can result from mitochondrial failure, which can damage neurones and release cytosolic components that activate astrocytes and microglia in the vicinity. Reactive oxygen species, reactive nitrogen species, and other pro-inflammatory cytokines will be released by these microglia and astrocytes in the vicinity. The inflammatory response is facilitated, and neuronal injury is exacerbated by the secretion of these cytokines.

Consequently, chronic glial cell activation establishes a vicious cycle that exacerbates and prolongs long-term neurodegenerative processes (Rekatsina M et al., 2020).

ETIOLOGY AND PATHOGENESIS OF ALZHIEMER'S DISEASE

Neurons in AD patients become disabled. The neuron's capacity to generate the energy (via metabolism) necessary for effective coordination between them is inhibited in the early stages of AD. Additionally, they become unable of self-healing, which eventually results in the death of neuron cells. It is still unclear exactly what disrupts the neuron's normal function, but three pathological characteristics are being proposed as possible targets in light of recent advancements in medical research (Figure 1)

Figure 1. Alzheimer's progression

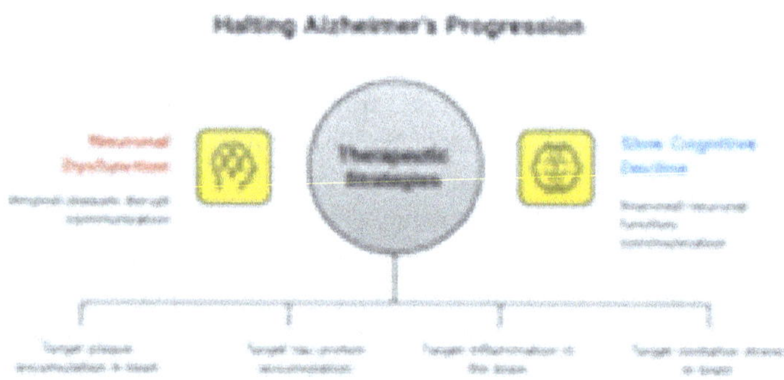

B-AMYLOID PLAQUES

A protein known as β-amyloid (Aβ) forms thick, sticky deposits of plaques that are tucked into the gaps between neurons. Other protein fragments, neurogenesis, and immune cells—specifically, microglia—encircle these plaques as well. These cells then break down the injured neurons and induce neuro-inflammation. Aβ is a 39–43 amino acid peptide that aggregates spontaneously. It is a fragment of a bigger protein known as the amyloid precursor protein (APP). APP is crucial for the production of neurones, which are present both within and outside of cells. The sequential proteolytic cleavage of APP by β- and γ-secretases results in the production of Aβ, (Lacham-Hartman et al., 2025). The membrane-anchored aspartic protease β-secretase (β-site of APP cleaving enzyme; BACE) generates a soluble N-terminal fragment and a C-terminal fragment that is affixed to the membrane during the initial cleavage. Subsequently, γ-secretase cuts the C-terminal region to generate Aβ peptides, which subsequently adhere to form plaques that are incapable of being degraded (Zhang et al., 2025). In accordance with the "β-amyloid cascade,"

the accumulation of Aβ plaques initiates a chain reaction that is detrimental to neurones leading to in neuroinflammation, which in turn leads to neurodegeneration.

NEUROFIBRILLARY TANGLES

Neurofibrillary tangles (NFTs) are a significant neuropathological characteristic of Alzheimer's disease (AD). The absence of cytoskeletal microtubules and tubulin-associated proteins has been identified in neurones that carry NFTs. Neurofibrillary lesions are most likely formed by signal transduction pathways involving protein phosphorylation and de-phosphorylation, even if the precise molecular mechanisms connecting cytoskeletal element loss to NFT development are still unknown. One example is the aberrant phosphorylation (hyperphosphorylation) of the microtubule-associated protein tau (Mapt), the main component of NFTs, in the brains of Alzheimer's disease (AD) patients when compared to non-demented persons. The process of amyotrophic lateral neuropathy (AD) involves epitope-specific hyperphosphorylation, which is thought to be the foundation for tau's mislocalization from axonal to somatodendritic neurones. According to Alonso et al. (2008), this change is believed to play a role in tau polymerisation and aggregation in addition to deregulating microtubule dynamics.

LOSS OF CHOLINERGIC NEURONS

When we learn, the cholinergic system is involved. Memory is another area where ACh has been linked in published studies. Additional research has shown that endogenous acetylcholine has a significant role in modulating learning and memory processes including acquisition, encoding, consolidation, reconsolidation, extinction, and retrieval. The memory loss seen in Alzheimer's disease (AD) patients is partly caused by the particular degeneration of these neurones, which highlights the role of the cholinergic neurones from the nucleus basalis of Meynert on memory. Another factor that can control ACh release in the forebrain is stress, which can alter biological and emotional outcomes through its effects on the hypothalamic-pituitary-adrenal (HPA) system. The activation of the HPA axis in response to a stressor agent is reduced in rats treated with the nicotinic receptor antagonist mecamylamine, according to research that assessed the role of the cholinergic system in mediating the stress response. In a similar vein, nicotine can activate nicotinic receptors to simulate ACh's actions on the HPA axis.

The cholinergic system also plays a crucial role in controlling when we sleep. Research has shown that stimulating certain areas of the brainstem with cholinergic neurones can enhance rapid eye movement (REM) sleep in a dose-dependent manner. The sensory cortex also employs ACh for a variety of modulatory tasks. By easing communication between the thalamus and the brain, ACh aids in auditory synaptic transmission. The visual cortex also relies on ACh for organisation and neuronal responsiveness. There is mounting evidence that ACh has a role in adult neurogenesis, (Bhattacharjee et al., 2020).

PHYTOMEDICINES IN ALZHEIMER'S DISEASE (AD)

For centuries, Traditional Chinese medicine (TCM) and Traditional Indian medicine (Ayurveda) have employed methods that involve the use of medicinal and other alternatives to drugs, (Sharma et al., 2019). Unusual treatment processes that have been passed down through the centuries and refined by extended use and experiences are still being implemented, based on a vast amount of data regarding the beneficial properties of a variety of plants, chemical substances, and innovative treatments. (Figure 2) It has also been shown that certain common household spices, such as ginger, cinnamon, rosemary, sage, garlic, and curcuma, can help prevent AD, (Gregory et al., 2021).

Figure 2. Exploring phytomedicines for parkinson disease

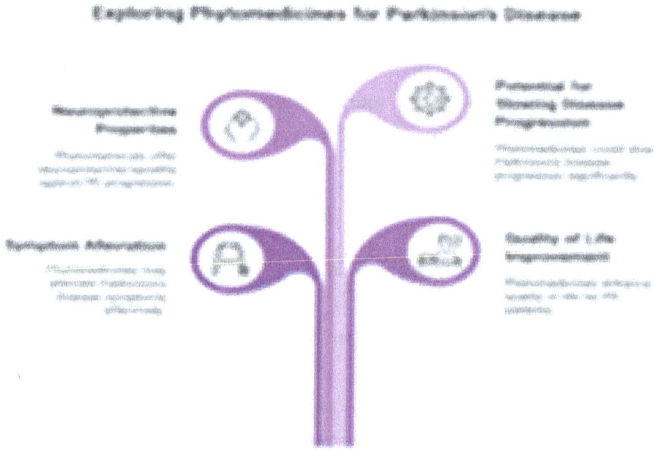

AYURVEDIC APPROACHES FOR THE TREATMENT OF AD

By observing the neuroprotective qualities of several extracts, the most recent scientific study has validated the effectiveness of Ayurvedic medicines in preventing AD. Asiatic pennywort (*Centella asiatica (L.)*) is one such herb, which can lower blood pressure, purify blood, and improve memory. In Ayurveda, its hydrophilic extracts are often employed to treat insomnia and stimulate the regeneration and healing of nerve cells, (Singh et al., 2021). Asiatic acid and asiaticoside are the two metabolites of Asiatic pennywort, are strong antioxidants, (Kushwah et al., 2023). Asiatic pennywort can effectively inhibit Aβ in mouse brains, as per as in vitro study. By preventing free radical formation, protecting against DNA damage, and inhibiting lipid peroxidation, it was also an antioxidant. Jatamansi root preparations in alcohol have been demonstrated by Lyle et al. to enhance learning and maintenance abilities and mitigate chronic fatigue syndrome effects in rats. Another herb, guggul (*Commiphora*), contains phenols, ferulic acid, and nonphenolic aromatic acids, among other very potent antioxidants that can be employed to treat AD. Neuroprotective

effects of guggul and Jatamansi and brain oxidative stress reduction are similar to those of Asiatic pennywort. Cat's claw (*Uncaria tomentosa*), a tropical vine, is recommended for the prevention and treatment of AD and pre-AD due to its immunomodulating and anti-inflammatory properties. Its ability to prevent aggregation and degradation of previously existing tau protein tangles and Aβ fibrils was indicated by the in vitro tests, (Snow et al., 2019). Curcuma longa, a most popular herb in this group, reduces Aβ levels and inflammation within cells, (Sivaraman et al., 2019). It regulates the cellular signal pathway and prevents formation of Aβ aggregates, (Sahiner et al., 2023). Three curcuminoids-curcumin, desmethoxycurcumin, and bisdemethoxycurcumin-fended normal human endothelial cells of the umbilical vein (HUVEC) and rat pheochromocytoma PC12 off Aβ attack. Many bioactive compounds under various headings are found in its extracts. There were twenty different phytochemicals identified in Brahmi ethanol extracts in total (Pramanik R et al., 2024). Ashwagandha (*Withania somnifera*) or winter cherry or Indian ginseng is one of the most prominent herbs with proven effectiveness for AD, (Menghani et al., 2021). Its alkaloids regulate ACh levels and reduce Aβ aggregation, which improves cognitive function. In vivo and in vitro experiments have indicated that ginseng possesses anti-inflammatory properties that involve reducing COX-2 enzyme levels, the key mediator in the inflammation process, and inhibiting inflammatory mediators like TNF-α, NF-κB, IL-1β, and IL6, (Ahn et al., 2017). Ethanol extracts from the roots as well as aerial parts of *Clitoria ternatea* plant (CT), commonly known as Shankpushpi, were evaluated by Taranalli and Cheeramkuzhy. When rats with amnesia produced by electroshock received a lower dose (300 mg/kg) of the extract, they demonstrated that memory function improved and the level of ACh in the brain increased. Both the root extract dosages (300 and 500 mg/kg) showed similar, but modestly greater, effects. Rosemary, or *Rosmarinus ofiicinalis*, has been found to be beneficial in AD-related disorders because it possesses cyclooxygenase-2 (COX-2) inhibitors such as apigenin and eugenol, which are likely to exert anti-inflammatory actions. The root extract of *Oroxylum indicum* has many principal constituents in which baicalein exert a range of effects on significant pathway associated with AD including reduced tau protein hyperphosphorylation, inhibition of Aβ generation, reduction of oxidative stress, and regulation of AChE activity, (Baranowska-Wójcik et al., 2025).

TRADITIONAL CHINESE MEDICINES APPROACH FOR THE TREATMENT OF AD

Many active compounds used in TCM may make treating AD patients easier, (Zhang et al., 2015). Clinical testing has shown their value in the early prevention of the illness as well as in helping afflicted individuals' brain activity and cognitive abilities, (Zhang et al., 2019). For example, it has been demonstrated that extracts from *Coptis chinensis* Franch (Huang Lian), (Chen et al., 2020), *Polygonum multiflorum* Thunb. (He Shou Wu), (Ning et al., 2021), and *Polygala tenuifolia* Willd. (Yuan Zhi) reduce cognitive deficiencies and help heal pathological damage in AD, (Park et al., 2019). The traditional oriental herbal compound Soshiho-tang (SST), or Xiaochaihu-tangin in Chinese and Sho-saiko-to in Japanese, was found by Sohn et al., 2021 to inhibit AChE activation and Aβ aggregation in vivo in a mouse model of AD. As per Jin et al. (2019), Baicalin (BAI), a natural flavonoid isolated from *Scutelaria baicalensis* Georgi (Huang Qin), may suppress neuro-inflammatory reactions induced by microglia in AD mice brain via inhibiting TLR4/NF-κB signal pathway and inflammasome NLRP3 activation. Sesame oil (SO),

which is rich in *Sesamum indicum* L. (Zhi Ma), was shown by Mohamed EA et al., 2021 to significantly improve learning capacity and reduce memory loss in rats administered AlCl3 (100 mg/kg) alone or combined with SO. Furthermore, it was shown that injection of AlCl3 caused histopathological changes, reduction in cerebral oxidative stress, and elevation in interleukin-1 beta (IL-1β) and tumour necrosis factor-alpha (TNF α). Cuya Tet al., 2018 report that 1-(3,4 dihydroxy-5-methoxyphenyl)-7-(4-hydroxy-3-ethoxyphenyl) heptane-3,5-diyl diacetate and (E)-1,7-bis (4-hydroxy-3-methoxyphenyl) hept-4-en-3-on, which are compounds present in ginger root extract, could potentially inhibit AChE in humans. By stimulating the glucagon-like peptide-1 receptor (GLP-1R), geniposide, an iridoid compound present in gardenia fruit (*Gardenia jasminoides* ElLis), protects against the neurotoxicity induced by Aβ, (Liu et al., 2015).

PHYTOMEDICINES IN PARKINSON'S DISEASE (PD)

Parkinson's disease (PD) is the second most common neurologic disorder in the world which is a neurologic disorder that primarily affects motor function, (Khan et al., 2019). It is characterized by stiffness, tremors, and difficulty with balancing and coordinating. The disease is caused by the loss of brain cells that produce dopamine, which disrupts nerve cell-to-nerve transmission, (Rewar, 2015). Use of Traditional Chinese Medicine (TCM) as an adjunct or alternative therapy has been researched. Although Western medicine has primarily utilized drugs such as levodopa, TCM depends on the overall body functioning to cure PD symptoms by restoring harmony in the functioning of the body and equilibrium of Qi (energy).

ANTIOXIDANT PROPERTIES OF PHYTOMEDICINES USED IN TCM IN THE TREATMENT OF PD

TCM has been used as the alternative medicine because it possesses neuroprotective effects. It has been proved that neuroprotective compounds obtained from TCM, including β-asaron, chrysin, cannabidiol, and toonasinoids, are highly efficient in curing Parkinson's disease. These TCM have also exhibited anti-inflammatory, anti-oxidative, anti-tumour, analgesic, and antiseptic effects along with neuroprotective advantages. From a recent study, it was found that reduction in reactive oxygen species enhanced dopaminergic neuron regeneration and reduced α-synuclein toxicity, two of the prime indicators of Parkinson's disease, (Muhammad et al., 2022). The treatment methods currently used for neurological disorders are inefficient because they primarily benefit a small number of patients and merely reduce the symptoms to some extent without halting the disease process. Levodopa, selegiline, and carbidopa are among the medications approved by the US Food and Drug Administration to treat Parkinson's disease (PD). These medications successfully lessen PD symptoms and slow the illness's progression. However, because to safety concerns, they are not advised for prolonged use. For example, even though Levodopa administration caused the frequent onset of motor issues, it improved the relief of motor symptoms in the majority of PD patients. Numerous studies have demonstrated that TCM treatment is linked to mRNA-level post-transcriptional changes, (Bhushan et al., 2024). In the context of Parkinson's disease, these changes may be advantageous or extremely dangerous.

THERAPEUTICAL HERBS IN THE TREATMENT OF PD

Alpinia

The plant *Alpiniae oxyphyllae Fructus* (AOF) named as YizhiRen in Chinese, is the completely developed and dehydrated seed of the *Alpinia oxyphylla Miq*. plant. According to Zhang et al. (2018), it is commonly used in medicine to treat symptoms such as diarrhoea, vomiting, abdominal pain, and excessive salivation, and to improve the function of the kidneys, stomach, and spleen. Research on zebrafish models of Parkinson's disease has shown that an ethanol extract of AOF might mitigate the impairment of psychomotor performance and potentially halt the degeneration of dopaminergic neurones caused by 6-hydroxydopamine (6-OHDA).This is achieved by reducing inflammation (by downregulating the expression of interleukin-1 beta and tumour necrosis factor-alpha) and oxidative stress (by preventing the synthesis of nitrous oxide). Alpiniae oxyphyllae possess anti-inflammatory and antioxidant activities which are necessary in the prevention of the neuroinflammation and oxidative stress associated with the progression of Parkinson's disease. Additionally, extracts of Alpiniae oxyphyllae have been proved that it has the property of inhibiting alpha-synuclein aggregation, which is a protein misfolding and aggregation, targetting pathophysiology of Parkinson's disease. In addition, Alphaniae oxyphyllae extracts have been observed to modify neurotransmitter systems like serotonin, glutamate, and dopamine, which become dysregulated in Parkinson's disease. Through enhanced dopaminergic transmission and modulation of glutamatergic and serotonergic transmission, Alpiniae oxyphyllae can potentially treat the motor symptoms and alleviate depression and anxiety, significant non-motor symptoms of PD, (Zhang et al., 2019).

Astragalus

The dried root of *Astragalus membranaceus (Fisch.)* is referred to as *Astragali Radix*, or Huangqi in Chinese. In TCM, it is widely acknowledged and utilized as a therapeutic agent. At least three bioactive substances with neuroprotective properties have currently been identified in Astragali Radix: astragaloside IV, astraisoflavan, and astragalus polysaccharides. It is clear that oxidative stress, especially the existence of free radicals, plays a major role in the development of Parkinson's disease (PD), even though the precise mechanism of neuron loss in these individuals is still unknown. According to recent research (Yin et al., 2021), astragalus polysaccharides may be an effective method for reducing oxidative stress in dopaminergic neurones. Astragali Radix exhibits potential as a treatment for Parkinson's disease (Cui et al., 2023). It has the potential to function as an antioxidant, reduce inflammation, and defend neurones that produce dopamine. Its immunomodulatory properties and capacity to modulate neurotransmitter systems may alleviate Parkinson's disease symptoms.

Baicalein and Baicalin

Natural chemical baicalein affects levels of microRNAs (miRNAs) (18), which are potential new regulators of cell metabolism, proliferation, and death. Significantly, a multitude of microRNAs play a role in the identification, development, and management of PD. One example is the crucial function that hsa-miR-30b-5p plays in neurodegenerative illnesses, including Parkinson's

disease. MiR-30b-5p is highly expressed in PD patients who have received treatment. But how miR-30b-5p contributes to mitochondrial autophagy in PD is still unclear. At the molecular level, SIRT1 activation triggers mitochondrial autophagy. Control of mitochondrial autophagy in neural stem cells is regulated by the Bhlhe40/SIRT1 axis. The induction of mitochondrial autophagy is facilitated by SIRT1 through the AMPK/mTOR pathway. Very less is known about baicalein's potential to protect against PD by modulating miR-30b-5p and mitochondrial autophagy via the SIRT1/AMPK/mTOR axis. apoptosis was halted and oxidative stress was reduced by inhibiting the p38 mitogen-activated protein kinase signalling pathway, (Ma et al., 2021).

Camellia

Camellia sinensis L. Kuntze plant leaf is in the Theaceae family, are used to make green and black tea. Camellia, which is often called "green tea" in Chinese, is a plant that has minerals, polyphenols, and it contains small amounts of vitamins, amino acids, and carbohydrate. In the past, Infusions of camellia were frequently used as sleep aids or purifying agents to alleviate anxiety, migraines, and stomach problems, (Malar et al., 2020). Neuroprotective, anti-inflammatory, and antioxidant characteristics are some of the other pharmacological effects. Green tea polyphenols have long been recognized for their neuroprotective properties against Parkinson's disease pathogenesis. By inhibiting the Jun N-terminal kinase/Myosin light chain kinase pathway, green tea can prevent the breakdown of nerve cells in the hippocampal region, (Xu et al., 2021). Camellia sinensis extract was shown to have antioxidant properties and to correct immunohistochemical alterations caused by 6-OHDA lesions in male Wistar rats. According to a study by Bitu Pinto, Natalia et al., Camellia sinensis has neuroprotective potential, and its catechins are a powerful component of its anti-inflammatory and antioxidant qualities.

Licorice

Glycyrrhiza glabra is a very useful medicinal plant that comes from the Fabaceae family (sometimes called Leguminosae). It is also used a lot for food for both people and animals. A randomised double-blind clinical study that looked at liquorice as an extra treatment for Parkinson's disease patients found that it helped their symptoms a lot and didn't have any bad affects that could be seen. Glabridin is a naturally occurring flavonoid that is found in Glycyrrhiza glabra. Glabbridin can protect neurones from PD-like symptoms caused by 1-methyl-4-phenyl-1, 2, 3, 6-tetrahydropyridine (MPTP) by blocking the ERK signalling pathway and lowering inflammation, (Zhao et al., 2017).

Morusalba

Morus alba L. is a plant that is highly beneficial and is frequently used in traditional medicine and Ayurveda. Morus alba is low in fat, but it is rich in essential nutrients, such as carbohydrates, protein, vitamins, and minerals. Mulberry fruit extract has been discovered by researchers to protect neurones from damage by enhancing the performance of dopaminergic neurones. This could potentially help individuals with chronic illnesses recover and prevent the onset of Parkinson's disease. A study conducted by Rebai Olfa et al. (2017) demonstrated that an extract from Morus alba leaves significantly reduced oxidative stress and mitigated the adverse effects of glyphosate

on the brain. The leaf extract also appears to have the capacity to reduce H2O2 levels, maintain stable iron and Ca2+ levels, and enhance SOD activity. As a result, the in vivo results suggest that mulberry leaf extract may serve as a herbal treatment for glyphosate-induced toxicity. The neuroprotective properties of Morus alba leaf extract may be attributed to the synergistic or antagonistic interactions among the numerous active phenolic compounds (Table 1).

Table 1. Therapeutic herbs for Parkinson's disease

Herb (common / scientific)	Part / extract used	Major active compound(s)	Proposed mechanisms relevant to PD	Reference
Alpinia / *Alpiniae oxyphyllae* (YizhiRen)	Ethanol extract of seed (AOF)	(complex mixture; anti-inflammatory & antioxidant constituents)	↓Neuroinflammation (↓ IL-1β, ↓ TNF-α), ↓ oxidative stress (↓ NO), inhibition of α-synucleinaggregation, modulation of dopaminergic, glutamatergic and serotonergic transmission	Zhang Q et al., 2018; Zhang Z et al., 2019
Astragalus / *Astragalus membranaceus* (Huangqi)	Dried root (Astragali Radix); extracts / isolated constituents	Astragaloside IV, astraisoflavan, astragalus polysaccharides	Antioxidant (scavenges ROS), anti-inflammatory, immunomodulation; protection of dopaminergic neurons; neurotransmitter regulation	Yin R et al., 2021; Cui D et al., 2023
Baicalein & baicalin (from *Scutellaria baicalensis*)	Root extracts; purified baicalein / baicalin	Baicalein, baicalin (flavones)	Anti-inflammatory (↓ NLRP3, ↓ caspase-1), anti-apoptotic, mitochondrial protection (via CREB / GSK-3β), inhibition of p38 MAPK; reduces microglial activation and proinflammatory cytokines	Rui W et al., 2020; Zhang X et al., 2017; Ma J et al., 2021
Camellia / *Camellia sinensis* (green/ black tea)	Leaf infusion / polyphenol extracts (catechins)	Epigallocatechin gallate (EGCG) and other catechins	Antioxidant, anti-inflammatory, inhibition of JNK/MLCK pathway, neuroprotection against toxin-induced degeneration	Malar DS et al., 2020; Xu Y et al., 2021; Jurado-Coronel et al., 2016
Licorice / *Glycyrrhiza glabra*	Root extract; glabridin (flavonoid)	Glabridin and other flavonoids	Anti-inflammatory (↓ ERK signalling), neuroprotection against MPTP toxicity	Zhao Y et al., 2017
Mulberry / *Morus alba*	Leaf or fruit extract (phenolic-rich)	Various phenolic compounds (flavonoids, phenolic acids)	Antioxidant (↑ SOD), reduces H_2O_2, stabilizes Fe^{2+}/Ca^{2+}, mitigates oxidative stress	Rebai Olfa et al., 2017

DELIVERY SYSTEMS AND BIOAVAILABILITY CHALLENGES

Neurological disorders such as Alzheimer's disease (AD), Parkinson's disease (PD), epilepsy, and stroke remain among the leading causes of disability and mortality worldwide. Current pharmacotherapies are often symptomatic, limited by side effects, or ineffective in halting disease progression. In this context, phytomedicines—bioactive compounds derived from plants—have emerged as promising alternatives due to their multitargeted mechanisms, antioxidant properties, and relatively favorable safety profiles, (Howes et. al., 2011). However, their clinical application is hindered by poor bioavailability, instability, and limited penetration across the blood–brain barrier (BBB). Recent advances in enzymology and drug delivery systems are offering solutions to these challenges.

ENZYMOLOGY IN NEUROLOGICAL DISORDERS

In the central nervous system (CNS), enzymes control important biochemical processes that affect neurotransmitter metabolism, oxidative stress, and neuroinflammation. A lot of neurological diseases have been caused by problems with how enzymes work. Acetylcholinesterase (AChE), for instance, is increased in Alzheimer's disease, which speeds up the breakdown of acetylcholine and makes it harder to think coherently. Alkaloids found in plants, like galantamine and huperzine A, naturally block AChE, which makes cholinergic signalling better, (Ma et.al., 2007). In the same way, monoamine oxidase (MAO) enzymes change how dopamine, serotonin, and norepinephrine are used, and too much of them can lead to Parkinson's disease. Flavonoids, such as quercetin and resveratrol, have weak MAO-inhibitory actions that make monoaminergic transmission robust, (de la Torre R et al., 2006).

Enzymes that neutralise free radicals are regulated by phytochemicals. To mitigate oxidative stress, a critical factor in neuronal mortality, polyphenols boost the activity of antioxidant enzymes such as glutathione peroxidase, superoxide dismutase (SOD), and catalase, (Uttara et al., 2009). In addition, terpenoids and phenolics decrease neuroinflammation by inhibiting pro-inflammatory enzymes such cyclooxygenase (COX), lipoxygenase (LOX), and inducible nitric oxide synthase (iNOS), (Venkatesan et.al., 2017) (Table 2). The significance of enzymology in natural neurotherapeutics is shown by these interactions between enzymes and phytomedicine.

Table 2. Enzymology in neurological disorders

Neurological Condition	Enzyme(s) Involved	Role / Pathophysiology	Clinical/Therapeutic Insights	Reference
Parkinson's & Depression	Monoamine oxidase (MAO-A/MAO-B)	Degrades dopamine, serotonin, norepinephrine	MAO-B inhibitors (selegiline, rasagiline) are neuroprotective	Youdim & Bakhle, Br J Pharmacol, 2006
Gaucher's Disease & PD risk	Glucocerebrosidase (GBA)	Deficient lysosomal degradation of glucocerebroside	Mutations increase risk of Parkinson's	Sidransky et al., N Engl J Med, 2009
Alzheimer's & PD	Asparagine endopeptidase (AEP)	Cleaves tau, APP, α-synuclein under acidic stress	AEP inhibition proposed as therapy	Zhang et al., Nature, 2014
ALS (familial)	Superoxide dismutase 1 (SOD1)	Mutations → oxidative stress, motor neuron death	Basis for SOD1-targeted gene therapy	Rosen et al., Nature, 1993
Tay–Sachs / Sandhoff	Hexosaminidases A & B	Deficiency causes GM2 ganglioside accumulation	Enzyme deficiency defines GM2 gangliosidoses	Gravel et al., The Metabolic Basis of Inherited Disease, 2001
Niemann–Pick Disease	Acid sphingomyelinase	Deficiency → sphingomyelin accumulation	Causes neurodegeneration, hepatosplenomegaly	Schuchman & Desnick, J Inherit Metab Dis, 2017
Homocystinuria	Cystathionine β-synthase (CBS)	Converts homocysteine → cystathionine	Deficiency → homocysteine buildup; B6 responsive	Mudd et al., N Engl J Med, 1985
Mitochondrial Encephalopathies	Pyruvate dehydrogenase (PDH)	Converts pyruvate → acetyl-CoA	Deficiency causes lactic acidosis, neurodeficits	Patel & Korotchkina, J Biol Chem, 2006

continued on following page

Table 2. Continued

Neurological Condition	Enzyme(s) Involved	Role / Pathophysiology	Clinical/Therapeutic Insights	Reference
Maple Syrup Urine Disease	Branched-chain α-ketoacid dehydrogenase (BCKDH)	Deficient catabolism of BCAAs	Causes neurotoxicity; dietary control is therapy	Chuang et al., J Inherit Metab Dis, 2006
Epilepsy, AD, ALS	Glutamine synthetase (GS)	Converts glutamate + ammonia → glutamine	Dysfunction → excitotoxicity, seizures	Eid et al., Neurochem Int, 2013

BIOAVAILABILITY AND DELIVERY CHALLENGES

Despite promising neuroprotective effects, most phytochemicals face pharmacokinetic limitations. Their clinical translation is impeded by:

1. Blood–Brain Barrier (BBB): Lipophilic and high-molecular-weight compounds poorly cross the BBB, restricting CNS access, (Pardridge et al., 2005).
2. First-pass metabolism: Many phytochemicals undergo rapid hepatic and intestinal metabolism by cytochrome P450 enzymes and esterases, leading to low systemic concentrations (Manach C et.al., 2004).
3. Poor solubility and stability: Hydrophobic compounds such as curcumin and resveratrol degrade quickly in biological fluids, (Anand et al., 2007).
4. Efflux transporters: P-glycoprotein and other efflux pumps actively expel phytochemicals from endothelial cells of the BBB, (Löscher et al., 2005).

These limitations necessitate advanced delivery systems to optimize therapeutic efficacy.

Potentially crucial neurology treatments based on phytomedicine are being developed through the convergence of phytochemistry, enzymology, and nanotechnology. Research in the future should centre on biomimetic nanoparticles that can pass the blood-brain barrier (BBB) via receptor-mediated pathways, personalised medicine methods, and formulations that target many targets at once. By influencing key enzymatic pathways, phytomedicines offer a wealth of neurotherapeutic agents. Nevertheless, their limited clinical value is due to low absorption and BBB limitations.

CHALLENGES AND FUTURE DIRECTION

Numerous obstacles prevent phytomedicines from being used therapeutically in neurology. Due to their low solubility, poor gastrointestinal absorption, and quick metabolism, many phytochemicals, including curcumin, quercetin, and resveratrol, have low systemic concentrations, (Anand et al., 2007). This makes poor bioavailability the most important problem. Additionally, most phytochemicals cannot pass through the blood–brain barrier (BBB) into the central nervous

system, and efflux transporters such P-glycoprotein actively remove a lot of chemicals, which prevents buildup in the brain (Pardridge, 2005).

Enzymatic interactions are complicated, which presents another difficulty. Acetylcholinesterase, monoamine oxidase, cyclooxygenase, and inducible nitric oxide synthase are only a few of the enzymatic pathways involved in neurological diseases. Phytochemicals may affect these processes in a way that isn't specific, which makes us worry about effects that aren't meant to happen, (Venkatesan et al., 2017). Genetic polymorphisms that cause changes in enzyme activity between people make therapeutic consistency even more difficult, (Ingelman-Sundberg et al., 2001). Also, phytochemical composition changes because herbal extracts are not standardised, which makes them less accurate and predictable in clinical applications, (Ekor, 2014).

Regulatory Challenges

Complex compound mixes are frequently found in phytomedicines, making it challenging to identify the specific ingredients causing therapeutic effects as well as to evaluate possible interactions and adverse consequences. The standardisation and quality control required for regulatory approval may be hampered by this diversity.

Regulations for herbal remedies differ per nation, ranging from stricter restrictions for pharmaceutical drugs to categories for traditional treatments. For academics and businesses looking to develop and market phytomedicines for neurodegenerative illnesses, this lack of harmonisation adds uncertainty and complication. Due to variables including plant species, place of origin, and harvesting conditions, phytomedicines may exhibit variety in their chemical content. It is difficult to guarantee constant product efficacy and quality because of this unpredictability. Regulatory agencies have reservations because there is frequently a lack of long-term safety evidence on phytomedicines, especially when they are used together with other drugs.

REFERENCES

Aggarwal, A., Rajalekshmi, R., Aggarwal, A., & Agrawal, D. K. (2025). Plants, pills, and the brain: Exploring phytochemicals and neurological medicines. *International Journal of Plant, Animal and Environmental Sciences*, *15*, 90–114.

Ahn, S., Singh, P., Castro-Aceituno, V., Yesmin Simu, S., Kim, Y. J., Mathiyalagan, R., & Yang, D. C. (2017). Gold nanoparticles synthesized using *Panax ginseng* leaves suppress inflammatory-mediators production via blockade of NF-κB activation in macrophages. *Artificial Cells, Nanomedicine, and Biotechnology*, *45*(2), 270–276. DOI: 10.3109/21691401.2016.1146727

Anand, P., Kunnumakkara, A. B., Newman, R. A., & Aggarwal, B. B. (2007). Bioavailability of curcumin: Problems and promises. *Molecular Pharmaceutics*, *4*(6), 807–818. DOI: 10.1021/mp700113r

Baranowska-Wójcik, E., Gajowniczek-Ałasa, D., Pawlikowska-Pawlęga, B., & Szwajgier, D. (2025). The potential role of phytochemicals in Alzheimer's disease. *Nutrients*, *17*(4), Article 653. DOI: 10.3390/nu17040653

Bhattacharjee, A., Ramakrishna, A., & Obulesu, M. (Eds.). (2020). *Phytomedicine and Alzheimer's disease*. CRC Press., DOI: 10.1201/9780429318429

Bhushan, B., Singh, N. K., & Singh, R. (2024). Traditional Chinese medicine: Its growing potential in treating neurological disorders. *Pharmacological Research - Modern Chinese Medicine*, *11*. *Pharmacological Research. Modern Chinese Medicine*, *100422*, 100422. Advance online publication. DOI: 10.1016/j.prmcm.2024.100422

Chagas, M. D., Behrens, M. D., Moragas-Tellis, C. J., Penedo, G. X., Silva, A. R., & Gonçalves-de-Albuquerque, C. F. (2022). Flavonols and flavones as potential anti-inflammatory, antioxidant, and antibacterial compounds. *Oxidative Medicine and Cellular Longevity*, *2022*. *Oxidative Medicine and Cellular Longevity*, *9966750*(1), 9966750. Advance online publication. DOI: 10.1155/2022/9966750 PMID: 36111166

Chen, Y., Chen, Y., Liang, Y., Chen, H., Ji, X., & Huang, M. (2020). Berberine mitigates cognitive decline in an Alzheimer's disease mouse model by targeting both tau hyperphosphorylation and autophagic clearance. *Biomedicine & Pharmacotherapy*, *121*. *Biomedicine and Pharmacotherapy*, *109670*, 109670. Advance online publication. DOI: 10.1016/j.biopha.2019.109670 PMID: 31810131

Connolly, E. L., Sim, M., Travica, N., Marx, W., Beasy, G., Lynch, G. S., Bondonno, C. P., Lewis, J. R., Hodgson, J. M., & Blekkenhorst, L. C. (2021). Glucosinolates from cruciferous vegetables and their potential role in chronic disease: Investigating the preclinical and clinical evidence. *Frontiers in Pharmacology*, *12*. *Frontiers in Pharmacology*, *767975*, 767975. Advance online publication. DOI: 10.3389/fphar.2021.767975 PMID: 34764875

Cui, D., Chen, Y., Ye, B., Guo, W., Wang, D., & He, J. (2023). Natural products for the treatment of neurodegenerative diseases. *Phytomedicine*, *121*. *Phytomedicine*, *155101*, 155101. Advance online publication. DOI: 10.1016/j.phymed.2023.155101 PMID: 37778246

Cuya, T., Baptista, L., & Celmar Costa França, T. (2018). A molecular dynamics study of components of the ginger (*Zingiber officinale*) extract inside human acetylcholinesterase: Implications for Alzheimer disease. *Journal of Biomolecular Structure and Dynamics*, *36*(14), 3843–3855. DOI: 10.1080/07391102.2017.1401004

de la Torre, R., Alvira, D., Pagès, N., & others. (2006). Flavonoids and the brain: Modulation of monoamine oxidase (MAO) activity. *Current Topics in Medicinal Chemistry*, *6*(17), 1841–1851. DOI: 10.2174/156802606778249801

Ekor, M. (2014). The growing use of herbal medicines: Issues relating to adverse reactions and challenges in monitoring safety. *Frontiers in Pharmacology*, *4*. *Frontiers in Pharmacology, 177*. Advance online publication. DOI: 10.3389/fphar.2013.00177 PMID: 24454289

Gregory, J., Vengalasetti, Y. V., Bredesen, D. E., & Rao, R. V. (2021). Neuroprotective herbs for the management of Alzheimer's disease. *Biomolecules*, *11*(4), Article 543. DOI: 10.3390/biom11040543

Hossain, M. S., Wazed, M. A., Asha, S., Amin, M. R., & Shimul, I. M. (2025). Dietary phytochemicals in health and disease: Mechanisms, clinical evidence, and applications—A comprehensive review. *Food Science & Nutrition*, *13*(3), Article e70101. DOI: 10.1002/fsn3.70101

Howes, M. J., & Perry, E. (2011). The role of phytochemicals in the treatment and prevention of dementia. *Drugs & Aging*, *28*(6), 439–468. DOI: 10.2165/11591310-000000000-00000

Ingelman-Sundberg, M. (2001). Pharmacogenomics of cytochrome P450 and its applications in drug therapy. *The Pharmacogenomics Journal*, *1*(2), 47–64. DOI: 10.1038/sj.tpj.6500017

Jin, X., Liu, M. Y., Zhang, D. F., Zhong, X., Du, K., Qian, P., Yao, W. F., Gao, H., & Wei, M. J. (2019). Baicalin mitigates cognitive impairment and protects neurons from microglia-mediated neuroinflammation via suppressing NLRP3 inflammasomes and TLR4/NF-κB signaling pathway. *CNS Neuroscience & Therapeutics*, *25*(5), 575–590. DOI: 10.1111/cns.13086

Jurado-Coronel, J. C., Echeverria, V., Hidalgo, O. A., Gonzalez, J., Aliev, G., & Barreto, G. E. (2016). Implication of green tea as a possible therapeutic approach for Parkinson disease. *CNS & Neurological Disorders - Drug Targets*, *15*(3), 292–300. https://doi.org/DOI: 10.2174/1871527315666160201115350

Kakoti, B. B., Bezbaruah, R., & Ahmed, N. (2022). Therapeutic drug repositioning with special emphasis on neurodegenerative diseases: Threats and issues. *Frontiers in Pharmacology*, *13*. *Frontiers in Pharmacology, 1007315*, 1007315. Advance online publication. DOI: 10.3389/fphar.2022.1007315 PMID: 36263141

Khan, A. U., Akram, M., Daniyal, M., & Zainab, R. (2019). Awareness and current knowledge of Parkinson's disease: A neurodegenerative disorder. *International Journal of Neuroscience*, *129*(1), 55–93. https://doi.org/DOI: 10.1080/00207454.2018.1501452

Kumar, A., P, N., Kumar, M., Jose, A., Tomer, V., Oz, E., Proestos, C., Zeng, M., Elobeid, T., K, S., & Oz, F. (2023). Major phytochemicals: Recent advances in health benefits and extraction method. *Molecules*, *28*(2), Article 887. DOI: 10.3390/molecules28020887

Kumar, R., Pal, O. P., Kamboj, N., & Jaiswal, A. (2025). Phytonutrients in neuroprotection and neurodegenerative disorders. *Current Research in Nutrition and Food Science Journal*, *13*(Special Issue Phytonutrients June 2025).

Kushwah, S., Maurya, N. S., Kushwaha, S., Scotti, L., Chawade, A., & Mani, A. (2023). Herbal therapeutics for Alzheimer's disease: Ancient Indian medicine system from the modern viewpoint. *Current Neuropharmacology*, *21*(4), 764–776. https://doi.org/DOI: 10.2174/1570159X21666230315162353

Lacham-Hartman, S., Oren, O., Rabinovitch, M., & Papo, N. (2025). Neuroprotective functions of the APPI domain of amyloid precursor protein (APP): Reducing KLK6-mediated APP cleavage and Aβ42 formation and aggregation. *International Journal of Biological Macromolecules*, *278*. *International Journal of Biological Macromolecules, 146066*, 146066. Advance online publication. DOI: 10.1016/j.ijbiomac.2025.146066 PMID: 40680950

Li, S., Han, Q., Qiao, C., Song, J., Cheng, C. L., & Xu, H. (2008). Chemical markers for the quality control of herbal medicines: An overview. *Chinese Medicine*, *3*. *Chinese Medicine*, 7(1), 7. Advance online publication. DOI: 10.1186/1749-8546-3-7 PMID: 18588699

Liu, J., Yin, F., Guo, L., Zhang, J., & Zidichouski, J. (2015). Molecular mechanisms of geniposide and genipin against Alzheimer's disease. In *Bioactive nutraceuticals and dietary supplements in neurological and brain disease* (pp. 221–227). Academic Press. https://doi.org/DOI: 10.1016/B978-0-12-411462-3.00023-7

Löscher, W., & Potschka, H. (2005). Blood-brain barrier active efflux transporters: ATP-binding cassette gene family. *NeuroRx*, *2*(1), 86–98. DOI: 10.1602/neurorx.2.1.86

Ma, J., Wang, R., Chen, T., Jiang, S., & Xu, A. (2021). Protective effects of baicalin in a *Caenorhabditis elegans* model of Parkinson's disease. *Toxicology Research*, *10*(3), 409–417. DOI: 10.1093/toxres/tfab021

Ma, X., Tan, C., Zhu, D., Gang, D. R., & Xiao, P. (2007). Huperzine A from *Huperzia* species—An ethnopharmacological review. *Journal of Ethnopharmacology*, *113*(1), 15–34. DOI: 10.1016/j.jep.2007.05.030

Malar, D. S., Prasanth, M. I., Brimson, J. M., Sharika, R., Sivamaruthi, B. S., Chaiyasut, C., & Tencomnao, T. (2020). Neuroprotective properties of green tea (*Camellia sinensis*) in Parkinson's disease: A review. *Molecules*, *25*(17), Article 3926. DOI: 10.3390/molecules25173926

Manach, C., Scalbert, A., Morand, C., Rémésy, C., & Jiménez, L. (2004). Bioavailability of polyphenols and flavonoids in humans. *The American Journal of Clinical Nutrition*, *79*(5), 727–747. DOI: 10.1093/ajcn/79.5.727

Menghani, Y. R., Bhattad, D. M., Chandak, K. K., Taksande, J. R., & Umekar, M. J. (2021). Review: Pharmacological and herbal remedies in the management of neurodegenerative disorder (Alzheimer's). *International Journal of Pharmacognosy and Life Science*, *2*(1), 18–27. DOI: 10.33545/27072827.2021.v2.i1a.21

Misrani, A., Tabassum, S., & Yang, L. (2021). Mitochondrial dysfunction and oxidative stress in Alzheimer's disease. *Frontiers in Aging Neuroscience*, *13*. *Frontiers in Aging Neuroscience, 617588*, 617588. Advance online publication. DOI: 10.3389/fnagi.2021.617588 PMID: 33679375

Mohamed, E. A., Ahmed, H. I., Zaky, H. S., & Badr, A. M. (2021). Sesame oil mitigates memory impairment, oxidative stress, and neurodegeneration in a rat model of Alzheimer's disease: A pivotal role of NF-κB/p38MAPK/BDNF/PPAR-γ pathways. *Journal of Ethnopharmacology*, *267*. *Journal of Ethnopharmacology, 113468*, 113468. Advance online publication. DOI: 10.1016/j.jep.2020.113468 PMID: 33049345

Muhammad, F., Liu, Y., Zhou, Y., Yang, H., & Li, H. (2022). Antioxidative role of traditional Chinese medicine in Parkinson's disease. *Journal of Ethnopharmacology*, *285*. *Journal of Ethnopharmacology, 114821*, 114821. Advance online publication. DOI: 10.1016/j.jep.2021.114821 PMID: 34838943

Ning, F., Chen, L., Chen, L., Liu, X., Zhu, Y., Hu, J., Xie, G., Xia, J., Shi, K., Lan, Z., & Wang, P. (2021). Combination of *Polygoni multiflori* radix praeparata and *Acori tatarinowii* rhizoma alleviates learning and memory impairment in scopolamine-treated mice by regulating synaptic-related proteins. *Frontiers in Pharmacology*, *12*. *Frontiers in Pharmacology, 679573*, 679573. Advance online publication. DOI: 10.3389/fphar.2021.679573 PMID: 34393775

Pardridge, W. M. (2005). The blood-brain barrier: Bottleneck in brain drug development. *NeuroRx*, *2*(1), 3–14. DOI: 10.1602/neurorx.2.1.3

Park, H., Kang, S., Nam, E., Suh, Y. H., & Chang, K. A. (2019). The protective effects of PSM-04 against beta amyloid-induced neurotoxicity in primary cortical neurons and an animal model of Alzheimer's disease. *Frontiers in Pharmacology*, *10*. *Frontiers in Pharmacology, 2*, 2. Advance online publication. DOI: 10.3389/fphar.2019.00002 PMID: 30733674

Pramanik, R., Dey, A., Chakrabarty, A. K., Banerjee, D., Narwaria, A., Sharma, S., Rai, R. K., Katiyar, C. K., & Dubey, S. K. (2024). Diabetes mellitus and Alzheimer's disease: Understanding disease mechanisms, their correlation, and promising dual activity of selected herbs. *Journal of Ethnopharmacology*, *333*. *Journal of Ethnopharmacology, 118402*, 118402. Advance online publication. DOI: 10.1016/j.jep.2024.118402 PMID: 38821139

Rebai, O., Belkhir, M., Boujelben, A., Fattouch, S., & Amri, M. (2017). *Morus alba* leaf extract mediates neuroprotection against glyphosate-induced toxicity and biochemical alterations in the brain. *Environmental Science and Pollution Research*, *24*(10), 9605–9613. https://doi.org/ DOI: 10.1007/s11356-017-8606-8

Rekatsina, M., Paladini, A., Piroli, A., Zis, P., Pergolizzi, J. V., & Varrassi, G. (2020). Pathophysiology and therapeutic perspectives of oxidative stress and neurodegenerative diseases: A narrative review. *Advances in Therapy*, *37*(1), 113–139. DOI: 10.1007/s12325-019-01148-5

Rewar, S. (2015). A systematic review on Parkinson's disease (PD). *Indian Journal of Research in Pharmacy and Biotechnology*, *3*(2), 176–182.

Rui, W., Li, S., Xiao, H., Xiao, M., & Shi, J. (2020). Baicalein attenuates neuroinflammation by inhibiting NLRP3/caspase-1/GSDMD pathway in MPTP-induced mice model of Parkinson's disease. *International Journal of Neuropsychopharmacology*, *23*(11), 762–773. DOI: 10.1093/ijnp/pyaa060

Sahiner, M., Yilmaz, A. S., Gungor, B., & Sahiner, N. (2023). A review on phyto-therapeutic approaches in Alzheimer's disease. *Journal of Functional Biomaterials*, *14*(1), Article 50. DOI: 10.3390/jfb14010050

Sharma, R., Kuca, K., Nepovimova, E., Kabra, A., Rao, M. M., & Prajapati, P. K. (2019). Traditional Ayurvedic and herbal remedies for Alzheimer's disease: From bench to bedside. *Expert Review of Neurotherapeutics*, *19*(5), 359–374. DOI: 10.1080/14737175.2019.1596803

Singh, A. K., Rai, S. N., Maurya, A., Mishra, G., Awasthi, R., Shakya, A., Chellappan, D. K., Dua, K., Vamanu, E., Chaudhary, S. K., & Singh, M. P. (2021). Therapeutic potential of phytoconstituents in management of Alzheimer's disease. *Evidence-Based Complementary and Alternative Medicine*, *2021*. *Evidence-Based Complementary and Alternative Medicine : eCAM, 5578574*, 1–19. Advance online publication. DOI: 10.1155/2021/5578574 PMID: 34211570

Sivaraman, D., Anbu, N., Kabilan, N., Kumar, M. P., Shanmugapriya, P., & Christian, G. J. (2019). Review on current treatment strategy in Alzheimer's disease and role of herbs in treating neurological disorders. *International Journal of Translational Research in Indian Medicine*, *1*(1), 33–43.

Snow, A. D., Castillo, G. M., Nguyen, B. P., Choi, P. Y., Cummings, J. A., Cam, J., Hu, Q., Lake, T., Pan, W., Kastin, A. J., & Kirschner, D. A. (2019). The Amazon rain forest plant *Uncaria tomentosa* (cat's claw) and its specific proanthocyanidin constituents are potent inhibitors and reducers of both brain plaques and tangles. *Scientific Reports*, *9*(1), Article 561. DOI: 10.1038/s41598-019-38645-0

Sohn, E., Kim, Y. J., & Jeong, S. J. (2021). Korean traditional herbal formula Soshiho-tang attenuates memory impairment and neuronal damage in mice with amyloid-beta-induced Alzheimer's disease. *Integrative Medicine Research*, *10*(3), Article 100723. DOI: 10.1016/j.imr.2021.100723

Thakur, M., Singh, K., & Khedkar, R. (2020). Phytochemicals: Extraction process, safety assessment, toxicological evaluations, and regulatory issues. In *Functional and preservative properties of phytochemicals* (pp. 341–361). Academic Press., DOI: 10.1016/B978-0-12-818593-3.00011-7

Uttara, B., Singh, A. V., Zamboni, P., & Mahajan, R. T. (2009). Oxidative stress and neurodegenerative diseases: A review. *International Journal of Molecular Sciences*, *10*(3), 781–796. https://doi.org/DOI: 10.3390/ijms10030781

Venkatesan, R., Ji, E., & Kim, S. Y. (2017). Phytochemicals that regulate neuroinflammation. *Current Pharmaceutical Design*, *23*(44), 6685–6700. https://doi.org/DOI: 10.2174/1381612823666170215164852

Xu, Y., Liu, S., Zhu, L., Dai, L., Qian, W., Zhang, J., Li, X., & Pan, W. (2021). Green tea protects against hippocampal neuronal apoptosis in diabetic encephalopathy by inhibiting JNK/MLCK signaling. *Molecular Medicine Reports*, *24*(2), Article 575. DOI: 10.3892/mmr.2021.12214

Yin, R., Xue, J., Tan, Y., Fang, C., Hu, C., Yang, Q., Mei, X., & Qi, D. (2021). The positive role and mechanism of herbal medicine in Parkinson's disease. *Oxidative Medicine and Cellular Longevity*, *2021*. *Oxidative Medicine and Cellular Longevity, 9923331*(1), 9923331. Advance online publication. DOI: 10.1155/2021/9923331 PMID: 34567415

Zhang, J., Yang, C., Wei, D., Li, H., Leung, E. L., Deng, Q., Liu, Z., Fan, X. X., & Zhang, Z. (2019). Long-term efficacy of Chinese medicine Bushen Capsule on cognition and brain activity in patients with amnestic mild cognitive impairment. *Pharmacological Research*, *146*. *Pharmacological Research, 104319*, 104319. Advance online publication. DOI: 10.1016/j.phrs.2019.104319 PMID: 31220560

Zhang, Q., Zheng, Y., Hu, X., Hu, X., Lv, W., Lv, D., Chen, J., Wu, M., Song, Q., & Shentu, J. (2018). Ethnopharmacological uses, phytochemistry, biological activities, and therapeutic applications of *Alpinia oxyphylla* Miquel: A review. *Journal of Ethnopharmacology*, *224*, 149–168. DOI: 10.1016/j.jep.2018.05.002

Zhang, X., Du, L., Zhang, W., Yang, Y., Zhou, Q., & Du, G. (2017). Therapeutic effects of baicalein on rotenone-induced Parkinson's disease through protecting mitochondrial function and biogenesis. *Scientific Reports*, *7*(1), Article 9968. https://doi.org/DOI: 10.1038/s41598-017-09824-0

Zhang, Y., Lin, C., Zhang, L., Cui, Y., Gu, Y., Guo, J., Wu, D., Li, Q., & Song, W. (2015). Cognitive improvement during treatment for mild Alzheimer's disease with a Chinese herbal formula: A randomized controlled trial. *PLoS ONE*, *10*(6), Article e0130353. DOI: 10.1371/journal.pone.0130353

Zhang, Y., Qian, C., Chen, Y., He, W., & Guo, Z. (2025). Phototherapy via modulation of β-amyloid in combating Alzheimer's disease. *Aggregate*, *6*(5), Article e70020. DOI: 10.1002/agt2.70020

Zhang, Z., Chen, J., Li, C., & others. (2014). Intranasal huperzine A-loaded nanostructured lipid carriers for brain delivery to treat Alzheimer's disease. *International Journal of Pharmaceutics*, *474*(1–2), 113–122. DOI: 10.1016/j.ijpharm.2014.08.003

Zhang, Z., Zhang, S., Lui, C. N., Zhu, P., Zhang, Z., Lin, K., Dai, Y., & Yung, K. K. (2019). Traditional Chinese medicine-based neurorestorative therapy for Alzheimer's and Parkinson's disease. *Journal of Neurorestoratology*, *7*(4), 207–222. DOI: 10.26599/JNR.2019.9040023

Zhao, Y., & Lu, Z. N. (2017). Glabridin attenuates MPTP-induced Parkinson disease by inhibiting extracellular regulated protein kinases signaling pathway. *Zhonghua Yi Xue Za Zhi*, *97*(26), 2050–2054. https://doi.org/DOI: 10.3760/cma.j.issn.0376-2491.2017.26.010

Chapter 14

Exploring the Role of Phytomedicines in Ameliorating the Manifestation of Brain Disorders

Odangowei Inetiminebi Ogidi
https://orcid.org/0000-0002-9961-893X
Bayelsa Medical University, Yenagoa, Nigeria

Mukul Machhindra Barwant
https://orcid.org/0000-0002-5639-4251
Sanjivani Arts Commerce and Science College, Kopargaon, India

Anamika Singh
Department of Pharmaceutical Chemistry, Mats School of Pharmacy, Mats University, India

ABSTRACT

Neurological and neurodegenerative disorders present a significant global health burden, often characterized by complex pathophysiology and limited therapeutic options. This chapter explores the potential of phytomedicines, which are bioactive substances derived from plants, as a means to prevent and treat neurological diseases and conditions such as epilepsy, depression, anxiety, Parkinson's disease, and Alzheimer's disease. Phytochemicals including polyphenols, flavonoids, alkaloids, and terpenoids have the ability to modulate neuroplasticity, neuroinflammatory pathways, oxidative stress, and the balance of neurotransmitters. The chapter also discusses recent preclinical and clinical findings, mechanisms of action, challenges in bioavailability, and prospects of integrating phytomedicines into mainstream neurological treatment. By drawing on interdisciplinary research, this work emphasizes the potential of phytomedicines as complementary or alternative therapies in mitigating the progression and symptomatology of brain disorders.

DOI: 10.4018/979-8-3373-4627-4.ch014

INTRODUCTION

Neurones and neuroglia make up the human brain, which is frequently said to be the most complex organ in the body. The job of neurones is to send and receive signals in the form of nerve impulses. After neurones experience damage or stress, microglia and astrocytes quickly step in to help, becoming crucial for guaranteeing the efficient working of neurones. Any disruption in the proper functioning of microglia or astrocytes, which are responsible for preserving the health of neurones, could have serious consequences for how the brain works. Acutely injured neurones send signals to the neuroglia to let them know how they are functioning. The neuroglia either aid the cancerous neurones in their regenerative process or destroy them if they are determined to be non-viable, depending on the severity of the damage (Ogidi et al., 2025a; Halliwell, 1992; Commenges et al., 2000).

Both age-related brain decline and neuropathological diseases include neurodegeneration. It is well-known that neurological and cerebrovascular diseases account for a disproportionate share of deaths worldwide. Both acute and chronic age-related brain disorders involve inflammation and oxidative stress, which are components of the normal ageing process. Phytochemicals are active substances that exist naturally in plants; they are present in some medicinal plants, edible fruits, and vegetables which can be seen in various studies (Ogidi et al., 2025d, f; 2024b). In terms of supporting cellular activity, they pale in comparison to minerals and vitamins. Inflammation and oxidative stress are linked to a wide variety of neurological disorders, including neuroprotection, anxiety, depression, and Alzheimer's disease (AD) (Kumar, 2006; Andrade et al., 2019).

From prehistoric times to now, plants have played an integral role in human culture, serving as food, medicine, and ornamentation. Despite this, there is a lot of uncharted territory in the potentially fruitful and potentially hazardous connection between plants and the human brain. It is of paramount interest to investigate neuroprotective and neurotoxic chemicals derived from plants since the brain, a wonder of intricacy and fragility, is prone to deterioration with age (Rehman et al., 2019; Ogidi & Ajoko, 2024). In the same way that the human brain's complex network of neurones and neurotransmitters necessitates careful maintenance for peak performance, plants' wide variety of bioactive phytoconstituents can have the opposite effect (Wojtunik-Kulesza, 2022). The identification of new neuroprotective drugs to fight neurodegenerative illnesses and improve cognitive function is the reason why studying plants with neurological effects is important (Kim et al., 2006). Research has shown that certain chemicals present in plants have the potential to mitigate neuroinflammation, protect neurones against neurotoxins, and enhance cognitive functions and memory (Vauzour, 2012).

Numerous chemicals found in plants have been found to have strong neuroprotective properties, meaning they can help prevent brain diseases and improve cognitive performance (Nadege et al., 2017). They aid in systemic strengthening and fight against different forms of nerve cell damage, which in turn promotes healthy brain function and promotes regeneration of damaged brain cells (Lahane & Katekar, 2024). Hypericum perforatum, more commonly known as St. John's Wort, is one plant compound that has demonstrated promise in protecting neurones from destruction and offering relief to those with neurological illnesses such as Alzheimer's and Parkinson's (Oliveira et al., 2016; Khalil et al., 2023). Research on the antioxidant properties of plants such as Cymbopogon cit ratus, Melissa officinalis, and Matricaria recutita has also shown promise in reducing brain oxidative stress. Because these plants contain antioxidants, which may have neuroprotective effects, we can see how oxidative stress contributes to the development

of neurological diseases. Because of their ability to scavenge free radicals and decrease lipid peroxidation, plant extracts have a dual role in neurological outcomes that help to maintain the health and function of neurones (Pereira et al., 2008).

By modulating the function of neurotransmitter receptors, phytocompounds derived from food and therapeutic herbs keep the brain's chemical equilibrium stable (Kumar et al., 2014). Fruits, vegetables, herbs, and nuts contain chemicals called polyphenols that have neuroprotective qualities and can improve cognitive function and memory (Turkez et al., 2020). Most diseases are caused by reactive oxygen species, which can be protected from by plant polyphenolic chemicals (Ogidi & Emaikwu, 2024; Popescu et al., 2016). Neurodegenerative illnesses are among the many health problems that triterpenic acids, a group of phytocompounds with a wide range of therapeutic actions, have been investigated in depth for their possible ability to treat (Mioc et al., 2022). Neuroprotective benefits are at least in part due to the presence of phytocompounds in plants like Gentiana olivieri, which include gentiopicroside and isoorientin (Dereli-Caliskan et al., 2021). To better protect against oxidative stress and damage, compounds with an antioxidant function are superior (Daliborca et al., 2015).

Lipid peroxidation follows oxidative stress, which is why this happens. Furthermore, studies have shown that red grapes' polyphenolic compound resveratrol can activate SIRT1, therefore shielding neurones from oxidative stress and toxicity brought on by amyloid-β peptides (Codecedo et al., 2012). Additional research has demonstrated the neuroprotective effects of phytoconstituents derived from plants, such as Calligonum polygonoides. Apigenin triacetate is one such compound that has interacted with important brain enzymes and receptors, which has improved hypercholesterolaemia and prevented neurodegenerative changes in areas of the brain like the cortex and hippocampus (Sakarwal et al., 2024). The primary goal of this chapter is to summarise the most current findings on the neuroprotective effects of herbal products on different NDs and to identify the possible mechanisms by which these products work, with a focus on phytochemicals formulated at the nanoscale (Ogidi & Emaikwu, 2023a,b).

NEURODEGENERATIVE DISEASES AND THEIR PROGRESSION

The loss of either cognitive or physical functions is a defining feature of NDs, as mentioned before. All of these neurological disorders AD, PD, HD, ALS, trauma, and ischaemic stroke fall under the same category (Figure 1). According to Sampson et al. (2009), the pathological features of these diseases mostly include neuronal loss and protein misfolding and aggregation, which in turn cause various symptoms such as motor abnormalities and dementia.

Figure 1. Types of neurodegenerative diseases

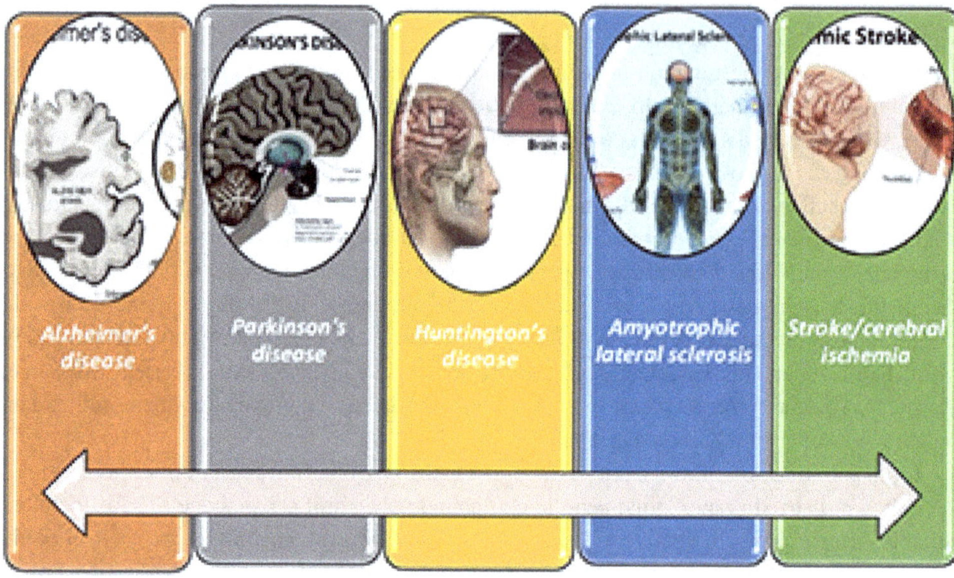

Alzheimer's Disease

According to Reitz and Mayeux (2014), Alzheimer's disease is the leading cause of permanent brain damage. Environmental and genetic variables both contribute to this illness, as stated by Iqbal and Grundke-Iqbal (2010), highlighting its complexity. According to Macdonald et al. (2014), the primary neuropathological indicators of Alzheimer's disease include neurofibrillary tangles, amyloid plaque, and neuronal loss. The development of the illness is influenced by multiple interrelated processes. Among these are oxidative stress, inflammation, cholinergic system loss, hyperphosphorylation and aggregation of tau, amyloid accumulation, and apoptosis (Webber et al., 2005). It comes as a surprise that there is now no remedy available for these symptoms that works completely. Doneprezil, rivastigmine, and galantamine are the only acetyl cholinesterase inhibitors that have received official approval for the treatment of Alzheimer's disease (AD) thus far. According to Kumar et al. (2015), these treatments may provide temporary relief from symptoms, but they will not address the root cause. Given the complexity of AD, it would be naïve to think that a panacea medication could eliminate the disease totally. Scientists are scouring the medical literature for potential illness targets and efficient treatments that can slow the disease's advancement (Kumar et al., 2015). According to Hosseinkhani et al. (2017), there may be multiple uses for nutraceuticals and herbal treatments.

Parkinson's Disease

The striatum and the substantia nigra pars compacta region are the primary sites of dopaminergic neurone loss in Parkinson's disease, the second most frequent form of the disease among

the elderly. Patients with PD experience a loss of motor control when the nigrostriatal pathway is disturbed. Lesverenz et al. (2009) cite tremors, stiffness, bradykinesia, weak muscles, and difficulty walking as the main symptoms of Parkinson's disease (PD). In the brains of individuals suffering from Parkinson's disease, there is pathological evidence such as α-synuclein aggregates known as Lewy Bodies and genetic mutation abnormalities. Cholinergic effect blocking and dopaminergic neural activity enhancement are the mainstays of Parkinson's disease treatment (Albin, 2006; Ogidi et al., 2025i). Despite the lack of a cure, there are drugs that can alleviate symptoms and increase survival rates for those with Parkinson's disease (Albin, 2006). Researchers are always looking for a novel medication that can help with symptoms or even cure the illness. Scientists are very interested in phytochemicals as a potential therapy for Parkinson's disease. What follows is a more in-depth discussion of this subject.

Huntington's Disease

Degenerative motor and cognitive abilities slowly worsen with the onset of HD, a genetic condition. A genetic disorder characterised by the progressive death of neurones in different brain regions. Symptoms most often experienced include a decline in cognitive abilities, changes in emotional stability, and unexplained tremors. While healthy persons typically have 6-35 CAG repeats in Exon 1 of the Huntingtin (HTT) gene on chromosome 4, patients with infections often have more than 36 repeats (Szlachcic et al., 2015). A neuronal accumulation of HTT protein follows from this. Degeneration of the brain's neural network and cell death are caused by this protein's lengthy polyglutamine region. Manoharan et al. (2016) listed depression, clumsiness, tumbling, short-term memory loss, lack of concentration, and concentration issues among the early symptoms. Loss of appetite, trouble swallowing, stuttering, itchiness, uncontrolled facial movements, and other late symptoms may also present. The area of HD prevention and therapy is quite active with research. In order to determine which medications work best, numerous experimental models have undergone experimental validation. Currently, medications can merely alleviate symptoms; there is currently no treatment or cure. The effectiveness of many natural chemicals against HD may hold the key to a successful treatment.

Amyotrophic Lateral Sclerosis

Motor neurone disease (MND), also known as amyotrophic lateral sclerosis (ALS) or Lou Gehrig's disease, is a neurodegenerative disease (ND) that causes motor symptoms. Some people have trouble swallowing or speaking (bulbar-onset sickness), while others have weak muscles in their arms and legs (spinal-onset illness) (Hardiman et al., 2017). Al-Chalabi et al. (2017) revealed that gene changes had a big effect in a small number of cases that were linked to family history. However, the specific cause of this illness is still unknown. Elamin et al. (2013) and Phukan et al. (2012) reported that 50% of people with amyotrophic lateral sclerosis (ALS) have movement problems, cognitive problems, and memory loss. These people may additionally have spasticity, sialorrhea, discomfort, muscle cramps, DVT, mood swings, and trouble breathing, in addition to the ones already mentioned. The FDA has only approved two medications for ALS: Riluzole (Rilutek) and Edaravone (Radicava). The basic goal is to make the symptoms better. These medications can only add three to six months to a person's life. This ND can kill you just like the others. Medical experts who care with amyotrophic lateral sclerosis (ALS) pay a lot

of attention to quality of life (QOL). Studies from all across the world have produced a lot of preclinical data, but it's still not clear if it can be used in human trials. Also, many human clinical trials have failed, which could be because people do not know enough about the disease or because it is naturally different in different people. Several research centres are now looking into how natural plants and the active ingredients they contain can help lessen the terrible symptoms of this disease. The plant chemicals' molecular processes and possible therapeutic effects need to be explored and put into practice.

Stroke/Cerebral Ischemia

Hicks & Jolkkonen (2009) reported that among brain illnesses, stroke ranks third in terms of mortality worldwide. Ischaemia strokes happen when blood flow to a region of the brain is abruptly and severely interrupted, either temporarily or permanently. Ischaemia mostly impacts the cornu ammonis 1 (CA1) region of the hippocampus. The term for the progressive loss of pyramidal neurones in the CA1 area four or five days following ischaemia is "delayed neuronal death" (DND). Park et al. (2017), Yousuf et al. (2009) and Ozbal et al. (2008) all found that during ischemia/reperfusion, the CA1 region experiences gliosis of astrocytes and microglia, excitotoxicity, oxidative stress, apoptosis, and inflammation. These alterations cause mitochondrial malfunction, which in turn causes a deficiency of ATP and, ultimately, neuronal death. With only a few number of effective neuroprotective pharmaceuticals on the market for stroke prevention, there is an urgent need for new medications with a multidisciplinary action that can ward off many symptoms. Many diseases, including stroke, have long been thought to be preventable by the use of specific herbs and nutraceuticals, according to traditional medicine. The anti-inflammatory and antioxidant properties are shared by many natural compounds, such as minerals, flavonoids, and polyphenols. What follows is an in-depth discussion of natural ingredients and their application to people suffering from ischaemia.

NEUROPROTECTIVE PHYTOCHEMICALS AND THEIR MODE OF ACTION ON NEURODEGENERATIVE DISORDERS

Neuroprotective phytochemicals such as curcumin, resveratrol, and quercetin exert their effects on neurodegenerative disorders by modulating oxidative stress, reducing neuroinflammation, and inhibiting the aggregation of toxic proteins like amyloid-beta and alpha-synuclein. These compounds activate cellular defense pathways, including Nrf2/ARE, SIRT1, and PI3K/Akt, thereby enhancing neuronal survival and maintaining synaptic integrity. For the purpose of ND prevention, "herbal medicines" are defined as phytochemicals derived from plants, fruits, and vegetables (Izah et al., 2023; Rahman & Chung, 2010; Bagli et al., 2004). Antioxidant activities are the primary mode of action for these compounds. The fact that they act on different enzymes and the products of those enzymes suggests that they may influence more than one signalling route (Harvey & Cree, 2010; Bagli et al., 2004). Ingesting these phytochemicals triggers the immune system and controls hormone levels (Farooqui, 2013). There is a lack of knowledge regarding the precise mechanism of action, while multiple pieces of supporting evidence have shown that phytochemicals functioning as nutraceuticals can improve ND symptoms. Table 1 shows the neuroprotective phytochemicals, their sources, targeted disorders, and modes of action.

Table 1. Neuroprotective phytochemicals, their sources, targeted disorders, and modes of action

Phytochemical	Source	Target Disorder(s)	Mode of Action	Reference
Curcumin	Turmeric (*Curcuma longa*)	Alzheimer's, Parkinson's, stroke	Antioxidant, anti-inflammatory (Inhibits NF-κB, activates PI3K/Akt/Nrf2, CREB/ BDNF, autophagy via PI3K/Akt/mTOR)	Kandezi et al. (2020); Cui et al. (2016)
Resveratrol	Grapes, berries, peanuts, red wine	Alzheimer's, Parkinson's, ALS	Activates SIRT1, antioxidant, anti-inflammatory, enhances mitochondrial biogenesis & mitophagy	Baur & Sinclair (2006); Zhao et al. (2024); Yao et al. (2022)
EGCG	Green tea	AD, PD	Scavenges ROS, inhibits apoptosis, stabilizes mitochondria	—
Quercetin	Onion, berries	AD, Huntington's	Reduces oxidative stress, anti-inflammatory, inhibits amyloid-beta toxicity	—
Luteolin	Celery, peppers	AD, PD, cognitive decline	Anti-inflammatory, modulates microglia, promotes mitophagy	Vongthip et al. (2024)
Berberine	*Coptis chinensis*, *Berberis aristata*	Alzheimer's	Enhances mitophagy via PINK1-Parkin, improves mitochondria	Wang et al. (2023)
Salidroside	*Rhodiola rosea*	Alzheimer's	Promotes NRF2–KEAP1 pathway, boosts SIRT3, enhances mitophagy	Yao et al. (2022)
Palmatine	*Coptis chinensis*, *Berberis aristata*	Alzheimer's	Improves mitochondrial potential, stimulates mitophagy	Lee et al. (2023)
Honokiol	*Magnolia officinalis*	Alzheimer's	Reduces amyloid-beta, enhances mitophagy, boosts synaptic proteins	Hou et al. (2022); Ogidi, 2025
Ampelopsin A	*Vitis vinifera*	Cognitive decline	Increases BDNF/CREB-driven LTP	—
Asiaticoside	*Centella asiatica*	Vascular dementia	Promotes autophagy via upregulating Beclin-1, LC3-II, inhibiting mTOR	—
Glycyrrhizic acid	Licorice root	Vascular dementia	Antioxidant, prevents apoptosis, preserves neuronal structure	—
Morin	*Morus* spp.	TBI, AD	Antioxidant, anti-inflammatory, anti-aggregation actions	—
Vitamin E (α-tocopherol)	Nuts, seeds, vegetable oils	Alzheimer's	Reduces Aβ deposition, tau phosphorylation; increases SOD & BDNF	—

Evidence of Effect of Phytochemicals in Memory, Cognition, And Alzheimer's Disease

Memory and cognitive abilities can be enhanced by some phytochemicals, which has been known for decades. Their future seems bright, according to emerging findings from in vivo, clinical, and in vitro investigations. Almonds are a natural memory booster because their oleic acid helps neurones build axons and dendrites (Polo-Hernández et al., 2014). Research by Park et al. (2006) indicates that the propyl endopeptidase enzyme, which is abundant in the brains of Alzheimer's disease patients, may have a significant reduction in its activity. Among the several active ingredients found in Withania somnifera are withanolide A, withanoside IV, and withanoside VI. These components were discovered to enhance neurotic outgrowth in research

carried out using the the SHSY5Y cell line from human neuroblastoma (Kuboyama et al., 2002). According to Zhu et al. (2011) and Asai et al. (2007), the rate of extracellular Aβ generation in HEK293 cells and H4 neuroglioma cells has reduced.

According to Xu et al. (2013) and Jia et al. (2012), berberine can reduce Aβ-induced neuroinflammation and protect against AD when pretreated with primary BV2 microglia cells and SK N-SH neuroblastoma cells. According to Kim et al. (2014), curcumin, a polyphenol extracted from the Curcuma longa plant's roots, has comparable anti-inflammatory, neuroprotective, anti-amyloid, and anti-tau characteristics. Reinke and Gestwicki (2007) found that it prevented amyloid beta, the main aggregating protein in Alzheimer's disease, from clumping together. Urbain et al. (2008) found that canscora de cussata magniferin elevated levels of the neurotransmitter acetylcholine, which is critical for learning and memory. Khan et al. (2012) and Thakuma et al. (2005) found that black seed oil's bioactive component, thymoquinone, significantly decreased oxidative stress and mitochondrial damages in PC12 cells treated with Aβ. Research conducted by Javed et al. (2015) demonstrated that hesperidin, a bioflavonoid present in citrus fruits, protected both cells treated with Aβ and an animal model of Alzheimer's disease produced by ICV-STZ. According to the findings, phytochemicals protect neurones from harm. Research conducted by Huang et al. (2017), Xu et al. (2017), and Jhang et al. (2017) has demonstrated that ginsenoside Rg1 from Panax notoginseng, Silibinin, hyperforin, resve ratrol, and capsaicin all exhibit comparable effects.

Evidence of Effect of Phytochemicals in Parkinson's Disease

One percent of the world's elderly population lives with PD, which exacerbates physical, psychological, and economical difficulties. A cluster of symptoms characterises the clinical disease known as Parkinsonism, which is similar to PD. Natural substances have been the subject of substantial investigation into potential therapeutics for parkinsonism and Parkinson's disease, with studies employing both in vitro and in vivo models. The main neurotoxic processes that cause this condition, according to multiple studies (Khan et al., 2012; Shrivastava et al., 2013; Khan et al., 2010), are mitochondrial dysfunctions. These dysfunctions lead to inflammatory cytokines, cell death, oxidative stress, and dopamine depletion. Several studies have shown that specific plant components can scavenge free radicals. These include Khan et al. (2012), Sharma et al. (2016), Shrivastava et al. (2013), and Khan et al. (2010). Ruthin, resveratrol, piperine, and quercetin are some of the components that make up this. The neuroprotective effects of carsonic acid in 6-hydroxydopamine-induced Parkinson's disease were studied by Wu et al. (2015). Hes peridin protected old mice from oxidative damage caused by 6-OHDA, according to study by Antunes et al. (2014).

Ahmad et al. (2012) found that mice were protected from 6-hydroxydopamine-induced neurotoxicity by using sesame seed oil, which acts as an antioxidant. The neuroprotective effects of these herbs were attributed by all of these PD models to their anti-oxidant characteristics. Zbarsky et al. (2005) found that in a 6-OHDA-induced PD model, naringenin increased dopamine levels and tyrosine hydroxylase positive cell numbers. Both Gan-Or et al. (2015) and Pan et al. (2008) shown that PD activates the autophagy-lysosome pathway (ALP). Gan-Or et al. (2015) and Pan et al. (2008) discovered that ALP deficiency causes neurodegeneration in PD, which is influenced by both hereditary and environmental variables. A disease-modifying treatment for Parkinson's disease may be possible with the help of a number of tiny chemicals discovered in plants. Research by Chen et al. (2014) and Song et al. (2014) established that the Chinese

plant Uncaria rhynchophylla contains the neurotoxic chemicals corynoxine B and corynoxine. The removal of α-synuclein from brain cells and fruit flies can be facilitated by corynoxine B, according to another discovery. The kaempferol, resveratrol, conophyl line, curcumin, celastrol, and a number of other nutraceuticals have demonstrated this quality (Ferretta et al., 2014; Song et al., 2016; Huang et al., 2013).

Evidence of Effect of Phytochemicals in Huntington's Disease

This genetic disorder can be identified in infants as early as one month of age. Deterioration in the cortex and striatum of the brain can lead to dyskinesia, cognitive failure, and early death. Regardless of gender, HD usually begins manifesting in individuals in their 40s or 50s, and half of all cases are in children of affected parents (Manoharan et al., 2016). As with all NDs, the exact reason for HD mortality is unknown; however, oxidative stress could be a clinical manifestation. Because of its high oxygen energy needs, oxidative stress can have a disproportionate impact on the brain (Walker, 2007). The effectiveness of natural plants as an HD treatment has been confirmed by researchers using a multitude of HD models. Researchers Wong et al. (2015) found that the Lotus plant's active component Neferine (Nelumbo nucifera) could autophagically clear PC12 cells treated with mutant HTT of neurotoxic protein aggregates. Khan et al. (2015) found that huperzine A, rosmarinic acid, curcumin, luteolin, and rosmarinic acid are among of the natural compounds that may inhibit caspases 1 and 3, hence preventing the development of NDs. The neuroprotective advantages of HD have been supported by histology investigations that show Ginkgo biloba has down-regulated striatal glyceraldehyde-3-phosphate dehydrogenase and unregulated Bcl-xl expression levels (Mahdy et al., 2011). As per Kumar and Kumar (2009), a commonly found plant known as Withania somnifera has the ability to affect HD through the GABAergic system. This mechanism is essential for HD.

Evidence of Effect of Phytochemicals in Amyotrophic Lateral Sclerosis

Supplemental and alternative medicine refers to the employment of non-mainstream methods in tandem with standard healthcare. A growing number of people with amyotrophic lateral sclerosis (ALS) are turning to alternative medicine practices including naturopathy, homoeopathy, and acupuncture in the hopes of finding a cure (Wasner et al., 2001). Gingsenosides, carbs, proteins, vitamins, and fatty acids are just a few of the components found in ginseng. A protective effect against amyotrophic lateral sclerosis has been demonstrated by reducing motor neurones (Cai & Yang, 2016). Evidence suggests that the Cu/Zn superoxide dismutase (SOD1) gene is mutated in amyotrophic lateral sclerosis (ALS) patients. The neurodegenerative disease amyotrophic lateral sclerosis (ALS) results from an imbalance between the brain's antioxidant defence system and an overabundance of reactive oxygen species (ROS) (Ogidi et al., 2025h). A transgenic SOD1 G93A mouse model of amyotrophic lateral sclerosis was found to have an increased lifetime in mice given madecassoside from Centella asiatica (Liu et al., 2006), which may indicate a protective effect against motor neurone degeneration.

Most people recognise epigallocatechin gallate (EGCG) as the main component in green tea. It protects neurones from damage, including amyotrophic lateral sclerosis, according to Mandel et al. (2004) and Koh et al. (2006). Garlic has the most powerful antioxidant, allicin. Dialyl trisulfide (DATS), the active monomer in allicin, has multiple physiological effects. Gly-

cal fibrillary acidic protein (GFAP) downregulation and heme oxygenase-1 (HO-1) activation were seen in a SOD1-G93A model of amyotrophic lateral sclerosis (ALS) (Guo et al., 2011). Research conducted by Kiaei et al. (2005) found that in the SOD1-G93A model of amyotrophic lateral sclerosis (ALS), celastrol had a substantial impact on motor capacity, survival duration, and the delay of illness start. According to research conducted by Sikora et al. (2010) and Ock et al. (2010), nutraceuticals such as paeonol, obovatol, curcumin, and resvera trol may be useful in preventing symptoms of amyotrophic lateral sclerosis (ALS).

Evidence of Effect of Phytochemicals in Cerebral Ischemia

In terms of global death rates, stroke ranks third, as reported by the World Health Organisation. The great majority of strokes, known as ischaemic strokes, occur when the brain's blood flow and oxygen supply are cut off. The pathogenic pathways linked to ischaemia include inflammation, excitotoxicity, apoptosis and oxidative stress (Yousuf et al., 2009). Although many studies have examined the causes of ischaemic brain injury, novel treatments are always being considered. Drug discovery relies on verifying the target as its most critical step in the search for viable therapeutic molecules (Ogidi et al., 2025b, c, g). Because oxidative stress is the principal aetiology, it is important to mention that naturally occurring compounds with antioxidant properties have shown remarkable efficacy in avoiding ischaemia. Khan et al. (2009) used the bioflavonoid rutin to shield neurones in rats against transient focal cerebral ischaemia.

Two separate studies conducted by Khan et al. (2010a, b) found that sesamin, an active ingredient in sesame seed oil, protected his brain from MCAO-induced harm. Quercetin offers substantial protection against the ischemia/reperfusion model because it reduces lipid peroxidation, caspase 3 activity, p53 activation, and enhances the body's antioxidant system (Ahmad et al., 2011). Raza et al. (2011) and hesperidin (Silymarin) have demonstrated that neurones in areas of cerebral ischaemia can be protected from oxidative damage. Hypoxia inducible factor-1 (HIF-1) is a transcription factor that becomes activated when atmospheric oxygen levels fall below a certain threshold. It plays an essential role in maintaining cellular oxygen homeostasis. Potentially protective against ischemia/reperfusion injury are agents with the capacity to activate HIF-1. Several cell lines have shown that the liquorice compound dibenzoylmethane can maintain HIF-1 protein levels (Mabjeesh et al., 2003). According to Wilson and Poellinger (2002), quercetin, another type of flavonoid, has been found to activate HIF-1 in HeLa cells.

MEDICINAL PLANTS COMMONLY USED FOR NEURODEGENERATIVE DISEASES

Medicinal plants have long served as foundational resources in traditional medicine systems and are now gaining scientific recognition for their potential in managing neurodegenerative diseases such as Alzheimer's disease (AD), Parkinson's disease (PD), and Huntington's disease (HD). Plants like *Bacopa monnieri*, *Withania somnifera* (Ashwagandha), and *Ginkgo biloba* are widely studied for their neuroprotective effects. These plants contain bioactive compounds such as bacosides, withanolides, and flavonoids, which contribute to reducing oxidative stress, improving mitochondrial function, modulating neurotransmitter activity, and enhancing synaptic plasticity. For instance, *Ginkgo biloba* extract has shown promise in improving cognitive function

and delaying the progression of dementia symptoms through its antioxidant and vasoregulatory effects (Nguyen & Alzahrani, 2025). Similarly, *Withania somnifera* is noted for its ability to modulate the hypothalamic-pituitary-adrenal (HPA) axis and inhibit acetylcholinesterase, which are relevant pathways in cognitive decline and neuroinflammation.

Other notable medicinal plants include *Rosmarinus officinalis* (rosemary), *Centella asiatica* (gotu kola), and *Mucuna pruriens*, which also play crucial roles in neurodegenerative therapy. *Rosmarinus officinalis* contains carnosic acid, a compound known to activate the Nrf2 pathway and protect dopaminergic neurons against oxidative damage (Giordano et al., 2011). *Centella asiatica*, rich in asiaticosides, supports mitochondrial function and promotes antioxidant defenses such as SOD and catalase, which are often compromised in AD and PD patients. Furthermore, *Mucuna pruriens*, a natural source of L-DOPA, is used in managing PD symptoms by replenishing dopamine levels and reducing motor deficits (Rai et al., 2017). The integration of these botanicals into therapeutic regimens represents a promising adjunct or alternative to conventional pharmacotherapies, especially given their multi-targeted mechanisms and lower toxicity profiles. Table 2 shows the medicinal plants commonly used in neurodegenerative diseases, along with their modes of action.

Table 2. Medicinal plants commonly used in neurodegenerative diseases, along with their modes of action

Plant	Active Components / Mechanisms	Targeted Disorders	Mode of Action	References
Rosmarinus officinalis	Carnosic acid; modulates PI3K/Akt, Nrf2; anti-apoptotic	PD, AD	Inhibits Bax/Bak/caspases, upregulates Bcl-2, reduces α-syn aggregation	Giordano et al. (2011)
Bacopa monnieri	Bacosides; antioxidant & anti-apoptotic	AD, PD	Bax/caspase-3, Bcl-2, enhances synaptic plasticity	Giordano et al. (2021); Smith et al. (2023)
Mucuna pruriens	L-DOPA; NF-κB/Akt modulation	PD	Reduces neuroinflammation, protects dopaminergic neurons	Giordano et al. (2021); Rai et al. (2017)
Glycyrrhiza glabra	Glycyrrhizin; enhances cholinergic transmission	AD	ACh signaling, antioxidant effects	Giordano et al. (2021)
Withania somnifera	Withanolides; antioxidant, AChE inhibition	AD, PD, general cognition	oxidative stress, modulates NMDA & AChE	Kumar et al. (2022); Patel et al. (2024)
Zingiber officinale	Gingerols; NGF-ERK/CREB pathway	AD, PD	NGF signaling, SOD activity, anti-inflammatory	Giordano et al. (2021); Rahman et al. (2024)
Centella asiatica	Asiaticosides; mitochondrial support	AD, PD	Protects complex I, SOD/catalase/GSH	Giordano et al. (2021); Lee et al. (2023)
Polygala tenuifolia	Tenuifolin; antioxidant, mitochondrial & Aβ modulation	AD	Aβ deposition, supports mitochondria	Deng et al. (2020)
Crocus sativus (Saffron)	Crocin/crocetin; Nrf2/HO-1, anti-amyloid	AD, PD, stroke	ROS, inhibits Aβ/tau aggregation	Lavandero et al. (2022)
Salvia officinalis (Sage)	Rosmarinic acid; antioxidant	AD	Cognitive improvement in RCTs	Akhondzadeh et al. (2003)
Vitis vinifera (Grape seed)	Resveratrol/polydatin; PI3K/Akt, mitochondrial protection	PD, Friedreich's	Improves motor and neurological function	Yiu et al. (2015); Chen et al. (2015)

continued on following page

Table 2. Continued

Plant	Active Components / Mechanisms	Targeted Disorders	Mode of Action	References
Ginkgo biloba	Flavonoids; antioxidant, BDNF increase	AD, PD	cognitive function, BDNF, free-radical scavenging	Savaskan et al. (2018); Nguyen & Alzahrani (2025)
Moringa oleifera	Kaempferol, myricetin; antioxidant, AChE modulation, Akt/ERK signaling	AD, PD, stroke	oxidative markers, neurogenesis	Ekong et al. (2017); Zeng et al. (2019)
Salvia miltiorrhiza	Tanshinones; Nrf2/HO-1, Akt pathway	PD	HO-1, reduces ROS	Zhang et al. (2021)

Withania somnifera (ashwagandha)

The plant Withania somnifera, more commonly referred to as Ashwagandha has been used for decades by Ayurvedic practitioners because to its memory-enhancing, immune-boosting effects, anti-inflammatory, anti-stress, anti-oxidant and neuroprotective (Jain et al., 2001; Khan et al., 2009). In their study of W. somnifera, Raut et al. (2012) evaluated its safety, activity, and dose tolerance; they found that 750–1250 mg daily was the sweet spot. Furthermore, the extract can reduce triglycerides and enhance muscular strength. The withanolides compounds found in ashwagandha were found to decrease cell proliferation in studies involving breast, CNS, and lung cancer cell lines. Some people also believe that eating withanolides can inhibit the growth of tumours (Ogidi et al., 2024a; Jayaprakasam et al., 2003).

Withania somnifera has a reducing effect on the stress-inducible NADPH-d activity. somnifera raises hippocampal serotonin levels by activating cholineacetyltransferase and decreasing corticosterone release, which in turn alters NADPH-d (Bhattacharya & Muruganandam, 2003). W. withanolide A, withanolide IV, and withanolide VI are withanolides produced from Withania somnifera that have the ability to regenerate neuronal axons, dendrites, pre- and post-synapses, and other neuronal components. Evidence suggests that extracts from several plant species, whether unprocessed or partially refined, can alleviate a variety of human health problems (Carlini, 2003). It was shown by Bhattacharya & Muruganandam (2003) that W. had anti-stress properties. When administered to Wistar rats, extracts from W. somnifera reduced the effects of chronic stress. serrata blossom.

Ginseng

An herb with both Korean and Chinese roots, ginseng (panax inseng) is used medicinally. The medicinal properties of this herb have garnered widespread fame for quite some time. Cancer, neurological disorders, high blood pressure, and diabetes are just some of the diseases that this plant can help alleviate. Ginseng helps keep you healthy because of its reputation for enhancing your immune system. Ginseng was studied by Kang & Min (2012) because of its capacity to inhibit voltage-dependent Ca2? pathways via a toxin-sensitive receptor linked to a G protein. A saponin ginsenoside, found in trace amounts, helps regulate Ca2? channels in neurones, according to the study. There has been study on the immune-modulatory effects of Ginseng (Kang & Min, 2012). It is anticipated that molecule K, a ginseng metabolite, will have a more potent inhibitory impact

compared to currently existing anti-allergy drugs on the market (Choo et al., 2003). Ginsenosides, or Ginseng's neuroprotective properties, make them an attractive therapeutic candidate for neurodegenerative diseases. By reducing ferroportin expression and preventing the elevation of nigral iron levels, research has demonstrated that the active component of P.ginseng can protect dopaminergic neurones from damage in Parkinson's disease (Wang et al., 2009). Reactive oxygen species (ROS) formation by dopamine, cytochrome c release into the cytosol, and suppression of caspase 3 activity are all reduced when Rg1 reduces NO synthesis, as stated by Chen et al. (2003). Through down-regulating the NF-KB signalling pathway and activating Akt and ERK, Rg1 has been discovered to reduce cell damage caused by hydrogen peroxide (Liu et al., 2011).

Curcumin

Curcumin, more often known as turmeric, is a popular Indian spice with deep roots in Ayurvedic medicine and traditional beauty practices. The spice is an excellent source of fibre, potassium, magnesium, and other minerals. This herb has numerous possible medical uses, including enhancing the immune system, reducing inflammation, and acting as an antioxidant. Many enzymes, cytokines, and transcription factors have their expression inhibited by curcumin (Aggarwal et al., 2013; Zhou et al., 2011). Increasing the activation of macrophages is one mechanism by which curcumin aids individuals with Alzheimer's disease. In Alzheimer's disease, amyloid plaque forms, and curcumin helps macrophages remove it. Curcumin was shown to have a role in the removal of amyloid plaque by Zhang et al. (2006) when it was first administered to macrophages of Alzheimer's disease patients and then exposed to amyloid plaque. Results demonstrated that macrophages treated with curcumin were more efficient at uptaking and consuming plaque than non-treated cells. Numerous studies have demonstrated that curcumin not only inhibits the formation of Ab oligomers and fibrils, but it also has anti-inflammatory characteristics (Ono et al., 2004; Yang et al., 2005).

Curcumin is useful for hypertension and the brain's microcirculatory function. Xia et al. (2016) investigated the possible ways in which curcumin reduces hypertension and its influence on cerebral microcirculation. Curcumin reduced blood pressure in mice compared to the control group. It altered open capillaries and circulating endothelial cells and increased blood flow and lactate dehydrogenase (LDF) velocity in both normal- and high-blood-pressure animals. In the setting of Alzheimer's disease, a 6-month pilot trial with curcumin was conducted by Baum et al. (2008). The study was double-blind, randomised, and placebo-controlled. Four or one gramme of curcumin, a placebo, or no treatment at all was given to twenty-two people at random. Of these, ten were given ten pills to take with meals, while twelve were given a packet of powder to add to their food. Curcumin actually increased vitamin E levels, and curcuminoids' antioxidant effects decreased both the need for and loss of vitamin E. Researchers also discovered that curcumin slowed the development of Alzheimer's disease. The levels of serum A[beta]40 did not change much between doses, but they did tend to rise while taking curcumin, which may be due to curcumin's ability to degrade A[beta] deposits in the brain and release the A[beta] for disposal in the bloodstream. It appears that curcumin had no significant side effects in Alzheimer's disease patients, and a tendency towards less adverse events was observed when 4 g was given.

Baccopa monnieri

Ayurvedic medicine places a great deal of importance on the use of Brahmi, which is known by its scientific name, Baccopa monnieri. Baccopa monnieri is a plant that is frequently discovered in both India and Australia. Additionally, it has the potential to revitalise nerve cells, which in turn can increase memory capacity. In addition to betulic acid and other alkaloids, Bacoside A and Bacoside B are two saponins that are derived from Brahmi. These saponins are made of sapogenins (Bacogenins A1-A4). According to reports, Bacoside A, one of the two main saponins, can improve memory power (Russo & Borrelli, 2005). Besides talent B, which enhances memory.

The several reported benefits of monnieri include its ability to relax smooth muscles, reduce inflammation, alleviate stress, and fight against microbes. The meaning of the statement made by Shinomol et al. (2012) about B. When it comes to the therapy of HD, the qualities of montnieri, which include an antioxidant and a protection against stress-induced nerve cell malfunction, are essential components. According to the findings of Mishra et al. (2006), the availability of glutathion (GSH) and the activity of glutathione reductase (GR) are both extremely important for B. monnieri to counteract oxidative stress caused by metals and improve detoxifying capacities. Two saponins derived from B., known as bacoside A and B, exhibit antistress characteristics. Sprague-Dawley rats were used in the study of monnieri by Chowdhuri et al. (2002). According to the results, B. Monnieri helps the brain fight off dangerous stress by activating superoxide dismutase, Hsp70, and P450.

Ginkgo biloba

Ginkgo biloba is another name for this ancient Chinese medicinal herb; some people call it a living fossil (Gao et al., 2016; Guan et al., 2016). Bilobalide is a trilactonic sesquiterpene and one of several chemical components found in the leaf, which also includes flavanoids and ginkgolides A-C and J-M. Shrunken form of G. The main component of ginkgo biloba is well-known for its antioxidant and anti-aggregation effects on platelets. The cardiovascular system and blood flow are both enhanced by this Chinese medicine, among its many benefits (McKenna et al., 2001).

In a study on Alzheimer's disease, Yao et al. (2004) looked at how well Ginkgo leaf extract inhibited the synthesis of Ab from b amyloid precursor protein. Supposedly, the extract's chemical components work by interacting with Ab to stop aggregation and competing with free cholesterol. An early indicator of neurodegenerative diseases, ginkgo can slow the pace of neuronal death, according to certain studies. Additionally, it has the ability to take in particular compounds that cause an overabundance of reactive oxygen species (ROS) (Bastianetto et al., 2000; Ergun et al., 2005). Ginkgo biloba extract contains bilobalide, which has potent anti-apoptotic and neuroprotective effects, according to Ahlemever & Krieglstein (2003). Researchers Abdou et al. found that rats given gingko bilobaand/or Trifolium had less sodium arsenite-induced neurotoxicity in many brain areas (including the cerebral cortex, hippocampus, stratum lucidum, and hindbrain) (Abdou et al., 2016).

Wolfberry

Chinese people often utilise wolfberry, scientifically known as Lycium barbarum (LB). The fruit's anti-aging and other medical properties have been known for a long time in Asian coun-

tries. Chinese medicine regards wolfberry as a "tonic herb" due to its anti-aging properties. The fruit's medical uses are varied and extensive. Wolfberry has a number of medical applications, including the treatment of diabetes and glaucoma. In recent times, dried wolfberry fruit has gained popularity as a dietary supplement. The fruit contains polysaccharides that are soluble in water. Wolfberry, of which barbarum makes up over 40% (Chiu et al., 2009; Ho et al., 2010a; 2009). Research on L.'s neuroprotective effects was carried out by Yu et al. (2005) shows toxic effects of barbarum on Alzheimer's illness.

Coronal neuronal pretreatment with L. lactate dehydrogenase release was inhibited by barbarum before exposure to Ab peptides. Additionally, the extract inhibited the activity of caspase-3 that had been activated by beta amyloid peptide. Research on wolfberry's effect on brain injury caused by plasma homocystein (Hcy) was conducted by Ho et al. (2010b). There is some evidence that the Lycium barbarum extract can inhibit Hcy-induced tau phosporylation and play a role in tau cleavage. The anti-ocular-hypertension effects of Lycium barbarum extract are well-documented. Researchers Chiu et al. (2009) proposed that L. The immune cells in the retina can be actively regulated by barbarum polysaccharide rides.

FUTURE PERSPECTIVE

The future of phytomedicine in addressing neurological disorders is promising, owing to advancements in biotechnology, pharmacognosy, and neuroscience. As our understanding of the brain's intricate biochemical and neurophysiological mechanisms expands, we concurrently gain greater opportunities to enhance phytomedicinal therapies. Future research are expected to employ high-throughput screening technologies and molecular docking simulations to identify novel plant-derived compounds that can safeguard the brain. This will initiate a new epoch of precise phytotherapy. Employing omics technologies such as genomics, proteomics, and metabolomics in phytomedicine research will enhance our understanding of the diverse effects of plant-derived compounds on human neurobiology (Ogidi, 2024; Ogidi et al., 2024c). These technologies will assist us in elucidating the molecular patterns of neurological disorders and how specific phytochemicals can alter the mechanisms of these conditions. Such discoveries will enhance the efficacy of medications and enable treatments to be customised according to individual genetic and metabolic profiles, thereby advancing personalised medicine in neurology. Simultaneously, advancements in nanotechnology and drug delivery systems may facilitate the absorption of phytochemicals into the body and enhance their ability to traverse the blood-brain barrier (Barwant et al., 2025). Nanocarriers and liposomal encapsulations could facilitate the targeted delivery of active plant compounds to specific regions of the brain, hence enhancing therapeutic efficacy (Ogidi et al., 2025e). This novel concept will be crucial for transitioning phytomedicines from experimental models to standard clinical application.

The future of phytomedicine will rely on collaboration among traditional medicine practitioners, neuroscientists, and regulatory agencies. Implementing standardised safety assessments, dosage guidelines, and protocols would enhance global trust and acceptance of these natural remedies among the medical community. Furthermore, developing comprehensive databases on phytochemicals and their neurological effects helps expedite medication discovery and facilitate subsequent clinical studies. The future of phytomedicines in the treatment of brain illnesses appears to be a synthesis of traditional knowledge and contemporary research. Phytomedicine may play a

pivotal role in the global pursuit of safer, more comprehensive therapies for neurological disorders through interdisciplinary research and innovative technology. If we continue to invest in it and maintain our curiosity, the natural world could fundamentally alter our approach to brain health.

CONCLUSION

The examination of phytomedicines in alleviating the symptoms of brain disorders such as huntington's disease, alzheimer's disease, amyotrophic lateral sclerosis, parkinson's disease, and age-related cerebral ischaemia, demonstrates the efficacy of plant-derived compounds in addressing various neurological issues. A comprehensive examination of phytochemicals and their mechanisms reveals that these natural compounds can modulate neuroinflammatory pathways, oxidative stress, and neurodegenerative processes, all of which are critical components in the development of neurological disorders. This demonstrates the continued relevance of ethnopharmacological knowledge in contemporary neuroscience and medicine. The chapter discusses the efficacy of phytomedicines in conjunction with other treatment modalities. Phytomedicines can enhance the efficacy of conventional pharmacological therapies and mitigate the likelihood of adverse effects; nonetheless, they should not serve as substitutes for these treatments.

This synergistic approach enhances therapeutic options and tailors treatment strategies for individuals with complex neurological disorders. Incorporating multiple case studies and experimental models into this concept enhances its credibility by demonstrating its applicability in real-world scenarios. It is essential to acknowledge the existing issues in the production and utilisation of phytomedicines. To ensure its safety and efficacy in clinical practice, issues such as dosage standardisation, bioavailability, and regulatory oversight must be addressed. The chapter asserts the necessity for more rigorous clinical trials and interdisciplinary collaboration to enhance these treatments, thereby bridging the divide between conventional remedies and contemporary scientific evidence. This chapter ultimately underscores nature's unexploited pharmacological potential and the imperative to address brain illnesses through a holistic, evidence-based approach. Researchers and physicians can enhance the prognosis and quality of life for those afflicted with debilitating neurological disorders by further investigating the therapeutic potential of phytomedicines.

ABBREVIATIONS

AD Alzheimer's disease
ALS amyotrophic lateral sclerosis
ATP Adenosine triphosphate
CA1 cornu ammonis 1
Cu Copper
DATS Dialyl trisulfide
DND delayed neuronal death
EGCG epigallocatechin gallate
HD Huntington Disease
HO-1 heme oxygenase-1

HPA hypothalamic-pituitary-adrenal
HTT Huntingtin
MND Motor neurone disease
NDs Neurodegenerative diseases
PD Parkinson's disease
QOL quality of life
ROS Reactive oxygen species
SOD superoxide dismutase
Zn Zinc
α Alpha
β Beta

REFERENCES

Abdou, H. M., Yousef, M. I., El Mekkawy, D. A., & Al-Shami, A. S. (2016). Prophylactic neuroprotective efficiency of co-administration of *Ginkgo biloba* and *Trifolium pretense* against sodium arsenite induced neurotoxicity and dementia in different regions of brain and spinal cord of rats. *Food and Chemical Toxicology, 94*, 112–127. DOI: 10.1016/j.fct.2016.05.015 PMID: 27234133

Aggarwal, B. B., Gupta, S. C., & Sung, B. (2013). Curcumin: An orally bioavailable blocker of TNF and other pro-inflammatory biomarkers. *British Journal of Pharmacology, 169*(8), 1672–1692. DOI: 10.1111/bph.12131 PMID: 23425071

Ahmad, A., Khan, M. M., Hoda, M. N., Raza, S. S., Khan, M. B., Javed, H., Ishrat, T., Ashafaq, M., Ahmad, M. E., Safhi, M. M., & Islam, F. (2011). Quercetin protects against oxidative stress associated damages in a rat model of transient focal cerebral ischemia and reperfusion. *Neurochemical Research, 36*(8), 1360–1371. DOI: 10.1007/s11064-011-0458-6 PMID: 21472457

Ahmad, S., Khan, M. B., Hoda, M. N., Bhatia, K., Haque, R., Fazili, I. S., Jamal, A., Khan, J. S., & Katare, D. P. (2012). Neuroprotective effect of sesame seed oil in 6-hydroxydopamine induced neurotoxicity in mice model: Cellular, biochemical and neurochemical evidence. *Neurochemical Research, 37*(3), 516–526. DOI: 10.1007/s11064-011-0638-4 PMID: 22089932

Akhondzadeh, S., Noroozian, M., Mohammadi, M., Ohadinia, S., Jamshidi, A. H., & Khani, M. (2003). Salvia officinalis extract and cognition in Alzheimer's disease: A randomized, controlled trial. *Journal of Clinical Pharmacy and Therapeutics, 28*(1), 53–58. DOI: 10.1046/j.1365-2710.2003.00463.x PMID: 12605619

Al-Chalabi, A., van den Berg, L. H., & Veldink, J. (2017). Gene discovery in amyotrophic lateral sclerosis: Implications for clinical management. *Nature Reviews. Neurology, 13*(2), 96–104. DOI: 10.1038/nrneurol.2016.182 PMID: 27982040

Albin, R. L. (2006). Parkinson's disease: Background, diagnosis, and initial management. *Clinics in Geriatric Medicine, 22*(4), 735–751. DOI: 10.1016/j.cger.2006.06.003 PMID: 17000333

Andrade, S., Ramalho, M. J., Loureiro, J. A., & Pereira, M. D. (2019). Natural compounds for Alzheimer's disease therapy: A systematic review of preclinical and clinical studies. *International Journal of Molecular Sciences, 20*(9), 2313. DOI: 10.3390/ijms20092313 PMID: 31083327

Antunes, M. S., Goes, A. T., Boeira, S. P., Prigol, M., & Jesse, C. R. (2014). Protective effect of hesperidin in a model of Parkinson's disease induced by 6-hydroxydopamine in aged mice. *Nutrition (Burbank, Los Angeles County, Calif.), 30*(11–12), 1415–1422. DOI: 10.1016/j.nut.2014.03.024 PMID: 25280422

Asai, M., Iwata, N., Yoshikawa, A., Aizaki, Y., Ishiura, S., Saido, T. C., & Maruyama, K. (2007). Berberine alters the processing of Alzheimer's amyloid precursor protein to decrease Abeta secretion. *Biochemical and Biophysical Research Communications, 352*(2), 498–502. DOI: 10.1016/j.bbrc.2006.11.043 PMID: 17125739

Bagli, E., Stefaniotou, M., Morbidelli, L., Ziche, M., Psillas, K., Murphy, C., & Fotsis, T. (2004). Luteolin inhibits vascular endothelial growth factor-induced angiogenesis: Inhibition of endothelial cell survival and proliferation by targeting phosphatidylinositol 3′-kinase activity. *Cancer Research*, *64*(21), 7936–7946. DOI: 10.1158/0008-5472.CAN-03-3104 PMID: 15520200

Barwant, M. M., Ogidi, O. I., Singh, S., & Singh, B. (2025). Novel Drug Delivery Methods for Herbal Medicine. In: Farid, A. (Ed.). (2025). Herbal Pharmacopeia: Nanotechnology and Advancing Drug Discovery (1st ed.). CRC Press. https://doi.org/DOI: 10.1201/9781003544418-15

Bastianetto, S., Ramassamy, C., Doré, S., Christen, Y., Poirier, J., & Quirion, R. (2000). The Ginkgo biloba extract (EGb 761) protects hippocampal neurons against cell death induced by β-amyloid. *The European Journal of Neuroscience*, *12*(6), 1882–1890. DOI: 10.1046/j.1460-9568.2000.00069.x PMID: 10886329

Baum, L., Lam, C. W., Cheung, S. K., Kwok, T., Lui, V., Tsoh, J., Lam, L., Leung, V., Hui, E., Ng, C., Woo, J., Chiu, H. F., Goggins, W. B., Zee, B. C., Cheng, K. F., Fong, C. Y., Wong, A., Mok, H., Chow, M. S., & Mok, V. (2008). Six-month randomized, placebo-controlled, double-blind, pilot clinical trial of curcumin in patients with Alzheimer disease. *Journal of Clinical Psychopharmacology*, *28*(1), 110–113. DOI: 10.1097/jcp.0b013e318160862c PMID: 18204357

Baur, J. A., & Sinclair, D. A. (2006). Resveratrol and life-span regulation. *Nature*, *444*(7117), 337–342. DOI: 10.1038/nature05354 PMID: 17086191

Bhattacharya, S. K., & Muruganandam, A. V. (2003). Adaptogenic activity of *Withania somnifera*: An experimental study using a rat model of chronic stress. *Pharmacology, Biochemistry, and Behavior*, *75*(3), 547–555. DOI: 10.1016/S0091-3057(03)00110-2 PMID: 12895672

Cai, M., & Yang, E. J. (2016). Ginsenoside Re attenuates neuroinflammation in a symptomatic ALS animal model. *The American Journal of Chinese Medicine*, *44*(2), 401–413. DOI: 10.1142/S0192415X16500233 PMID: 27080948

Carlini, E. A. (2003). Plants and the central nervous system. *Pharmacology, Biochemistry, and Behavior*, *75*(3), 501–512. DOI: 10.1016/S0091-3057(03)00112-6 PMID: 12895668

Chen, L. L., Song, J. X., Lu, J. H., Yuan, Z. W., Liu, L. F., Durairajan, S. S., & Li, M. (2014). Corynoxine, a natural autophagy enhancer, promotes the clearance of alpha-synuclein via Akt/mTOR pathway. *Journal of Neuroimmune Pharmacology*, *9*(3), 380–387. DOI: 10.1007/s11481-014-9528-2 PMID: 24522518

Chen, X., Zhang, Y., Zhu, J., Ma, L., Dong, Y., & Zhang, M. (2015). Polydatin attenuates nigrostriatal dopaminergic degeneration and motor deficits in a rat model of Parkinson's disease. *Neurochemistry International*, *89*, 49–58. DOI: 10.1016/j.neuint.2015.07.002

Chen, X. C., Zhu, Y. G., Zhu, L. A., Huang, C., Chen, Y., Chen, L. M., Fang, F., Zhou, Y. C., & Zhao, C. H. (2003). Ginsenoside Rg1 attenuates dopamine-induced apoptosis in PC12 cells by suppressing oxidative stress. *European Journal of Pharmacology*, *473*(1), 1–7. DOI: 10.1016/S0014-2999(03)01945-9 PMID: 12877931

Chiu, K., Chan, H. C., Yeung, S. C., Yuen, W. H., Zee, S. Y., Chang, R. C., & So, K. F. (2009). Erratum: Modulation of microglia by Wolfberry on the survival of retinal ganglion cells in a rat ocular hypertension model. *Journal of Ocular Biology, Diseases, and Informatics*, *2*(3), 127–136. DOI: 10.1007/s12177-009-9035-5 PMID: 20046845

Choo, M. K., Park, E. K., Han, M. J., & Kim, D. H. (2003). Antiallergic activity of ginseng and its ginsenosides. *Planta Medica*, *69*(6), 518–522. DOI: 10.1055/s-2003-40653 PMID: 12865969

Chowdhuri, D. K., Parmar, D., Kakkar, P., Shukla, R., Seth, P. K., & Srimal, R. C. (2002). Antistress effects of bacosides of *Bacopa monnieri*: Modulation of Hsp70 expression, superoxide dismutase and cytochrome P450 activity in rat. *Phytotherapy Research*, *16*(7), 639–645. DOI: 10.1002/ptr.1023 PMID: 12410544

Commenges, D., Scotet, V., Renaud, S., Jacqmin-Gadda, H., Barberger-Gateau, P., & Dartigues, J. F. (2000). Intake of flavonoids and risk of dementia. *European Journal of Epidemiology*, *16*(4), 357–363. DOI: 10.1023/A:1007614613771 PMID: 10959944

Cui, Q., Li, X., Zhu, H., & Tian, J. (2016). Curcumin ameliorates dopaminergic neuronal oxidative damage via activation of the Akt/Nrf2 pathway. *Molecular Medicine Reports*, *13*(2), 1381–1388. DOI: 10.3892/mmr.2015.4657 PMID: 26648392

Daliborca, C. V., Dumitrascu, V., Popescu, R., Cimporescu, A., Vlad, C. S., Flangea, C., Grecu, D. S., Vagvolgyi, C., Papp, T., & Horhat, F. (2015). Gas chromatography–mass spectrometry evidences for new chemical insights of *Momordica charantia*. *Revista de Chimie*, *66*, 1914–1920.

Deng, X., Zhao, S., Liu, X., Han, L., Wang, R., Hao, H., Jiao, Y., Han, S., & Bai, C. (2020). Polygala tenuifolia: A source for anti-Alzheimer's disease drugs. *Pharmaceutical Biology*, *58*(1), 73–85. DOI: 10.1080/13880209.2020.1758732 PMID: 32429787

Dereli-Caliskan, N., Husunet, M., Ila, H., & Karagoz, I. (2021). Determination of potential anti-Alzheimer activity of gentiopicroside and isoorientin using molecular docking studies. *Eurasia Proceedings of Science, Technology. Engineering and Mathematics*, *12*, 106–112.

Ekong, E. E., Akpanabiatu, M. I., Ndem, J. I., & Offor, S. J. (2017). Neuroprotective effects of Moringa oleifera leaf extract against aluminium-induced cortical degeneration in rats. *Environmental Toxicology*, *32*(5), 2033–2045. DOI: 10.1002/tox.22418

Elamin, M., Bede, P., Byrne, S., Jordan, N., Gallagher, L., Wynne, B., O'Brien, C., Phukan, J., Lynch, C., Pender, N., & Hardiman, O. (2013). Cognitive changes predict functional decline in ALS: A population-based longitudinal study. *Neurology*, *80*(17), 1590–1597. DOI: 10.1212/WNL.0b013e31828f18ac PMID: 23553481

Ergun, U., Yurtcu, E., & Ergun, M. A. (2005). Protective effect of *Ginkgo biloba* against gossypol-induced apoptosis in human lymphocytes. *Cell Biology International*, *29*(8), 717–720. DOI: 10.1016/j.cellbi.2005.04.005 PMID: 15949956

Farooqui, A. A. (2013). Effect of lifestyle, aging, and phytochemicals on the onset of neurological disorders. In *Phytochemicals, signal transduction, and neurological disorders* (pp. 1–23). Springer., DOI: 10.1007/978-1-4614-3804-5_1

Ferretta, A., Gaballo, A., Tanzarella, P., Piccoli, C., Capitanio, N., & Nico, B.. (2014). Effect of resveratrol on mitochondrial function: Implications in parkin-associated familial Parkinson's disease. *Biochimica et Biophysica Acta (BBA) -. Molecular Basis of Disease*, *1842*(7), 902–915. DOI: 10.1016/j.bbadis.2014.02.010 PMID: 24582596

Gan-Or, Z., Dion, P. A., & Rouleau, G. A. (2015). Genetic perspective on the role of the autophagy lysosome pathway in Parkinson disease. *Autophagy*, *11*(9), 1443–1457. DOI: 10.1080/15548627.2015.1067364 PMID: 26207393

Gao, N., Wadhwani, P., Muhlhauser, P., Liu, Q., Riemann, M., Ulrich, A. S., & Nick, P. (2016). An antifungal protein from *Ginkgo biloba* binds actin and can trigger cell death. *Protoplasma*, *253*(4), 1159–1174. DOI: 10.1007/s00709-015-0876-4 PMID: 26315821

Giordano, G., White, C. C., Mohar, I., Kavanagh, T. J., Costa, L. G., & Cole, T. B. (2011). Neuroprotective effects of rosemary (Rosmarinus officinalis): In vitro studies in human dopaminergic cells. *Journal of Ethnopharmacology*, *134*(2), 498–503. DOI: 10.1016/j.jep.2011.01.041

Guan, R., Zhao, Y., Zhang, H., Fan, G., Liu, X., Zhou, W., Shi, C., Wang, J., Liu, W., Liang, X., Fu, Y., Ma, K., Zhao, L., Zhang, F., Lu, Z., Lee, S. M., Xu, X., Wang, J., Yang, H., & Chen, W. (2016). Draft genome of the living fossil *Ginkgo biloba*. *GigaScience*, *5*(1), 49. DOI: 10.1186/s13742-016-0154-1 PMID: 27871309

Guo, Y., Zhang, K., Wang, Q., Li, Z., Yin, Y., Xu, Q., Duan, W., & Li, C. (2011). Neuroprotective effects of diallyl trisulfide in SOD1-G93A transgenic mouse model of amyotrophic lateral sclerosis. *Brain Research*, *1374*, 110–115. DOI: 10.1016/j.brainres.2010.12.014 PMID: 21147075

Halliwell, B. (1992). Reactive oxygen species and the central nervous system. *Journal of Neurochemistry*, *59*(5), 1609–1623. DOI: 10.1111/j.1471-4159.1992.tb10990.x PMID: 1402908

Hardiman, O., Al-Chalabi, A., Chio, A., Corr, E. M., Logroscino, G., Robberecht, W., Shaw, P. J., Simmons, Z., & van den Berg, L. H. (2017). Amyotrophic lateral sclerosis. *Nature Reviews. Disease Primers*, *3*(1), 17071. DOI: 10.1038/nrdp.2017.71 PMID: 28980624

Harvey, A. L., & Cree, I. A. (2010). High-throughput screening of natural products for cancer therapy. *Planta Medica*, *76*(11), 1080–1086. DOI: 10.1055/s-0030-1250162 PMID: 20635309

Hicks, A., & Jolkkonen, J. (2009). Challenges and possibilities of intravascular cell therapy in stroke. *Acta Neurobiologiae Experimentalis*, *69*(1), 1–11. DOI: 10.55782/ane-2009-1724 PMID: 19325636

Ho, Y. S., So, K. F., & Chang, R. C. C. (2010). Anti-aging herbal medicine—How and why can they be used in aging-associated neurodegenerative diseases? *Ageing Research Reviews*, *9*(3), 354–362. DOI: 10.1016/j.arr.2009.10.001 PMID: 19833234

Ho, Y. S., Yu, M. S., Yang, X. F., So, K. F., Yuen, W. H., & Chang, R. C. C. (2010). Neuroprotective effects of polysaccharides from wolfberry, the fruits of *Lycium barbarum*, against homocysteine-induced toxicity in rat cortical neurons. *Journal of Alzheimer's Disease*, *19*(3), 813–827. DOI: 10.3233/JAD-2010-1280 PMID: 20157238

Ho, Y. S., Yu, M. S., Yik, S. Y., So, K. F., Yuen, W. H., & Chang, R. C. C. (2009). Polysaccharides from wolfberry antagonizes glutamate excitotoxicity in rat cortical neurons. *Cellular and Molecular Neurobiology, 29*(8), 1233–1244. DOI: 10.1007/s10571-009-9419-x PMID: 19499323

Hosseinkhani, A., Sahragard, A., Namdari, A., & Zarshenas, M. M. (2017). Botanical sources for Alzheimer's: A review on reports from traditional Persian medicine. *American Journal of Alzheimer's Disease and Other Dementias, 32*(7), 429–437. DOI: 10.1177/1533317517717013 PMID: 28683559

Hou, X., Liu, Y., Li, C., Zhang, X., & Wu, X. (2022). Honokiol reduces amyloid-β levels and enhances synaptic markers by promoting mitophagy in Alzheimer's model mice. *Neuropharmacology, 201*, 108831. DOI: 10.1016/j.neuropharm.2021.108831

Huang, W., Cheng, P., Yu, K., Han, Y., Song, M., & Li, Y. (2017). Hyperforin attenuates aluminum-induced Aβ production and Tau phosphorylation via regulating Akt/GSK-3β signaling pathway in PC12 cells. *Biomedicine and Pharmacotherapy, 96*, 1–6. DOI: 10.1016/j.biopha.2017.09.114 PMID: 28961505

Huang, W. W., Tsai, S. C., Peng, S. F., Lin, M. W., Chiang, J. H., Chiu, Y. J., Fushiya, S., Tseng, M. T., & Yang, J.-S. (2013). Kaempferol induces autophagy through AMPK and AKT signaling molecules and causes G2/M arrest via downregulation of CDK1/cyclin B in SK-HEP-1 human hepatic cancer cells. *International Journal of Oncology, 42*(6), 2069–2077. DOI: 10.3892/ijo.2013.1909 PMID: 23591552

Iqbal, K., & Grundke-Iqbal, I. (2010). Alzheimer's disease, a multifactorial disorder seeking multi-therapies. *Alzheimer's & Dementia, 6*(5), 420–424. DOI: 10.1016/j.jalz.2010.04.006 PMID: 20813343

Izah, S., Ogidi, O. I., Ogwu, M., Salimon, S., Yusuf, Z., Akram, M., Raimi, M., & Iyingiala, A. (2023). Historical Perspectives and overview of the value of herbal medicine. In: Reference Series in Phytochemistry. Herbal Medicine Phytochemistry. *Springer Nature Singapore Pte Ltd.* DOI: 10.1007/978-3-031-21973-3_1-1

Jain, S., Shukla, S. D., Sharma, K., & Bhatnagar, M. (2001). Neuroprotective effects of *Withania somnifera* Dunal. in hippocampal subregions of female albino rat. *Phytotherapy Research, 15*(6), 544–548. DOI: 10.1002/ptr.802 PMID: 11536389

Javed, H., Vaibhav, K., Ahmed, M. E., Khan, A., Tabassum, R., Islam, F., Safhi, M. M., & Islam, F. (2015). Effect of hesperidin on neurobehavioral, neuroinflammation, oxidative stress and lipid alteration in intracerebroventricular streptozotocin-induced cognitive impairment in mice. *Journal of the Neurological Sciences, 348*(1–2), 51–59. DOI: 10.1016/j.jns.2014.10.044 PMID: 25434716

Jhang, K. A., Park, J. S., Kim, H. S., & Chong, Y. H. (2017). Resveratrol ameliorates tau hyperphosphorylation at Ser396 site and oxidative damage in rat hippocampal slices exposed to vanadate: Implication of ERK1/2 and GSK-3β signaling cascades. *Journal of Agricultural and Food Chemistry, 65*(44), 9626–9634. DOI: 10.1021/acs.jafc.7b03252 PMID: 29022339

Jia, L., Liu, J., Song, Z., Pan, X., Chen, L., & Cui, X.. (2012). Berberine suppresses amyloid β-induced inflammatory response in microglia by inhibiting NF-κB and MAPK signalling pathways. *The Journal of Pharmacy and Pharmacology*, *64*(10), 1510–1521. DOI: 10.1111/j.2042-7158.2012.01529.x PMID: 22943182

Kandezi, N., Mohammadi, M., Ghaffari, M., Gholami, M., Motaghinejad, M., & Safari, S. (2020). Novel insight to neuroprotective potential of curcumin: A mechanistic review of possible involvement of mitochondrial biogenesis and PI3/Akt/GSK3 or PI3/Akt/CREB/BDNF signaling pathways. *International Journal of Molecular and Cellular Medicine*, *9*(1), 1–32. DOI: 10.22088/IJMCM.BUMS.9.1.1 PMID: 32832482

Kang, S., & Min, H. (2012). Ginseng, the 'immunity boost': The effects of *Panax ginseng* on the immune system. *Journal of Ginseng Research*, *36*(4), 354–368. DOI: 10.5142/jgr.2012.36.4.354 PMID: 23717137

Khalil, H., Henafy, H., Khalil, I., Bakr, A., Fahmy, M., Younis, N., & El-Shiekh, R. (2023). *Hypericum perforatum* L. nanoemulsion mitigates cisplatin-induced chemobrain via reducing neurobehavioral alterations, oxidative stress, neuroinflammation, and apoptosis in adult rats. *Toxics*, *11*(159), 159. Advance online publication. DOI: 10.3390/toxics11020159 PMID: 36851034

Khan, A., Vaibhav, K., Javed, H., Khan, M. M., Tabassum, R., & Ahmed, M. E.. (2012). Attenuation of Aβ-induced neurotoxicity by thymoquinone via inhibition of mitochondrial dysfunction and oxidative stress. *Molecular and Cellular Biochemistry*, *369*(1–2), 55–65. DOI: 10.1007/s11010-012-1368-x PMID: 22752387

Khan, M. M., Ahmad, A., Ishrat, T., Khan, M. B., Hoda, M. N., Khuwaja, G., Raza, S. S., Khan, A., Javed, H., Vaibhav, K., & Islam, F. (2010a). Resveratrol attenuates 6-hydroxydopamine-induced oxidative damage and dopamine depletion in a rat model of Parkinson's disease. *Brain Research*, *1328*, 139–151. DOI: 10.1016/j.brainres.2010.02.031 PMID: 20167206

Khan, M. M., Ahmad, A., Ishrat, T., Khuwaja, G., Srivastawa, P., Khan, M. B., Raza, S. S., Javed, H., Vaibhav, K., Khan, A., & Islam, F. (2009). Rutin protects against neural damage induced by transient focal ischemia in rats. *Brain Research*, *1292*, 123–135. DOI: 10.1016/j.brainres.2009.07.026 PMID: 19631195

Khan, M. M., Ishrat, T., Ahmad, A., Hoda, M. N., Khan, M. B., Khuwaja, G., Srivastava, P., Raza, S. S., Islam, F., & Ahmad, S. (2010b). Sesamin attenuates behavioral, biochemical and histological alterations induced by reversible middle cerebral artery occlusion in rats. *Chemico-Biological Interactions*, *183*(1), 255–263. DOI: 10.1016/j.cbi.2009.10.003 PMID: 19835851

Khan, S., Malik, F., Suri, K. A., & Singh, J. (2009). Molecular insight into the immune up-regulatory properties of the leaf extract of Ashwagandha and identification of the Th1 immunostimulatory chemical entity. *Vaccine*, *27*(43), 6080–6087. DOI: 10.1016/j.vaccine.2009.07.011 PMID: 19628058

Kiaei, M., Kipiani, K., Petri, S., Chen, J., Calingasan, N. Y., & Beal, M. F. (2005). Celastrol blocks neuronal cell death and extends life in a transgenic mouse model of amyotrophic lateral sclerosis. *Neurodegenerative Diseases*, *2*(5), 246–254. DOI: 10.1159/000090364 PMID: 16909005

Kim, J., Lyu, Y., Lee, M., & Kang, H. (2006). Neuroprotective effect of some plant extracts in cultured CT105-induced PC12 cells. *Biological & Pharmaceutical Bulletin, 29*(10), 2021–2024. DOI: 10.1248/bpb.29.2021 PMID: 17015944

Kim, M. H., Kim, S. H., & Yang, W. M. (2014). Mechanisms of action of phytochemicals from medicinal herbs in the treatment of Alzheimer's disease. *Planta Medica, 80*(15), 1249–1258. DOI: 10.1055/s-0034-1383038 PMID: 25210998

Koh, S. H., Lee, S. M., Kim, H. Y., Lee, K. Y., Lee, Y. J., Kim, H. T., Kim, J., Kim, M.-H., Hwang, M. S., Song, C., Yang, K.-W., Lee, K. W., Kim, S. H., & Kim, O.-H. (2006). The effect of epigallocatechin gallate on suppressing disease progression of ALS model mice. *Neuroscience Letters, 395*(2), 103–107. DOI: 10.1016/j.neulet.2005.10.056 PMID: 16356650

Kuboyama, T., Tohda, C., Zhao, J., Nakamura, N., Hattori, M., & Komatsu, K. (2002). Axon- or dendrite-predominant outgrowth induced by constituents from Ashwagandha. *Neuroreport, 13*(14), 1715–1720. DOI: 10.1097/00001756-200210070-00005 PMID: 12395110

Kumar, A., Singh, A., & Ekavali, S. (2015). A review on Alzheimer's disease pathophysiology and its management: An update. *Pharmacological Reports, 67*(2), 195–203. DOI: 10.1016/j.pharep.2014.09.004 PMID: 25712639

Kumar, G., Raghavan, A., & Naveen, S. (2014). Phytochemicals having neuroprotective properties from dietary sources and medicinal herbs. *Pharmacognosy Journal, 7*(1), 1–17. DOI: 10.5530/pj.2015.1.1

Kumar, P., & Kumar, A. (2009). Possible neuroprotective effect of *Withania somnifera* root extract against 3-nitropropionic acid-induced behavioral, biochemical, and mitochondrial dysfunction in an animal model of Huntington's disease. *Journal of Medicinal Food, 12*(3), 591–600. DOI: 10.1089/jmf.2008.0028 PMID: 19627208

Kumar, V. (2006). Potential medicinal plants for CNS disorders: An overview. *Phytotherapy Research, 20*(12), 1023–1035. DOI: 10.1002/ptr.1970 PMID: 16909441

Lahane, V. D., & Katekar, L.Vishal D. LahaneVinayak A. Katekar. (2024). Exploring the neuroprotective potential of herbal plants: A comprehensive review. *GSC Biological and Pharmaceutical Sciences, 27*(3), 141–148. DOI: 10.30574/gscbps.2024.27.3.0175

Lavandero, S., Troncoso, R., Riquelme, J. A., & Vicencio, J. M. (2022). Redox modulation of stress resilience by Crocus sativus L. *Mechanisms of Ageing and Development, 205*, 111602. DOI: 10.1016/j.mad.2022.111602 PMID: 35609733

Lee, H., Kim, J. H., & Choi, Y. S. (2023). Palmatine enhances mitophagy and improves mitochondrial function in PS2APP mice. *Neurochemistry International, 155*, 105305. DOI: 10.1016/j.neuint.2023.105305

Liu, Q., Kou, J. P., & Yu, B. Y. (2011). Ginsenoside Rg1 protects against hydrogen peroxide-induced cell death in PC12 cells via inhibiting NF-κB activation. *Neurochemistry International, 58*(1), 119–125. DOI: 10.1016/j.neuint.2010.11.004 PMID: 21078355

Liu, Y. J., Kobayashi, Y., & Li, S. H.. (2006). Therapeutic potential of madecassoside in transgenic mice of amyotrophic lateral sclerosis. *Chinese Traditional and Herbal Drugs*, *37*, 718–720.

Mabjeesh, N. J., Willard, M. T., Harris, W. B., Sun, H. Y., Wang, R., Zhong, H., Umbreit, J. N., & Simons, J. W. (2003). Dibenzoylmethane, a natural dietary compound, induces HIF-1α and increases expression of VEGF. *Biochemical and Biophysical Research Communications*, *303*(1), 279–286. DOI: 10.1016/S0006-291X(03)00336-X PMID: 12646199

Macdonald, I. R., Rockwood, K., Martin, E., & Darvesh, S. (2014). Cholinesterase inhibition in Alzheimer's disease: Is specificity the answer? *Journal of Alzheimer's Disease*, *42*(2), 379–384. DOI: 10.3233/JAD-140219 PMID: 24898642

Mahdy, H. M., Tadros, M. G., Mohamed, M. R., Karim, A. M., & Khalifa, A. E. (2011). The effect of *Ginkgo biloba* extract on 3-nitropropionic acid-induced neurotoxicity in rats. *Neurochemistry International*, *59*(6), 770–778. DOI: 10.1016/j.neuint.2011.07.012 PMID: 21827809

Mandel, S., Weinreb, O., Amit, T., & Youdim, M. B. (2004). Cell signaling pathways in the neuroprotective actions of the green tea polyphenol (–)-epigallocatechin-3-gallate: Implications for neurodegenerative diseases. *Journal of Neurochemistry*, *88*(6), 1555–1569. DOI: 10.1046/j.1471-4159.2003.02291.x PMID: 15009657

Manoharan, S., Guillemin, G. J., Abiramasundari, R. S., Essa, M. M., Akbar, M., & Akbar, M. D. (2016). The role of reactive oxygen species in the pathogenesis of Alzheimer's disease, Parkinson's disease, and Huntington's disease: A mini review. *Oxidative Medicine and Cellular Longevity*, *8590578*(1), 8590578. Advance online publication. DOI: 10.1155/2016/8590578 PMID: 28116038

McKenna, D. J., Jones, K., & Hughes, K. (2001). Efficacy, safety, and use of *Ginkgo biloba* in clinical and preclinical applications. *Alternative Therapies in Health and Medicine*, *7*(5), 70–86. PMID: 11565403

Mioc, M., Prodea, A., Racoviceanu, R., Mioc, A., Ghiulai, R., Milan, A., Voicu, M., Mardale, G., & Soica, C. (2022). Recent advances regarding the molecular mechanisms of triterpenic acids: A review (part II). *International Journal of Molecular Sciences*, *23*(23), 8896. DOI: 10.3390/ijms23168896 PMID: 36012159

Mishra, S., Srivastava, S., Tripathi, R. D., Govindarajan, R., Kuriakose, S. V., & Prasad, M. N. V. (2006). Phytochelatin synthesis and response of antioxidants during cadmium stress in *Bacopa monnieri* L. *Plant Physiology and Biochemistry*, *44*(1), 25–37. DOI: 10.1016/j.plaphy.2006.01.007 PMID: 16545573

Nadège, K., Sylviane, D., Agathe, F., Clarisse, M., Germain, T., David, P., Simon, P., Stéphanie, M., & Élisabeth, N. (2017). Antioxidant properties of *Dichrocephala integrifolia* (Asteraceae) in a mouse model of monosodium glutamate-induced neurotoxicity. *African Journal of Traditional, Complementary, and Alternative Medicines : AJTCAM*, *14*(1), 147–155. DOI: 10.21010/ajtcam.v14i5.18

Nguyen, T., & Alzahrani, T. (2025). Ginkgo Biloba. In *StatPearls*. StatPearls Publishing., https://www.ncbi.nlm.nih.gov/books/NBK548425/

Ock, J., Han, H. S., Hong, S. H., Lee, S. Y., Han, Y. M., Kwon, B. M., & Suk, K. (2010). Obovatol attenuates microglia-mediated neuroinflammation by modulating redox regulation. *British Journal of Pharmacology, 159*(8), 1646–1662. DOI: 10.1111/j.1476-5381.2010.00659.x PMID: 20397299

Ogidi, O. I. (2024). Recent advances in anticancer activity and Bioinformatics Approach from Potential Plants. In: Computational Approaches in Biomaterials, Bioinformatics and Biomedical Engineering Applications. *CRC Press, Taylor and Francis Group, Florida, USA*. DOI: 10.1201/9781003354437-3

Ogidi, O. I. (2025). Natural Products Modulating Mitophagy: Implications for Cancer Therapy. In Pandurangan, A. (Ed.), *Roles of Mitophagy in Cancer Regulation* (pp. 325–358). IGI Global Scientific Publishing., DOI: 10.4018/979-8-3693-3836-0.ch012

Ogidi, O. I., & Ajoko, I. (2024). Neuroprotective Potentials of Phytochemicals. In: M.S. Rajput, T. Sarachana, P.D. Sarkar, M. Raval (eds) NeuroPhytomedicine. *CRC Press, Routledge Taylor and Francis Group.*

Ogidi, O. I., Ajoko, I. T., & Chukwudi, P. (2024b). Natural Antioxidant Compounds for Skin Care. In *Eco-Friendly Skin Solutions for Natural Cosmeceuticals*. IGI Global., DOI: 10.4018/979-8-3693-5473-5.ch008

Ogidi, O. I., Alfred-Ugbenbo, D., & Poripo, B. E. (2025g). AI-Driven Drug Discovery, Design, and Development in Immunological Disorders. In Chen, J. (Ed.), *AI-Assisted Computational Approaches for Immunological Disorders* (pp. 143–180). IGI Global Scientific Publishing., DOI: 10.4018/979-8-3693-9725-1.ch005

Ogidi, O. I., Aye, T., & Felagha, I. (2025c). Antiviral Therapeutics for Emerging Viruses. In Aslam, M., Yingngam, B., Javed, T., & Riaz, S. (Eds.), *Global Perspectives on Antiviral Drug Development* (pp. 217–260). IGI Global Scientific Publishing., DOI: 10.4018/979-8-3693-9276-8.ch006

Ogidi, O. I., Barwant, M. M., & Okara, E. (2024a). Biomarker Discovery: Protein Phosphorylation State. In *Spatially Variable Genes in Cancer: Development, Progression, and Treatment Response*. IGI Global., DOI: 10.4018/979-8-3693-7728-4.ch005

Ogidi, O. I., Christopher, E., & Orlu, H. A. (2025a). Environmental DNA and RNA Metabarcoding: Advancing Insights in Cancer Research. In Raghavan, R. (Ed.), *Cancer Exposomics and Environmental Influences on Carcinogenesis* (pp. 279–322). IGI Global Scientific Publishing., DOI: 10.4018/979-8-3373-2165-3.ch007

Ogidi, O. I., Chukwunonso, O. A., Afakwu-Adimoha, H. C., & Barwant, M. M. (2025b). Ethical Considerations in Generative Artificial Intelligence in Healthcare. In: Generative Artificial Intelligence in Healthcare: Current Practice and Future Development. *CRC Press, Taylor and Francis Group, Florida, USA*. https://doi.org/DOI: 10.1201/9781003488255-5

Ogidi, O. I., Ebong, C. U., & Ikimi, C. G. (2025d). Lifespan-Extending Natural Compounds. In Chen, J. (Ed.), *Drug Discovery and Antiaging Approaches for Human Longevity* (pp. 351–390). IGI Global Scientific Publishing., DOI: 10.4018/979-8-3693-9730-5.ch010

Ogidi, O. I., & Emaikwu, N. G. (2023a). Chapter 1: Adoption and Application of Biotechnology in Herbal Medicine Practices. In: Reference Series in Phytochemistry. Herbal Medicine Phytochemistry. *Springer Nature Singapore Pte Ltd.*

Ogidi, O. I., & Emaikwu, N. G. (2023b). Utilization methods and Practices of herbal Medicine in Africa. In: Reference Series in Phytochemistry. Herbal Medicine Phytochemistry. *Springer Nature Singapore Pte Ltd.* DOI: 10.1007/978-3-031-21973-3_7-1

Ogidi, O. I., & Emaikwu, N. G. (2024). Plant Phenolic compound isolation and its Bioinformatics Approaches of Molecular Mechanisms in Antimicrobial activities and Resistance. In: Computational Approaches in Biomaterials, Bioinformatics and Biomedical Engineering Applications. *CRC Press, Taylor and Francis Group, Florida, USA.* DOI: 10.1201/9781003354437-8

Ogidi, O. I., Erho, S. A., & Omu, O. (2025h). Reactive Oxygen Species in Cancer. In Prabhakar, P. (Ed.), *The Role of Reactive Oxygen Species in Human Health and Disease* (pp. 339–376). IGI Global Scientific Publishing., DOI: 10.4018/979-8-3693-7919-6.ch010

Ogidi, O. I., Ijere, N. D., & Sogoi, P. B. (2025i). Neural and Endocrine Regulation of Immunity. In Reddy, K. (Ed.), *Research Methodologies and Practical Applications in Psychoneuroimmunology* (pp. 17–42). IGI Global Scientific Publishing., DOI: 10.4018/979-8-3693-7432-0.ch002

Ogidi, O. I., Ogoun, T. R., Alex, E. I., Edward, R. B., Joshua, M. T., & Bunu, E. M. (2024c). Radiogenomics and Genetic Diversity of Glioblastoma Characterization. In: Radiomics and Radiogenomics in Neuro-Oncology: An Artificial Intelligence Paradigm- volume 2: Genetics and clinical applications. *Elsevier.* https://doi.org/DOI: 10.1016/B978-0-443-18509-0.00002-5

Ogidi, O. I., Okara, E., & Barwant, M. M. (2025e). Nanocarriers in Plant Genetic Engineering. In Chen, J. (Ed.), *Nanocarriers in Plant Science and Agriculture* (pp. 89–124). IGI Global Scientific Publishing., DOI: 10.4018/979-8-3693-9869-2.ch004

Ogidi, O. I., Orlu, H. A., & Ajoko, I. T. (2025f). Antimicrobial Properties of Secondary Metabolites. In Alexiou, A., Jha, S., & Pandey, R. (Eds.), *Secondary Metabolites and Their Applications in Various Diseases* (pp. 277–324). IGI Global Scientific Publishing., DOI: 10.4018/979-8-3693-9112-9.ch009

Oliveira, A., Pinho, C., Sarmento, B., & Dias, A. (2016). Neuroprotective activity of *Hypericum perforatum* and its major components. *Frontiers in Plant Science*, *7*, 1004. DOI: 10.3389/fpls.2016.01004 PMID: 27462333

Ono, K., Hasegawa, K., Naiki, H., & Yamada, M. (2004). Curcumin has potent anti-amyloidogenic effects for Alzheimer's β-amyloid fibrils in vitro. *Journal of Neuroscience Research*, *75*(6), 742–750. DOI: 10.1002/jnr.20025 PMID: 14994335

Ozbal, S., Erbil, G., Koçdor, H., Tuğyan, K., Pekçetin, C., & Ozoğul, C. (2008). The effects of selenium against cerebral ischemia–reperfusion injury in rats. *Neuroscience Letters*, *438*(3), 265–269. DOI: 10.1016/j.neulet.2008.03.091 PMID: 18490106

Pan, T., Kondo, S., Le, W., & Jankovic, J. (2008). The role of autophagy-lysosome pathway in neurodegeneration associated with Parkinson's disease. *Brain*, *131*(Pt 8), 1969–1978. DOI: 10.1093/brain/awm318 PMID: 18187492

Park, J. H., Lee, T. K., Ahn, J. H., Shin, B. N., Cho, J. H., Kim, I. H., Lee, J.-C., Kim, J.-D., Lee, Y. J., Kang, I. J., Hong, S., Kim, Y. H., Jeon, Y. H., Lee, Y. L., & Won, M.-H. (2017). Pre-treated *Populus tomentiglandulosa* extract inhibits neuronal loss and alleviates gliosis in the gerbil hippocampal CA1 area induced by transient global cerebral ischemia. *Anatomy & Cell Biology*, *50*(4), 284–292. DOI: 10.5115/acb.2017.50.4.284 PMID: 29354300

Park, Y. S., Jang, H. J., Lee, K. H., Hahn, T. R., & Paik, Y. S. (2006). Prolyl endopeptidase inhibitory activity of unsaturated fatty acids. *Journal of Agricultural and Food Chemistry*, *54*(4), 1238–1242. DOI: 10.1021/jf052521h PMID: 16478242

Patel, N., Rathi, D., & Desai, R. (2024). Ashwagandha (Withania somnifera): Cognitive benefits in neurodegenerative models. *Phytotherapy Research*, *38*(2), 1420–1432. DOI: 10.1002/ptr.7716

Pereira, R., Fachinetto, R., Prestes, A., Puntel, R., Silva, G., Heinzmann, B., Boschetti, T., Athayde, M., Burger, M., & Morel, A.. (2008). Antioxidant effects of different extracts from *Melissa officinalis, Matricaria recutita*, and *Cymbopogon citratus. Neurochemical Research*, *34*(5), 973–983. DOI: 10.1007/s11064-008-9861-z PMID: 18853256

Phukan, J., Elamin, M., Bede, P., Jordan, N., Gallagher, L., Byrne, S., Lynch, C., Pender, N., & Hardiman, O. (2012). The syndrome of cognitive impairment in amyotrophic lateral sclerosis: A population-based study. *Journal of Neurology, Neurosurgery, and Psychiatry*, *83*(1), 102–108. DOI: 10.1136/jnnp-2011-300188 PMID: 21836033

Polo-Hernández, E., Tello, V., Arroyo, A. A., Domínguez-Prieto, M., de Castro, F., Tabernero, A., & Medina, J. M. (2014). Oleic acid synthesized by stearoyl-CoA desaturase (SCD-1) in the lateral periventricular zone of the developing rat brain mediates neuronal growth, migration and the arrangement of prospective synapses. *Brain Research*, *1570*, 13–25. DOI: 10.1016/j.brainres.2014.04.038 PMID: 24836198

Popescu, R., Daliborca, C. V., Cimporescu, A., Vlad, C. S., Verdes, D., Botau, D., Filimon, M., Pauliuc, I., Citu, C., & Dumitrascu, V. (2016). Chemical properties and in vitro antitumor effects of *Momordica charantia* extracts in different solvents. *Revista de Chimie*, *67*, 69–73.

Rahman, I., & Chung, S. (2010). Dietary polyphenols, deacetylases and chromatin remodeling in inflammation. *Journal of Nutrigenetics and Nutrigenomics*, *3*(4–6), 220–230. DOI: 10.1159/000324358 PMID: 21474953

Rahman, M. M., Islam, M. T., & Hossain, S. (2024). Neuroprotective effects of ginger via NGF-mediated ERK/CREB activation. *Journal of Neurochemistry*, *151*(1), 95–107. DOI: 10.1111/jnc.16035

Rai, G., Behl, T., & Sehgal, A. (2017). Mucuna pruriens reduces neuroinflammation and protects dopaminergic neurons in MPTP-mice. *Behavioural Brain Research*, *333*, 183–191. DOI: 10.1016/j.bbr.2017.06.022

Raut, A. A., Rege, N. N., Tadvi, F. M., Solanki, P. V., Kene, K. R., Shirolkar, S. G., Pandey, S. N., Vaidya, R. A., & Vaidya, A. B. (2012). Exploratory study to evaluate tolerability, safety, and activity of Ashwagandha (*Withania somnifera*) in healthy volunteers. *Journal of Ayurveda and Integrative Medicine*, *3*(3), 111–114. DOI: 10.4103/0975-9476.100168 PMID: 23125505

Raza, S. S., Khan, M. M., Ahmad, A., Ashafaq, M., Khuwaja, G., Tabassum, R., Javed, H., Siddiqui, M. S., Safhi, M. M., & Islam, F. (2011). Hesperidin ameliorates functional and histological outcome and reduces neuroinflammation in experimental stroke. *Brain Research*, *1420*, 93–105. DOI: 10.1016/j.brainres.2011.08.047 PMID: 21959178

Rehman, M., Wali, A., Ahmad, A., Shakeel, S., Rasool, S., Ali, R., Rashid, S. M., Madkhali, H., Ganaie, M. A., & Khan, R. (2019). Neuroprotective strategies for neurological disorders by natural products: An update. *Current Neuropharmacology*, *17*(3), 247–267. DOI: 10.2174/1570159X16666180911124605 PMID: 30207234

Reinke, A. A., & Gestwicki, J. E. (2007). Structure–activity relationships of amyloid beta-aggregation inhibitors based on curcumin: Influence of linker length and flexibility. *Chemical Biology & Drug Design*, *70*(3), 206–215. DOI: 10.1111/j.1747-0285.2007.00557.x PMID: 17718715

Reitz, C., & Mayeux, R. (2014). Alzheimer disease: Epidemiology, diagnostic criteria, risk factors and biomarkers. *Biochemical Pharmacology*, *88*(4), 640–651. DOI: 10.1016/j.bcp.2013.12.024 PMID: 24398425

Russo, A., & Borrelli, F. (2005). *Bacopa monniera*, a reputed nootropic plant: An overview. *Phytomedicine*, *12*(4), 305–317. DOI: 10.1016/j.phymed.2003.12.008 PMID: 15898709

Sakarwal, A., Sen, K., Ram, H., Chowdhury, S., Kashyap, P., Shukla, S., & Panwar, A. (2024). Neuroprotective efficacy of phytoconstituents of methanolic shoots extract of *Calligonum polygonoides* L. in hypercholesterolemia-associated neurodegenerations. [replace with actual DOI if available]. *Endocrine, Metabolic & Immune Disorders Drug Targets*, *24*, e020424228551. DOI: 10.2174/187153032466624021512 PMID: 38571361

Sampson, E. L., Blanchard, M. R., Jones, L., Tookman, A., & King, M. (2009). Dementia in the acute hospital: Prospective cohort study of prevalence and mortality. *The British Journal of Psychiatry*, *195*(1), 61–66. DOI: 10.1192/bjp.bp.108.055335 PMID: 19567898

Savaskan, E., Olivieri, G., Meier, F., Seifritz, E., & Wirz-Justice, A. (2018). Ginkgo biloba extract EGb 761 improves behavioral and psychological symptoms of dementia: A meta-analysis. *International Psychogeriatrics*, *30*(3), 429–437. DOI: 10.1017/S1041610217001892 PMID: 28931444

Sharma, D. R., Wani, W. Y., Sunkaria, A., Kandimalla, R. J., Sharma, R. K., Verma, D., Bal, A., & Gill, K. D. (2016). Quercetin attenuates neuronal death against aluminum-induced neurodegeneration in the rat hippocampus. *Neuroscience*, *324*, 163–176. DOI: 10.1016/j.neuroscience.2016.02.055 PMID: 26944603

Shinomol, G. K., Mythri, R. B., Srinivas Bharath, M. M., & Muralidhara, H. (2012). *Bacopa monnieri* extract offsets rotenone-induced cytotoxicity in dopaminergic cells and oxidative impairments in mice brain. *Cellular and Molecular Neurobiology*, *32*(3), 455–465. DOI: 10.1007/s10571-011-9776-0 PMID: 22160863

Shrivastava, P., Vaibhav, K., Tabassum, R., Khan, A., Ishrat, T., Khan, M. M., Ahmad, A., Islam, F., Safhi, M. M., & Islam, F. (2013). Anti-apoptotic and anti-inflammatory effect of piperine on 6-OHDA-induced Parkinson's rat model. *The Journal of Nutritional Biochemistry*, *24*(4), 680–687. DOI: 10.1016/j.jnutbio.2012.03.018 PMID: 22819561

Sikora, E., Scapagnini, G., & Barbagallo, M. (2010). Curcumin, inflammation, ageing and age-related diseases. *Immunity & Ageing*, *7*(1), 1. DOI: 10.1186/1742-4933-7-1 PMID: 20205886

Smith, J. A., Luo, Y., & Thomas, M. (2023). Bacopa monnieri supplementation enhances memory and cellular antioxidant defenses in older adults. *Journal of Ethnopharmacology*, *279*, 114482. DOI: 10.1016/j.jep.2021.114482

Song, J. X., Lu, J. H., Liu, L. F., Chen, L. L., Durairajan, S. S., Yue, Z., Zhang, H.-Q., & Li, M. (2014). HMGB1 is involved in autophagy inhibition caused by SNCA/α-synuclein overexpression: A process modulated by the natural autophagy inducer corynoxine B. *Autophagy*, *10*(1), 144–154. DOI: 10.4161/auto.26751 PMID: 24178442

Song, J. X., Sun, Y. R., Peluso, I., Zeng, Y., Yu, X., Lu, J. H., Xu, Z., Wang, M.-Z., Liu, L.-F., Huang, Y.-Y., Chen, L.-L., Durairajan, S. S. K., Zhang, H.-J., Zhou, B., Zhang, H.-Q., Lu, A., Ballabio, A., Medina, D. L., Guo, Z., & Li, M. (2016). A novel curcumin analog binds to and activates TFEB in vitro and in vivo independent of MTOR inhibition. *Autophagy*, *12*(8), 1372–1389. DOI: 10.1080/15548627.2016.1179404 PMID: 27172265

Szlachcic, W. J., Switonski, P. M., Krzyzosiak, W. J., Figlerowicz, M., & Figiel, M. (2015). Huntington disease iPSCs show early molecular changes in intracellular signaling, the expression of oxidative stress proteins and the p53 pathway. *Disease Models & Mechanisms*, *8*(9), 1047–1057. DOI: 10.1242/dmm.019406 PMID: 26092128

Turkez, H., Arslan, M., Stefano, A., Cacciatore, I., & Mardinoglu, A. (2020). Nonpharmacological treatment options for Alzheimer's disease: From animal testing to clinical studies. *Turkish Journal of Zoology*, *44*(2), 81–89. DOI: 10.3906/zoo-1911-32

Urbain, A., Marston, A., Grilo, L. S., Bravo, J., Purev, O., Purevsuren, B., Batsuren, D., Reist, M., Carrupt, P.-A., & Hostettmann, K. (2008). Xanthones from *Gentianella amarella* ssp. *acuta* with acetylcholinesterase and monoamine oxidase inhibitory activities. *Journal of Natural Products*, *71*(5), 895–897. DOI: 10.1021/np070690l PMID: 18336006

Vauzour, D. (2012). Dietary polyphenols as modulators of brain functions: Biological actions and molecular mechanisms underpinning their beneficial effects. *Oxidative Medicine and Cellular Longevity*, *914273*, 1–16. Advance online publication. DOI: 10.1155/2012/914273 PMID: 22701758

Vongthip, S., Suksamrarn, A., & Phuttharak, W. (2024). Luteolin regulates mitophagy and reduces oxidative stress in HT-22 cells exposed to amyloid-beta. *Journal of Cellular Biochemistry*, *125*(2), 209–221. DOI: 10.1002/jcb.30234

Walker, F. O. (2007). Huntington's disease. *Lancet*, *369*(9557), 218–228. DOI: 10.1016/S0140-6736(07)60111-1 PMID: 17240289

Wang, J., Xu, H. M., Yang, H. D., Du, X. X., Jiang, H., & Xie, J. X. (2009). Rg1 reduces nigral iron levels of MPTP-treated C57BL/6 mice by regulating certain iron transport proteins. *Neurochemistry International*, *54*(1), 43–48. DOI: 10.1016/j.neuint.2008.10.003 PMID: 19000728

Wang, X., Yang, Y., Liu, Q., & Zhao, W. (2023). Berberine promotes mitophagy and reduces neuroinflammation in APP/PS1 mice. *Neurobiology of Aging*, *126*, 56–65. DOI: 10.1016/j.neurobiolaging.2023.04.002

Wasner, M., Klier, H., & Borasio, G. D. (2001). The use of alternative medicine by patients with amyotrophic lateral sclerosis. *Journal of the Neurological Sciences*, *191*(1–2), 151–154. DOI: 10.1016/S0022-510X(01)00615-3 PMID: 11677007

Webber, K. M., Raina, A. K., Marlatt, M. W., Zhu, X., Prat, M. I., Morelli, L., Casadesus, G., Perry, G., & Smith, M. A. (2005). The cell cycle in Alzheimer disease: A unique target for neuropharmacology. *Mechanisms of Ageing and Development*, *126*(10), 1019–1025. DOI: 10.1016/j.mad.2005.03.024 PMID: 15936057

Wilson, W. J., & Poellinger, L. (2002). The dietary flavonoid quercetin modulates HIF-1 alpha activity in endothelial cells. *Biochemical and Biophysical Research Communications*, *293*(1), 446–450. DOI: 10.1016/S0006-291X(02)00244-9 PMID: 12054621

Wojtunik-Kulesza, K. (2022). Toxicity of selected monoterpenes and essential oils rich in these compounds. *Molecules (Basel, Switzerland)*, *27*(6), 1716. DOI: 10.3390/molecules27051716 PMID: 35268817

Wong, V. K., Wu, A. G., Wang, J. R., Liu, L., & Law, B. Y. (2015). Neferine attenuates the protein level and toxicity of mutant huntingtin in PC-12 cells via induction of autophagy. *Molecules (Basel, Switzerland)*, *20*(3), 3496–3514. DOI: 10.3390/molecules20033496 PMID: 25699594

Wu, C. R., Tsai, C. W., Chang, S. W., Lin, C. Y., Huang, L. C., & Tsai, C. W. (2015). Carnosic acid protects against 6-hydroxydopamine-induced neurotoxicity in in vivo and in vitro model of Parkinson's disease: Involvement of antioxidative enzymes induction. *Chemico-Biological Interactions*, *225*, 40–46. DOI: 10.1016/j.cbi.2014.11.011 PMID: 25446857

Xia, J., Wang, H., Zhang, Q. M., Zheng, Z., & Han, Z. M. (2016). The therapeutic effect of curcumin in male albino rats and its putative mechanisms on cerebral microvascular flow. *Brain Research*, *1642*, 131–135. DOI: 10.1016/j.brainres.2016.03.022 PMID: 27017961

Xu, J., Zhang, H., Yang, F., & Yu, J. X. (2013). Intervention effect of berberine on expressions of TNF-alpha and receptor type I in Abeta25-35-induced inflammatory reaction in SH-SY5Y cell lines. *Zhongguo Zhongyao Zazhi*, *38*(9), 1327–1330. PMID: 23944062

Xu, W., Liu, J., Ma, D., Yuan, G., Lu, Y., & Yang, Y. (2017). Capsaicin reduces Alzheimer-associated tau changes in the hippocampus of type 2 diabetes rats. *PLoS One*, *12*(2), e0172477. DOI: 10.1371/journal.pone.0172477 PMID: 28225806

Yang, F., Lim, G. P., Begum, A. N., Ubeda, O. J., Simmons, M. R., Ambegaokar, S. S., Chen, P., Kayed, R., Glabe, C. G., Frautschy, S. A., & Cole, G. M. (2005). Curcumin inhibits formation of amyloid β oligomers and fibrils, binds plaques, and reduces amyloid in vivo. *The Journal of Biological Chemistry*, *280*(7), 5892–5901. DOI: 10.1074/jbc.M404751200 PMID: 15590663

Yao, Y., Liu, T., Zhuang, Z., & Zhang, H. (2022). Salidroside improves mitochondrial function and induces mitophagy through SIRT3 in Alzheimer's model mice. *Journal of Alzheimer's Disease*, *88*(3), 917–932. DOI: 10.3233/JAD-220389

Yao, Z. X., Han, Z., Drieu, K., & Papadopoulos, V. (2004). *Ginkgo biloba* extract (EGb 761) inhibits beta-amyloid production by lowering free cholesterol levels. *The Journal of Nutritional Biochemistry*, *15*(12), 749–756. DOI: 10.1016/j.jnutbio.2004.06.008 PMID: 15607648

Yiu, E. M., Tai, G., Peverill, R. E., Lee, K. J., Croft, K. D., Mori, T. A., & Corben, L. A. (2015). Resveratrol improves neurological function in Friedreich's ataxia patients: A randomized, open-label study. *Journal of Neurology*, *262*(5), 1139–1147. DOI: 10.1007/s00415-015-7689-y PMID: 25845763

Yousuf, S., Atif, F., Ahmad, M., Hoda, N., Ishrat, T., Khan, B., & Islam, F. (2009). Resveratrol exerts its neuroprotective effect by modulating mitochondrial dysfunctions and associated cell death during cerebral ischemia. *Brain Research*, *1250*, 242–253. DOI: 10.1016/j.brainres.2008.10.068 PMID: 19027723

Yu, M. S., Leung, S. K. Y., Lai, S. W., Che, C. M., Zee, S. Y., So, K. F., Yuen, W. H., & Chang, R. C. C. (2005). Neuroprotective effects of anti-aging oriental medicine *Lycium barbarum* against β-amyloid peptide neurotoxicity. *Experimental Gerontology*, *40*(8–9), 716–727. DOI: 10.1016/j.exger.2005.06.010 PMID: 16139464

Zbarsky, V., Datla, K. P., Parkar, S., Rai, D. K., Aruoma, O. I., & Dexter, D. T. (2005). Neuroprotective properties of the natural phenolic antioxidants curcumin and naringenin but not quercetin and fisetin in a 6-OHDA model of Parkinson's disease. *Free Radical Research*, *39*(10), 1119–1125. DOI: 10.1080/10715760500233113 PMID: 16298737

Zhang, L., Fiala, M., Cashman, J., Sayre, J., Espinosa, A., Mahanian, M., Zaghi, J., Badmaev, V., Graves, M. C., Bernard, G., & Rosenthal, M. (2006). Curcuminoids enhance amyloid-beta uptake by macrophages of Alzheimer's disease patients. *Journal of Alzheimer's Disease*, *10*(1), 1–7. DOI: 10.3233/JAD-2006-10101 PMID: 16988474

Zhang, Y., Wang, Y., & Zhao, M. (2021). Tanshinone IIA activates Nrf2/HO-1 and enhances survival of dopaminergic neurons. *Phytomedicine*, *80*, 153372. DOI: 10.1016/j.phymed.2020.153372

Zhao, R., Wang, X., Zhang, Q., & Li, M. (2024). Resveratrol activates the SIRT1–PGC1α pathway to regulate mitophagy in an ALS mouse model. *Journal of Neurochemistry*, *169*(1), 99–113. DOI: 10.1111/jnc.15984

Zhou, H., Beevers, C. S., & Huang, S. (2011). Targets of curcumin. *Current Drug Targets*, *12*(3), 332–347. DOI: 10.2174/138945011794815356 PMID: 20955148

Zhu, F., Wu, F., Ma, Y., Liu, G., Li, Z., Sun, Y., & Pei, Z. (2011). Decrease in the production of β-amyloid by berberine inhibition of the expression of β-secretase in HEK293 cells. *BMC Neuroscience*, *12*(1), 125. DOI: 10.1186/1471-2202-12-125 PMID: 22152059

Chapter 15 Phytomedicinal Approaches to Mitigating Neurological Disorder: A Promising Avenue

Tahniyat Ansari
https://orcid.org/0009-0008-5474-0852
CMP College, University of Allahabad, Prayagraj, India

Rupal Shukla
https://orcid.org/0009-0007-5153-1636
CMP College, University of Allahabad, Prayagraj, India

Sudhi Shrivastava
https://orcid.org/0009-0008-5474-0852
CMP College, University of Allahabad, Prayagraj, India

Ratnesh Kumar Soni
https://orcid.org/0000-0002-5774-8664
K.N. Government P.G. College, Gyanpur Bhadohi, India

ABSTRACT

Neurodegenerative disorder such as Parkinson's disease, Alzheimer's disease, Huntington's disease, and ALS, increasing globally; marked by progressive neuronal damage, severe impairments such as cognitive, learning, memory loss, and motor functions. Pharmaceutical drugs have limited success due to side effects and inefficacy. Phytomedicines, plant-based therapies recognize for their many bioactive components with neuroprotective, anti-inflammatory, antioxidant, and neurogenic qualities. Over 80% of people globally use herbal remedies for health issues and traditional Indian texts emphasizes rich source for such treatments. Plant like Withania somnifera, Bacopa monnieri, Curcuma longa, Centella asiatica, Ocimum sanctum, and others contain complex phytochemical substances with medicinal qualities, such as alkaloids, phenylpropanoids, and isoprenoids. The chapter examine how phytomedicines contribute in managing neurodegenerative diseases. Herbal remedies offer a promising, holistic alternative to synthetic drugs.

DOI: 10.4018/979-8-3373-4627-4.ch015

INTRODUCTION

Information is conveyed throughout the entire human body via a specific network of neurons. Neurons facilitate the coordination of all fundamental aspects of life by using chemical and electrical impulses. An electrical or chemical signal is sent from a neuron passes to the adjoining cell via its axon. Each neuron is linked to a thousand others, creating a vast communication network (Fields et al., 2020; Heiney et al., 2021). The rapid loss of brain components, such as cognitive and motor neuron function can be lost rapidly due to neurodegenerative illnesses, posing a serious challenge for the elderly (Puri et al., 2022).

The phrase "neurodegenerative disorders" refers to a group of ailments that arise from the gradual loss of normal neuronal structure and function, primarily in the central nervous system (Srivastava et al., 2016).

These disorders linked to Neurological Diseases (NDs) in various anatomical regions of the brain through multiple pathways, such as neuroinflammation, protein aggregation, mitochondrial damage, and oxidative stress (Di et al., 2019; Harischandra et al., 2019; Fu et al., 2018). There are common characteristics and causes among neurodegenerative disorders, despite their diverse clinical manifestations. These features include nuclear or cytosolic protein aggregation at the regional level. Intracellular hyperphosphorylated tau inclusions that bind microtubules and external amyloid-beta (Aβ) plaques are form in Alzheimer Disease (Katsumoto et al., 2019; Roda et al., 2022). The presence of TAR DNA-binding protein (TDP)-43 transactive response in ALS, frontotemporal dementia, and other associated conditions; the intracellular storage of α-synuclein in Parkinson's disease; and the accumulation of polyglutamine protein aggregates in Huntington's Disease (HD) and other repeat CAG-polyglutamine diseases (Arnold et al., 2013; Toyoshima and Takahashi, 2014). These disorders account for 3% of the global burden of disease (Puri et al., 2022).

People with NDs have a wide range of symptoms that frequently overlap, from cognitive and memory impairment to problems walking, talking, and breathing. Advancing age and certain genetic variants are recognized risk factors for neurological disorders. Gender, low educational attainment, endocrine disorders, oxidative stress, inflammation, stroke, hypertension, diabetes, smoking, head trauma, depression, infections, malignancies, vitamin deficiencies, immunological and metabolic disorders, and chemical exposure are some of the more likely causes of NDs (Brown et al., 2005). In the fight against NDs, a great deal of research has tried to elucidate the procedure and possible therapeutic goals. Although a number of strategies have been employed to manage NDs, none of them have been proven to be an effective treatment, even if the majority of them improve health status (Moise et al., 2024). Plant derived components or phytomedicines such as alkaloids and flavonoids have been extensively used as remedies for NDs since ancient times (Srivastava et al., 2019). This chapter gives a broad overview of current scientific understanding and clinical evidence demonstrating the effectiveness of phytomedicines to treat and cure a range of neurodegenerative illnesses in ameliorating the manifestations of brain disorders.

A Brief Account of NDs

Neurological diseases (NDs) significantly affect health around the world. When neurons in the brain and spinal cord start to deteriorate, NDs arise (Vellingiri et al., 2024). A total of 12% of deaths worldwide are caused by neurological conditions. Cerebrovascular disorders account

for 85% of these deaths, making them a major contributing factor to mortality from neurological disorders (Wahid et al., 2020). NDs can be categorized on the basis of pathogenic protein deposited (such as tau, amyloid, alpha-synuclein, and TDP-43) or by the clinical symptoms present (such as cognitive decline, hyperkinetic, and hypokinetic movements disorder) (Khatri et al., 2021). The highly observed NDs depicted in Figure 1 in India. NDs are of several types.

Figure 1. Diagram showing the common type of neurological disorders

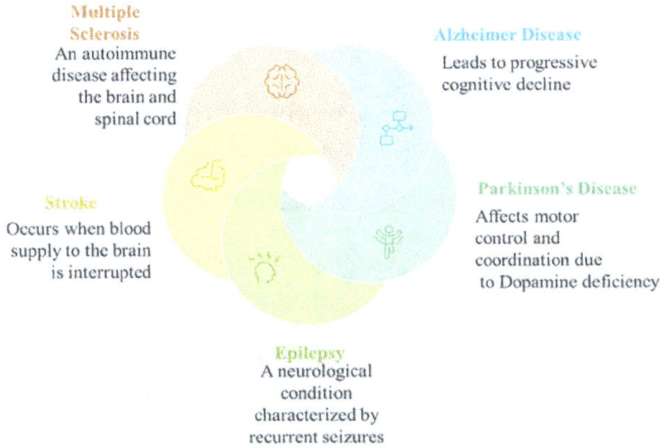

Alzheimer's Disease

Alzheimer's disease (AD) named in honor of Alois Alzheimer, the German psychiatrist, is the most prevalent kind of dementia; which is a gradually progressive neurodegenerative conditions marked by neuritic plaques and neurofibrillary tangles brought on by the buildup of amyloid-beta peptide in the brain's most affected region, the medial temporal lobe, as well as neocortical structures (De-Paula et al., 2012). AD or other conditions like intoxication, infections, abnormalities in the pulmonary and circulatory systems that reduce the amount of oxygen reaching the brain, vitamin B12 deficiency, tumors, and nutritional deficiencies can all contribute to a progressive loss of cognitive abilities (Terry et al., 1980; Rathmann et al., 1984). AD is the sixth most common cause of mortality in the US and is a deadly type of dementia (Taylor et al., 2017). Recent data indicates that around 14.2% of people over 60 who live in underdeveloped countries account for nearly 70% of the disease's overall prevalence (Ravindranath et al., 2021). Gene mutation or inheritance is a major risk factor for the development of AD (Giri et al., 2016). AD is primarily caused by the gradual decline of cognitive function brought on by the degeneration of synapses and neurons. In Figure 2 diagram showing the cause of AD. The precise mechanisms underlying AD remain unclear. According to the AD hypothesis, tau aggregation is linked to A1 in a neurotoxic form called A oligomers (Ao), not amyloid plaques, and abnormal amyloid peptide production is what initiates a series of detrimental events. Most research suggests that upregulating amyloid precursor protein (APP) improves cell proliferation and health. Concurrently, tau protein experiences hyperphosphorylation, which modifies the protein and impairs its regulatory

capabilities, ultimately resulting in neuronal death (Venugopal et al., 2020); resulting in cell death and neurological dysfunction. As a result, it is evident that hereditary variables account for more than 70% of AD prevalence (Agarwal & Tripathi, 2014).

Figure 2. Diagram showing the causes of Alzheimer's disease

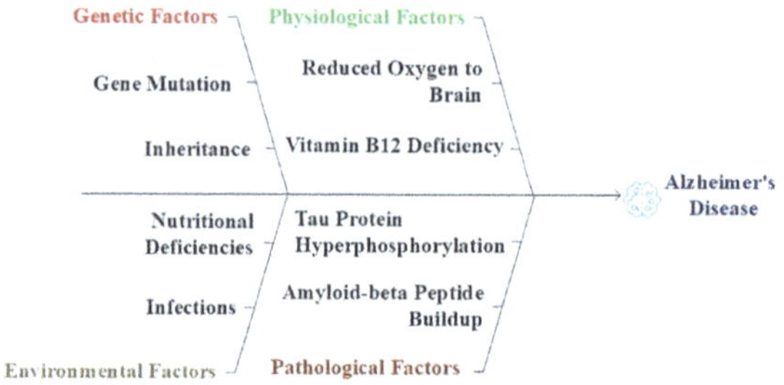

Parkinson's Disease

Roughly 1% of people over 65 have Parkinson's Disease (PD), which is acknowledged as the second most common neurological illness after AD (Lotharius and Brundin, 2002). PD is a degenerative neurological disorder characterized by the death of dopaminergic neurons and the buildup of alpha synuclein protein (Venkatesan et al., 2021; Venkatesan et al., 2022). The intracellular aggregates and aberrant accumulations of the neuronal protein alpha-synuclein are known as Lewy bodies. Parkinson's disease that causes stiffness and slow mobility in the body. Along with non-motor symptoms like depression and autonomic psychosis disorder, the psychiatric diagnosis includes bradykinesia, rest tremors, hypokinesia, and rigidity. Facial rigidity, gait, psychological changes, repetitive motions, lack of blinking, autonomic dysfunction, micrography, neurological and sensory consequences, and muscle atrophy are additional warning signs (Kalia and Lang, 2015). In Figure 3 diagram unveiling the multifaceted nature of PD. PD exact cause is still unknown, but mounting data indicates that intraneuronal alpha synuclein inclusions impair neurons' ability to function normally, ultimately leading to their demise. Numerous mechanisms, including as mitochondrial malfunction, lysosomal impairment, membrane disruption, endoplasmic reticulum stress, and synaptic dysfunction, have been shown to cause neuronal toxicity and neuronal death when alpha synuclein aggregates build up (Roberts and Brown, 2015; Xu and Pu, 2016; Zhang et al., 2018; Zhang et al., 2019).

Figure 3. Diagram unveiling the multifaceted nature of Parkinson's disease

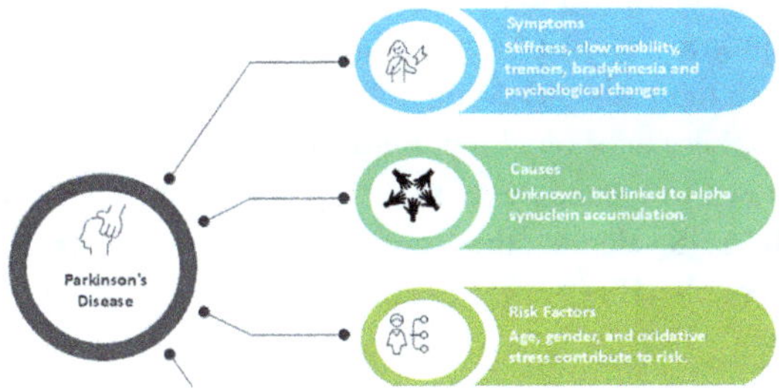

Because estrogen, a sexual hormone, is believed to protect against the onset of Parkinson's disease, men are more likely than women to get the disease (Baldereschi et al., 2000; Eeden et al., 2003). PD progression has been connected to a number of possible oxidative stressors, such as dopamine, mitochondria, endoplasmic reticulum, and α synuclein (Puspita et al., 2017).

Huntington's Disease

Huntington's disease (HD), a rare ND of the central nervous system with a genetic autosomal-dominant inheritance that initially affects the basal ganglia (caudate nucleus and putamen). In HD autonomic nervous system dysfunction, sleep and circadian rhythm abnormalities, and weight damage. The diagram in Figure 4 represents HD: symptoms, genetic factor, and pathological factor. Genetically, HD is caused by an expanded CAG repeat, which encodes abnormally long polyglutamine delayed onset, selective neuronal vulnerability, abnormal protein aggregation and processing, and cellular toxic effects involving both cell autonomous and cell interaction (Begum & Fathima, 2020).

Figure 4. Represents Huntington's disease: symptoms, genetic factor, and pathological factor

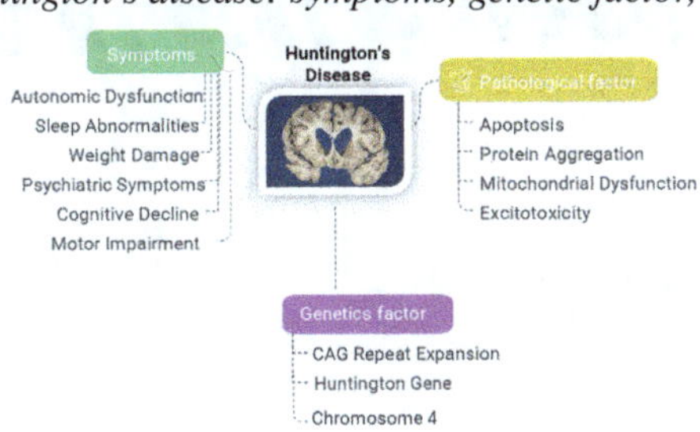

HD is characterized by psychiatric symptoms, cognitive decline, and motor impairment (Martin and Gusella, 1986). The defining feature of HD is a unique choreic movement disease that usually manifests subtly and in the fourth to fifth decade of life and progressively worsens throughout the ten to twenty years leading up to death. There is currently no medication that

can effectively postpone or stop the start and progression of HD because molecular basis for neuronal loss in this debilitating condition has not been identified. The genetic defect causing HD was assigned to chromosome 4 in 1983 (MacDonald et al., 1993). Potential mechanisms that may be connected to the pathophysiology of HD, such as increased apoptosis, detrimental protein aggregation, trophic factor blocking, mitochondrial dysfunction, and excitotoxicity, all of which have been shown to reduce the onset and progression of HD (Vonsattel et al., 2011). According to the NIMHANS scientist, there are around 40,000-70,000 HD patients in India, or 3-5 cases per 100,000 people (Hussain et al., 2020; Gupta et al., 2021).

Epilepsy

The primary characteristic of epilepsy is the recurrence of spontaneous seizures brought on by hyperactivity in the brain. The diagram in Figure 5 showing seizures generation. People with epilepsy may experience crises that affect their ability to function physically, mentally, or behaviorally (Beyhan et al., 2017; Thijs et al., 2019). Individuals with epilepsy have a persistent propensity to have seizures, which impacts their social conduct, mental health, and cognitive abilities (Neri et al., 2022). The prevalence of epilepsy is believed to be 5-9 per 1,000 persons worldwide, and an estimated 70 million people suffer from the condition (Amudhan et al., 2015). Epilepsy is classified as either acquired or idiopathic based on its cause. Childhood is the onset age for idiopathic epilepsy, which has no neurological signs. An aberrant "seizure," a symptomatic disturbance of neurologic function, is caused by the brain's neurons firing abnormally and hypersynchronously (Shorvon et al., 2011; Stafstrom et al., 2015). Due to seizure-related trauma, people with epilepsy are more likely to experience physical issues and to suffer from psychosocial illnesses including sadness and anxiety. Significantly, the risk of dying young is up to three times greater than that of people in the general population (Beghi, 2020).

Figure 5. Showing the seizures generation

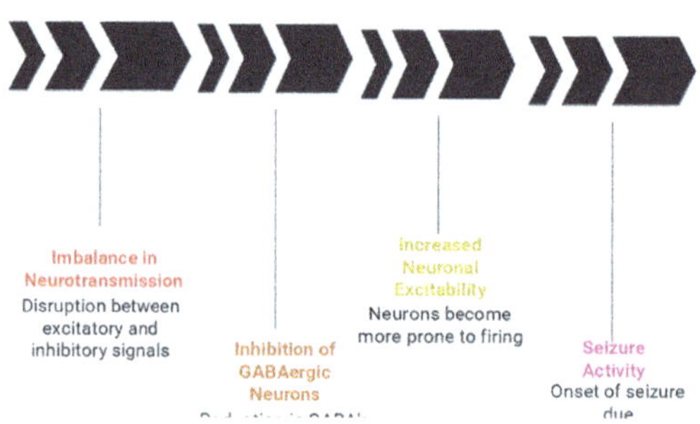

Headache

A headache is a very common complaint, and with a prevalence of 48.9% in the general population, among the most prevalent of the nervous system disorders. Headaches are more common in women. Certain types of headaches are incredibly incapacitating and negatively affect a

person's quality of life, resulting in enormous expenses for healthcare and, consequently, for the overall economy. Nearly 98% of all headaches are primary headache disorders, such as migraine, tension headache, and cluster headache; however, secondary headaches should be recognized since they are dangerous and can even be fatal (Ahmed, 2012). According to the 2010 Global Burden of condition study, tension-type headache (TTH) is the second most frequent condition globally, despite migraine being the primary cause of disability (GBD 2010) (Steiner et al., 2015). Many extrinsic and intrinsic causes, including menstruation, menstrual pains, hunger, thirst, and fatigue from food and drink as well as weather changes, have been shown to cause headaches (Goadsby et al., 2017). Effective treatment relies on educating patients about what triggers migraines (Chakravarty, 2006). The diagram in Figure 6 depicted the clinical characteristics and pathophysiology of headache.

Figure 6. Represents headache pathophysiology and clinical characteristics

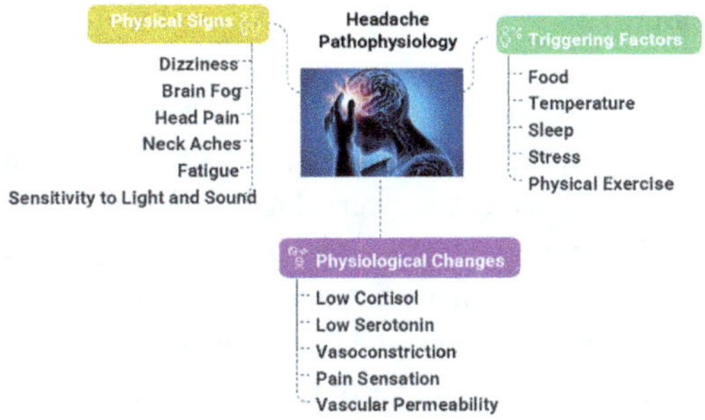

Stroke

Stroke is a dangerous illness that occurs when there is a disruption in the blood supply to the brain, usually due to a blood artery rupturing or a clot blocking it (Tater et al., 2021). This damages brain tissue by cutting off the brain's supply of nutrients and oxygen. The pathophysiology of stroke is defined by two main categories, which are clinical syndromes:

- Ischaemic strokes are caused by an abrupt blockage of the arteries that supply the brain, either because of a thrombus that forms in another area of the circulation or at the location of the blockage. Between 50% and 85% of all strokes globally are caused by it.
- The two main causes of hemorrhagic strokes are intra-cerebral hemorrhage, which is arterial bleeding in the gap between meninges, and subarachnoid hemorrhage, which is bleeding from one of the brain's arteries into the brain tissue. About 1% to 7% and 7% to 27% of all strokes globally fall into this category (Taylor et al., 2012). It ranks fourth globally in terms of disability and is the second most prevalent cause of death (Strong et al., 2007). To date, there have been relatively few reliable estimates of stroke morbidity and mortality in India (Kamalakannan et al., 2015). The diagram in Figure 7 showing a comparative analysis between Ischemic stroke and Hemorrhagic stroke.

Figure 7. Showing a comparative analysis between ischemic stroke and hemorrhagic stroke

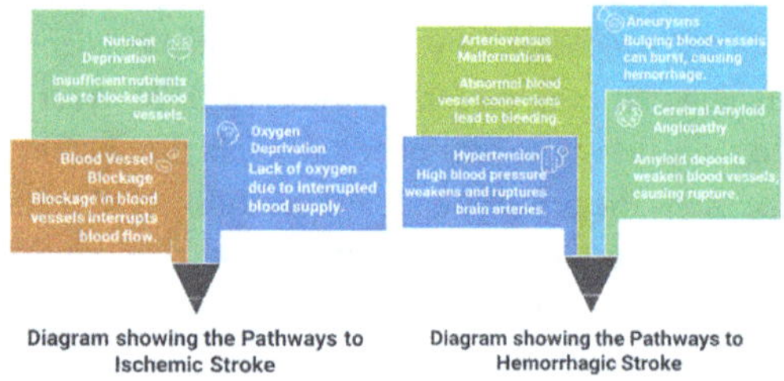

Amyotropic Lateral Sclerosis

The degeneration of both upper motor neurons, or neurons that project from the cortex to the brainstem and spinal cord, and lower motor neurons, or neurons that project from the brainstem or spinal cord to muscle, is a hallmark of amyotrophic lateral sclerosis (ALS), a heterogeneous neurodegenerative disease that causes both motor and extra-motor symptoms. A range of nonmotor symptoms, such as neuropsychiatric symptoms, pain, exhaustion, and sleep difficulties, are also brought on by ALS through direct (related to the involvement of nonmotor neurons) and indirect (secondary to weakening) pathways. As the leading cause of disabilities and illness worldwide in recent decades, neurological illnesses, of which ALS is an example, produce a wide range of disability (Taga et al., 2024). A hexanucleotide repeat increase in C9orf72 (encoding the guanine nucleotide exchange protein C9orf72) has been found, along with frontotemporal dementia FTD5,6, and ALS has been reclassified as a neurological ailment instead of a neuromuscular disease. An increasing body of research indicates that alterations in the structure and biochemistry of the mitochondria impact the pathogenesis of ALS (Chung & Suh, 2002). Patients with ALS can present differently at first; some may have spinal-onset disease, which is characterized by the onset of limb muscle weakness, while others may have bulbar-onset disease, which is characterized by dysphagia (difficulty swallowing) and dysarthria (difficulty speaking). (Keon et al., 2021).

Etiology

The following are the main causes of neurodegenerative diseases (NGDs):

Oxidative Stress

Oxidative stress, which damages cells and compromises the DNA repair pathway, is caused by an imbalanced formation of reactive oxygen species (ROS) and an insufficient antioxidant defence system. Neurodegenerative disease results from either an increase or decrease in oxygen production.

Neuroinflammation

Neurodegeneration is a direct result of an inflammatory process that affects the neurological system, which includes the brain and spinal cord, and both the innate and adaptive immune systems. The process of neuroinflammation may have a role in both neuropathological and normal brain development. Microglia are the main immune defense component in the central nervous system. Microglia quickly acquire the altered shape and activate in response to pathogenic changes in the nervous system. A number of inflammatory mediators, including cytokines, chemokines, and cytotoxic substances like glutamate, prostaglandins, ROS, and cyclo-oxygenase 2 (COX-2), are secreted by microglia. In addition to triggering the neuron to react for its life, these inflammatory mediators will also activate astrocytes to produce a secondary inflammatory or growth factor repair response (Leng & Edison, 2021).

Excitotoxicity

In the central nervous system, excitotoxicity is a degenerative process that leads to neuronal death when excitatory amino acids or excitotoxins excessively or persistently activate glutamate receptors. In addition to binding to glutamate receptors, pathologically elevated glutamate release levels can cause serious excitotoxicity by facilitating the rapid entry of calcium ions into cells. Inducible Nitric Oxide Synthase (iNOS), phospholipases, lipases, protein phosphatases, protein kinases, xanthine oxidases, and endonucleases are a number of calcium-dependent enzymes that are triggered when calcium ions readily pass through. These enzymes eventually damage cell structures linked to the cytoskeleton, membrane, and DNA. Moreover, the production of ROS, defective mitochondria, oxidative stress, and inflammatory responses may all be facilitated by the excessive calcium influx. These processes eventually cause neuronal cells to die.

Abnormal Proteins

NGDs have also been reported to be associated with the aberrant protein in the brain. The brain nerve cells could be destroyed by these abnormal proteins. Research has linked the amyloid protein to the onset of Alzheimer's disease. Synuclein is another abnormal protein linked to multiple system atrophy, Parkinson's disease, and Lewy body dementia (Ross et al., 2004).

Environmental and Genetic Variables

It is believed that a combination of environmental factors, such as frequent exposure to toxins and certain chemicals, and genetic factors causes the majority of neurological problems. In some cases, neurological diseases might arise as a result of defective genes inherited from family members (Armstrong, 2020).

Neuronal Damage or Apoptosis

Neurons are the building blocks of the nervous system, which includes the brain and spinal cord, any damage or loss to these neurons in the brain is assumed to be the cause of NGDs. Damage to some bodily areas prevents neurons from self-replicating. The brain shrinks and

neurons are damaged as people age. Membrane cell death, chromatin condensation, DNA fragmentation, and cell shrinkage are all associated with neuronal apoptosis, a highly structured kind of cell death. ATP is required for the activation, protein synthesis, and signal transmission of this energy-dependent function. Both internal and external stimuli can initiate the complex process of apoptosis. The activation of death receptors upon ligand binding and subsequent signaling via a series of protein-protein interactions comprise the extrinsic route. The intrinsic process propels the change in mitochondrial permeability, which in turn triggers either caspase-dependent or caspase-independent apoptosis to release proapoptotic materials into the cytosol from the mitochondrial intermembrane gaps (Kamboj et al., 2024).

Mitochondrial Dysfunction

The mitochondria help to keep the calcium levels in the cytosol low since they are the locations of oxidative phosphorylation and cellular respiration. Overabundance of calcium absorption and the generation of reactive oxygen species (ROS) are the main causes of the mitochondrial membrane's potential collapse and the opening of the mitochondrial permeability transition pores. Through the mitochondrial permeability transition pores, apoptosis-inducing factor and cytochrome-C are liberated from the mitochondrial intermembrane space and enter the cytosol, causing the outer membrane of the mitochondria to rupture and the mitochondrial matrix to expand. Cytochrome-C forms a large quaternary protein structure with procaspase-9 and apoptotic protease-activating factor-1 in a caspase-related mechanism, which triggers the apoptotic death of nerve cells. The result is the disaggregation of essential cellular substrates, particularly poly (ADP-ribose) polymerase-1 (PARP-1). These changes in mitochondrial function could be a sign that neural cells are about to die (Nissanka et al., 2018). The diagram in Figure 8 showing the complex cause of NDs.

Figure 8. Diagram showing the complex cause of neurodegenerative disease

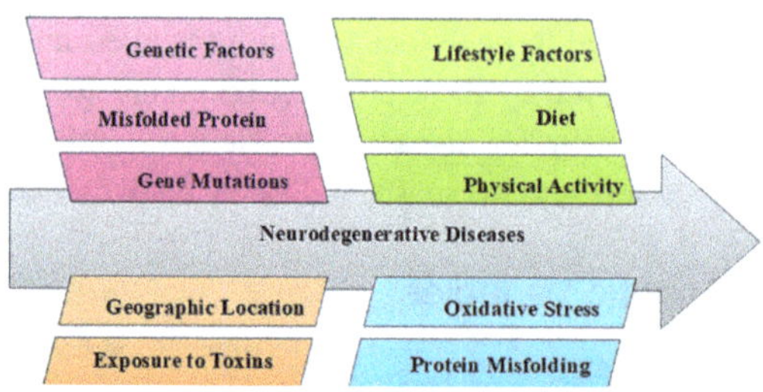

NGDs Symptoms

NGDs can cause damage to the brain and neurological system over time, which can affect a person's temperament, personality, and mental health. These conditions, which take time to develop, impair thinking and memory. As the disease worsens, the symptoms get more severe.

The illustration shown in Figure 9 depicts the symptoms of NDs. The aforementioned symptoms are also common:

- Forgetfulness,
- Apathy,
- Anxiety,
- Agitation,
- Lack of inhibition,
- Memory loss, and
- Behavioral elevation (Kamboj et al., 2024).

Figure 9. Exposing neurodegenerative disease symptoms

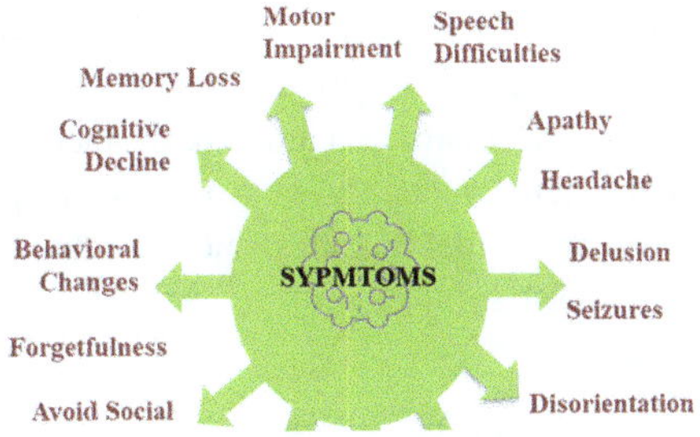

PHYTOMEDICINES IN BRAIN HEALTH

Herbal medicine having therapeutic and healing qualities is known as phytomedicine (Oniyangi et al., 2020). An herbal medicine or a phytopharmaceutical preparation occasionally defined as a medicine are made from whole plants or plant parts and can be produced in a pure pharmaceutical formulation or in a crude form (Andrade et al., 2018). The brain, a marvel of complexity and fragility, is prone to deterioration over time making the investigation of neuroprotective chemicals derived from plants is matter of essential importance. With its complex web of neurons and neurotransmitters, the human brain needs meticulous care to perform at its optimal level and plants, with their wide range of bioactive phytoconstituents, have the power to support this function (Kulesza & Karolina, 2022).

Historical Background and Ethnobotanical Perspective

Phytomedicines has existed from the beginning of human society. Herbal remedies have been used for ages to promote mental and neurological health in traditional medical systems including Ayurveda, Traditional Chinese Medicine (TCM), and Indigenous healing practices in the form of sacred texts such as Rigveda, Yajurveda, Samaveda, and Atharvanaveda (Srivastava & Yadav, 2016). Dating back to approximately 3000 BC, Sheng Nongs Herbal Book is known as one of the

earliest sources of traditional folk knowledge in China based on the usage of herbs. It includes information on about 365 different plants, animals, and minerals that find a place in medication. There are around 420,000 different plant species on Earth, but not much is known about them or their many applications (Pandey et al., 2011; Srivastava et al., 2019). Plants and human civilization have been intertwined with since prehistoric period. Researching plants that have neurological effects is important because it may lead to the identification of new neuroprotective compounds that can improve cognitive function and fight neurodegenerative disorders. Numerous research has been conducted to identify the active molecules that provide the neuroprotective benefits of herbal remedies owing to their promise in the treatment of a variety of disorders (Rehman et al., 2019). Phytoconstituents, such as polyphenolic antioxidants, are present in herbs, fruits, nuts, and vegetables, in addition to freshwater and marine plants. These phytoconstituents have the potential to enhance cognitive function and mind memory while halting neurodegeneration. Additionally, they are believed to be essential in the prevention and treatment of neurodegenerative diseases like AD, epilepsy, and Parkinson's disease (Türkez et al., 2020).

In Figure 10 shows plants that have long been valued for their emotional and cognitive advantages include Ginkgo biloba, Bacopa monnieri (Brahmi), and Withania somnifera (Ashwagandha), Curcuma longa, Centella asiatica, Ocimum sanctum, Nardostachys jatamansi, Emblica officinalis and others. Plant parts like stems, roots, leaves, fruits, flowers, and seeds contain complex phytochemical substances with medicinal qualities, such as alkaloids, phenylpropanoids, and isoprenoids (Srivastava & Yadav, 2016).

Figure 10. Represents role of different plant in improving neurological disorder

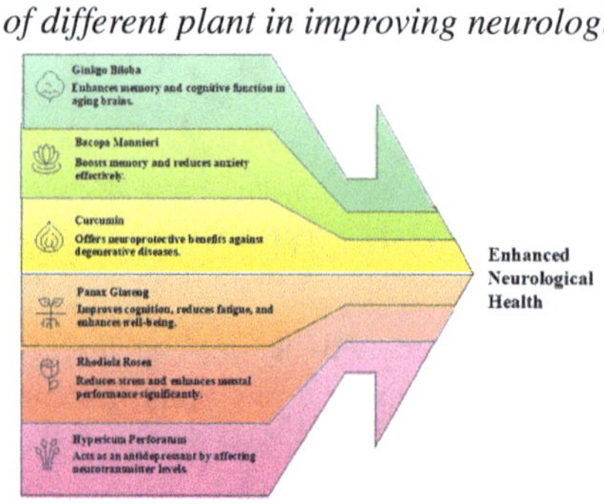

MODE OF ACTION OF PHYTOMEDICINE IN BRAIN DISORDER

Although they may include active chemical elements from various classes or families, botanicals from different families may nonetheless have an impact on the same or different receptors. Figure 11 displays the impacts of phytomedicines on brain function. Multiple mechanisms through which phytomedicines exert their therapeutic effects are:

Figure 11. Showing the phytomedicine's impact on brain function.

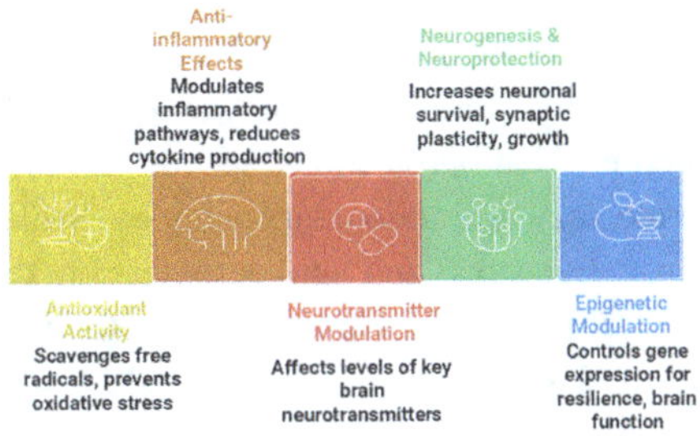

1. **Antioxidant activity:** Prevents oxidative stress, a major contributor to neurodegeneration, by scavenging free radicals.
2. **Anti-inflammatory effects:** Changing inflammatory pathways and cytokine production has anti-inflammatory effects.
3. **Neurotransmitter modulation:** Affecting the levels of acetylcholine, GABA, dopamine, and serotonin.
4. **Neurogenesis and neuroprotection:** Increasing synaptic plasticity, growth, and neuronal survival.
5. **Epigenetic modulation:** Controlling the expression of genes related to resilience and brain function.

KEY PHYTOMEDICINES AND THEIR APPLICATION

Withania somnifera (WS)

It has long been used in Indian traditional medicine, frequently known as ashwagandha (Grandhi et al. 1994) and member of the family Solanaceae. The plant's Sanskrit name, Ashwagandha (Kulkarni and Dhir 2008), comes from the fact that it smells like a sweating horse. The word somnifera comes from Latin name, which means "sleep inducer" which highlight plant's soothing qualities. Furthermore, ashwagandha root powder scavenges free radicals (Sankar et al., 2007).

Active Compounds

The primary chemical components of the plant are alkaloids and steroidal lactones, with a small number of flavonoids, tannins, and other substances. More than a dozen alkaloids, such as withananine, pseudo-withanine, somniferine, and somniferinine, have been identified. Additionally, 40 subtypes of steroidal lactones, also known as withanolides, were identified (Mirjalili et al. 2009; Srivastava et al., 2016).

Mechanism of Action

Withania somnifera's diverse chemical makeup adds to its neuroprotective properties. The plant contains withanolides, alkaloids, steroidal lactones, and glycosides, all of which are essential to its pharmacological properties. Neuroprotection depends on these bioactive substances' immunomodulatory, anti-inflammatory, and antioxidant qualities (Sankar et al., 2007). Antioxidant activity of WS, preventing oxidative stress and lipid peroxidation, therefore preventing damage to erythrocytes (Sandhu et al., 2010). Its neuroprotective potential is further increased by its capacity to alter pathways such as MAP kinase signaling and JAK-STAT (Moise et al., 2024).

Application

Clinical uses for Withania somnifera include investigation as a supplemental therapy for ailments such as Parkinson's disease. Research has demonstrated that Withania somnifera's neuroprotective properties, which result in increased dopamine activity, can help Parkinson's sufferers with their motor symptoms (Nakajima et al., 2011). Animal studies and clinical trials further support the use of WS for a variety of illnesses, including AD, senile dementia, anxiety, and neurological and cognitive impairments. In rats, W. somnifera also has neuroprotective properties against Parkinsonism brought on by 6-OHDA. (Ahmad et al., 2005). Withania somnifera may be useful in treating inflammation, aging, healthy aging, and fertility issues, according to a number of preclinical and clinical research (Basudkar et al., 2024). The steroidal lactone withanolide IV, who's active aglycone ingredient sominone, has been shown to reduce Aβ (25–35)-induced axonal, dendritic, and synaptic losses as well as memory deficits in mice (Kuboyama et al., 2006).

Bacopa monnieri (BM)

Bacopa monnieri **(BM)**, also known asl **Brahmi** a name stemming from Brahma, the creator god of Hinduism. This perennial creeping plant, member of the Scrophulariaceae family, grows in moist, marshy places (Aguiar and Borowski 2013).

Active Compound

Alkaloids like nicotine, herpestine, and brahmine; monnierin, and D-mannitol; hersaponin and other are the chemical components in **BM**. Additionally, BM had significant levels of beta-sitosterol, stigmastarol, betulic acid, bacopaside I, bacopaside II, bacopaside X, bacopasaponin C, and bacopaside N2. The more minor components included bacopasaponin F, bacopasaponin E, bacopaside N1, bacopaside III, bacopaside IV, and bacopaside V.

Mechanisms of Action

The bacosides found in **BM** are typically nonpolar glycosides, which allow them to pass through the blood-brain barrier (BBB) through simple lipid-mediated passive diffusion (Abdul Manap et al., 2019). By preventing a formation of free radicals in the brain, bacosides or extract strengthen the body's defenses against oxidative stress. As a medicinal antioxidant, BM may be able to lower oxidative stress, which could improve cognitive function and provide neuropro-

tection (Simpson et al., 2015). **BM** may enhance memory through various signaling routes and mechanisms in addition to its various active chemical constituents revealed that bacopasides cause membrane dephosphorylation and a rise in protein and RNA turnover in particular brain regions. **BM** demonstrated a protective effect against ischemia-induced memory impairment in the plus maze task, inhibited the shortened transfer latency in ischemic rats in a step through test, and decreased the number of infarcts in the ischemic brain. Significantly increased catalase activity and decreased nitrite, nitrate, and lipid peroxidation were indicators of free radical scavenging, the mechanism underlying this action (Siesjo 1992).

Application

The use of BM for a number of mental health issues, including anxiety, impaired cognition, and lack of focus. Furthermore, research has indicated that it may be used to treat epilepsy and mental disease. Enhancement of the body's antioxidant defense system was attributed to Bacoside A (Anbarsi, et al. 2006) where its optical isomer, bacoside B, exhibits memory-enhancing properties. Bacosides also shield neurons from Aβ-induced toxicity and stop Aβ from aggregating and forming fibril. They have served as anti-aging and traditional medicine (Abdul Manap et al., 2019). It has been demonstrated to improve lipid content, reduce alpha synuclein aggregation, and dopaminergic neurodegeneration in Caenorhabditis elegans (C. elegans) to demonstrate its protective impact against parkinsonian symptoms (Srivastava et al., 2016). It may also be utilized as a treatment for neurodegenerative illnesses, such as Parkinson's disease.

Curcuma longa (CL)

Commonly referred to as "turmeric," used around the world as a spice, food preservative, and coloring agent. *CL* is a plant in the Zingiberaceae family that is prized for both its unique flavor and vivid yellow color (Moise et al., 2024). Curcumin has been proven to be useful in treating Alzheimer's disease, tardive dyskinesia brought on by neuroleptics, and chemically induced neurotoxicity from lead and cadmium (Garcia-Alloza et al.2007; Bishnoi et al. 2008).

Active Compound

CL biological composition, especially its curcuminoids, has drawn attention due to its potential in medical uses. It has been demonstrated that curcumin, the main bioactive ingredient in curcuma longa, has antioxidant qualities and the capacity to alter a number of signaling pathways related to inflammation and cell viability.

Mechanisms of Action

Studies indicates that curcumin can decrease the activation of transcription factors like NF-kappa B, which are involved in neurodegenerative processes, as well as lessen oxidative stress and inflammation. Curcumin has also been shown to activate AMP-activated protein kinases and upregulate the expression of heme oxygenase-1, which are involved in energy metabolism and cellular stress responses (Moise et al., 2024). The phenolic hydroxyl group of curcumin may contribute to the antiamyloidogenic activity. The inhibition of Aβ42 and APP (amyloid precursor

protein) can be observed in phenyl-substituted methoxy groups, and hydrophobic interactions have also been implicated. In addition, phenyl ring elongation may have less of an impact on AD patients (Chainoglou and Hadjipavlou-Litina, 2020).

Application

The anti-inflammatory qualities of Curcuma longa have also been investigated for their possible use in treating diseases like arthritis, where they may help reduce symptoms and enhance joint function (Moise et al., 2024). Curcumin's anti-inflammatory, antimicrobial, and antioxidant properties, make it a promising candidate for the prevention and management of NDs.

Centella asiatica (CA)

CA, also referred to as gotu kola, member of the Apiaceae family and has been used traditionally for medicinal purposes for a long time (Johnson et al., 2023). CA is a perennial herb exerts a significant neuroprotective cardioprotective effect and antigastric ulcer activity. It is also used to treat a variety of conditions, including wound healing, dermatitis, ulcers, leprosy, and insanity (Srivastava et al., 2016).

Active Compound

The plant's primary chemical components are pentacyclic triterpenic acids and their corresponding glycosides, which are either ursane or oleanane in type. These include asiatic acid, asiaticoside, madecassic acid, madecassoside, brahmoside, brahmic acid, brahminoside, thankuniside, isothankuniside, centelloside, madasiatic acid, centic acid, cenellic acid, betulinic acid, and indocentic acid (Zheng et al., 2007). Triterpenes and flavonoids are among the plant's many chemical constituents, which enhance its medicinal potential in preserving the health and function of neurons.

Mechanisms of Action

By strengthening antioxidant defenses and lowering lipid peroxidation, it can control oxidative stress (Choi et al., 2016). Furthermore, Centella asiatica has been demonstrated to control inflammatory mediators such tumor necrosis factor and interleukins, reducing inflammation-induced neuronal damage (Kuswati, 2015). Especially asiaticoside, have anti-apoptotic qualities by blocking the brain's caspase-3 production and other cell death pathways (Ariani et al., 2024).

Application

CA viable option for treating age-related cognitive decline and memory impairment; and effective by lowering oxidative stress and enhancing cognitive function, in Parkinson's and Alzheimer's disease (Kannoor & Ramani, 2020). Additionally, CA has shown antiseizure qualities, which may help treat diseases like epilepsy (Jiang et al., 2016).

Ocimum sanctum (OS)

Known as "Tulsi" or "Tulasi" in Hindi or Holy Basil in English known for its medicinal value in various traditional system of medicine in India, particularly Ayurveda and Unani, belongs to the Labiatae (Lamiaceae) family and is a tiny, upright herb that is typically grown in gardens and temples.

Active Compound

The main chemical components of OS are Rosmarinic acid, oleanolic acid, eugenol, carvacrol, linalool, ursolic acid, and β-caryophyllene. Moreover, OS 15–25% aldehydes and 45–73% phenyl. The stable oil content of seeds is 17.8%. The plant also includes tannins, glycosides, and alkaloids. Carotene and ascorbic acid are present in the leaves (Srivastava et al., 2016).

Mechanisms of Action

Show antioxidant Activity and anti-inflammatory Effect.

Application

A week of treatment with an ethanol extract of OS leaves stopped the noise-induced alterations in the brain's cholinergic characteristics. According to reports, ursolic acid extracted from OS extract lowers free radicals (Srivastava et al., 2016).

Ginkgo biloba (GB)

GB, a well-known ancient Chinese tree in the Ginkgoaceae family, is renowned for its ability to promote health.

Active Compound

Terpenes, flavonoids, organic acids, and other substances are all present in GB. The most significant bioactive component is ginkgolide B.

Mechanisms of Action

The reason GB has neuroprotective properties is because it can (a) reverse the decreases caused by ischemia by reducing the bax/bcl-2 ratios in neurons before cell death. (b) prevent the formation of NO, which could result in cell damage from NO. (c) Scavenge free radicals to lessen the amount of lipid peroxidation (Wahid et al., 2020).

Application

GB was tested in clinical trials to see if it may help patients with dementia. Clinical studies carried out in China showed that GB considerably enhances cognitive performance and lowers

the prevalence of vascular illnesses, cerebral infarction dementia, and multi-infarct dementia, all of which enhance patients' quality of life (Wahid et al., 2020).

Cannabis sativa (CS)

Cannabis is a genus name that means "cane-like," and sativa means "sown," indicating that the plant is propagated from the seed rather than the roots. Cannabis refers to the products (drugs and essential oils) that are made from the annual herb CS and its varieties, which belong to the Cannabaceae family.

Active Compound

Cannabis, as herbal medicine, is a complex mixture of compounds, including cannabinoid phenols, non-cannabinoid phenols (stilbenoids, lignans, spiro-indans, and dihydrophenanthrenes), flavonoids, terpenoids, alcohols, aldehydes, n-alkanes, wax esters, steroids, and alkaloids. Over 550 chemical components have been found in cannabis, including over 100 phytocannabinoids, such as cannabidiol (CBD) and Δ^9-tetrahydrocannabinol (THC). In order to function, these phytocannabinoids bind to both cannabinoid receptors and other receptor systems (Rock et al., 2020).

Mechanisms of Action

Having antioxidant action similar to that of vitamins E and C, it can protect oxidation processes, reduce metal ions, and scavenge free radicals. The potential of cannabinoids as anti-emetics, hunger stimulants in debilitating conditions (such as cancer and AIDS), analgesics, and anti-inflammatory treatments for multiple sclerosis, spinal cord injuries, Tourette's syndrome, epilepsy, and glaucoma is intriguing (Kopustinskiene et al., 2022).

Application

In many medical problems, including pain, anxiety, epilepsy, nausea and vomiting, and post-traumatic stress disorder, cannabis and its constituents have been suggested as therapeutic agents. For the treatment of fever, inflammation, gout, arthritis, and joint pain, as well as skin burns, hard tumors, postpartum hemorrhage, difficult child labor, STDs, gastrointestinal disorders, and infections, the root of the cannabis plant has been suggested. Cannabis has also been used as a digestive aid, appetite stimulant, and to treat rheumatism, asthma, epilepsy, exhaustion, glaucoma, sleeplessness, nausea, and pain (Odieka et al., 2022).

Camella sinensis (Green Tea)

Camellia sinensis (the tea plant) belongs to the family Theaceae. Green tea, which is "non-fermented," has more catechins than oolong or black tea.

Active Compound

Tea is reported to contain polyphenols of which Flavonoids are the main components of tea. Plant chemical includes polyphenols contain catechins thought to be responsible for health benefits. In green tea, epigallocatechin-3-gallate (EGCG) is the most prevalent and active catechin.

Mechanisms of Action & Application

- **Anti Alzheimer Activity:** EGCG shows antioxidant activity by protecting beta- amyloid induced neurotoxicity in cultured hippocampal neuron.
- **Antiparkinson Activity:** EGCG prevent loss of dopaminergic neuron in substantia nigra pars compacta and also prevent accumulation of alpha-synuclein.
- **Antistroke Activity:** With increased consumption of green tea particularly in women reduced risk from cardiovascular disease especially from stroke.
- **Obesity and Weight Loss**
- **Antimicrobial properties**: Tea help heal wounds and infections (Namita et al., 2012).

Zingiber officinale (Ginger)

Ginger belongs to Zingiberaceae family is used as a condiment, cooking spice, and herbal cure all over the world.

Active Compound

The sesquiterpenes bisapolene, zingiberene, and zingiberol are the main active components of ginger oil.

Mechanisms of Action

- Anti-ulcer activity
- Anti-inflammatory activity
- Antioxidant activity

Application

Abdominal pain, anorexia, arthritis, atonic dyspepsia, bleeding, cancer, chest congestion, cholera, chronic bronchitis, cold extremities, colic, colitis, common cold, cough, cystic fibrosis, diarrhea, respiratory difficulties, dropsy, fever, flatulent, indigestion, gallbladder disorders, hyperacidity, hypercholesterolemia, hyperglycemia, indigestion, morning sickness, nausea, rheumatism, sore throat, throat ache, stomach ache, and vomiting are among the conditions for which it is said to be used (Moghaddasi et al., 2012).

Allium sativum (Garlic)

Garlic, belongs to the Alliaceae family and is extensively used as a valuable spice and a common treatment for a number of illnesses and physiological conditions.

Active Compound

There are at least 33 sulfur compounds, many enzymes, 17 amino acids, and minerals like selenium in garlic. Alliin, also known as diallyl thiosulfinate or diallyl disulfide, is one of the most physiologically active substances. Garlic does not contain it until it is crushed or chopped; damage to the garlic bulb triggers the enzyme allinase, which converts alliin to it. Vinyldithiines result from additional metabolism of allicin (Londhe et al., 2011).

Mechanisms of Action & Application

- Garlic's many chemical components, particularly its organosulfur compounds, have been demonstrated to have anti-Parkinsonian effects by focusing on mitochondrial dysfunction, oxidative stress, and signaling linked to inflammation (Rakshit et al., 2023).
- Anti-inflammatory Potential
- Antioxidant Potential (Londhe et al., 2011).

Hypericum perforatum (St. John's Wort)

St. John's wort, hypericum, or millepertuis, is indigenous to northern Africa, western Asia, and Europe belongs to the Hypericaceae family (Oliveira et al., 2016).

Active Compound

Hypericin, hyperforin, and many flavonoids like quercetin, rutin, and kaempferol are among the many bioactive substances found in St. John's wort (Rychlewski et al., 2023)

Mechanisms of Action & Application

- It's yet unknown exactly how H. perforatum works to reduce depression. Hypericin may have antidepressant effects via inhibiting the monoamine oxidase (MAO) enzyme, according to in vitro studies.
- In the prevention of neurodegenerative diseases by antioxidant activity.
- H. perforatum's main components have a protective impact against neurotoxicity, which suggests that they may have a positive effect on neurodegenerative diseases like Parkinson's and Alzheimer's.
- It has potential neuroprotective effect on β-amyloid-induced cell damage (Oliveira et al., 2016).

LIST OF MEDICINAL PLANT

The plants that demonstrate and validate their ability to treat neurological disorders are discussed in Table 1:

Table 1.

Botanical Name	Family	Used Parts	Secondary Metabolites	Mechanism Of Action	Outcome
Ginkgo biloba	Ginkgoaceae	Leaves	Flavonoids, terpene lactones	Antioxidant activity and anti-amyloid aggregation.	Improvement in cognitive function
Centella asiatica	Apiaceae	The aerial parts (leaves and stems)	Asiaticoside, asiaticoside, Madecassoside	Anti-inflammatory, anti-oxidant	Improvement in stress, anxiety, depression, adjustment, and attention.
Panax ginseng	Araliaceae	Roots	ginsenosides	antioxidant	significantly improved the learning and memory abilities
Withania somnifera	Solanaceae	Roots, leaves (occasionally)	withanolides, withaferin A, 12-deoxy Withastramonoli de	Antioxidant activity and anti-amyloid aggregation.	Play role in AD, PD, HD
Curcuma longa	Zingiberaceae	Rhizome	Curcumin	Anti-inflammatory, antioxidant, anti-cancer, neuro-protective.	Treatment of ADs
Zingiber officinale	Zingiberaceae	Rhizome	Gingerol	Anti-inflammatory, antiemetic, antioxidant	Treatment of ADs

LIMITATIONS

Despite the encouraging neuroprotective efficacy in preclinical settings, human clinical studies of neurodegenerative illnesses have not produced encouraging results, making the translation of promising preclinical investigations to clinical application challenging. Poor bioavailability and decreased water solubility, physical and chemical instabilities, fast metabolism, and BBB crossing are some of the issues and limitations that natural products and isolated natural chemicals encounter and can jeopardize their therapeutic efficacy. Their effectiveness is consequently diminished. Furthermore, natural chemicals are unable to enter the brain and reach their site of

action because of the BBB. As a result, their dispersion is restricted to brain tissue, and their bioavailability is minimal (Rahman et al., 2021).

CONSIDERATION

Natural products and their separated constituents can be delivered more effectively and with better therapeutic responses with the use of nanotechnology and nanocarriers, which will help address its limitations. To improve the bioavailability of natural goods and their components, nanoparticles could be incorporated into the delivery system. The most often utilized nanoparticles are micelles, dendrimer complexes, crystalline nanoparticles, hard lipid nanoparticles, polymeric nanoparticles, and nanogels.

FUTURE DIRECTIONS AND RESEARCH NEEDS

Recent studies have also looked into using herbal-based nanosystems to increase the potency of herbal treatments for neurodegenerative illnesses. By raising the concentration of the therapeutic ingredients in the targeted area, these nanosystems can be made to specifically target brain cells or tissues, hence enhancing therapy efficacy. Moving forward, future research directions in the field of phytomedicine based neuroprotection would need to cover the following topics: the discovery of new neuroactive substances; investigation of plant-based formulations that work well together; clarification of molecular mechanisms of action; investigation of plant-rich diets, targeting of neuroinflammation and neuroplasticity; interaction with neurotransmitter systems; blood-brain barrier integrity; mitochondrial function; and epigenetic regulation. To fully understand their mechanisms of action and prove their safety and effectiveness, more research is needed.

CONCLUSION

For millennia, medicinal plants have been utilized to produce therapeutic compounds that can be used to prevent and treat a wide range of illnesses. Study into how plants affect human brain function has shown the complex relationship between botanical species and brain health, emphasizing the potential of plants to be neuroprotective. The current chapter has covered the active ingredients in plants that are used to treat neurodegenerative disorders. The plant's active ingredients, which include flavonoids, alkaloids, polysaccharides, vitamins, tannins, and phenolic acid, are potent antioxidants that can shield neurons in the substantia nigra and other areas of the brain cortex from oxidative damage. In addition to avoiding neuronal damage, certain plant components can improve dopamine and acetylcholine synthesis and secretion, which are necessary in AD and PD. Given that the main issue for the treatment of neurological illnesses is the existence of bioactive chemicals, it is important to determine the precise method by which medicinal plants protect neurons. Research should be planned to determine how they actually prevent neurodegeneration. The dream of a healthy world may soon come true given the widespread use and efficacy of herbal remedies.

REFERENCES

Abdul Manap, A. S., Vijayabalan, S., Madhavan, P., Chia, Y. Y., Arya, A., Wong, E. H., Rizwan, F., Bindal, U., & Koshy, S. (2019). Bacopa monnieri, a neuroprotective lead in Alzheimer disease: A review on its properties, mechanisms of action, and preclinical and clinical studies. *Drug Target Insights, 13*, 1177392819866412. DOI: 10.1177/1177392819866412 PMID: 31391778

Agarwal, R., & Tripathi, C. B. (2014). Association of apolipoprotein E genetic variation in Alzheimer's disease in Indian population: A meta-analysis. *American Journal of Alzheimer's Disease and Other Dementias, 29*(7), 575–582. DOI: 10.1177/1533317514531443 PMID: 25551132

Aguiar, S., & Borowski, T. (2013). Neuropharmacological review of the nootropic herb Bacopa monnieri. *Rejuvenation Research, 16*(4), 313–326. DOI: 10.1089/rej.2013.1431 PMID: 23772955

Ahmad, M., Saleem, S., Ahmad, A. S., Ansari, M. A., Yousuf, S., Hoda, M. N., & Islam, F. (2005). Neuroprotective effects of Withania somnifera on 6-hydroxydopamine induced Parkinsonism in rats. *Human and Experimental Toxicology, 24*(3), 137–147. DOI: 10.1191/0960327105ht509oa PMID: 15901053

Ahmed, F. (2012). Headache disorders: Differentiating and managing the common subtypes. *British Journal of Pain, 6*(3), 124–132. DOI: 10.1177/2049463712459691 PMID: 26516483

Amudhan, S., Gururaj, G., & Satishchandra, P. (2015). Epilepsy in India I: Epidemiology and public health. *Annals of Indian Academy of Neurology, 18*(3), 263–277. DOI: 10.4103/0972-2327.160093 PMID: 26425001

Andrade, J. M., Faustino, C., Garcia, C., Ladeiras, D., Reis, C. P., & Rijo, P. (2018). Rosmarinus officinalis L.: An update review of its phytochemistry and biological activity. *Future Science OA, 4*(4), FSO283. Advance online publication. DOI: 10.4155/fsoa-2017-0124 PMID: 29682318

Ariani, A., Khotimah, H., Sulistyarini, A., & Daniaridevi, A. S. (2024). Centella asiatica extract ameliorates deoxygenation-induced neurological dysfunction in zebrafish larvae. *Open Veterinary Journal, 14*(5), 1154. DOI: 10.5455/OVJ.2024.v14.i5.9 PMID: 38938421

Armstrong, R. (2020). What causes neurodegenerative disease? *Folia Neuropathologica, 58*(2), 93–112. DOI: 10.5114/fn.2020.96707 PMID: 32729289

Arnold, S. J., Dugger, B. N., & Beach, T. G. (2013). TDP-43 deposition in prospectively followed, cognitively normal elderly individuals: Correlation with argyrophilic grains but not other concomitant pathologies. *Acta Neuropathologica, 126*(1), 51–57. DOI: 10.1007/s00401-013-1110-0 PMID: 23604587

Baldereschi, M., Di Carlo, A., Rocca, W. A., Vanni, P., Maggi, S., Perissinotto, E., Grigoletto, F., Amaducci, L., & Inzitari, D. (2000). Parkinson's disease and parkinsonism in a longitudinal study: Two-fold higher incidence in men. *Neurology, 55*(9), 1358–1363. DOI: 10.1212/WNL.55.9.1358 PMID: 11087781

Basudkar, V., Gujrati, G., Ajgaonkar, S., Gandhi, M., Mehta, D., & Nair, S. (2024). Emerging vistas for the nutraceutical Withania somnifera in inflammaging. *Pharmaceuticals (Basel, Switzerland)*, *17*(5), 597. DOI: 10.3390/ph17050597 PMID: 38794167

Beghi, E. (2020). The epidemiology of epilepsy. *Neuroepidemiology*, *54*(2), 185–191. DOI: 10.1159/000503831 PMID: 31852003

Begum, A. U., & Fathima, J. (2020). Huntington's disease: A rare Neurodegernative disorder. *World Journal of Pharmaceutical Research*, *9*, 353–435. DOI: 10.20959/wjpr20206-17470

Beyhan, N., Kocyigit-Kaymakcioglu, B., Gümrü, S., & Aricioglu, F. (2017). Synthesis and anticonvulsant activity of some 2-pyrazolines derived from chalcones. *Arabian Journal of Chemistry*, *10*, S2073–S2081. DOI: 10.1016/j.arabjc.2013.07.037

Bishnoi, M., Chopra, K., & Kulkarni, S. K. (2008). Protective effect of Curcumin, the active principle of turmeric (Curcuma longa) in haloperidol-induced orofacial dyskinesia and associated behavioural, biochemical and neurochemical changes in rat brain. *Pharmacology, Biochemistry, and Behavior*, *88*(4), 511–522. DOI: 10.1016/j.pbb.2007.10.009 PMID: 18022680

Brown, R. C., Lockwood, A. H., & Sonawane, B. R. (2005). Neurodegenerative diseases: An overview of environmental risk factors. *Environmental Health Perspectives*, *113*(9), 1250–1256. DOI: 10.1289/ehp.7567 PMID: 16140637

Chainoglou, E., & Hadjipavlou-Litina, D. (2020). Curcumin in health and diseases: Alzheimer's disease and curcumin analogues, derivatives, and hybrids. *International Journal of Molecular Sciences*, *21*(6), 1975. DOI: 10.3390/ijms21061975 PMID: 32183162

Chakravarty, A. (2006). Primary headaches associated with sexual activity—Some observations in Indian patients. *Cephalalgia*, *26*(2), 202–207. DOI: 10.1111/j.1468-2982.2005.01027.x PMID: 16426276

Choi, M. J., Zheng, H. M., Kim, J. M., Lee, K. W., Park, Y. H., & Lee, D. H. (2016). Protective effects of Centella asiatica leaf extract on dimethylnitrosamine-induced liver injury in rats. *Molecular Medicine Reports*, *14*(5), 4521–4528. DOI: 10.3892/mmr.2016.5809 PMID: 27748812

Chung, M. J., & Suh, Y. L. (2002). Ultrastructural changes of mitochondria in the skeletal muscle of patients with amyotrophic lateral sclerosis. *Ultrastructural Pathology*, *26*(1), 3–7. DOI: 10.1080/01913120252934260 PMID: 12028652

De-Paula, V. J., Radanovic, M., & Diniz, B. S. (2012). and Orestes V. Forlenza. *Protein Aggregation and Fibrillogenesis in Cerebral and Systemic Amyloid Disease, 65*, 329.

Fields, C., Bischof, J., & Levin, M. (2020). Morphological coordination: A common ancestral function unifying neural and non-neural signaling. *Physiology (Bethesda, MD)*, *35*(1), 16–30. DOI: 10.1152/physiol.00027.2019 PMID: 31799909

Fu, H., Hardy, J., & Duff, K. E. (2018). Selective vulnerability in neurodegenerative diseases. *Nature Neuroscience*, *21*(10), 1350–1358. DOI: 10.1038/s41593-018-0221-2 PMID: 30250262

Garcia-Alloza, M., Borrelli, L. A., Rozkalne, A., Hyman, B. T., & Bacskai, B. J. (2007). Curcumin labels amyloid pathology in vivo, disrupts existing plaques, and partially restores distorted neurites in an Alzheimer mouse model. *Journal of Neurochemistry*, *102*(4), 1095–1104. DOI: 10.1111/j.1471-4159.2007.04613.x PMID: 17472706

Giri, M., Zhang, M., & Lü, Y. (2016). Genes associated with Alzheimer's disease: An overview and current status. *Clinical Interventions in Aging*, ●●●, 665–681. DOI: 10.2147/CIA.S105769 PMID: 27274215

Goadsby, P. J., Holland, P. R., Martins-Oliveira, M., Hoffmann, J., Schankin, C., & Akerman, S. (2017). Pathophysiology of migraine: A disorder of sensory processing. *Physiological Reviews*, *97*(2), 553–622. Advance online publication. DOI: 10.1152/physrev.00034.2015 PMID: 28179394

Grandhi, A., Mujumdar, A. M., & Patwardhan, B. (1994). A comparative pharmacological investigation of Ashwagandha and Ginseng. *Journal of Ethnopharmacology*, *44*(3), 131–135. DOI: 10.1016/0378-8741(94)01119-2 PMID: 7898119

Gupta, S., Khan, A., Vishwas, S., Gulati, M., Singh, T. G., Dua, K., & Abdel-Daim, M. M. (2021). Demethyleneberberine: A possible treatment for Huntington's disease. *Medical Hypotheses*, *153*, 110639. DOI: 10.1016/j.mehy.2021.110639 PMID: 34229236

Harischandra, D. S., Ghaisas, S., Zenitsky, G., Jin, H., Kanthasamy, A., Anantharam, V., & Kanthasamy, A. G. (2019). Manganese-induced neurotoxicity: New insights into the triad of protein misfolding, mitochondrial impairment, and neuroinflammation. *Frontiers in Neuroscience*, *13*, 654. DOI: 10.3389/fnins.2019.00654 PMID: 31293375

Heiney, S. A., Wojaczynski, G. J., & Medina, J. F. (2021). Action-based organization of a cerebellar module specialized for predictive control of multiple body parts. *Neuron*, *109*(18), 2981–2994. e5. DOI: 10.1016/j.neuron.2021.08.017 PMID: 34534455

Hussain, Z., Mukherjee, A., Ganguly, G., Joardar, A., Roy, S., Guin, D. S., & Das, S. K. (2020). Clinical profile of genetically proven huntington's disease patients from Eastern India. *Annals of Indian Academy of Neurology*, *23*(2), 195–200. DOI: 10.4103/aian.AIAN_505_19 PMID: 32189861

Jiang, H., Zheng, G., Lv, J., Chen, H., Lin, J., Li, Y., Fan, G., & Ding, X. (2016). Identification of Centella asiatica's effective ingredients for inducing the neuronal differentiation. *Evidence-Based Complementary and Alternative Medicine : eCAM*, *2016*(1), 9634750. DOI: 10.1155/2016/9634750 PMID: 27446228

Johnson, W.Jr, Bergfeld, W. F., Belsito, D. V., Hill, R. A., Klaassen, C. D., Liebler, D. C., Marks, J. G.Jr, Shank, R. C., Slaga, T. J., Snyder, P. W., Gill, L. J., & Heldreth, B. (2023). Safety assessment of Centella asiatica-derived ingredients as used in cosmetics. *International Journal of Toxicology*, *42*(1, suppl), 5S–22S. DOI: 10.1177/10915818231158272 PMID: 36812692

Kalia, L. V., & Lang, A. E. (2015). Parkinson's disease. *Lancet*, *386*(9996), 896–912. DOI: 10.1016/S0140-6736(14)61393-3 PMID: 25904081

Kamalakannan, S. K., Gudlavalleti, A. S., Gudlavalleti, V. S. M., Goenka, S., & Kuper, H. (2015). Challenges in understanding the epidemiology of acquired brain injury in India. *Annals of Indian Academy of Neurology*, *18*(1), 66–70. DOI: 10.4103/0972-2327.151047 PMID: 25745314

Kamboj, S., Sharma, P., Kamboj, R., Kamboj, S., Hariom, , Girija, , Guarve, K., Dutt, R., Verma, I., Dua, K., & Rani, N. (2024). Exploring the therapeutic potential of phytoconstituents for addressing neurodegenerative disorders. *Central Nervous System Agents in Medicinal Chemistry*, *24*(2), 129–144. DOI: 10.2174/0118715249273015231225091339 PMID: 38265386

Kannoor, A., & Ramani, P. (2020). Effect of ethanolic extract of Centella asiatica on pentylene tetrazol induced seizure in albino mice. *International Journal of Basic and Clinical Pharmacology*, *9*(1583), 2319–2003. DOI: 10.18203/2319-2003.ijbcp20204101

Katsumoto, A., Takeuchi, H., & Tanaka, F. (2019). Tau pathology in chronic traumatic encephalopathy and Alzheimer's disease: Similarities and differences. *Frontiers in Neurology*, *10*, 980. DOI: 10.3389/fneur.2019.00980 PMID: 31551922

Keon, M., Musrie, B., Dinger, M., Brennan, S. E., Santos, J., & Saksena, N. K. (2021). Destination amyotrophic lateral sclerosis. *Frontiers in Neurology*, *12*, 596006. DOI: 10.3389/fneur.2021.596006 PMID: 33854469

Khatri, D. K., Kadbhane, A., Patel, M., Nene, S., Atmakuri, S., Srivastava, S., & Singh, S. B. (2021). Gauging the role and impact of drug interactions and repurposing in neurodegenerative disorders. *Current Research in Pharmacology and Drug Discovery*, *2*, 100022. DOI: 10.1016/j.crphar.2021.100022 PMID: 34909657

Kopustinskiene, D. M., Masteikova, R., Lazauskas, R., & Bernatoniene, J. (2022). Cannabis sativa L. bioactive compounds and their protective role in oxidative stress and inflammation. *Antioxidants*, *11*(4), 660. DOI: 10.3390/antiox11040660 PMID: 35453344

Kuboyama, T., Tohda, C., & Komatsu, K. (2006). Withanoside IV and its active metabolite, sominone, attenuate Aβ (25–35)-induced neurodegeneration. *The European Journal of Neuroscience*, *23*(6), 1417–1426. DOI: 10.1111/j.1460-9568.2006.04664.x PMID: 16553605

Kulkarni, S. K., & Dhir, A. (2008). Withania somnifera: An Indian ginseng. *Progress in Neuro-Psychopharmacology & Biological Psychiatry*, *32*(5), 1093–1105. DOI: 10.1016/j.pnpbp.2007.09.011 PMID: 17959291

Kuswati, K. (2015). The effect of centella asiatica ethanolic extract on caspase-3 expression in prefrontal cortex of chronic restraint stress induced sprague dawley rat. *JKKI: Jurnal Kedokteran dan Kesehatan Indonesia*, 65-72. https://doi.org/DOI: 10.20885/JKKI.Vol7.Iss2.art6

Leng, F., & Edison, P. (2021). Neuroinflammation and microglial activation in Alzheimer disease: Where do we go from here? *Nature Reviews. Neurology*, *17*(3), 157–172. DOI: 10.1038/s41582-020-00435-y PMID: 33318676

Londhe, V. P., Gavasane, A. T., Nipate, S. S., Bandawane, D. D., & Chaudhari, P. D. (2011). Role of garlic (Allium sativum) in various diseases: An overview. *Angiogenesis*, *12*(13), 129–134.

Lotharius, J., & Brundin, P. (2002). Pathogenesis of Parkinson's disease: Dopamine, vesicles and α-synuclein. *Nature Reviews. Neuroscience*, *3*(12), 932–942. DOI: 10.1038/nrn983 PMID: 12461550

MacDonald, M. E., Ambrose, C. M., Duyao, M. P., Myers, R. H., Lin, C., Srinidhi, L., & Harper, P. S. (1993). A novel gene containing a trinucleotide repeat that is expanded and unstable on Huntington's disease chromosomes. *Cell, 72*(6), 971–983. DOI: 10.1016/0092-8674(93)90585-E PMID: 8458085

Martin, J. B., & Gusella, J. F. (1986). Huntingtons disease. *The New England Journal of Medicine, 315*(20), 1267–1276. DOI: 10.1056/NEJM198611133152006 PMID: 2877396

Mirjalili, M. H., Moyano, E., Bonfill, M., Cusido, R. M., & Palazón, J. (2009). Steroidal lactones from Withania somnifera, an ancient plant for novel medicine. *Molecules (Basel, Switzerland), 14*(7), 2373–2393. DOI: 10.3390/molecules14072373 PMID: 19633611

Moghaddasi, M. S., & Kashani, H. H. (2012). Ginger (Zingiber officinale): A review. *Journal of Medicinal Plants Research, 6*(26), 4255–4258. DOI: 10.5897/JMPR11.787

Moise, G., Jîjie, A. R., Moacă, E. A., Predescu, I. A., Dehelean, C. A., Heghe , A., Vlad, D. C., Popescu, R., & Vlad, C. S. (2024). Plants' Impact on the Human Brain—Exploring the Neuroprotective and Neurotoxic Potential of Plants. *Pharmaceuticals (Basel, Switzerland), 17*(10), 1339. DOI: 10.3390/ph17101339 PMID: 39458980

Nakajima, H., Wakabayashi, Y., Wakamatsu, K., & Imokawa, G. (2011). An extract of withania somnifera attenuates endothelin-1-stimulated pigmentation in human epidermal equivalents through the interruption of pkc activity within melanocytes. *Phytotherapy Research, 25*(9), 1398–1411. DOI: 10.1002/ptr.3552 PMID: 21678520

Namita, P., Mukesh, R., & Vijay, K. J. (2012). Camellia sinensis (green tea): A review. *Global Journal of Pharmacology, 6*(2), 52–59.

Neri, S., Mastroianni, G., Gardella, E., Aguglia, U., & Rubboli, G. (2022). Epilepsy in neurodegenerative diseases. *Epileptic Disorders, 24*(2), 249–273. DOI: 10.1684/epd.2021.1406 PMID: 35596580

Nissanka, N., & Moraes, C. T. (2018). Mitochondrial DNA damage and reactive oxygen species in neurodegenerative disease. *FEBS Letters, 592*(5), 728–742. DOI: 10.1002/1873-3468.12956 PMID: 29281123

Odieka, A. E., Obuzor, G. U., Oyedeji, O. O., Gondwe, M., Hosu, Y. S., & Oyedeji, A. O. (2022). The medicinal natural products of Cannabis sativa Linn.: A review. *Molecules (Basel, Switzerland), 27*(5), 1689. DOI: 10.3390/molecules27051689 PMID: 35268790

Oliveira, A. I., Pinho, C., Sarmento, B., & Dias, A. C. (2016). Neuroprotective activity of Hypericum perforatum and its major components. *Frontiers in Plant Science, 7*, 1004. DOI: 10.3389/fpls.2016.01004 PMID: 27462333

Oniyangi, O., & Cohall, D. H. (2020). Phytomedicines (medicines derived from plants) for sickle cell disease. *Cochrane Database of Systematic Reviews*, (9). Advance online publication. DOI: 10.1002/14651858.CD004448.pub7 PMID: 32977351

Pandey, M., Debnath, M., Gupta, S., & Chikara, S. K. (2011). Phytomedicine: An ancient approach turning into future potential source of therapeutics. *Journal of Pharmacognosy and Phytotherapy*, *3*(3), 27–37.

Puri, V., Kanojia, N., Sharma, A., Huanbutta, K., Dheer, D., & Sangnim, T. (2022). Natural product-based pharmacological studies for neurological disorders. *Frontiers in Pharmacology*, *13*, 1011740. DOI: 10.3389/fphar.2022.1011740 PMID: 36419628

Puspita, L., Chung, S. Y., & Shim, J. W. (2017). Oxidative stress and cellular pathologies in Parkinson's disease. *Molecular Brain*, *10*(1), 1–12. DOI: 10.1186/s13041-017-0340-9 PMID: 29183391

Rahman, M. H., Bajgai, J., Fadriquela, A., Sharma, S., Trinh, T. T., Akter, R., Jeong, Y. J., Goh, S. H., Kim, C.-S., & Lee, K. J. (2021). Therapeutic potential of natural products in treating neurodegenerative disorders and their future prospects and challenges. *Molecules (Basel, Switzerland)*, *26*(17), 5327. DOI: 10.3390/molecules26175327 PMID: 34500759

Rakshit, D., Nayak, S., Kundu, S., Angelopoulou, E., Pyrgelis, E. S., Piperi, C., & Mishra, A. (2023). The pharmacological activity of garlic (Allium sativum) in Parkinson's disease: From molecular mechanisms to the therapeutic potential. *ACS Chemical Neuroscience*, *14*(6), 1033–1044. DOI: 10.1021/acschemneuro.2c00789 PMID: 36861262

Rathmann, K. L., & Conner, C. S. (1984). Alzheimer's disease: Clinical features, pathogenesis, and treatment. *Drug Intelligence & Clinical Pharmacy*, *18*(9), 684–691. DOI: 10.1177/106002808401800902 PMID: 6383752

Ravindranath, V., & Sundarakumar, J. S. (2021). Changing demography and the challenge of dementia in India. *Nature Reviews. Neurology*, *17*(12), 747–758. DOI: 10.1038/s41582-021-00565-x PMID: 34663985

Rehman, M. U., Wali, A. F., Ahmad, A., Shakeel, S., Rasool, S., Ali, R., Rashid, S. M., Madkhali, H., Ganaie, M. A., & Khan, R. (2019). Neuroprotective strategies for neurological disorders by natural products: An update. *Current Neuropharmacology*, *17*(3), 247–267. DOI: 10.2174/1570159X16666180911124605 PMID: 30207234

Roberts, H. L., & Brown, D. R. (2015). Seeking a mechanism for the toxicity of oligomeric α-synuclein. *Biomolecules*, *5*(2), 282–305. DOI: 10.3390/biom5020282 PMID: 25816357

Rock, E. M., & Parker, L. A. (2020). Constituents of Cannabis sativa. *Cannabinoids and neuropsychiatric disorders*, 1-13.

Roda, A. R., Serra-Mir, G., Montoliu-Gaya, L., Tiessler, L., & Villegas, S. (2022). Amyloid-beta peptide and tau protein crosstalk in Alzheimer's disease. *Neural Regeneration Research*, *17*(8), 1666–1674. DOI: 10.4103/1673-5374.332127 PMID: 35017413

Ross, C. A., & Poirier, M. A. (2004). Protein aggregation and neurodegenerative disease. *Nature Medicine*, *10*(S7, Suppl 7), S10–S17. DOI: 10.1038/nm1066 PMID: 15272267

Rychlewski, P., Kamgar, E., Mildner-Szkudlarz, S., Kowalczewski, P. Ł., & Zembrzuska, J. (2023). Determination of the contents of bioactive compounds in St. John's wort (Hypericum perforatum): Comparison of commercial and wild samples. *Open Chemistry*, *21*(1), 20220347. DOI: 10.1515/chem-2022-0347

Sandhu, J. S., Shah, B., Shenoy, S., Chauhan, S., Lavekar, G. S., & Padhi, M. M. (2010). Effects of Withania somnifera (Ashwagandha) and Terminalia arjuna (Arjuna) on physical performance and cardiorespiratory endurance in healthy young adults. *International Journal of Ayurveda Research*, *1*(3), 144. DOI: 10.4103/0974-7788.72485 PMID: 21170205

Sankar, S., Manivasagam, T., Krishnamurti, A., & Ramanathan, M. (2007). The neuroprotective effect of Withania somnifera root extract in MPTP-intoxicated mice: An analysis of behavioral and biochemical varibles. *Cellular & Molecular Biology Letters*, *12*(4), 473–481. DOI: 10.2478/s11658-007-0015-0 PMID: 17415533

Shorvon, S. D., Andermann, F., & Guerrini, R. (Eds.). (2011). *The causes of epilepsy: common and uncommon causes in adults and children.* Cambridge University Press. DOI: 10.1017/CBO9780511921001

Siesjö, B. K. (1992). Pathophysiology and treatment of focal cerebral ischemia: Part II: mechanisms of damage and treatment. *Journal of Neurosurgery*, *77*(3), 337–354. DOI: 10.3171/jns.1992.77.3.0337 PMID: 1506880

Simpson, T., Pase, M., & Stough, C. (2015). Bacopa monnieri as an antioxidant therapy to reduce oxidative stress in the aging brain. *Evidence-Based Complementary and Alternative Medicine : eCAM*, *2015*(1), 615384. DOI: 10.1155/2015/615384 PMID: 26413126

Srivastava, A., Srivastava, P., Pandey, A., Khanna, V. K., & Pant, A. B. (2019). Phytomedicine: A potential alternative medicine in controlling neurological disorders. In *New look to phytomedicine* (pp. 625-655). Academic Press. https://doi.org/DOI: 10.1016/B978-0-12-814619-4.00025-2

Srivastava, P., & Yadav, R. S. (2016). Efficacy of natural compounds in neurodegenerative disorders. *The Benefits of Natural Products for Neurodegenerative Diseases*, 107-123. https://doi.org/DOI: 10.1007/978-3-319-28383-8_7

Srivastava, P., & Yadav, R. S. (2016). Efficacy of natural compounds in neurodegenerative disorders. *The Benefits of Natural Products for Neurodegenerative Diseases*, 107-123. https://doi.org/DOI: 10.1007/978-3-319-28383-8_7

Stafstrom, C. E., & Carmant, L. (2015). Seizures and epilepsy: An overview for neuroscientists. *Cold Spring Harbor Perspectives in Medicine*, *5*(6), a022426. DOI: 10.1101/cshperspect.a022426 PMID: 26033084

Steiner, T. J., Birbeck, G. L., Jensen, R. H., Katsarava, Z., Stovner, L. J., & Martelletti, P. (2015). Headache disorders are third cause of disability worldwide. *The Journal of Headache and Pain*, *16*(1), 1–3. DOI: 10.1186/s10194-015-0544-2 PMID: 26109437

Strong, K., Mathers, C., & Bonita, R. (2007). Preventing stroke: Saving lives around the world. *Lancet Neurology*, *6*(2), 182–187. DOI: 10.1016/S1474-4422(07)70031-5 PMID: 17239805

Taga, A., Charalampopoulou, A., & Sari, M. C. (2024). Amyotrophic Lateral Sclerosis: Exploring Disability Beyond Motor Weakness. In *The Palgrave Encyclopedia of Disability* (pp. 1-15). Cham: Springer Nature Switzerland. https://doi.org/DOI: 10.1007/978-3-031-40858-8_218-1

Tater, P., & Pandey, S. (2021). Post-stroke movement disorders: Clinical spectrum, pathogenesis, and management. *Neurology India, 69*(2), 272–283. DOI: 10.4103/0028-3886.314574 PMID: 33904435

Taylor, C. A. (2017). Deaths from alzheimer's disease—United States, 1999–2014. *MMWR. Morbidity and Mortality Weekly Report*, •••, 66. PMID: 28542120

Taylor, F. C., & Suresh Kumar, K. (2012). *Stroke in India fact sheet (updated 2012). South Asia Network for Chronic Disease*. IIPH Hyderabad, Public Health Foundation of India.

Terry, R. D., & Davies, P. (1980). Dementia of the Alzheimer type. *Annual Review of Neuroscience, 3*(1), 77–95. DOI: 10.1146/annurev.ne.03.030180.000453 PMID: 6251745

Thijs, R. D., Surges, R., O'Brien, T. J., & Sander, J. W. (2019). Epilepsy in adults. *Lancet, 393*(10172), 689–701. DOI: 10.1016/S0140-6736(18)32596-0 PMID: 30686584

Toyoshima, Y., & Takahashi, H. (2014). TDP-43 pathology in polyglutamine diseases: With reference to amyotrphic lateral sclerosis. *Neuropathology, 34*(1), 77–82. DOI: 10.1111/neup.12053 PMID: 23889603

Türkez, H., Arslan, M. E., Stefano, A. D., Cacciatore, I., & Mardînoğlu, A. (2020). Nonpharmacological treatment options for Alzheimer's disease: From animal testing toclinical studies. *Turkish Journal of Zoology, 44*(2), 81–89. DOI: 10.3906/zoo-1911-32

Van Den Eeden, S. K., Tanner, C. M., Bernstein, A. L., Fross, R. D., Leimpeter, A., Bloch, D. A., & Nelson, L. M. (2003). Incidence of Parkinson's disease: Variation by age, gender, and race/ethnicity. *American Journal of Epidemiology, 157*(11), 1015–1022. DOI: 10.1093/aje/kwg068 PMID: 12777365

Vellingiri, B. (2024). An overview about neurological diseases in India–A theranostics approach. *Aging and Health Research, 4*(1), 100177. DOI: 10.1016/j.ahr.2023.100177

Venkatesan, D., Iyer, M., S, R. W., Narayanasamy, A., Kamalakannan, S., Valsala Gopalakrishnan, A., & Vellingiri, B. (2022). Genotypic-phenotypic analysis, metabolic profiling and clinical correlations in Parkinson's disease patients from Tamil Nadu population, India. *Journal of Molecular Neuroscience, 72*(8), 1724–1737. DOI: 10.1007/s12031-022-02028-4 PMID: 35676593

Venkatesan, D., Iyer, M., Wilson, R., & Vellingiri, B. (2021). The association between multiple risk factors, clinical correlations and molecular insights in Parkinson's disease patients from Tamil Nadu population, India. *Neuroscience Letters, 755*, 135903. DOI: 10.1016/j.neulet.2021.135903 PMID: 33894333

Venugopal, A., Iyer, M., Balasubramanian, V., & Vellingiri, B. (2020). Mitochondrial calcium uniporter as a potential therapeutic strategy for Alzheimer's disease. *Acta Neuropsychiatrica, 32*(2), 65–71. DOI: 10.1017/neu.2019.39 PMID: 31556366

Vonsattel, J. P. G., Keller, C., & Ramirez, E. P. C. (2011). Huntington's disease–neuropathology. *Handbook of Clinical Neurology, 100*, 83–100. DOI: 10.1016/B978-0-444-52014-2.00004-5 PMID: 21496571

Wahid, M., Ali, A., Saqib, F., Aleem, A., Bibi, S., Afzal, K., Ali, A., Baig, A., Khan, S. A., & Bin Asad, M. H. H. (2020). Pharmacological exploration of traditional plants for the treatment of neurodegenerative disorders. *Phytotherapy Research, 34*(12), 3089–3112. DOI: 10.1002/ptr.6742 PMID: 32478964

Wojtunik-Kulesza, K. A. (2022). Toxicity of selected monoterpenes and essential oils rich in these compounds. *Molecules (Basel, Switzerland), 27*(5), 1716. DOI: 10.3390/molecules27051716 PMID: 35268817

Xu, L., & Pu, J. (2016). Alpha-Synuclein in Parkinson's Disease: From Pathogenetic Dysfunction to Potential Clinical Application. *Parkinson's Disease, 2016*(1), 1720621. DOI: 10.1155/2016/1720621 PMID: 27610264

Zhang, G., Xia, Y., Wan, F., Ma, K., Guo, X., Kou, L., Yin, S., Han, C., Liu, L., Huang, J., Xiong, N., & Wang, T. (2018). New perspectives on roles of alpha-synuclein in Parkinson's disease. *Frontiers in Aging Neuroscience, 10*, 370. DOI: 10.3389/fnagi.2018.00370 PMID: 30524265

Zhang, J., Li, X., & Li, J. D. (2019). The Roles of Post-translational Modifications on α-Synuclein in the Pathogenesis of Parkinson's Diseases. *Frontiers in Neuroscience, 13*, 381. DOI: 10.3389/fnins.2019.00381 PMID: 31057362

Zheng, C. J., & Qin, L. P. (2007). Chemical components of Centella asiatica and their bioactivities. *Zhong xi yi jie he xue bao=. Journal of Chinese Integrative Medicine, 5*(3), 348–351. DOI: 10.3736/jcim20070324 PMID: 17498500

Chapter 16

Traditional Phytomedicine and Enzymatic Modulation in Neurodegenerative Disorder Prevention:

Ethnobotanical Evidence From Talassemtane National Park (Morocco)

Mariam Rhattas
https://orcid.org/0009-0003-9484-5863
Department of Biology, Faculty of Sciences, Ibn Tofaïl University, Kénitra, Morocco

Rajaa Kaddar
Department of Geology, Faculty of Sciences, Ibn Tofaïl University, Kénitra, Morocco

Karima Rhattas
Department of Chemistry, Faculty of Sciences, Ibn Tofaïl University, Kénitra, Morocco

Yassine Mouniane
https://orcid.org/0000-0002-6037-5301
Faculty of Sciences, Ibn Tofail University, Kenitra, Morocco

Brahim El Ouardi
https://orcid.org/0009-0000-4559-6141
Faculty of Sciences, Ibn Tofail University, Kenitra, Morocco

Imane Aitouhanni
https://orcid.org/0009-0004-1400-8027
ENSIAS, SSLAB, Mohammed V University, Rabat, Morocco

Ouafae El Yahyaoui
Faculty of Sciences, Ibn Tofail University, Kenitra, Morocco

Sanae Masmoudi
Institut Supérieur des Professions Infirmières et Techniques de la Santé, Kenitra, Morocco

Mohamed Belomaria
Institut Supérieur des Professions Infirmières et Techniques de la Santé, Kenitra, Morocco

Mohamed El Bakkali
Institut Supérieur des Professions Infirmières et Techniques de la Santé, Kenitra, Morocco

DOI: 10.4018/979-8-3373-4627-4.ch016

ABSTRACT

Recent pharmacological strategies have begun to explore the role of enzymatic pathways in slowing or reversing disease progression. Alongside modern drug development, traditional phytomedicine offers a largely untapped reservoir of bioactive compounds that may influence key enzymes implicated in neurodegeneration. This chapter presents an ethnobotanical study conducted in Talassemtane National Park (Northern Morocco), documenting medicinal plants traditionally used for the treatment of nervous system disorders. Through a pharmacological review of selected species, we highlight their potential to modulate enzymatic and oxidative pathways particularly through antioxidant, anti-inflammatory, and neuroprotective mechanisms. In addition, they are capable of interacting with targets such as acetylcholinesterase and neuroinflammatory mediators. By integrating traditional knowledge with pharmacological and biochemical analysis, we propose that phytomedicines from Mediterranean biodiversity can contribute to enzyme-based therapeutic strategies in neurodegeneration.

INTRODUCTION

Neurodegenerative diseases such as Alzheimer's, Parkinson's, and amyotrophic lateral sclerosis (ALS) represent a major medical and societal challenge due to their progressive nature, the lack of curative treatments, and their growing impact on aging populations (Pathak et al., 2022; Ciurea et al., 2023). These diseases share common pathophysiological mechanisms, including oxidative stress, the accumulation of misfolded proteins, neurogenic inflammation, and mitochondrial dysfunction (Sharifi-Rad et al., 2020; Chaudhary et al., 2023). Scleroderma in plaques This is an auto-immune disease of the white matter of the central nervous system that primarily affects women, with a sex ratio of about one man for every three women (Jankowska et al., 2023). It often strikes young adults between the ages of 20 and 30. Its prevalence appears to be rising in light of recent epidemiological investigations (Wong et al., 2023). Huntington's disease is thought to be a degenerative disease, so treating it requires careful consideration of the severity of the symptoms and the rate of progression of the affected individuals as well as the possibility or confirmation of a genetic origin that affects the descendents and ancestors even more (Ivy, 2021). However, for other seemingly less severe pathologies like pain, migraines (which are most frequently associated with the brain), and crises, symptoms may include nausea, vomiting, photophobia, phonophobia, hypotension, irritability (Masereel, 2018). Additionally, daily headaches, headaches, or nerve-related depressions, which most frequently manifest as insomnia or anxiety (Goetz, 2011). Emerging therapeutic targets include enzymes involved in protein degradation pathways, neuronal signaling, and the regulation of oxidative metabolism. In this context, medicinal plants appear to be a promising source of natural compounds with neuroprotective and enzyme-modulating activity involved in these processes. Ethnobotany offers a valuable starting point for identifying these plants, leveraging traditional knowledge in a rigorous scientific approach.

Similar to many developing nations, medicinal plants have long been the primary source of medical care in the absence of appropriate medical supervision (Tabuti et al., 2003). Due to its biogeographic location, Morocco offers a high degree of ecosystemological diversity, which translates to floristic diversity. As a result, it is one of the Mediterranean countries whose popu-

lations have long been accustomed to traditional medical practices and have developed a level of expertise in this area through the use of medicinal plants (Scherrer et al., 2005). As a matter of fact, the knowledge contributed by the various ethnic groups that have migrated to Morocco from various regions has helped to develop and deepen the Moroccan pharmacopée (Bellakhdar, 1997). Therefore, medicinal plants are a wealth of knowledge for those who have chosen to approach their daily lives in a different way by turning their backs on the chemical arsenal of modern medicine (Hseini, et al., 2007). Due to their effectiveness in a variety of therapeutic procedures, medicinal plants are still widely used today despite advancements in synthetic chemistry (Lazli et al., 2019).

Owing to the active ingredients in medicinal plants' impact on their therapeutic efficacy, these plants interact with the human body in a variety of ways. These uses are more common in rural areas than elsewhere, which can be attributed to knowledge accumulated over many years and the various experiences of their ancestors that have been passed down through the generations (Ghourri et al., 2014). Additionally, one is invited to learn about the various neurological diseases found in the PNTL and to enumerate the most commonly used plants in this regard, so that it can serve as a reference for future scientific research. Based on comparable scientific research, such as that conducted by Togo et al. (2022). Additionally, to (Bayali & Dami, 2019), who conducted research on clinical phytotherapy in neurological disorders.

Morocco boasts exceptional biodiversity and a rich medicinal tradition passed down orally through generations. The Talassemtane National Park, located in the Rif Mountains, is renowned for its endemic flora and ethnobotanical significance. A field survey was conducted among local populations and herbalists in the region to identify plants used in the treatment of nervous system disorders. Data was collected using semi-structured questionnaires, documenting vernacular names, parts used, methods of preparation, and therapeutic indications. The methodological approach is based on quantitative indices such as the use value index (UV) and frequency of citation.

With this in mind, the main objective of this study is to highlight the pharmacological potential of medicinal plants traditionally used in Talassemtane National Park for the treatment of nervous system disorders, with a particular focus on their effects on enzymes involved in neurodegenerative processes. By promoting local knowledge through a rigorous scientific approach, this work aims to identify plant species capable of modulating key enzymatic targets such as acetylcholinesterase (AChE), monoamine oxidase (MAO), or mediators of neuronal inflammation. This contribution is part of a bioprospecting and development effort for alternative or complementary therapies based on natural compounds of interest for the treatment or prevention of neurodegenerative diseases.

LITERATURE REVIEW

Neurodegenerative Disorders: Mechanisms and Therapeutic Challenges

Neurodegenerative diseases (NDD), including Alzheimer's disease (AD), Parkinson's disease (PD), amyotrophic lateral sclerosis (ALS), and Huntington's disease, are marked by progressively irreversible degeneration of neurons in the CNS (Lamptey et al., 2022; Giri et al., 2024). These diseases have overlapping pathogenic mechanisms, such as oxidative stress, mitochondrial dysfunction, neuroinflammation, and inappropriately folded proteins like β-amyloid plaques or tau aggregates. What's more, these interconnected biological pathways are clearly complicating single-target therapeutic options, thus rendering traditional therapeutic strategies suboptimal.

With few exceptions, contemporary medical therapies for NDD are symptomatic, and do not preserve or revert disease progression (Doroszkiewicz et al., 2022). Therefore, discovering new therapeutic options that target innate molecular dysfunctions and processes, especially those involving enzymatic processes, is warranted (Anwar et al., 2024).

Enzyme Therapy in Neurodegenerative Diseases

Enzyme therapy is a new modality for neurodegenerative diseases which provides excitement, enthusiasm, and hope in terms of a new potential intervention and a new potential treatment. Enzyme therapy as an intervention for neurodegenerative diseases is any pharmacological approach which modulates (i.e., inhibiting, activating, or replacing) enzymes that can restore biochemical homeostatic states that maintain the functional status of neurodegenerative targets (De La Fuente et al., 2021; Choi et al., 2024). Enzymes such as acetylcholinesterase (AChE), monoamine oxidase (MAO) and butyrylcholinesterase (BuChE) have emerged as a significant intervention target. AChE has demonstrated clinical utility in AD, providing clinical assessment improvement (i.e., cognitive function) by enhancing cholinergic neurotransmission (Nasso et al., 2021). More broadly, AChE inhibitors administered to persons with AD, improve cholinergic neurotransmission through selective inhibition of AChE in the brain (Moreta et al., 2021). Specifically, MAO is inhibited which increases, and maintains, dopamine levels in persons with Parkinson's disease (PD). In the forward-facing future, emerging genetic technologies will be available to investigate interventions that can modify a patient's genetic code (gene-editing CRISPR/cas9) and employ nano-carrier systems to deliver enzymes directly to the central nervous system. Enzyme therapy ultimately can be viewed as an interdisciplinary methodology that parallels areas of biological science, pharmacological sciences, and biotechnology, that could culminate in discovery of drugs and disease modifying interventions (Torres-Herrero et al., 2024).

Potential of Natural Products in Enzyme Modulation

Natural products, in particular plant-based compounds, are great sources of bioactive molecules which are capable of modulating activity of relevant enzymes in neurodegeneration (Shoaib et al., 2023). Flavonoids such as quercetin and luteolin have shown the ability to inhibit acetylcholinesterase activity while demonstrating both great antioxidant or free radical scavenging capabilities (Calderaro et al., 2022). Alkaloids such as galantamine and harmine have dual inhibition of receive both AChE and MAO activity thereby mediating increased levels of neurotransmitters; both flavonoids and alkaloids, much like terpenes, exhibit a wide spectrum of phenolic based pharmacologic activity (Larit & León, 2023). Terpenes such as linalool or rosmarinic acid provide anti-inflammatory, antioxidant, and neuroprotective properties. Polyphenols and tannins also influence redox status and regultion of inflammatory pathways contributing to cellular protection. The pharmacologic spectrum of phytochemicals and their synergistic contributions support their use in multi-target therapeutic applications against the complex pathology of neurodegenerative diseases (Sahakyan et al., 2022; Dzah et al., 2024).

Growing Interest in Traditional Phytomedicine in Neuropharmacology

In recent years, there has been a growing recognition of how ethnopharmacological knowledge can be integrated into contemporary drug discovery (Tan et al., 2025). Traditional medicinal systems provided the bulk of knowledge that is based upon empirical observations regarding the use of plants to treat nervous system disorders, including anxiety, epilepsy, insomnia, and memory loss, which can be associated with neurodegenerative processes (Yuan et al., 2016). North Africa and the Mediterranean, for example, have a history of using selected plants for neurological health. Many species, such as *Ginkgo biloba*, *Salvia officinalis*, *Curcuma longa*, and *Bacopa monnieri*, have been thoroughly studied, thereby corroborating the scientific validity, which is consistent with ethnopharmacological methods to treat and modulate conditions associated with oxidative stress, inflammation, and enzyme regulating activity. The combination of traditional knowledge systems and scientific methods is an unimaginatively instructive approach to finding novel phytomedicinal therapies for treating neurodegenerative conditions (Jensen et al. 2024; Rodrigues et al., 2024).

Growing Interest in Traditional Phytomedicine in Neuropharmacology

Despite the encouraging contribution of traditional healing plants, some deficits have been identified in the literature (Sibeko & Johns, 2021). The bulk of ethnobotanical literature has not tracked the use of endemic species in Morocco with respect to their enzymatic capabilities, particularly in the context of potential therapeutic interventions related to neurodegenerative concerns. Transition between traditional and clinical bioactivity is often limited by a lack of standardization, chemical profiling, and determinative validation of bioactivity (Barba-Ostria et al., 2022). Additional efforts should be concentrated on bio-guided fractionation, *in vitro* and *in vivo* models, and the elucidation of the mechanism of action for traditional plants targeting particular enzymes involved in cognitive decline and neuronal degeneration. Communicating the purpose of ethnobotany to molecular neuroscience and enzyme pharmacology could suggest new pathways toward preventive and/or curative medicine and pharmacology in neurodegenerative interventions (Ribaudo et al., 2021; Dai et al., 2022).

MATERIALS AND METHODS

Study Area Description

The area chosen to conduct this inquiry is the 58 900 hectare national park of Talassemtane (PNTL), which is situated in the far northeastern and southwest of Morocco. The provincial authorities in charge of water and forest management, as well as the fight against the desertion of Chefchaouen and Tétouan, are responsible for overseeing the management of the PNTL forest area. The park consists of ten rural communes that are divided into three cercles (Bab Taza, Bou Ahmed, and Tétouan) and two provinces (Chefchaouen and Tétouan) (tableau 1) (Salohi, 2012).

Table 1. Territory of the Parc de Talassemtane is divided into several administrative units

Province	Circle	Municipality	Superficie (in hectares)
Tétouan	**Tétouan**	Al Ouad	3177
		Al Hamra	1090
		Bni Said	15
		Oulad Ali Mansour	7260
Chefchaouen	**Bou Ahmed**	Beni Selmane	9395
		Tizgane	17
		Talambote	16072
		Stehat	2809
		Tassift	16684
	Bab Taza	Bni Darkoul	1195
		Bab Taza	6887
Total			64601

Salohi (2012)

The Paleozoic Zone and the Calabi-Maya Chain comprise the PNTL's territory, which is the northern portion of the median domain of the Rifaine Chain, also known as the Septentrional Rif. (Benabid A., 1982). The majority of the park's geological and geomorphological features are made up of the dorsale calcareous portion that runs the length of this region of the Rif. The highest points on the Western Ridge are found in the Park. It concerns the mountains Lakraâ (2.159 m), Tissouka (2.122 m), and Taloussisse (2.005 m). According to El Gharbaoui (1981), the calcaro-dolomitic dorsale relief is composed of aiguë-shaped ridges that almost always correlate to the affleurement of the original écailles' fronts since they are directly derived from the dolomitic structure. Durable roches and sub-vertical pendages are characteristics of this relief. Views from the fronts are directed towards the interior of the dolomitic-calcarous chain. The PNTL is drained by the Oueds Laou, El Kanar, and partially by Bouhaya, Ahrosse, and Ihikkaman, which only cover a small fraction of the park. With the meridional forces of the Talassemtane massif, his intervention in the Atlantic Versants is minor. In fact, the only massifs partially drained by Oued Ouergha affluents that flow into Oued Sebou are the Est of Jbels Bouslimane and Bou Halla.

We base our analysis of climate factors on data provided by Benabid (1982). These data do not differ significantly from those of Maurer (1968) and two previous series of calculations, one from 1925 to 1945 by the Rabat Scientific Institute (Salohi, 2012) and the other from 1933 to 1963 by the Hydraulic Service.

The geological and geomorphological formations have a significant impact on the climate in Talassemtane National Park. According to Benabid (1982), the park is recognized by:

- An oceanization and general warming of the climate, resulting in a reduction in thermal differences.
- An abundance of precipitation (pluies and occulted precipitations).
- A stark contrast exists between the atlantic, rather wet façade and the Mediterranean, relatively dry façade.

Figure 1. Shows the administrative boundaries of the PNTL, as well as the provincial directions for water, forests, and desertification prevention in Chefchaouen and Tétouan (Salohi, 2012)

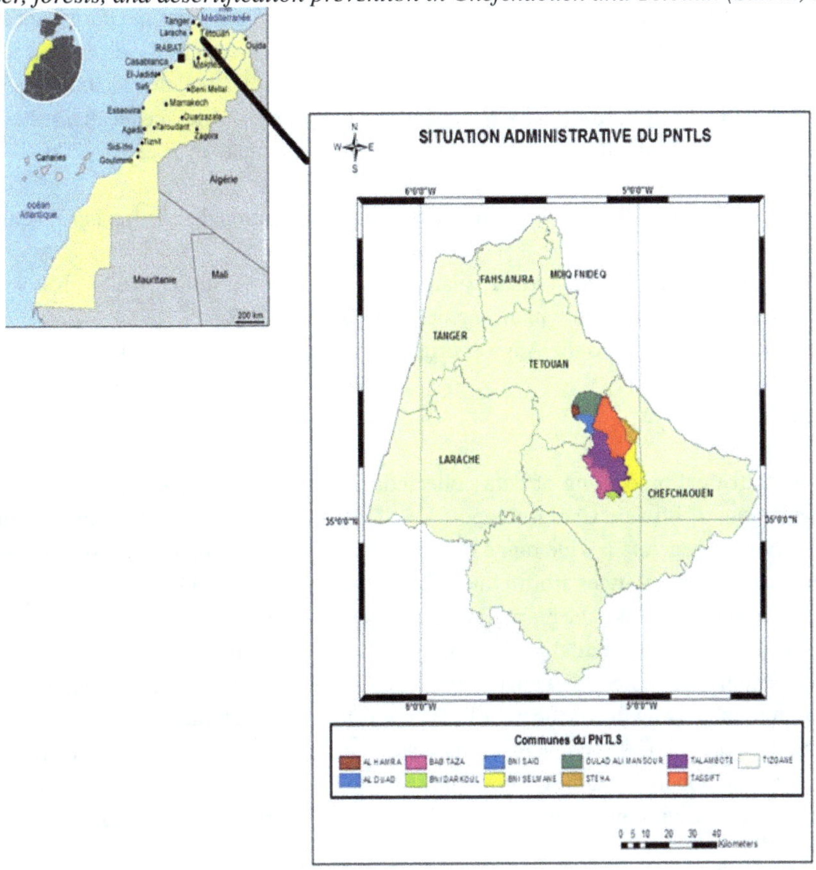

Methodology

To conduct this pharmacological study on medicinal plants used to treat neurological disorders in the PNTL, we used stratified sampling (11 rural communes). And, using questionnaires, a series of ethnobotanical surveys were conducted at the level of 31 communities, with 30 people each village, for a total of 930 questionnaires.

The population who reported using neurological phytotherapy consisted of 144 people polled between March and August 2014 during five 5-day field missions (April, May, June, July, and August) (tableau 2). The choice of this period is related to the printanière period, which is distinguished by the flowering of the various plant species found in the region.

We began our field research by conducting open interviews with the park's local people, which is a crucial category for our investigation. To become acquainted with the surrounding environment and the local language.

During our conversation with them, we focused on general information about medicinal plants. Following that, we asked them to collect samples with us and discuss the various uses of plants and their medicinal properties. We were able to collect data about the informant's profile (sex, age group) as well as information about local phytotherapy, such as the diseases treated, the method of preparation, the form of use, the dose, and the portion used, thanks to this technique.

The traditional Moroccan pharmacopée was used to identify wild species harvested on the land. - The Practical Flora of Morocco, Volumes 1 and 2 (Fennane et al., 1999, 2005, 2007).

- Nouvelle flore d'Algérie et des régions désertiques méridionales, Tome I et II (Querzel et al., 1962);
- Moroccan medicinal and aromatic plants: An economic feasibility study for investing in the medicinal and aromatic plant sector (Hmamouchi, 1999).
- Plant families belong to the Angiosperm Phylogeny Group IV (APG IV 2016).

Statistical Analysis

The biostatistical processing of data collected during our field expedition was carried out using the computer software Cristal Reaport V.9. This is a decision-making computer program that allows you to generate a wide range of reports from computer data. It enables the creation of connections to data sources from Oracle databases, Microsoft SQL Server databases, and Microsoft Access databases. The graphs presented in this study were generated using the Python programming language. Quantitative data analysis methods in ethnobotany rely in particular on the use of quantitative indices that enable an objective assessment of plant knowledge and uses within a community. Drawing on the work of Prance et al. (1987), Tardio and Pardo-de-Santayana (2008) and Gueye et al. (2012), it is recommended to use certain indices considered particularly relevant for ethnobotanical studies. These indices allow for the rigorous synthesis and analysis of collected data, providing valuable objectivity to the interpretation of results.

Fidelity Level Indicator (FL)

The percentage of informants who cited the use of a given species to treat a disease was calculated according to (Gueye et al., 2012).

$$FL\,(\%) = \frac{I_p}{I_u} \times 100$$

With:

I_p: Number of informants who confirmed the use of a specific species to treat a disease;
I_u: Total number of informants interviewed.

Citation Frequency (FC)

The frequency of citation allows us to assess the credibility of the information received as well as the level of knowledge of the plants in the study population. This is the number of informants who mentioned a specific species (Prance et al., 1987).

Consensual Factor of Information (FCI) (Heinrich et al., 1998)

$$FCI = \frac{N_{ur-N_t}}{N_{ur-1}}$$

N_{ur}: the number of times a specific category of attachment has been mentioned.

N_t: the number of plant(s) mentioned for the treatment of this particular affection.

This is an index that is frequently used to determine the medicinal uses of plants.

If FCI < 0.5, it indicates a low level of consensus on the information.

If FCI > 0.5, it indicates a high level of unanimity on the information.

Relative Frequency of Citation (FRC)

This index was calculated to assess each species' local relevance. It is the result of the citation frequency (FC), or the number of citations for a species divided by the total number of informants.

This indice varies from 0 to 1. When it is close to 1, the species is considered useful (Tardio & Pardo-de-Santayana, 2008).

Number of Usage (NUs)

This is the total number of utilisations for each species in the dataset.

NC is the number of use categories (Prance et al., 1987).

Table 2. Distribution of questionnaires based on species used for therapeutic purposes against neurological disorders

Villages	Number of persons surveyed	Frequence de fidélité FL (%)
Ain Erami	10	6
Akchour - cascades	15	10
Akchour - Talambot	10	7
Aqujiouen	5	3
Ben Qarich	42	29
Cascades	5	3
JBEL LAKRÂA	26	18
Oued Laou	15	10
Tisouka	5	3
ZAOUIA - Bab Taz	6	4

continued on following page

Table 2. Continued

Villages	Number of persons surveyed	Frequence de fidélité FL (%)
ZAOUIA - JBEL TISOUKA	5	3
Grand total	144	100

The study was conducted in a remote rural area and provided us with valuable information on practices that are frequently overlooked by contemporary medicine.

RESULTS AND DISCUSSION

Informator Profile

144 of the 930 people interviewed reported using medicinal plants to treat a variety of neurological conditions. The majority of women aged [40 to 59] and [20 to 39] use traditional pharmaceuticals to treat neurological disorders, with 31% and 26%, respectively, compared to men aged [20 to 39] and 7% [40 to 59]. This difference in frequency indicates that women have a greater understanding of the various plants that can be used to treat neurological infections, and it is they who prepare the phytotherapeutic recipes. Several studies have demonstrated this trend using percentages of (63%; 57%; 65.60%; 60%) (Benkhnigue et al., 2014; Rhattas et al., 2016a; Rhattas et al., 2016b; El hilah et al., 2016). These findings are consistent with those of Addoun (2017), who reported that women are the most active users of plants in the Tlemcen region. Talbi et al. (2020) observed a similar result in Sefrou (Northern Morocco). Women's predominance in health care can be explained by their responsibility to their families (Miara et al., 2018).

Figure 2. Distribution of questionnaires using traditional medication for neurological disorders according on gender and age group

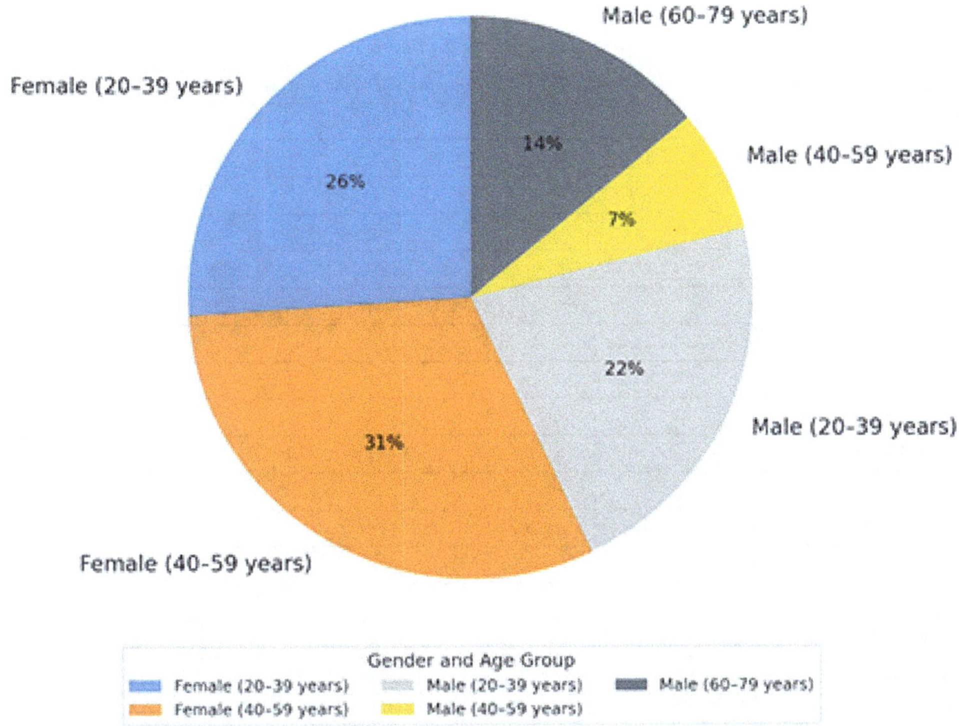

Women and men are equally responsible for collecting medicinal plants, drying them, and storing them on the research site. However, only men collect in reputedly dangerous areas. Women prepare recipes for family members.

These findings enabled the reclassification of 22 species for the treatment of 15 nervous system problems identified in the Talassemtane National Park (PNTL). The examination of Table 3 reveals that 144 of those interviewed suffer from neurological disorders of the type; fièvre (FL=15%) and (FL=10%) confirm that they are prone to (migraine, stress, and cerebral affections). These findings are consistent with those of Bayali & Dami (2019), who reported that in 15 to 25% of migraineurs, the headache is frequently preceded by an aura. Thus, migraine can be described as a neuronal sensitization and neurogenic inflammation in the context of numerous neurochemical stimuli (Lipton, 2000). Then come the diseases, which are classified into two kinds (anxiety and vertigo) (FL=8%). Finally, people who suffer from céphalée, sleep problems, anxiety, mild nerve disorders, and headaches are represented by (FL=7%). The majority of these diseases can be linked to an altered environment (excessive cannabis and other drug use), a stressful event, or another medical condition.

Insomnia is the most common sleep disturbance. It affects one-third of the adult population and ten percent of children. In France, over 30% of the adult population suffers from insomnia.

Nearly 20% experience chronic insomnia. Other studies have shown only 10% of chronic insomnia (Morin et al, 2006; Léger, 2010).

Table 3. Various sorts of neurological diseases encountered in the national park of Talassemtane

Types of neurological diseases	Number of informants (Ip)	frequency of reference FL (%)
Fever	21	15%
Cerebral affection	15	10%
Migraines	15	10%
Stress	15	10%
Anxiety, and vertigo	11	8%
Headache	10	7%
Sleep disorders, anxiety, mild nervous breakdown	10	7%
Cephalea	10	7%
Alzheimer's	6	4%
Fever, headache	6	4%
Anxiety, agitation, insomnia,	5	3%
Frequent nervous disorders, depression, anxiety and migraines.	5	3%
Anxiety and nervous tension	5	3%
Neurological condition	5	3%
Vertigo	5	3%
grand total	**144**	**100%**

The majority of these various illnesses found are treated (tableau n°4) by 22 species belonging to 16 families, the most commonly used plants being Tetraclinis articulata (FL=9,97%), which is used to treat head and cervical injuries. In many parts of Morocco, Tetraclinis articulata is a plant that is well-known for its therapeutic uses (Mehdioui & Kahouadji, 2007; Benkhnigue et al., 2011). This plant is mostly used to treat intestinal and respiratory infections, diabetes, and hypertension (Ziyyat et al., 1997). Its use is explained by its intriguing biological and therapeutic properties, which result from its rich chemical composition of several bioactive constituents. For example, Bourkhiss et al. (2007) reported the presence of 28 compounds in the essential oil of leaves, which are the most commonly used for healing, with the main constituents being limonène, α-pinène, and acétate de bornyle. According to our study, those surveyed confirmed that Tetraclinis articulata has a new therapeutic use in addition to that mentioned above, namely the treatment of brain and spinal disorders. However, clinical evidence of this therapeutic efficacy is required.

Verbena officinalis also represents it (FL=8%), and is used for its effects on the nervous system, specifically on anxiety, vertigo, agitation, and insomnia. Next up are *Matricaria chamomilla* (FL = 7%), which treats sleep disorders, anxiety, mild depressive disorders, *Nerium oleander* (FL = 7%), which is used as a therapeutic agent against cephalopathy, and *Myrtus communis* (FL = 7%), which is also used to treat migraines.

Table 4. Most commonly used spermaceous extracts in neurology phytotherapy (PNTL)

Scientific name (Family + Specie)		Frequency of citation FL (%)
Asteraceae	*Achillea millefolium*	3
	Centaurea clementei	3
	Matricaria chamomilla	7
Brassicaceae	*Alyssum spinosum*	4
Anacardiaceae	*Pistacia lentiscus*	3
Apocynaceae	*Nerium oleander*	7
Boraginaceae	*Anchusa italica*	4
Cannabaceae	*Canabis Sativa*	3
Capparidaceae	*Cleome violacea*	3
Cupressaceae	*Juniperus Communis*	3
	Juniperus oxycedrus	3
	Tetraclinis articulata	10
Fabaceae	*Anthyllis vulneraria*	3
Lamiaceae	*Origanum majorana*	3
	Rosmarinus officinalis	4
Lythraceae	*Lythrum hyssopifolia*	3
Myrtaceae	*Myrtus communis*	7
Oleaceae	*Jasminum officinale*	3
Papaveraceae	*Papaver rhoeas*	3
Solanaceae	*Atropa baetica*	3
	Atropa belladona	3
Verbenaceae	*Verbena officinalis*	8
Total		100

As indicated by Table 5 on the cataloging of medicinal plants used in the national Talassemtane park to treat neurological system disorders. They are arranged by family, species, French and colloquial names, portion used, mode of employment, and forms of diseases. By indicating the quantitative indicators (FC, FRC, NU, and FCI) to analyze each species' medicinal significance.

Table 5. Catalogue of medicinal plants used for the treatment of neurological system pathologies in Talassemtane National Park, their FC, FRC, NU and FCI

Family	Specie	French name	Common name	Part used	Form of employment	Disease types	FC	FRC	NU	FCI
Anacardiaceae	*Pistacia lentiscus*	Pistachier lentisque	Drou - Fadid	Leaves	Powder	Antimigraine	5	0,034	1	0,714
Apocynaceae	*Nerium oleander*	Laurier rose	Dafla	Roots	Another form of employment	Cephalea	10	0,048	1	0
Asteraceae	*Achillea millefolium*	verveine de rocher	Louiza lehjar	Leaves	Tisane	Treats fever	5	0,116	1	0,8
	Centaurea clementei	Centaurée	El kantouryoune	Plante entière	Another form of employment	Fever-reducing	5		1	0,8
	Matricaria chamomilla	Camomille	Amlal/Babounej	Leaves	Herbal tea and essential oil	Sleep disorders, anxiety, mild nervous breakdown	10		3	0
Brassicaceae	*Alyssum spinosum*	Passerage épineux	Alousen - Hachichat soulahfat	Sems, Flowers	Another form of employment	Fever, headache	6	0,027	2	0
Boraginaceae	*Anchusa italica*	Buglosse bleue		Leaves, Roots	Another form of employment	Fièvre.	6	0,027	1	0,75
Cannabaceae	*Canabis Sativa*	Chanvre cultivé	Kif	Flower, Leaves, Seeds	Powder	Stress	5	0,034	3	0,714
Capparidaceae	*Cleome violacea*	Cleome d'Arabie	Mkhinza	Leaves	Tisane	Fever-reducing	5	0,034	1	0,8
Cupressaceae	*Juniperus Communis*	Genévrier commun	Elarâr - Amzi	Leaves	Tisane	Brain disease	5	0,138	1	0,714
	Juniperus oxycedrus	Genévrier oxycédre	El arâar - el gadi	Leaves	Tisane	Brain disease	5		1	0,714
	Tetraclinis articulata	Thuya de Berbérie	El arâar - Azougaâ	Whole plant/ leaves	Tisane	Brain condition/ headache	15		2	0,714
Fabaceae	*Anthyllis vulneraria*	Vulnéraire	Enafla	roots	Another form of employment	For dizziness	5	0,034	1	0
Lamiaceae	*Origanum majorana*	Marjolen origano	Merdadouch= Merdekouch	Leaves	Tisane	Frequent nervous disorders, depression, anxiety and migraines.	5	0,061	4	0
	Rosmarinus officinalis	Romarin	Azir	Leaves	Powder	Cured Alzheimer's	6		1	0
Lythraceae	*Lythrum hyssopifolia*	Lythrum	Rayhan elmaa - sabon elmaa	Flowers	Another form of employment	Neurological condition	5	0,034	1	0
Myrtaceae	*Myrtus communis*	Myrte commum	Elhbak-Arayhan- Ass	Leaves/ Flowers	Powder	Used for migraine pain	10	0,048	1	0,357
Oleaceae	*Jasminum officinale*		Jawhar edar	Leaves	Tisane	Anxiety, agitation, insomnia,	5	0,034	3	0
Papaveraceae	*Papaver rhoeas*	Grand Coquelicot	El khachkhach - Belnaâman	Seeds, Petals	Essential oils	Anxiety and nervous tension	5	0,034	2	0

continued on following page

Table 5. Continued

Family	Specie	French name	Common name	Part used	Form of employment	Disease types	FC	FRC	NU	FCI
Solanaceae	*Atropa baetica*	Belladone bétique	Bleydour	Fruits, seeds	Powder	Relieves pain and stress	5	0,068	2	0,714
	Atropa belladona	Belladone	Bleydour	Fruits, seeds	Powder	Relieves pain and stress	5		2	0,714
Verbenaceae	*Verbena officinalis*	Verveine	Elouiza	Leaves	Tisane	Nervous system action: anxiety, dizziness	11	0,055	2	0

Analysis of Specific Botanical Families and Species, Including Quantitative Analysis Using the FRC and FCI Indices

The cataloging allowed us to identify 22 species belonging to 16 botanical families. The most commonly used families are Cupressaceae (3 species), Asteraceae (3 species), and Lamiaceae (2 species), while the remaining families were represented by a single species (Table 5). Based on the FRC index, we identified four most often cited families: Asteraceae (FRC = 0.116) with FCI = 0.8 > 0.5, representing the two species (achillea millefolium and *Centaurea clementei*), which have a high level of citation in the treatment of fever. The Cupressaceae family (FRC = 0,138) with FCI = 0,714 > 0,5 represents the three species (*Juniperus communis, Juniperus oxycedrus,* and *Tetraclinis articulata*), which are also highly cited in the treatment of cérébral diseases. Finally, the Lamiaceae family (FRC = 0.061) with FCI = 0 < 0.5 represents the two species (*Origanum majorana* and *Rosmarinus officinalis*), which have a low level of citation in the treatment of nerve problems, depression, anxiety, frequent migraines, and Alzheimer's. These plant species, whether natural or cultivated, require phytochemical and pharmaceutical research to identify their chemical constituents and active principles (Benkhnigue et al., 2022).

Recipes, Posology, and Other Common Therapeutic Uses in Traditional Medicine for Neurological Disorders

A plant is considered medicinal when it has a therapeutic effect on humans. As a result (figuren°3), 86% of the species included in the PNTL are therapeutic in nature, compared to 14% that are therapeutic/cosmetic in nature. These findings indicate that the use of traditional pharmacopeia against neurological disorders is more therapeutic than cosmetic, owing to the most common disorders encountered in the region, which include fever, headache, and migraine.

Figure 3. Therapeutic use against neurological disorders

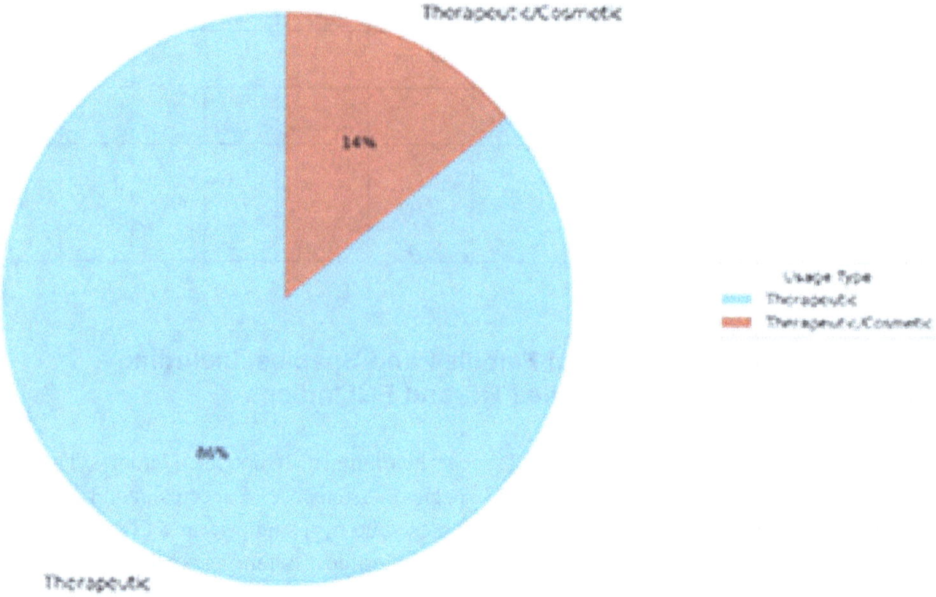

To determine the therapeutic value of a plant, you must first understand its medicinal properties, the composition of the cueillette, the portion that has all of the active constituents that have a therapeutic effect on the body, and the duration of storage. The herb can also be toxic, depending on the dose and how it was used. For this reason, there is a high use of leaves (53% vs. 10% racines) (figure 4); this is due to the plant's active constituents, which are found in its leaves. The ease and speed with which leaves are harvested can explain their high frequency of use. However, they are also the site of photosynthesis and, in some cases, the storage of secondary metabolites responsible for the plant's biological properties (Bigendako-Polygenis & Lejoly, 1990). The use of leaves poses no threat to plant regeneration and will ensure the preservation of botanical diversity.

According to Rhattas et al. (2016b), medicinal plants lose their activity with time; so, flower actives should not be used for more than a year; leaves for more than two years; and roots for three or four years.

Figure 4. Part of the plant most commonly used in traditional medicine to treat neurological disorders

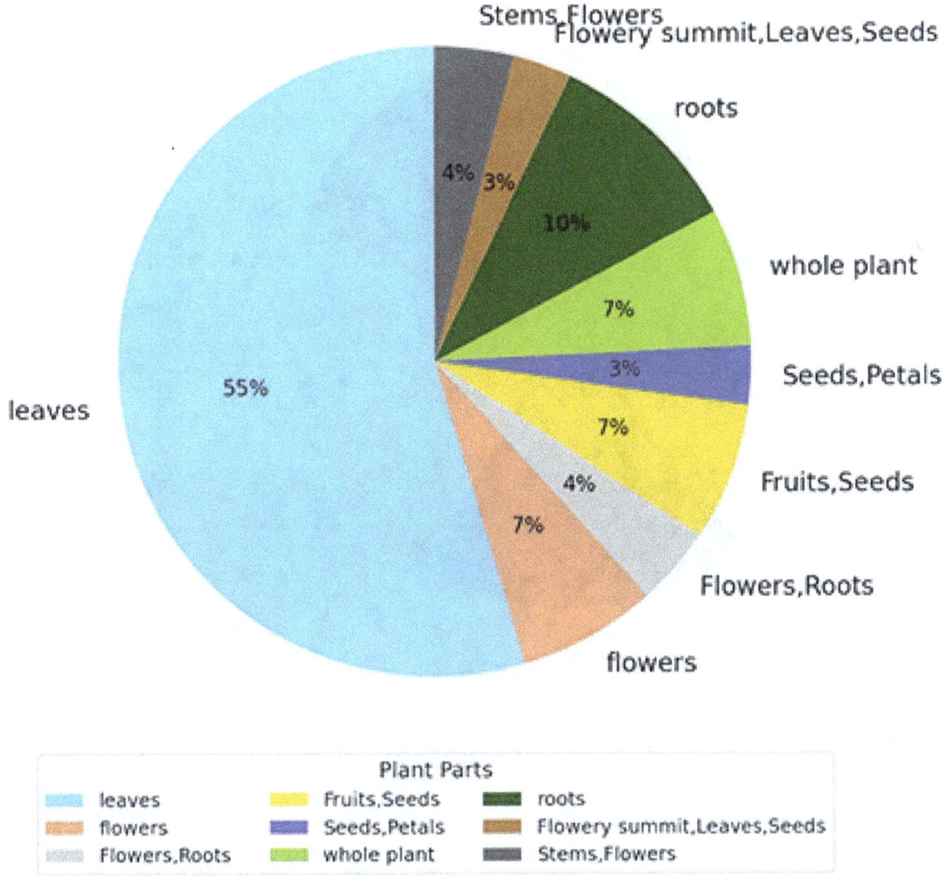

Plant's cueillies must be used in an appropriate manner. According to Figures 5 and 6, there are three modes of use: infusion (39%), extraction (19%), and maceration (14%), which are used in the following three ways (Figure 6), tea (39%), and powder (25%). Tisanes are used to extract the active material from plants: aromatic plants should not be boiled since their active principles dissolve in vapor, and flowers should not be boiled either (WIchtl & Anton, 1999). The infusion is suitable for fragile drugs such as most fragile leaves, flowers, and organs that are high in essential oils (WIchtl & Anton, 1999). This method is appropriate for dry or very dry drogues (bois, racines, écorces, tige, grains, or baies) (WIchtl & Anton, 1999). This method of preparation is particularly applicable to mucilaginous drugs (guimauve or lin...) (WIchtl & Anton, 1999).

According to Rhattas et al. (2016b), the most common and oldest example is tisane, which can be obtained through an infusion, a decoction, or a macération, depending on how long the plant is immersed in bouillante water. However, the plant can also appear as a powder after being broyed, pulvérized, or tamed; this allows it to be absorbed directly into cells.

Figure 5. Most commonly used preparation method in traditional pharmacopeia for neurological disorders

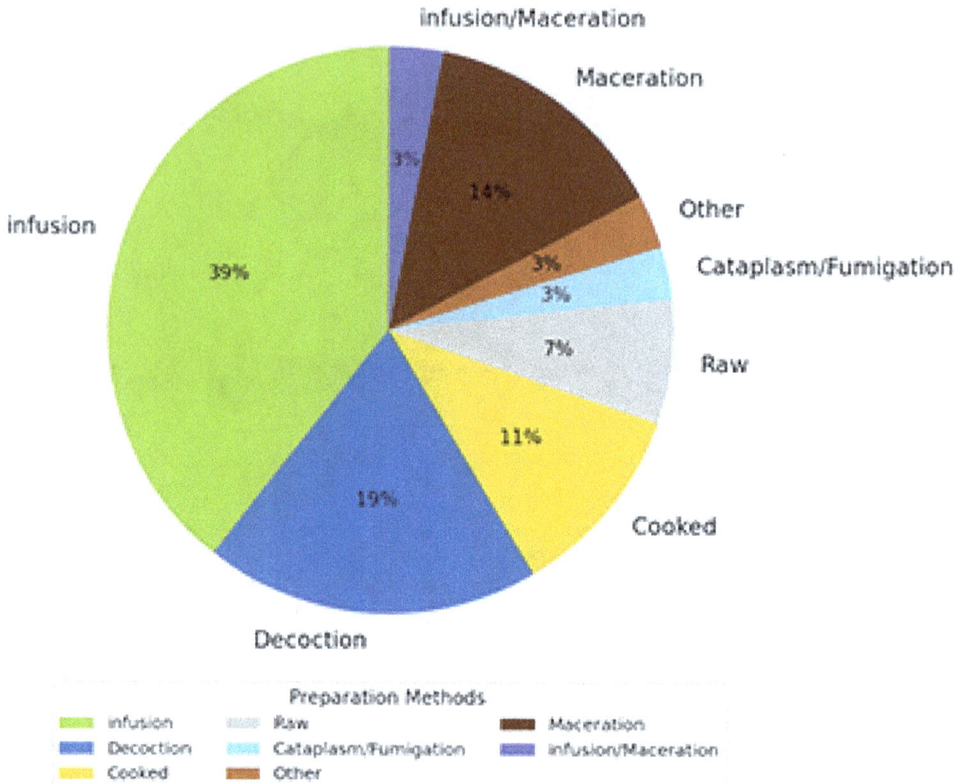

Figure 6. Most common use of traditional pharmaceuticals against neurological disorders

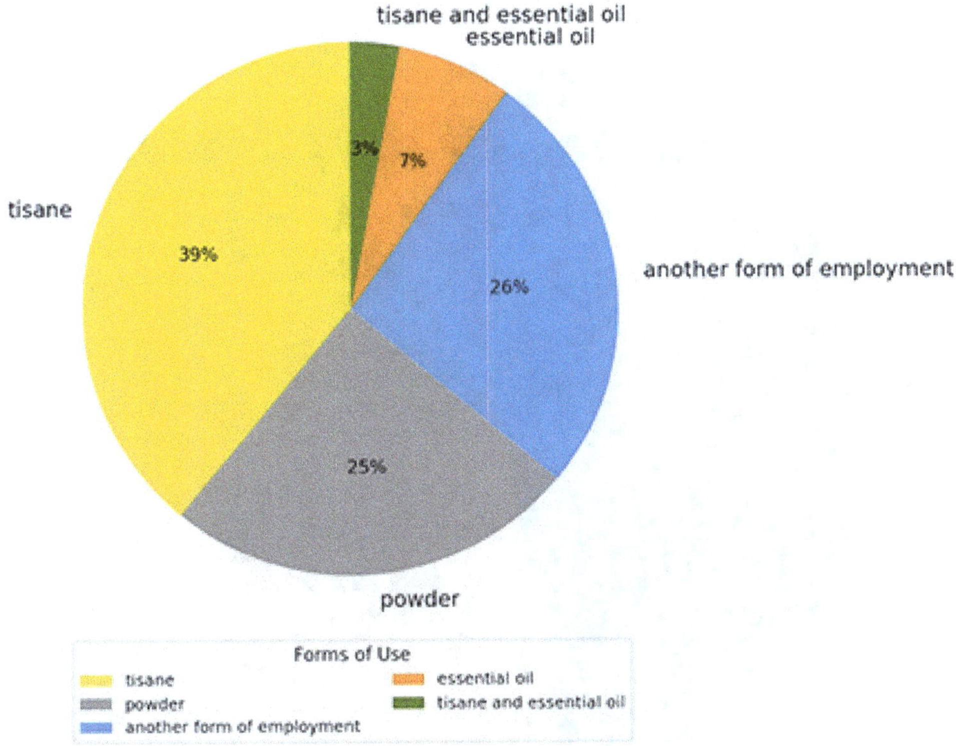

The recommended doses (Figure 7) for taking these recipes are measured by a vers (47%) or a cuillère (29%), to ensure the effectiveness of the remedies and to avoid the risks of intoxication.

Figure 7. Shows the dose used in neurological herbal medication

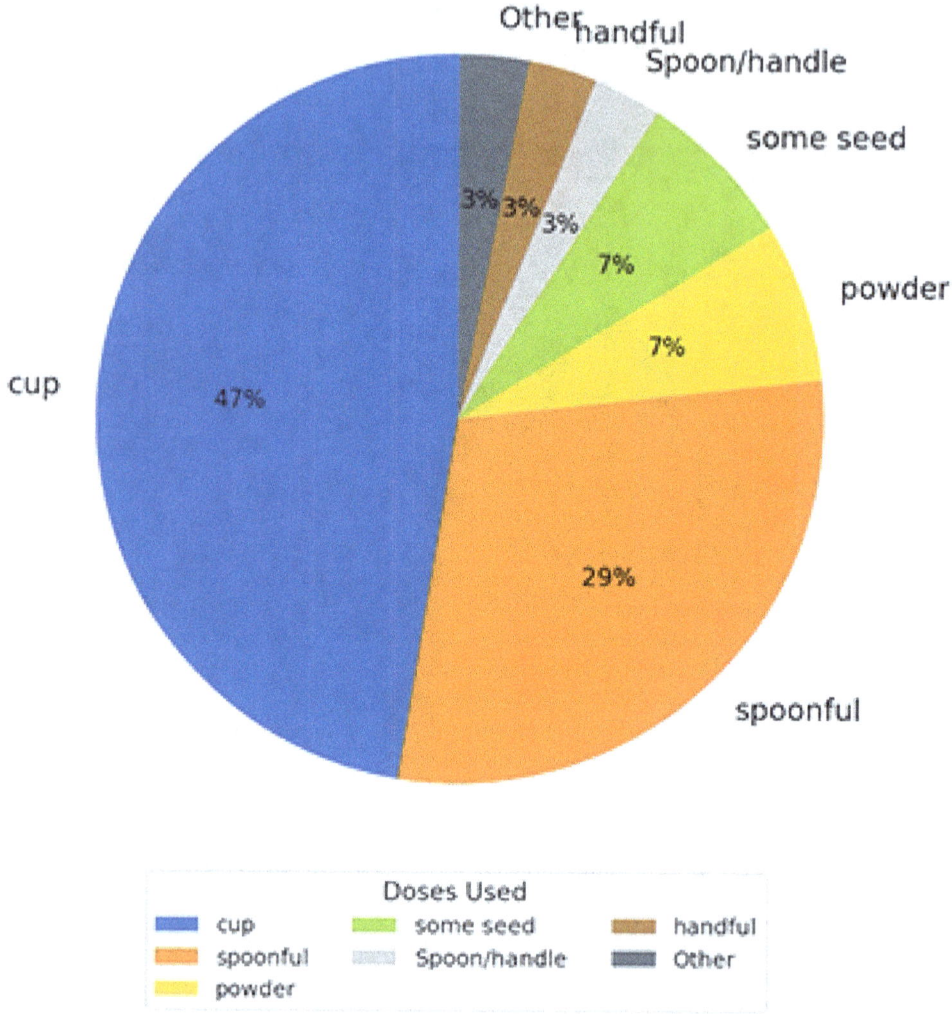

The form and mode of administration specify how to take a pante-based medication that is prepared traditionally according to the knowledge of traditional practitioners. And it is clear that taking a plant extract-based medication via intravenous route runs the risk of intoxication due to ignorance. However, the doses, methods, and routes of administration of plant-based preparations must always be respected (Grünwald & Jänicke, 2007; Debuigne et al., 2013; Fleurentin, 2013; Minker, 2013). According to Rhattas et al. (2016b), self-medication has its limitations, both in terms of effectiveness and risk. The diagnosis of the underlying disease must be precise, the selection of a phytotherapeutic remedy must be based on adequate botanical and pharmacological knowledge, and the preparation of the remedy must adhere to strict protocols. Furthermore, nature is not always benign: the history of poisons is similar to that of medicinal plants. Posadzki et al.

(2013) conducted a synthesis of 50 systematic reviews, each focusing on a different medicinal plant, highlighting that the majority of these plants were associated with adverse effects, most often minor or moderate.

Phytomedicine and Enzyme-Based Therapies

The convergence of historical ethnobotanical knowledge and contemporary pharmacological science provides an exciting avenue for elucidating new enzyme-modulating agents from medicinal plants (Kumar et al., 2021). In many alternative healing traditions, phytomedicines offer several benefits that can be especially relevant to the study of neurodegenerative diseases. Compounds derived from plants often exhibit multi-functional biological activities, effectively modulating several pathological targets at the same time: for example, oxidative stress, neuroinflammation, mitochondrial dysfunction, and dysregulation of enzymes (Rashid et al., 2021; Koppula et al., 2025). This multi-target approach aligns naturally with the complex and multifactorial features of neurodegenerative diseases.

Phytochemicals have a high degree of biocompatibility and low toxicity, especially when compared to synthetic medicines, from a therapeutic perspective. Their long history of use in traditional medicine systems suggests they have acceptable safety profiles, though this claim must be able to be supported through toxicity data from modern toxicological testing (Imam et al., 2021; Mittal & Banerjee, 2021). In addition, many cameral classes found in plants (flavonoids, alkaloids, terpenoids and phenolic acids) provide a very broad structural library for identifying new enzyme inhibitors or activators. For example, many plant bioactive compounds have been shown to inhibit the enzymatic activity of acetylcholinesterase and monoamine oxidase at potencies comparable to pharmaceutical drugs while also exhibiting antioxidant and antiinflammatory activity.

Nonetheless, translating these natural products into clinically useful enzyme-based therapeutics has proven to be difficult (Narayanan, 2025). One of the underlying reasons is the large variability in plant extracts, which can arise due to geographic provenance, processing methods, harvesting specifications, and plant chemotypes. This variability complicates reproducibility of pharmacological results while making standardized formulation development more difficult. Another major limitation is the lack of product standardization and quality control in virtually all phytomedicinal research. Without accurately identifying and quantifying active constituents, it is impossible to link biological activities and chemical structures or determine what constitutes appropriate dosing (Heim et al., 2002; Ebetino et al., 2022). Moreover, most research studies involving plants only utilize *in vitro* assays involving enzyme inhibition - valuable information but limited in its understanding of how a compound behaves in biologically complex systems.

To address these challenges, a multidisciplinary research approach is necessary. Ethnobotanical surveys must be matched with bioactivity-guided fractionation, in silico molecular docking, and enzyme kinetics to identify and optimize active compounds. Once lead candidates are identified, they should enter preclinical testing in animal models for efficacy and toxicity studies and receive eventual human clinical trials to evaluate safety, bioavailability, and therapeutic intent. The extent of technology and innovation in recent years in computational biology and AI has also provided new pathways for faster timeframes in drug discovery from natural sources. For instance, AI and machine learning algorithms can now estimate enzyme binding affinities, toxicity, and pharmacokinetics, decreasing the amount of time and money spent on compound portfolios. Therefore,

the addition of omics data (e.g., metabolomics, proteomics) from the studies of medicinal plants may enhance the understanding of their bioactivity and synergistic properties.

From both ethical and conservation perspectives, the valorisation of traditional knowledge must be attentive to cultural heritage and biodiversity conservation. Sustainable harvesting principles and benefit-sharing provisions, should be a part of any bioprospecting process. Phytomedicine represents an important potential source of additional information to enhance the enzyme therapy sphere of neurodegeneration. But this application is contingent on marrying traditional practices with modern pharmacological tasks, computational tools, and regulatory conditions. At best, an integration could lead to safer, more effective, and culturally relevant therapeutic options for diseases which currently have no solution.

Limitations and Future Perspectives

Notwithstanding the helpful insights of this ethnobotanical-pharmacological study, we need to be cognizant of several limitations. First, most of the data we collected on the use of medicinal plants comes from traditional knowledge and self-reported uses. Although these data provide robust information to indicate potential pathways for scientific exploration, they are subjective and may vary due to local cultural context, memory bias, or interpretation by the informant. Thus, the therapeutic claims made in regards to the listed plants require further experimental validation through proper pharmacological studies. Another limiting factor is the underdeveloped phytochemical characterization and the lack of dose standardization. Most traditional preparations are aqueous or hydroalcoholic decoctions, whose chemical constituents could vary widely based on plant maturity, climate factors, and method of preparation. It would be difficult to achieve the reproducibility and well-defined therapeutic outcomes without precise measurement of active constituents. None of the plant species cited have been formally tested using appropriate in vivo models of neurodegeneration, and nearly all of the plant species have not had clinical trials to represent the first objective step along the pathway toward evidence-based integration into therapy. Most of the enzyme inhibition data in the available literature is pharmacological in nature, meaning that it is in vitro data. In vitro data can be informative, but in vivo it does not always result in efficacy due to the potential impact of poor absorption, metabolism, and penetration across the blood-brain barrier. In addition, there is still a lack of knowledge regarding how multiple phytochemicals within the same extract may work relative to each other to produce synergistic or antagonistic interactions.

To further the progress of the studies in this area, we recommend future studies should now focus on the bio-guided fractionation and phytochemical evaluation of the top ranking medicinal plants. This work will help to be able to successfully isolate and identify actual bioactive compounds that modulate the enzymes at question. More specifically, once isolated, the bioactive compound should then be used to conduct molecular docking and computational simulations, in order to determine binding affinities, specificity for the appropriate enzymatic target, as well as off target predictions. Once in silico predictions have been made regarding bioactive compounds using biomolecular modelling, a strong next step for validation would include using the compounds in animal models for neurodegenerative diseases. Some examples include: Alzheimer's disease, Parkinson's disease, or amyotrophic lateral sclerosis (ALS), This would allow a rigorous biological assessment for efficacy and safety as well as determine how to use the bioactive compounds in a biological context. Would also need to perform any pharmacokinetic

work to assess bioavailability and to see how long it would take to sub-stantiate any binding at the enzyme level, as well as assess absorption, metabolism, and how to cross the blood-brain barrier for therapeutic efficacy.

Additionally, we need standardized formulations of whole plant extracts and/or purified compounds for reproducibility and clinical application. Research should also consider the possibilities of synergistic interactions among phytochemicals in mixtures as multi-component therapies could produce a more potent therapeutic benefit than providing a single agent. Beyond the science and technology there are ethical, environmental, and regulatory concerns, including the sustainable use of plant resources, respect for indigenous knowledge systems, and compliance with bioprospecting and intellectual property laws. Researchers can harness the strengths of ethnopharmaceutical, neuroscience, pharmacology, and bioinformatics to develop a robust interdisciplinary paradigm for the identification of new neuroprotective agents. An integrated strategy is a powerful tool for growing the pool of enzyme-targeted therapies and allowing sustainable biodiversity conservation and respectful inclusion of cultural knowledge into alternative neurodegenerative disease treatments.

CONCLUSION

Neurodegenerative diseases are still one of the most difficult situations facing contemporary medicine today because of their multi-factorial aetiology, progressive nature, and a lack of disease-modifying treatments. Indigenous ethnobotanical knowledge (particularly knowledge of the medicinal plants of Morocco's Talassemtane National Park) has the potential to be a source of multi-target drugs capable of modulating the key enzymatic processes involved in neuronal cell deterioration. In this chapter we have illustrated the efficacy of phytochemicals from a number of structural classes (including flavonoids, alkaloids, terpenoids and polyphenols) inhibiting enzymes including acetylcholinesterase and monoamine oxidase and exerting antioxidant and anti-inflammatory action. The results discussed in this chapter demonstrate that there is potential from plant-derived products. But ultimately, would require rigorous phytochemical standardisation, in vivo validation, and clinical trials. The fieldwork demonstrated both the extent of local knowledge about plants, as well as its practicality. Based on 144 recorded interviews, it is evident that medicinal plants are used regularly for many neurological symptoms and ailments, including fever, vertigo, minor nerve disorders, anxiety, insomnia, and headaches. Overall, we documented 22 neuroactive species from 16 plant families, with the most represented families being Cupressaceae, Asteraceae, Lamiaceae, and Verbenaceae. The species that were most often recorded as treatments for neurological ailments were Tetraclinis articulata (Cupressaceae), Verbena officinalis (Verbenaceae), and Matricaria chamomilla (Asteraceae). Collectively, leaves were the plant part used most often (which have the least processing) and infusion, decoction, or maceration (to be taken as herbal tea or powder) were the dominant methods of preparation. Women were identified as the dominant custodians of this pharmacopoeia, which reinforces the importance of gender to traditional medical knowledge. The socio-economic context further emphasizes the significance of these findings: in a continent where 80% of the population cannot afford regular medical treatment, accessible medicinal plants can serve as an essential line of approach. Realizing their community's global potential for pharmacy and biotechnology purposes requires two approaches: (i) a scientific approach—isolating, characterizing, and optimizing

active constituents for safety and standardization for use; and (ii) a socio-ecological approach—protecting the percentage of floristic, genetic and cultural diversity through sustainable harvesting and education to communities generally. Moving forward with broad-scale sensitization of local stakeholders can assist in conserving these resources while making sure they are contextualized within a modern approach to neuropharmacology. By linking ethnopharmacology through the the lens of molecular neuroscience and biotechnology, we can convert traditional remedies for neurodegenerative disease into scientifically validated and enzyme-directed interventions, thus simultaneously enhancing both global health and the conservation of biodiversity.

REFERENCES

Addoun, A. B. S. (2017). *Étude ethnobotanique sur les plantes toxiques dans la région de la ville de Tlemcen.*

Anwar, S., Alrumaihi, F., Sarwar, T., Babiker, A. Y., Khan, A. A., Prabhu, S. V., & Rahmani, A. H. (2024). Exploring therapeutic potential of catalase: Strategies in disease prevention and management. *Biomolecules*, *14*(6), 697. DOI: 10.3390/biom14060697 PMID: 38927099

Barba-Ostria, C., Carrera-Pacheco, S. E., Gonzalez-Pastor, R., Heredia-Moya, J., Mayorga-Ramos, A., Rodríguez-Pólit, C., Zúñiga-Miranda, J., Arias-Almeida, B., & Guamán, L. P. (2022). Evaluation of biological activity of natural compounds: Current trends and methods. *Molecules (Basel, Switzerland)*, *27*(14), 4490. DOI: 10.3390/molecules27144490 PMID: 35889361

Bayali, N., Dami, A. (2019). Phytothérapies cliniques dans les affections neurologiques [Thèse de doctorat en pharmacie, Université Mohammed V de Rabat, Faculté de médecine et de pharmacie de Rabat].

Bellakhdar, J. (1997). *La pharmacopée marocaine traditionnelle: Médecine arabe ancienne et savoirs populaires*. Ibis Press.

Benabid, A. (1982). Études phytoécologique, biogéographique et dynamique des associations et séries sylvatiques du Rif Occidental (Maroc) [Thèse de doctorat, Université Aix-Marseille III, France] (199 p.).

Benkhnigue, O., Ben Akka, F., Salhi, S., Fadli, M., Douira, A., & Zidane, L. (2014). Catalogue des plantes médicinales utilisées dans le traitement du diabète dans la région d'Al Haouz-Rhamna (Maroc). *Journal of Animal & Plant Sciences*, *23*(1), 3539–3568.

Benkhnigue, O., Chaachouay, N., Khamar, H., El Azzouzi, F., Douira, A., & Zidane, L. (2022). Ethnobotanical and ethnopharmacological study of medicinal plants used in the treatment of anemia in the region of Haouz-Rehamna (Morocco). *Journal of Pharmacy & Pharmacognosy Research*, *10*(2), 279–302. DOI: 10.56499/jppres21.1196_10.2.279

Benkhnigue, O., Zidane, Z., Fadli, M., Elyacoubi, H., Rochdi, A., & Douira, A. (2011). Étude ethnobotanique des plantes médicinales dans la région de Mechraâ Bel Ksiri (Région du Gharb du Maroc). *Acta Botanica Barcinonensis*, *53*, 191–216.

Bigendako-Polygenis, M. J., & Lejoly, J. (1990). La pharmacopée traditionnelle au Burundi. Pesticides et médicaments en santé animale. In *Pres* (pp. 425–442). Univ.

Bourkhiss, M., Hnach, M., Bourkhiss, B., Ouhssine, M., & Chaouch, A. (2007). Composition chimique et propriétés antimicrobiennes de l'huile essentielle extraite des feuilles de Tetraclinis articulata (Vahl) du Maroc. *Afrique SCIENCE*, *3*, 232–242.

Calderaro, A., Patanè, G. T., Tellone, E., Barreca, D., Ficarra, S., Misiti, F., & Laganà, G. (2022). The neuroprotective potentiality of flavonoids on Alzheimer's disease. *International Journal of Molecular Sciences*, *23*(14835), 14835. Advance online publication. DOI: 10.3390/ijms232314835 PMID: 36499159

Chaudhary, P., Janmeda, P., Docea, A. O., Yeskaliyeva, B., Abdull Razis, A. F., Modu, B., Calina, D., & Sharifi-Rad, J. (2023). Oxidative stress, free radicals and antioxidants: Potential crosstalk in the pathophysiology of human diseases. *Frontiers in Chemistry, 11*, 1158198. Advance online publication. DOI: 10.3389/fchem.2023.1158198 PMID: 37234200

Choi, H. K., Chen, M., Goldston, L. L., & Lee, K.-B. (2024). Extracellular vesicles as nanotheranostic platforms for targeted neurological disorder interventions. *Nano Convergence, 11*(1), 19. Advance online publication. DOI: 10.1186/s40580-024-00426-5 PMID: 38739358

Ciurea, A. V., Mohan, A. G., Covache-Busuioc, R. A., Costin, H. P., Glavan, L. A., Corlatescu, A. D., & Saceleanu, V. M. (2023). Unraveling molecular and genetic insights into neurodegenerative diseases: Advances in understanding Alzheimer's, Parkinson's, and Huntington's diseases and amyotrophic lateral sclerosis. *International Journal of Molecular Sciences, 24*(13), 10809. DOI: 10.3390/ijms241310809 PMID: 37445986

Dai, R., Sun, Y., Su, R., & Gao, H. (2022). Anti-Alzheimer's disease potential of traditional Chinese medicinal herbs as inhibitors of BACE1 and AChE enzymes. *Biomedicine and Pharmacotherapy, 154*, 113576. DOI: 10.1016/j.biopha.2022.113576 PMID: 36007279

De La Fuente, M., Lombardero, L., Gómez-González, A., Solari, C., Angulo-Barturen, I., Acera, A., Vecino, E., Astigarraga, E., & Barreda-Gómez, G. (2021). Enzyme therapy: Current challenges and future perspectives. *International Journal of Molecular Sciences, 22*(17), 9181. DOI: 10.3390/ijms22179181 PMID: 34502086

Debuigne, G., & Couplan, F. (2013). *Petit Larousse des plantes médicinales*. Editions Larousse.

Doroszkiewicz, J., Groblewska, M., & Mroczko, B. (2022). Molecular biomarkers and their implications for the early diagnosis of selected neurodegenerative diseases. *International Journal of Molecular Sciences, 23*(9), 4610. DOI: 10.3390/ijms23094610 PMID: 35563001

Dzah, C. S., Zhang, H., Gobe, V., Asante-Donyinah, D., & Duan, Y. (2024). Anti- and pro-oxidant properties of polyphenols and their role in modulating glutathione synthesis, activity and cellular redox potential: Potential synergies for disease management. *Advances in Redox Research : an Official Journal of the Society for Redox Biology and Medicine and the Society for Free Radical Research-Europe, 11*, 100099. DOI: 10.1016/j.arres.2024.100099

Ebetino, F. H., Sun, S., Cherian, P., Roshandel, S., Neighbors, J. D., Hu, E., Dunford, J. E., Sedghizadeh, P. P., McKenna, C. E., Srinivasan, V., Boeckman, R. K., & Russell, R. G. G. (2022). Bisphosphonates: The role of chemistry in understanding their biological actions and structure-activity relationships, and new directions for their therapeutic use. *Bone, 156*, 116289. DOI: 10.1016/j.bone.2021.116289 PMID: 34896359

El Gharbaoui, A. (1981). La Terre et l'Homme dans la Péninsule Tingitane: étude sur l'homme et le milieu naturel dans le Rif Occidental. Travaux de l'Institut Scientifique, Rabat, série Géologie Géographie Physique, 15, 1–439.

El Hilah, F., Ben Akka, F., Bengueddour, R., Rochdi, A., & Zidane, L. (2016). Étude ethnobotanique des plantes médicinales utilisées dans le traitement des affections dermatologiques dans le plateau central marocain. *Journal of Applied Biosciences, 98*(0), 9252–9260. DOI: 10.4314/jab.v98i1.2

Fennane, M., & Ibn Tattou, M. (2005). Flore vasculaire du Maroc: Inventaire et chorologie (Vol. 1). Travaux de l'Institut Scientifique, Rabat, Série Botanique No. 37, 483 pages.

Fennane, M., Ibn Tattou, M., Mathez, J., Ouyahya, A., & Eloualidi, J. (1999). Flore pratique du Maroc, manuel de détermination des plantes vasculaires. Volume 1: Ptéridophytes - Gymnospermes, Angiospermes (Lauraceae - Neuradaceae). Travaux de l'Institut Scientifique, Rabat, Série Botanique No. 36, 558 pages.

Fennane, M., Ibn Tattou, M., Mathez, J., Ouyahya, A., & Eloualidi, J. (2007). Flore pratique du Maroc, manuel de détermination des plantes vasculaires. Volume 2: Angiospermes (Leguminoseae - Lentibulariaceae). Travaux de l'Institut Scientifique, Rabat, Série Botanique No. 38, 636 pages.

Fleurentin, J. (2013). Du bon usage des plantes qui soignent. Éditions Ouest-France.

Ghourri, M., Zidane, L., & Douira, A. (2014). La phytothérapie et les infections urinaires (la pyélonéphrite et la cystite) au Sahara Marocain (Tan-Tan). *Journal of Animal & Plant Sciences*, *20*(3), 3171–3193.

Giri, P. M., Banerjee, A., Ghosal, A., & Layek, B. (2024). Neuroinflammation in neurodegenerative disorders: Current knowledge and therapeutic implications. *International Journal of Molecular Sciences*, *25*(7), 3995. DOI: 10.3390/ijms25073995 PMID: 38612804

Goetz, P. (2011). Phytothérapie de l'insomnie. *Phytothérapie*, *9*(1), 38–41. DOI: 10.1007/s10298-010-0605-2

Grünwald, J., & Jänicke, C. (2007). *Guide de la phytothérapie*. Editions Marabout.

Gueye, M., Cisse, A., Diatta, C. D., Diop, S., & Koma, S. (2012). Étude ethnobotanique des plantes utilisées contre la constipation chez les Malinké de la communauté rurale de Tomboronkoto, Kédougou (Sénégal). *International Journal of Biological and Chemical Sciences*, *6*(2), 773–781. DOI: 10.4314/ijbcs.v6i2.19

Heim, K. E., Tagliaferro, A. R., & Bobilya, D. J. (2002). Flavonoid antioxidants: Chemistry, metabolism and structure-activity relationships. *The Journal of Nutritional Biochemistry*, *13*(10), 572–584. DOI: 10.1016/S0955-2863(02)00208-5 PMID: 12550068

Heinrich, M., Ankli, A., Frei, B., Weimann, C., & Sticher, O. (1998). Medicinal plants in Mexico: Healers' consensus and cultural importance. *Social Science & Medicine*, *47*(11), 1859–1871. DOI: 10.1016/S0277-9536(98)00181-6 PMID: 9877354

Hmamouchi, M. (1999). Les plantes médicinales et aromatiques marocaines, étude de faisabilité économique pour investir dans le secteur des plantes médicinales et aromatiques. Fedalla (ed.), 5 pages.

Hseini, S., & Kahouadji, A. (2007). Étude ethnobotanique de la flore médicinale dans la région de Rabat (Maroc occidental). *Lazaroa*, *28*, 79–93.

Imam, S. S., Alshehri, S., Ghoneim, M. M., Zafar, A., Alsaidan, O. A., Alruwaili, N. K., Gilani, S. J., & Rizwanullah, M. (2021). Recent advancement in chitosan-based nanoparticles for improved oral bioavailability and bioactivity of phytochemicals: Challenges and perspectives. *Polymers, 13*(22), 4036. DOI: 10.3390/polym13224036 PMID: 34833334

Ivy, D. (2021). Les maladies neurodégénératives s'invitent et les pertes se succèdent. Le Journal des psychologues, 6(388), 14–19.

Jankowska, A., Chwojnicki, K., Grzywińska, M., Trzonkowski, P., & Szurowska, E. (2023). Choroid plexus volume change—A candidate for a new radiological marker of MS progression. *Diagnostics (Basel), 13*(16), 2668. DOI: 10.3390/diagnostics13162668 PMID: 37627928

Jensen, M. G., Goode, M., & Heinrich, M. (2024). Herbal medicines and botanicals for managing insomnia, stress, anxiety, and depression: A critical review of the emerging evidence focusing on the Middle East and Africa. *PharmaNutrition, 29*, 100399. DOI: 10.1016/j.phanu.2024.100399

Koppula, S., Shaik, B., & Maddi, S. (2025). Phytosomes as a new frontier and emerging nanotechnology platform for phytopharmaceuticals: Therapeutic and clinical applications. *Phytotherapy Research, 39*(5), 2217–2249. DOI: 10.1002/ptr.8465 PMID: 40110760

Kumar, A., Kumar, S., Komal, , Ramchiary, N., & Singh, P. (2021). Role of traditional ethnobotanical knowledge and indigenous communities in achieving sustainable development goals. *Sustainability (Basel), 13*(6), 3062. DOI: 10.3390/su13063062

Lamptey, R. N. L., Chaulagain, B., Trivedi, R., Gothwal, A., Layek, B., & Singh, J. (2022). A review of the common neurodegenerative disorders: Current therapeutic approaches and the potential role of nanotherapeutics. *International Journal of Molecular Sciences, 23*(3), 1851. DOI: 10.3390/ijms23031851 PMID: 35163773

Larit, F., & León, F. (2023). Therapeutics to treat psychiatric and neurological disorders: A promising perspective from Algerian traditional medicine. *Plants, 12*(22), 3860. DOI: 10.3390/plants12223860 PMID: 38005756

Lazli, A., Beldi, M., Ghouri, L., & Nouri, N. H. (2019). Étude ethnobotanique et inventaire des plantes médicinales dans la région de Bougous (Parc National d'El Kala, - Nord-est algérien). *Bulletin de la Société Royale des Sciences de Liège, 88*, 22–43. DOI: 10.25518/0037-9565.8429

Léger, D. (2010). *Le sommeil dans tous ses états*. Plon.

Lipton, R. B. (2000). American Migraine Study II. Presented at the *42nd Annual Scientific Meeting of the American Headache Society*, June 23, 2000.

Masereel, B. Histoire de la Pharmacie. Cours d'Introduction aux sciences pharmaceutiques. Université de Namur Webcampus. Consulté le 28 septembre 2018, p. 5.

Maurer, G. (1968). *Les montagnes du Rif central. Étude géomorphologique. Travaux de Doctorat ès-lettres*. Faculté des Lettres et Sciences Humaines.

Mehdioui, R., & Kahouadji, A. (2007). Étude ethnobotanique auprès de la population riveraine de la forêt d'Amsittène: Cas de la Commune d'Imi n'Tlit (Province d'Essaouira). Bulletin de l'Institut Scientifique, Rabat. *Section Sciences de la Vie*, *29*, 11–20.

Miara, M. D., Bendif, H., Ait Hammou, M., & Teixidor-Toneu, I. (2018). Ethnobotanical survey of medicinal plants used by nomadic peoples in the Algerian steppe. *Journal of Ethnopharmacology*, *219*, 248–256. DOI: 10.1016/j.jep.2018.03.011 PMID: 29548971

Minker, C. (2013). *200 plantes qui vous veulent du bien*. Editions Larousse.

Mittal, A. K., & Banerjee, U. C. (2021). In vivo safety, toxicity, biocompatibility and anti-tumour efficacy of bioinspired silver and selenium nanoparticles. *Materials Today. Communications*, *26*, 102001. DOI: 10.1016/j.mtcomm.2020.102001

Moreta, M. P.-G., Burgos-Alonso, N., Torrecilla, M., Marco-Contelles, J., & Bruzos-Cidón, C. (2021). Efficacy of Acetylcholinesterase Inhibitors on Cognitive Function in Alzheimer's Disease: Review of Reviews. *Biomedicines*, *9*(11), 1689. DOI: 10.3390/biomedicines9111689 PMID: 34829917

Morin, C. M., Leblanc, M., Daley, M., Grégoire, J. P., & Mérette, C. (2006). Epidemiology of insomnia: Prevalence, self-help treatments, consultations, and determinants of help-seeking behaviors. *Sleep Medicine*, *7*(2), 123–130. DOI: 10.1016/j.sleep.2005.08.008 PMID: 16459140

Narayanan, K. B. (2025). Enzyme-based anti-inflammatory therapeutics for inflammatory diseases. *Pharmaceutics*, *17*(5), 606. DOI: 10.3390/pharmaceutics17050606 PMID: 40430897

Nasso, R., Pagliara, V., D'Angelo, S., Rullo, R., Masullo, M., & Arcone, R. (2021). Annurca Apple Polyphenol Extract Affects Acetyl-Cholinesterase and Mono-Amine Oxidase In Vitro Enzyme Activity. *Pharmaceuticals (Basel, Switzerland)*, *14*(1), 62. DOI: 10.3390/ph14010062 PMID: 33466604

Pathak, N., Vimal, S. K., Tandon, I., Agrawal, L., Hongyi, C., & Bhattacharyya, S. (2022). Neurodegenerative disorders of Alzheimer, Parkinsonism, amyotrophic lateral sclerosis and multiple sclerosis: An early diagnostic approach for precision treatment. *Metabolic Brain Disease*, *37*(1), 67–104. DOI: 10.1007/s11011-021-00800-w PMID: 34719771

Posadzki, P., Watson, L. K., & Ernst, E. (2013). Adverse effects of herbal medicines: An overview of systematic reviews. *Clinical Medicine*, *13*(1), 7–12. DOI: 10.7861/clinmedicine.13-1-7 PMID: 23472485

Prance, G. T., Balee, W., Boom, B. M., & Carneiro, R. L. (1987). Quantitative ethnobotany and the case for conservation in Amazonia. *Conservation Biology*, *1*(4), 296–310. DOI: 10.1111/j.1523-1739.1987.tb00050.x

Querzel, P., & Santa, S. (1962). *Nouvelle flore de l'Algérie et des Régions désertiques méridionales* (Vol. I). Centre National de la Recherche Scientifique.

Rashid, S., Majeed, L. R., Nisar, B., Nisar, H., Bhat, A. A., & Ganai, B. A. (2021). Phytomedicines: Diversity, extraction, and conservation strategies. In Phytomedicine: A treasure of pharmacologically active products from plants (pp. 1–33). https://doi.org/DOI: 10.1016/B978-0-12-824109-7.00009-1

Rhattas, M., Douira, A., & Zidane, L. (2016). Étude ethnobotanique des plantes médicinales dans le Parc National de Talassemtane (Rif occidental du Maroc). *Journal of Applied Biosciences, 97*(0), 9187–9211. DOI: 10.4314/jab.v97i1.5

Rhattas, M., Douira, A., & Zidane, L. (2016). Phytothérapie épidermique utilisée par la population du parc national de Talassemtane. *International Journal of Innovation and Scientific Research, 24*(1), 20–31.

Ribaudo, G., Memo, M., & Gianoncelli, A. (2021). Multi-target natural and nature-inspired compounds against neurodegeneration: A focus on dual cholinesterase and phosphodiesterase inhibitors. *Applied Sciences (Basel, Switzerland), 11*(11), 5044. DOI: 10.3390/app11115044

Rodrigues, M. J., Pereira, C. G., & Custódio, L. (2024). Neuroprotective and mental health benefits of salt-tolerant plants: A comprehensive review of traditional uses and biological properties. *Applied Sciences (Basel, Switzerland), 14*(13), 5534. DOI: 10.3390/app14135534

Sahakyan, G., Vejux, A., & Sahakyan, N. (2022). The role of oxidative stress-mediated inflammation in the development of T2DM-induced diabetic nephropathy: Possible preventive action of tannins and other oligomeric polyphenols. *Molecules (Basel, Switzerland), 27*(24), 9035. DOI: 10.3390/molecules27249035 PMID: 36558167

Salohi, S. (2012). *Mémoire de fin d'étude: la Réserve de Biosphère Intercontinentale de la Méditerranée (RBIM). École Nationale Forestière d'Ingénieurs, Rabat–Salé.* ENFI.

Scherrer, A. M., Motti, R., & Weckerle, C. S. (2005). Traditional plant use in the areas of Monte Vesole and Ascea, Cilento National Park (Campania, Southern Italy). *Journal of Ethnopharmacology, 97*(1), 129–143. DOI: 10.1016/j.jep.2004.11.002 PMID: 15652287

Sharifi-Rad, M., Anil Kumar, N. V., Zucca, P., Varoni, E. M., Dini, L., Panzarini, E., Rajkovic, J., Tsouh Fokou, P. V., Azzini, E., Peluso, I., Prakash Mishra, A., Nigam, M., El Rayess, Y., Beyrouthy, M. E., Polito, L., Iriti, M., Martins, N., Martorell, M., Docea, A. O., & Sharifi-Rad, J. (2020). Lifestyle, oxidative stress, and antioxidants: Back and forth in the pathophysiology of chronic diseases. *Frontiers in Physiology, 11*, 694. Advance online publication. DOI: 10.3389/fphys.2020.00694 PMID: 32714204

Shoaib, S., Ansari, M. A., Fatease, A. A., Safhi, A. Y., Hani, U., Jahan, R., Alomary, M. N., Ansari, M. N., Ahmed, N., Wahab, S., Ahmad, W., Yusuf, N., & Islam, N. (2023). Plant-Derived Bioactive Compounds in the Management of Neurodegenerative Disorders: Challenges, Future Directions and Molecular Mechanisms Involved in Neuroprotection. *Pharmaceutics, 15*(3), 749. DOI: 10.3390/pharmaceutics15030749 PMID: 36986610

Sibeko, L., & Johns, T. (2021). Global survey of medicinal plants during lactation and postpartum recovery: Evolutionary perspectives and contemporary health implications. *Journal of Ethnopharmacology, 270*, 113812. DOI: 10.1016/j.jep.2021.113812 PMID: 33450288

Tabuti, J. R. S., Lye, K. A., & Dhillion, S. S. (2003). Traditional herbal drugs of Bulamogi, Uganda: Plants, use and administration. *Journal of Ethnopharmacology*, *88*(1), 19–44. DOI: 10.1016/S0378-8741(03)00161-2 PMID: 12902048

Talbi, S., Rojas, J. A., Sahrawy, M., Rodríguez-Serrano, M., Cárdenas, K. E., Debouba, M., & Sandalio, L. M. (2020). Effect of drought on growth, photosynthesis and total antioxidant capacity of the Saharan plant Oudeneya africana. *Environmental and Experimental Botany*, *176*, 104099. DOI: 10.1016/j.envexpbot.2020.104099

Tan, E. W., Low, L. H., Atanasov, A. G., & Goh, B. H. (2025). Bridging traditions and technology: The role of ethnopharmacology in shaping next-generation multidisciplinary researchers. *Pharmacology Research & Perspectives*, *13*(1), e70074. DOI: 10.1002/prp2.70074 PMID: 39929745

Tardío, J., & Pardo-de-Santayana, M. (2008). Cultural importance indices: A comparative analysis based on the useful wild plants of Southern Cantabria (Northern Spain). *Economic Botany*, *62*(1), 24–39. DOI: 10.1007/s12231-007-9004-5

Togo, M., Maïga, Y. M., & Guinto, C. O. (2022). *Impact de la médecine traditionnelle dans la prise en charge des pathologies neurologiques au Mali (Mémoire de D.E.S en Neurologie). Faculté de Médecine et d'Odonto-Stomatologie, Université des Sciences, des Techniques et des Technologies de Bamako (USTTB)*. République du Mali.

Torres-Herrero, B., Armenia, I., Ortiz, C., Martinez de la Fuente, J., Betancor, L., & Grazú, V. (2024). Opportunities for nanomaterials in enzyme therapy. *Journal of Controlled Release*, *372*, 619–647. DOI: 10.1016/j.jconrel.2024.06.035 PMID: 38909702

Wichtl, M., & Anton, R. (1999). *Plantes thérapeutiques: traditions, pratiques officinales, science et thérapeutique*. Tec & Doc.

Wong, V. W. S., Ekstedt, M., Wong, G. L. H., & Hagström, H. (2023). Changing epidemiology, global trends and implications for outcomes of NAFLD. *Journal of Hepatology*, *79*(3), 842–852. DOI: 10.1016/j.jhep.2023.04.036 PMID: 37169151

Yuan, H., Ma, Q., Ye, L., & Piao, G. (2016). The traditional medicine and modern medicine from natural products. *Molecules (Basel, Switzerland)*, *21*(5), 559. DOI: 10.3390/molecules21050559 PMID: 27136524

Ziyyat, A., Legssyer, A., Mekhfi, H., Dassouli, A., Serhrouchni, M., & Benjelloun, W. (1997). Phytotherapy of hypertension and diabetes in oriental Morocco. *Journal of Ethnopharmacology*, *58*(1), 45–54. DOI: 10.1016/S0378-8741(97)00077-9 PMID: 9324004

Chapter 17
Cognitive Revival Through Nature by Investigating the Neuroactive Potential of Phytomedicines

Vivek Pazhamalai
https://orcid.org/0000-0003-2088-7545
Department of Bioengineering, Vels Institute of Science, Technology, and Advanced Studies, India

M. Suriya
https://orcid.org/0009-0008-5398-0221
Department of Bioengineering, Vels Institute of Science, Technology, and Advanced Studies, India

V. Aarthi
https://orcid.org/0009-0004-0177-7716
Department of Bioengineering, Vels Institute of Science, Technology, and Advanced Studies, India

S. Ivo Romauld
https://orcid.org/0000-0003-0610-0646
Department of Bioengineering, Vels Institute of Science, Technology, and Advanced Studies, India

S. S. Meenambiga
https://orcid.org/0000-0002-5445-525X
Department of Bioengineering, Vels Institute of Science, Technology, and Advanced Studies, India

R. Chandrasekaran
Department of Biomedical Engineering, Vels Institute of Science, Technology, and Advanced Studies, India

N. M. Hariharan
Department of Biotechnology, Vel Tech Rangarajan Dr. Sagunthala R&D Institute of Science and Technology, India

ABSTRACT

This chapter explores the growing challenge posed by neurodegenerative and psychiatric disorders, which have underscored the limitations of conventional treatments. It focuses on the therapeutic potential of phytomedicines, particularly their antioxidant, anti-inflammatory, and neurotransmitter-modulating effects. Specifically, it examines the role of plant-derived compounds, such as terpenoids, alkaloids, and flavonoids, in mitigating symptoms of depression, anxiety, Parkinson's disease, and Alzheimer's disease. This chapter discusses the fusion of traditional

DOI: 10.4018/979-8-3373-4627-4.ch017

wisdom with contemporary scientific methods, highlighting the need for rigorous standards and regulatory frameworks that prioritize ethical considerations. The integration of nanotechnology, AI, and personalized medicine is transforming phytomedicine, paving the way for innovative approaches to brain health and wellness.

INTRODUCTION

There is an increase in severity and prevalence of both neurodegenerative diseases like Alzheimer's and Parkinson's, as well as depression, anxiety, schizophrenia and other neuropsychiatric disorders. The complex nature of these disorders, their chronic progression, coupled with existing pharmaceutical treatment's limited effectiveness presents significant problems. Most conventional drugs tend to focus on singular pathways. This is coupled with undesirable side effects and limited long-term benefits (Przedborski, Vila, & Jackson-Lewis, 2003). In recent years, there has been an increase in focus towards nature- rooted and alternative therapies. Such herbal medicines are used in Ayurveda and Traditional Chinese Medicine, and are gaining recognition for their ability to target several neurological pathways at once with their neuroprotective, antioxidant, anti-inflammatory, and cognitive abilities, thus providing multi-faceted phytomedicinal support (Howes, Perry, & Houghton, 2003).

Some phytochemicals open new therapeutic avenues for neuroprotection and treatment of cognitive disorders. Flavonoids, alkaloids, terpenoids and polyphenols have shown the ability to modulate critical neurotransmitter systems, reduce oxidative stress, and enhance neurogenesis and synaptic plasticity (Goyal, Nagori & Sasmal, 2011). Such compounds have a marked ability to cross the blood brain barrier which is crucial for almost all neurological interventions (Aguiar & Borowski, 2013). With the increasing trust in efficacy of such compounds, focus has shifted to incorporate such and other natural compounds into contemporary neurotherapeutic approaches. This chapter focuses on the changing paradigm of brain disorder treatment by phytomedicine, analysing the pathophysiological phytomedicinal mechanisms, therapeutic possibilities, as well as problems dealing standardization, regulation and ethical issues. Phytomedicines may provide the integration of ancient knowledge and modern science into neural and mental health as well as offer more balanced and green solutions.

Overview of Neurological and Neuropsychiatric Disorders

The term neurological and neuropsychiatric disorders include a wide range of diseases that affect the central nervous system and the peripheral nervous system. They may be related to structural, biochemical, or electrical changes in the tissues making up the brain, spinal cord, or peripheral nerves, and are accompanied by symptoms such as amnesia, dementia, movement disorders, and affective disorders (Feigin et al., 2020). There is, however, a rising global burden of these conditions, adding markedly to the existing disability and mortality burden. Alzheimer's and Parkinson's disease, major depressive disorder, schizophrenia, and stroke are commonly encountered disorders that each pose distinct diagnostic and therapeutic hurdles (Nestler & Hyman, 2010).

With consideration of these overlapping symptoms and the multifactorial etiology of these disorders, their classification and understanding needs an integrated clinical perspective, one that

takes all factors into account. As an illustration, one differential feature for most neurodegenerative diseases is the progressive loss of neurons, whereas neuropsychiatric disorders tend to be associated with neurotransmitter shifts and changed brain circuitry connections (Gorelick et al., 2011). In **Table 1**, included summarizing classification of the major brain disorders with their salient clinical features and the most up-to-date treatment approaches available to show their shortcomings. Also, provided the structural overview of the brain in relation to some disorders (shown in **Figure 1.** Summary of the brain disorders and affected areas) like Alzheimer's (which affects the hippocampus), Parkinson's (which affects the substantia nigra), and depression (which affects the prefrontal cortex), thus reinforcing the anatomical basis of their clinical manifestations. Both structural and functional aspects have to be understood to develop effective and complete strategies focused on the integration of various treatment modalities.

Neurodegenerative Disorders

Neurodegenerative diseases, or disorders of the neuron, consist of a range of progressive conditions characterized by the gradual degeneration, which involves the death or malfunction of neurons. Of the finest among the most prominent are Alzheimer's disease (AD), Parkinson's disease (PD), Huntington's disease (HD) and amyotrophic lateral sclerosis3 (ALS). These diseases share in common a pathological including protein aggregation, mitochondrial dysfunction, oxidative stress, and gradual neuronal loss (Kovacs, 2016). In Alzheimer's, the beta-amyloid plaques accumulating neurofibrillary tangles lead to synaptic dysfunction and cognitive decline, particularly affecting brain areas such as the hippocampus. Parkinson's disease is around characterized by the death of dopaminergic neurons in the substantia nigra, resulting in motor symptoms bradykinesia, tremors, and rigidity often blamed on synuclein aggregation forming Lewy bodies (Kalia & Lang, 2015). Huntington's disease, a genetic disorder due to CAG trinucleotide repeat expansion in the HTT gene, causes extensive brain. Atrophy, especially in the striatum, and manifests with choreiform movements, dementia, and psychiatric conditions. ALS causes motor neurons to slowly deteriorate in the brain and spinal cord resulting in muscle weakness, atrophy and eventually respiratory failure (Hardiman et al, 2017). These disorders have fun with intersecting mechanisms of neurodegeneration, still incompletely-understood and poorly treated by current medications.

Neuropsychiatric Disorders

Neuropsychiatric disorders are a category of mental illness that arise from issues with the brain function, typically involving neurotransmitter dysregulation, neuroinflammation and altered these are MDD, anxiety such as GAD, panic disorder, and phobias, and schizophrenia and bipolar MDD is associated with low serotonin, norepinephrine, and dopamine, resulting in persistent sadness, anhedonia, and cognitive dysfunction (Malhi & Mann, 2018). Anxiety disorders hijack the amygdala. HPA dysregulation, leading to too much fear autonomic arousal responses. Dopaminergic hallucinations are central to schizophrenia and glutamatergic signalling, producing hallucinations, delusions and compromised executive functioning, linked to synaptic pruning and cortical thinning. Manic-depressive bipolar illness, with its manic and depressive phases, is change. monoamine neurotransmitters and inflammatory markers plus brain abnormalities circuits regulating emotion and impulse control (Grande et al., 2016). Pharmacotherapy remains

the foundation of treatment including antidepressants, antipsychotics and mood stabilizers, many patients experience partial remission or side effects, highlighting requirement for more concentrated and synergistic therapies.

Neurodevelopmental Disorders

The neurodevelopmental disorders are the class of disorders that emerge in the initial developmental periods and are characterized by deficiencies in personal, social, academic, or occupational functioning. Most prominent among them are autism spectrum disorder (ASD), Attention-Deficit/Hyperactivity Disorder (ADHD), and intellectual disabilities. These disorders often result from multiple interactions between genetic, epigenetic, and environmental factors that produce disruptions in usual brain activity and maturation. Abnormalities of maturation of the synapses, connectivity, and neurotransmitter signalling underlie the deficits in social interaction, communication, and repetitive behaviors (Lord et al., 2020). ADHD is associated with dysregulation of dopaminergic and noradrenergic systems, most notably with the cortex, the area dealing with attention, impulse regulation, and executive function. Intellectual disabilities, that is, having serious impairments in intellectual functioning and adaptive behavior, are frequently linked with chromosome defects, disease of metabolism, and premature brain injury, and genetic mutations that affect the pathways of neurodevelopment (Rosenberg et al., 2019). Recent research centers on the synaptic dysregulation and altered neuronal plasticity underlying the disorders, and consequences for the timing of diagnosis and treatment. Present treatment is primarily symptomatic and includes behavior therapy, educational interventions, and pharmacologic help, but don't address the core processes of neurobiology, highlighting the need for novel therapeutic methods.

Cerebrovascular and Traumatic Disorders

Cerebrovascular and traumatic disorders comprise a range of disorders due to vascular or mechanical injury to the brain, stroke, Traumatic Brain Injury (TBI), and vascular dementia being the most prominent examples. They very frequently share common pathological characteristics such as cerebral ischemia, neuroinflammation, excitotoxicity, and disruption of the blood-brain barrier. Stroke, either ischemic or hemorrhagic, leads to the rapid brain dysfunction due to interrupted supply of blood, which triggers the series of events including oxidative stress, cell death, and activation of the immune response (Doyle et al., 2008). TBI, resulting from external mechanical forces, causes both acute and delayed brain injury characterized by axonal injury, edema, and longstanding neuroinflammation, and able to cause impairment in cognitive and motor performance in the long term (Loane & Kumar, 2016). Vascular dementia, the second most common form of dementia after Alzheimer's disease, is caused by long-standing reduced cerebral blood flow and repeated microinfarcts, with accompanying slow loss of memory, judgment, and reasoning (Kalaria, 2016). The diseases emphasize the significance of cerebrovascular brain health integrity and the necessity of neuroprotective interventions that are able to decrease inflammation and preserve neuronal function following vascular injury.

Common Issues in Diagnosis and Management

The recognition and treatment of neurological and neuropsychiatric ailments provide specific clinical complexities with overlapping symptoms, delayed identification of the disease, and the limitations of treatments available. Most of the disorders share common features such as cognitive impairment, disturbances of mood, and behavior changes which often complicated differential diagnosis, particularly during the initial periods (Arciniegas & Beresford, 2001). Furthermore, the lack of clear biomarkers and reliance upon the individual clinical judgment explain proximal muscle weakness, delayed or misdiagnosis, particularly in diseases such as Parkinson's disease and others dementia (Postuma et al., 2015). Long-term pharmacologic therapy, while central to symptom management, is frequently associated with undesirable side effects such as cognitive blunting, metabolic disturbances, and drug tolerance, that lower quality of life and patient compliance (Haddad & Sharma, 2007). And the current therapy is still mainly symptomatic, offering limited reversal or disease modification, particularly for chronic neurodegenerative disorders. These kinds of problems underscore the need for holistically oriented and innovative techniques that enhance diagnostic precision, lower treatment-related complications, and the multifactorial character of brain disorders.

Figure 1. Summary of the brain disorders and affected areas

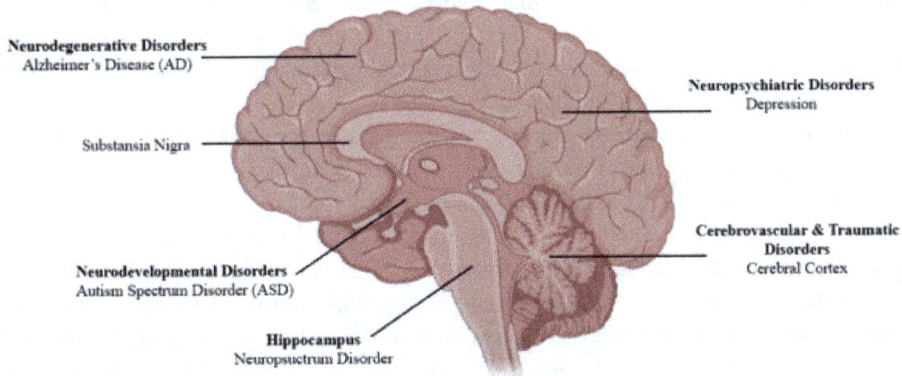

Table 1. Classification of major brain disorders

Category	Examples	Key Features	Current Limitations
Neurodegenerative	Parkinson's disease	Memory loss, motor dysfunction	Symptomatic treatment, no cure
Neuropsychiatric	Depression, Schizophrenia, Anxiety	Mood swings, delusions, anxiety	Drug resistance, relapse, side effects
Neurodevelopmental	Autism, ADHD	Communication problems, inattention	Restricted pharmacotherapy, behavioural focus
Traumatic	Stroke, TBI	Paralysis, cognitive impairment	Postponed neuro regeneration, rehabilitation is needed

Global Burden and its Effect on Quality of Life

These neuropsychiatric and neurological disorders are rapidly becoming an extremely serious worldwide public health problem, immensely contributing to the level of disability and mortality all over the world. Neurological disorders are the largest single source of Disability-Adjusted Life Years (DALYs) and the second most common cause of death, primarily due to stroke, Alzheimer's disease, and dementia (Feigin et al., 2019) Mental health conditions, including depression and anxiety, are among the most common causes of Years Lived with Disability (YLDs) too. They often begin at a very young age and remain undertreated over several years, mainly because of stigma and restricted care accessibility (Rehm & Shield, 2019). An aging population, changes in lifestyles, and higher exposure to environmental and psychological stressors have all helped increase the prevalence of the disorders.

The issue is most pronounced among Low- and Middle-Income Countries (LMICs), with under-resourced health systems that cannot provide timely diagnosis or effective care, driving burgeoning health inequities globally. Beyond physical symptoms, the disorders significantly compromise quality of life, with long-term cognitive, emotional, and social sequelae. This means loss of autonomy, increased burdens on caregivers, increased likelihood of unemployment, and alienation from society. Economically, the cost is twofold: countries and families pay both the direct costs such as long-term care and medications, and the indirect costs such as loss of productivity and home care costs. Emotionally and socially, the consequences like stigma, depression, and lowered well-being are too often overlooked in clinical visits as well. Management of the complex and growing crisis necessitates an integrated worldwide response of early identification, integrated care, and preventive public health methods (Dua et al., 2011).

Epidemiological Trends of Brain Disorders

The prevalence of neurological and neuropsychiatric disorders has grown substantially in the past couple of decades, and it is now a significant public health threat globally. Neurological diseases are known to affect over one billion people worldwide, and the most common among them are stroke, dementia, epilepsy, and migraine. Mental health disorders, including depression, anxiety, and schizophrenia, are still leading causes of global disability (GBD 2019 Diseases and Injuries Collaborators, 2020). The burden is unequally shared. LMICs are unduly affected due to weak health infrastructure, sparse mental health care, and higher exposure to dangers like malnutrition,

infectious illness, and trauma (Patel et al., 2018). Additionally, population shifts urbanization, physical inactivity, and higher psychological stress are driving the increase in prevalence of the disorders. This trend, which is occasionally referred to as the "epidemiological transition," and the ineffectiveness of available preventive techniques signify the need to adopt national and global health policies with an attitude of awareness, early management, and integrated care.

Disability and Mortality due to Brain Disorders

Brain disorders are among the most important causes of DALYs and YLDs and are most prevalent among the elderly and young adults. Mental and neurological disorders like depression, schizophrenia, stroke, Alzheimer's disease, and epilepsy account for more than 10% of total worldwide DALYs, and neuropsychiatric disorders alone account for nearly one-third of total worldwide YLDs (Whiteford et al., 2013). Apart from lowering life expectancy, the disorders increase the risk of acquiring secondary health issues such as heart disease, diabetes, and drug or alcohol abuse, and consequently raise their overall intensity. One of the major challenges is underdiagnosis, especially in the poor areas, where the stigma, ignorance, and lack of clinical experience exacerbate the challenge of properly identifying the disorders. There is still a huge treatment gap existing even at the level of diagnosis. 75% of the people with mental illness in LMICs still lack any sort of treatment (Kohn et al., 2004). Addressing the gap will require enhanced diagnostic infrastructure, community-level mental health services, and community-level education to avoid long-term disability and premature death.

Socioeconomic Consequences

The economic and societal costs of neurological and neuropsychiatric disorders are significant and multi-dimensional. The direct costs include hospitalization, medications, diagnostic tests, and long-term care. Indirect costs are due to lowered productivity, premature retirement, and premature death. These ailments often result in chronic disability, which decreases the patient's ability to work and independence most problematic in resource-poor regions. Caregivers, often the patient's own relatives, become physically, emotionally, and financially overwhelmed, if professional care is unattainable or beyond their financial reach. Most health systems worldwide are unprepared to meet the rising demand for neurological and psychiatric care, and this leads to stressed services and sparse availability of specialist care (Bloom et al., 2011). This is the experience in rural areas and LMICs, which are bedevilled with inadequacies in healthcare infrastructure, mental health literacy, and trained manpower (Bloom et al., 2011). These inequities perpetuate the disease and poverty cycle, and it is clear that there is a compelling need to supply equitable health policies and long-term investment in brain health services globally.

Conventional Pharmacological Therapy Limits

Though there has been considerable progress in the pathophysiology of brain disease, conventional pharmacologic therapy rarely provides long-term and holistic cures. Most available drugs are symptomatic and do not intend to cure or reverse disease course. For example, in neurodegenerative disease like Alzheimer's and Parkinson's disease, drugs may briefly reverse or enhance cognition or motor skill but cannot reverse the loss of the underlying neurones. Psy-

chiatric medications such as antidepressants and antipsychotics, despite being helpful in select patients, take many weeks before their effectiveness becomes obvious and possess undesirable side effects from sedation and weight gain to metabolic impairment and flattening of emotion.

Additionally, the response to therapy is highly individual and locale-specific, and clinical therapy is primarily based on hit-or-miss therapy techniques. Long-term therapy with available drugs is frequently followed by tolerance, dependency, or withdrawal symptoms. Additionally, multiple medications or polypharmacy specific among elderly patients make the regimens of therapy cumbersome and increase the risk of drug interactions. There is an added concern also about the lack of innovation in the pipeline of neuropharmacology, and most pharma corporations are cutting investments in research because of the very huge number of failures during clinical trials and entry into regulation (Cummings et al., 2014). These inadequacies necessitate the unfolding of novel, multimodal, and patient-specific therapy techniques, including the ones based on natural and customary systems of therapy.

Rise in Demand for Plant-Based and Alternative Remedies

The expanding limitations and side effects of conventional pharmacologic therapies have driven the world toward plant and alternative therapies, primarily in the management of chronic neurological and neuropsychiatric disorders. As health consciousness increases and the population turns to holistically based therapies, interest in phytomedicine—natural plant-derived molecules with therapeutic value continues to expand. Many of these therapies possess multi-targeted mechanisms of action, improved safety profiles, and higher cultural acceptability. Historical traditional systems of medicine, such as Ayurveda, Traditional Chinese Medicine (TCM), and ethnomedicine, have long used herbs such as *Bacopa monnieri, Withania somnifera*, and *Ginkgo biloba* for the enhancement of cognition and the regulation of mood.

Contemporary pharmacologic research is now, however, fully documenting many of the historical uses of the herbal sector based on evidence-based techniques, and this has contributed to the renewed interest in incorporating herbal therapy into mainstream medical treatment. Additionally, the consumer may view the natural product as safer and body-compatible, making it more attractive, especially among patients disenchanted with the synthetically based medications. The World Health Organization has acknowledged the importance of customary therapeutics and has called for its incorporation into the nation's health systems as an integral component of the overall plan to advance the health endpoints (World Health Organization, 2013). This paradigm shift is more than merely an attitude adjustment, however, for it represents an increased recognition of the therapeutic value of nature in the management of the complex brain disorders.

Objectives and Scope of the Present Chapter

The chapter examines the neuroactive activity of phytomedicines in the management of neurological and neuropsychiatric disease. Set against the background of the global trend towards plant-based and holistic therapeutic approaches, the world faces an acute need to critically assess the therapeutic value of phytochemicals in brain health and disease. The chapter hopes to provide an overview of the major brain disorders and the limitations of the conventional pharmacological remedy. It goes on to outline the molecular pathways wherein plant-derived molecules might occasion their neuroprotective, antioxidant, anti-inflammatory, and neuromodulatory effects. In-

dividual herbs and their bioactive molecules are examined under the lenses of both the preclinical and clinical literature, with an eye towards their efficacy and safety profiles. The chapter goes on to address the regulatory, moral, and scientific barriers that militate against the standardization and admission of phytomedicines into evidence-based clinical practice. The bigger picture is the coming together of the world's traditional systems of knowledge and the modern science of neuroscience, with the aim to developing sustainably feasible and culturally acceptable and clinically relevant therapeutic modalities based on an integrated approach to therapy.

UNDERSTANDING PHYTOMEDICINES AND THEIR NEUROACTIVE PROPERTIES

Derived from different plant parts including bark, roots, seeds, and leaves, phytomedicines used for millennia in conventional medical systems including Ayurveda, Traditional Chinese Medicine (TCM) and native healing modalities. These plant-based treatments are coming back fame resulting from their wide variety of bioactive chemicals with therapeutic possibilities for sophisticated illnesses, especially those influencing the Central Nervous System (CNS) (Ekor, 2014). Unlike traditional single-target synthesized pharmaceuticals, phytomedicines usually several phytochemicals interacting synergistically on several biological processes. Addressing the multifactorial nature is especially beneficial with poly-pharmacological impact. of brain disorders, where oxidative stress, inflammatory reaction, neurotransmitter imbalances and often concurrent with mitochondrial dysfunction.

Among other types of phytochemicals include flavonoids, alkaloids, terpenoids, saponins, and significant neuroprotective, anti-inflammatory, antioxidant, and phenolic acids have been found. Neuro modulatory activities in preclinical and clinical trials (Kennedy & Wightman, 2011). These substances control a number of neuronal processes including scavenging reactive oxygen. species (ROS), regulating and improving Brain-Derived Neurotrophic Factor (BDNF) signalling pathways of neurotransmitters including dopaminergic, serotonergic, and cholinergic systems. The ability of certain phytochemicals to cross the blood-brain barrier is noteworthy. transforming them into potential candidates for treating central nervous system disorders (Aguiar & Borowski, 2013) There is a chance of phytomedicines being harmless, safe and effective. Enhanced therapies for brain disorders, or as an adjunct to existing pharmacological treatments.

Definition, History, and Traditional Uses of Phytomedicines

Therapeutic items produced from medicinal plants, phytomedicines include whole plants, portions of plants, or standardized extracts with bioactive phytochemicals. Traditionally, these natural chemicals have been used to cure a great number of ailments. including central nervous system disorders. Unlike artificial medicines that usually target because of their complex nature, phytomedicines often act on multiple targets single molecular pathways. chemical composition makes them especially good for treating multifactorial illnesses like neurological and neuropsychiatric diseases (Mukherjee et al., 2007). Traditionally, plant-based medicines have been employed thousands of years.

Ancient medical systems like Ayurveda in India, Traditional Chinese Medicine (TCM), Unani, and several other long acknowledged the therapeutic possibilities of indigenous customs

throughout the Americas and Africa. of herbs. Ayurvedic medicine has utilized plants like *Bacopa monnieri* and *Withania somnifera* for its therapeutic benefits. improve stress resilience, cognition, and memory. Likewise, TCM has included ginseng and *Ginkgo biloba* for brain function and mental clarity (Patwardhan et al., 2005). Importantly, certain phytochemicals show the capacity to traverse the blood-brain barrier only for symptom relief but also for disease prevention and restoration of health. Modern pharmacological studies are progressively confirming these customary applications, therefore pointing the therapeutic value of phytomedicines in modern neurotherapeutics (Heinrich & Gibbons, 2001).

Classes of Bioactive Phytochemicals with Neuroactivity

Neuroactive phytochemicals cover many different chemical groups, each showing particular methods of action on the neurological system. These chemicals react with Neurotransmitters regulate neuroinflammation, offer antioxidant capabilities, and advance neuroprotection. Knowing the main categories of neuroactive plant-based substances clarifies their therapeutic capacity in diseases of the nervous and neuropsychiatric systems.

The main categories are glycosides, phenolic acids, terpenoids, alkaloids, and flavonoids. Many bioactive substances extracted from several medical plants make up every class. Helping to improve cognition, neuroprotection, anxiolytic, and antidepressant effects.

Major Classes of Neuroactive Phytochemicals

Neuroactive bioactive phytochemicals include many important chemical groups, each using several processes to generate particular effects on the nervous system. Principally known for alkaloids, nitrogen-containing molecules like galantamine and berberine neuroprotection and acetylcholinesterase inhibition found in plants like *Galanthus* species found in *nivalis* and *Berberi*. Among polyphenols are flavonoids, including luteolin and quercetin. Substances with potent anti-inflammatory, antioxidant, and neuroprotective characteristics, often found *in Ginkgo biloba*, vegetables, and fruits. Terpenoids include ginkgolides derived from Ginkgo biloba and limonene derived from citrus peels help to control neurotransmitter systems and lower neuroinflammation. Found in coffee, cereals, and phenolic acids include caffeic acid and ferulic acid because of their antioxidant activity, fruits provide significantly to neuroprotection. Finally, well are glycosides bacosides from *Bacopa monnieri* and ginsenosides from *Panax ginseng* among others. Recorded for their cognitive improvement and advocacy of neuroplasticity (Santos & Ferreira, 2020) Along with these courses and their representative chemicals, their sources and **Table 2** is the basis for the historical application of medicinal plants in the treatment of neurological illnesses as well their developing role in contemporary neurotherapeutics.

Table 2. Major classes of neuroactive phytochemicals and their neuropharmacological effects

Class of Phytochemical	Representative Compounds	Primary Neuroactivity	Plant Sources
Alkaloids	Galantamine, Berberine	Neuroprotection, Acetylcholinesterase inhibition	*Galanthus nivalis, Berberi*'s species
Flavonoids	Luteolin, Quercetin	Antioxidant, Anti-inflammatory, Neuroprotection	Various fruits, vegetables, *Ginkgo biloba*
Terpenoids	Limonene, Ginkgolides	Anti-inflammatory, Neurotransmitter modulation	*Ginkgo biloba*, citrus peels
Phenolic acids	Ferulic acid, Caffeic acid	Neuroprotection, Anti-oxidant.	Coffee, cereals, fruits
Glycosides	Ginsenosides, Bacosides	Neuroplasticity, Cognitive enhancement	*Bacopa monnieri, Panax ginseng*

Mechanisms of Action on the Central Nervous System

These neuroactive phytochemicals act through several mechanisms to produce their prophylactic effects. Aimed at the Central Nervous System (CNS). Unlike synthetic drugs, which usually target one single receptor, the canonical TRPs are particularly interesting as they can be activated by diverse natural chemicals and mediate various physiological responses. Molecules, phytochemicals commonly influence cross-linked pathways multimodal strategy in the management of the sophisticated neurological and polytrauma injured, neurodegenerative conditions. Key mechanisms are a modulation of neurotransmitter systems, antioxidant effects, anti-inflammatory properties, inhibition neurotoxic enzyme, and the induction of neurogenesis and synaptic plasticity. These cooperative effects contribute to improvement of cognition, prevention of neural injury, modulate neurotransmission, and maintain brain repair mechanisms. Figure 2 illustrates the complex molecular interactions through which phytochemicals influence central nervous system (CNS) activity.

Figure 2. Mode of action of phytochemicals in the brain

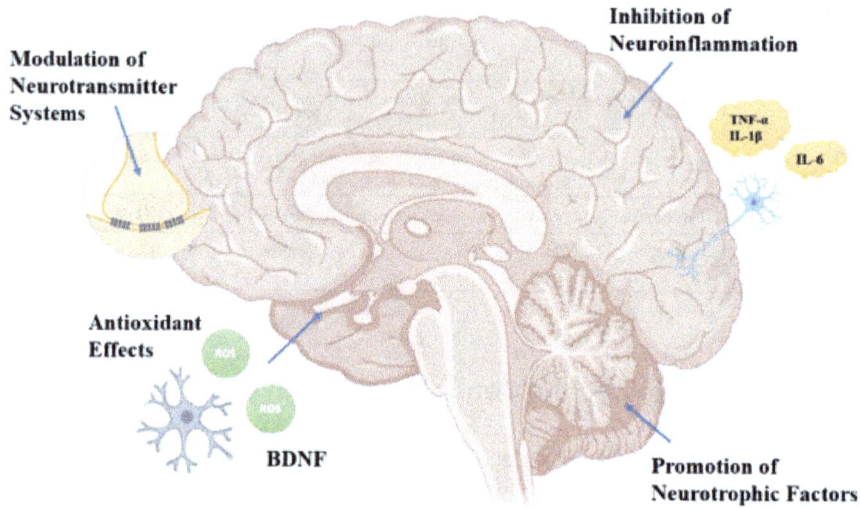

Figure 2. Mechanisms of Action of Phytochemicals on the Brain

Neurotransmitter Modulation

A number of the phytochemicals that are neuroactive exert their therapeutic activities through neurotransmitter functional modulation systems of the central nervous system. Such compounds act to modulate the levels of either-or receptor sensitivity to their respective neurotransmitters, to modulate synaptic transmission and neuronal signalling. For instance, alkaloids like galantamine function as acetylcholinesterase inhibitors, resulting in an increased concentration of acetylcholine in the synaptic cleft and increased cholinergic neurotransmission this latter action particularly useful in the treatment of Alzheimer's disease. Hyphenated to techniques in Environmental Analysis Similarly, flavonoids and terpenoids have been found to the effects of their inhibition. GABAA/serotonin receptor, exerting anxiolytic and antidepressant activities. Phytochemical-mediated dopaminergic regulation such as curcumin and berberine also participates in lifted mood, better cognition, and increased evidence of motor coordination. (Kennedy & Wightman, 2011) These multisided activities emphasize the importance of plant-origin molecules for the reversion neurotransmitter equilibrium and the improvement in brain conditions in a range of neuropsychiatric disorders.

Antioxidant Effects in Neurons

Oxidative stress plays a pivotal role in neuronal injury, neurodegeneration, and brain aging. Phytochemicals such as quercetin, curcumin, and caffeic acid permeate the blood–brain barrier

and can efficiently remove Reactive Oxygen Species (ROS) such as superoxide and hydroxyl radicals, within neuronal tissues. Additionally, these compounds upregulate endogenous radical scavenging enzymes SOD, catalase, and glutathione peroxidase, which together helps to protect neuronal the mitochondria, maintain the integrity of the membrane, and lower lipid peroxidation. By these ways phytochemicals act neuroprotective by RTVF reinforces our current understanding of drug discovery approach and mechanism of action. Stabilizing redox state and reducing oxidative damage of brain cells (Rehman et al., 2019).

Inhibition of Neuroinflammation

The chronic neuroinflammation is a key player in the neuroprogression of neurodegenerative conditions including Alzheimer's and Parkinson's. Phytochemicals like flavonoids, saponins, and phenolic acids has been shown to have the ability to inhibit the activation of microglia the immune cells in the central nervous system. By inhibiting microglial overactivation, the production and release of pro-inflammatory compounds are decreased by these compounds' inflammatory cytokines (tumor necrosis factor-alpha (TNF-α), interleukin-1 beta (IL-1β) and interleukin-6 (IL-6). This anti-inflammatory effect prevents any further damage to the neurons, maintains synaptic integrity and cognitive resilience (Vauzour et al., 2008).

Enhancement of Neurotrophic Factors and Neurogenesis

Phytochemicals, bacosides (*Bacopa monniera*), ginsenosides (*panax ginseng*) such substances interacting collectively have a synergistic therapeutic effect known as synergism and resveratrol (polyphenol found in grapes and berries) neurotrophins (as Brain-Derived Neurotrophic Factor (BDNF), and Nerve Growth Factor (NGF). These neurotrophins are crucial for the survival, synaptic growth, and plasticity of neurons basic mechanisms mediating learning, memory, and control of emotion. Enhanced BDNF, signalling is particularly tightly linked to the strongly associated with hippocampal, cognitive function. Through these pathways, the phytochemicals can be potential inhibitors of neurodegeneration and damage. Also, enhanced neuronal repair under conditions of aging and disease (Pallas et al., 2009).

Regulation of Intracellular Signalling Pathways

Many neuroactive phytochemicals harness their therapeutic potential through modulating. Cellular signalling cascades, including the PI3K/Akt, MAPK/ERK, and Nrf2/ARE. These pathways contribute to the regulation of neuronal survival, plasticity, and resistance to cellular stress. PI3K/Akt and MAPK/ERK Signalling Activation Contribute to the Neuroprotection via upregulation of anti-apoptotic gene expression and maintaining synaptic reorganization. At the same time, activation of Nrf2/ARE results in the up-regulation of antioxidant- and cytoprotective-related genes that oppose oxidative and inflammatory-mediated insults. Phytochemicals are thus, by these molecular pathways, involved in preserving neuronal integrity and function in both normal and disease states (de Oliveira et al., 2020).

Enzyme Inhibition Relevant to Neurodegeneration

Some plant-made chemicals protect the brain by stopping certain enzymes tied to brain diseases. Items like curcumin, resveratrol, and rosmarinic acid slow down Monoamine oxidase (MAO), this way cutting down harmful side products like hydrogen peroxide. Other substances, such as catechins and ferulic acid, go after β-secretase (BACE1), a main player in making amyloid-beta bits linked with Alzheimer's disease. Also, by holding back tyrosinase with flavonoids, it might stop too much bad dopamine which hurts nerve cells in Parkinson's disease. These actions by the chemicals help stop harmful build-ups and stress, slowing the disease (Figueira et al., 2017).

Blood-Brain Barrier Permeability of Plant Compounds

The Blood-Brain Barrier (BBB) acts as a careful screen that shields the brain, letting only needed stuff in and keeping bad things out. For plant chemicals to work on the brain, they need to get past this barrier. Some, like curcumin, resveratrol, quercetin, and ginsenosides can cross the BBB, helped by their design or special carriers. Features like their love for fats, size, and how they deal with exit proteins affect how well they cross. New tech in drugs, like wrapping them in small fat or plant-based capsules, is tested to better their entry and effect (Wohlfart et al., 2012). Knowing and boosting how well these can cross the BBB is key to making good plant treatments for brain issues.

Synergistic Effects in Polyherbal Formulations

Mixes of two or more plants for healing are key in old health ways like Ayurveda and Chinese Medicine. These mixes show strong shared effects, where the total health outcome is more than each plant on its own. This lift can start from many spots: better work of active parts, mixed health effects, changes in body paths, or fewer bad effects. For instance, mixing *Withania somnifera* with *Bacopa monnieri* has had better results on brain and mind boost in tests than using only one herb. This method also allows for using less of each herb, reducing the risk of harm while improving effectiveness. The complete impact on various brain systems with these herb combos provides a solid approach to tackle major brain issues like Alzheimer's and depression (Dhanani et al., 2013). More often, new drug studies find that these old combos work well using full-body and network drug methods.

PHYTOMEDICINAL INTERVENTIONS IN SPECIFIC BRAIN DISORDERS

Mind issues like Alzheimer's, Parkinson's, big sad times, fits, and worry are big head health problems all over the world. They often come with many causes like cell harm, brain swelling, messed-up brain signals, and bad nerve links. Usual drugs work, but can also have bad side effects or may not be enough in tough cases. In this light, plant meds give a full and many-way fix. They mix healing bits with power to guard against cell harm, lower swelling, protect nerves, and help fix them. Old plant cures like *Bacopa monnieri*, *Ginkgo biloba*, *Curcuma longa*, and *Withania somnifera* work well in fixing brain signals, stopping bad brain stuff, and helping nerve health. New drug studies back up these old uses, showing that plant bits like bacosides, curcumin,

quercetin, ginsenosides, and galantamine hit key points tied to each mind issue. The next parts look into these plant fixes with more focus, sorted by uses in certain brain problems, going over how they work and their help backed by science.

Alzheimer's Disease and Memory-Enhancing Botanicals

Alzheimer's disease (AD) is a neurodegenerative disorder characterized by a progressive cognitive deficit, deterioration, memory deficits, and behavioural deficits. The pathology involves β-amyloid plaque deposits, tau hyperphosphorylation, cholinergic impairment, mitochondrial impairment, oxidative damage, and chronic neuroinflammation. Conventional treatments like acetylcholinesterase inhibitors and NMDA receptor antagonists offer symptomatic treatment only are frequently associated with side effects. This has raised more concern about herbal drugs that have multi-target treatment effects and better safety properties. Several botanicals have shown very promising effects in improving memory and containing the progression of AD.

An Ayurvedic supplement Bacopa monnieri that is enriched with bacosides, has strengthen synaptic signalling, induce dendritic branching, and increase expression of brain-derived neurotrophic factor (BDNF), which sustains neurogenesis and cognitive resistance. Ginkgo biloba contains flavonoids, and terpenoids such as ginkgolides, which exhibit antioxidant, anti-inflammatory, and anti-apoptotic activity, as well as increasing cerebral blood flow and cholinergic transmission. Curcuma longa (turmeric) provides curcumin, which has been shown to inhibit amyloid aggregation inhibit free radicals, and inhibit neuroinflammation via the inhibition of NF-κB. Panax ginseng have also been found to possess memory augmenting potential through the modulation of ACH, the reduction of oxidative stress, and the improvement of synaptic plasticity (Howes & Perry, 2011).

Parkinson's Disease and Neuroprotective Plant Extracts

Parkinsons disease is a term condition that affects the nervous system and progresses, the condition is identified by the breakdown of dopamine producing neurons, in a region of the brain called the substantia nigra pars compact. The decrease, in dopamine levels results in motor symptoms like slowed movement and tremors while at rest. Rigidity and balance issues, along, with decline are symptoms to watch for depression and autonomic dysfunction are issues, in Parkinsons disease that are characterized by stress, among other pathophysiological factors. Pharmacological therapies, like levodopa and dopamine agonists along, with MAOB inhibitors present treatment options. Medications can provide relief from symptoms. They do not stop the progression of the disease and can sometimes result in motor issues over time.

Phytomedicines offer an approach, for protecting against neurodegeneration in Parkinsons disease. As an illustration, the leguminous plant *Mucuna pruriens* is known to contain natural levodopa, which works as well as synthetic forms. It also has less associated dyskinesia side effects. Green tea containing polyphenols like EGCG and *Curcuma Longa* (curcumin) also have antioxidant properties as well as anti-aggregatory actions that help conserve dopaminergic neurons. Moreover, Ginsenosides from *Panax ginseng* along with resveratrol, a polyphenol found in grapes that activates SIRT1 signalling, improve mitochondrial biogenesis and bolster the survival of dopaminergic neurons.

Additionally, Baicalein from Scutellaria baicalensis is recognized for lessening the α-synuclein associated microglial activation and fibrillation linked to the progression of Parkinson's disease. These phytochemicals target through various neuroprotective mechanisms i.e. inhibition of monoamine oxidase (MAO-B), reduction in the level of reactive oxygen species, downregulation of pro-inflammatory cytokines, and enhancement of the neurotrophic signalling i.e. BDNF. (Wang et al., 2021) this multiform action is not only useful for symptom relief but also promising to change the disease progression in Parkinson's Disease (PD).

Depression and Anxiety Treatment with Adaptogenic Herbs

Depression and anxiety are two of the most common mood disorders, which stem from dysfunctions of neurotransmitters involved in the regulation of mood (serotonin, dopamine, GABA), chronic stress, oxidative stress, and involvement of the hypothalamic-pituitary-adrenal (HPA) axis. While traditional medicine (e.g., SSRIs, benzodiazepines) for symptom relief but the results are almost always varied. Related to late onset, side effects and treatment resistance in a large proportion of patients.

This has renewed interest in adaptogenic herbs, which help the body resist stress and the challenges of maintaining physiological balance while avoiding over-sedation and over-stimulation. A number of aphrodisiac and adaptogenic herbs have been found to be useful in mood disorders. *Withania sominera* (Ashwagandha) is one of the most excitingly studied one with an anxiolytic and antidepressant properties. It normalizes cortisol levels, can up-regulate GABAergic transmission, and improves resilience to stress-induced neurotoxicity. *Rhodiola rosea*, another well-established adaptogen, mood and cognitive function could be improved through monoamine regulation and inhibiting monoamine oxidase (MAO) enzymes.

Active compounds the active constituents of Rhodiola are the rosavin and salidroside are involved in neuroprotection and stress resistance. *Panax ginseng*, which is abundant in ginsenosides, restores mood and energy by maintaining HPA-axis activity and by increasing brain-derived neurotrophic factor (BDNF). In addition, *Ocimum sanctum* (Holy basil) and *Bacopa monnieri* show antidepressant-like effects by modulation of serotonergic and dopaminergic transmission and it decreasing oxidative and inflammatory pressure on the brain (Sarris et al., 2013). These herbs act via a neuroendocrine, anti-oxidant, anti-inflammatory measures, facilitating neural balance and emotion equilibrium stability. Their holistic effects make them especially useful in the treatment of the chronic stress-associated conditions and mood as changes with lesser side effects than conventional drugs (Panossian & Wikman, 2010).

Epilepsy and Anticonvulsant Phytocompounds

Epilepsy is a serious, chronic neurological disorder marked by recurrent, unprovoked seizures caused by unusual electrical activity in the brain. Affecting approximately 50 million people around the world, epilepsy has a serious impact on quality of life and cause cognitive disorder, distress, and endured social stigma. While conventional antiepileptic drugs (AEDs) can seizure-free many, approximately 30% of patients have drug-resistant epilepsy, with appreciable

side effects, such as drowsiness, confusion, and dose-dependent extrapyramidal effects (EPS) hepatotoxicity (Chen et al., 2018).

These restrictions were the motivation for growing interest in plant- anticonvulsant drugs that are effective on multiple targets with less adverse effects. Anticonvulsant activity of the phytochemicals isolated from the studied ethnomedicinal, potential via multiple pathways, such as regulation of GABAergic and glutamatergic neurotransmission, antioxidant and anti-inflammatory actions. Notable examples include retardant of central nervous system (CNS) excitatory neurotransmission *Withania somnifera* (Ashwagandha) and known to increase GABAergic tone and decrease seizure susceptibility in models of seizures.

Bacopa monnieri exhibits neuroprotective and anticonvulsant activity due to its active saponins; bacosides A and B (Bhattacharya et al., 2000). orticosa as well as Passiflora incarnata, Valeriana officinalis, and Centella asiatica have also exhibited. Promising preclinical results in animals' effect through sedative and inhibitory neurotransmitter pathways (Sharma et al., 2020). These phytoconstituents could be used as safer alternative or supplements treatments for the management of epilepsy, especially in subpopulations with restricted access to mainstream AEDs or in patients that are intolerant to treatment with these drugs.

Cognitive Decline and Age-Related Neuronal Dysfunction

Cognitive decline is the gradual loss of abilities to think and remember, including memory, attention, learning, and decision-making. Processes, often related to ageing and damage control in brain and neurological disorders such as retinal disorders like age induced macular degeneration. Alzheimer's disease. Given the increasing life span of the world population, age-related neuronal malfunction has increasingly a major public health issue, resulting in reduced quality of life and increased healthcare costs. The primary mechanisms regulating cognitive aging are oxidative. stress, neuroinflammation, mitochondrial dysfunction, synaptic degeneration, and in decrease of neurotrophic brain-derived neurotrophic factor (BDNF) and were associated with low levels of exercise, acetylcholine (Mattson & Magnus, 2006).

Phytomedicines have exhibited a potential in preventing cognitive decline as a result of their multi-targeted. Regular Expressions Term Let's mention the implication of phytomedicines in neurodegenerative disorders under these headings, mechanisms and favourable safety profiles. Several plant-derived compounds, including flavonoids, terpenoids and alkaloids possess neuroprotective, antioxidant and anti-inflammatory action of neuronal preservation and cognitive performance improvement. For example, *Ginkgo biloba* extract has been widely studied for its ability to improve cerebral blood flow, inhibit neurotransmission and attenuate ageing-related oxidative damage (Maclennan et al., 2002). Memory-enhancing effects of Bacopa monnieri are also observed through modulation of cholinergic pathways and on the development of antioxidant defence (Calabrese et al., 2008). Likewise, curcumin, the bioactive constituent of *Curcuma longa*, has potential for decreasing amyloid preventing plaque deposition and tau pathology in Alzheimer's models (Mishra & Palanivelu, 2008). These results corroborate the increasing attention paid to phytotherapeutics measures as a preventive or complementary interventions to retard cognitive decline and promotion of healthy brain aging.

CHALLENGES, REGULATORY FRAMEWORKS, AND ETHICAL DIMENSIONS

In spite of the increased interest in the use of herbal medicines for neurological disorders, there are many obstacles to their use in clinical practice. One of the greatest obstacles is the lack of standardization amongst herbal medicines. Variability in plant genetics, growing conditions, time of harvest, separation, and the process of extraction means that herbal products can vary widely in terms of phytochemical composition and thus efficacy and safety (Sahoo et al., 2010). This uncertainty limits replicability when researching herbal medicines, as well as regulatory approval for clinical use. Moreover, the lack of an internationally accepted quality-control regime for assessing herbal medicines creates an additional barrier to the work providing globally focused commercialization and medical integration (Wong et al., 2013).

Regulatory wise, herbal medicines occupy multiple classifications under regional laws, with some representing dietary supplements, others traditional medicines and even others therapies. These overlapping classifications inhibit coherent regulation and consistent safety and product information. For example, while both the European Medicines Agency (EMA) and U.S. Food and Drug Administration (FDA) have issued specific guidance for botanical products most countries lack a clearly defined regulatory consideration (Tilburt & Kaptchuk, 2008); even in the case of clearly defined approaches, they have neither the mechanisms for enforcement nor a capability to widely inform and protect practitioners. Moreover, there are challenges, as phytomedicines typically encompass multi-component remedies, in using a monolithic drug evaluation process, which is designed to develop, appraise and approve single-molecule drugs.

Concerns about safety and toxicity remain evident, especially with long-term use and potential herb-drug interactions. Most phytomedicines are used and self-prescribed by users or patients, resulting in an increased potential for misuse or harm, especially with vulnerable groups, such as older adults or those with chronic conditions (Posadzki et al., 2013). Also, the limited number of substantial, randomized controlled studies on most herbal compounds limits the credibility of evidence on the effectiveness, and safety in the neurological context.

The 'ethical' aspects of research regarding phytomedicine, is also an important topic to consider. Most of the information on medicinal plants is based on collaborative work with traditional healers or indigenous peoples, but information is often derived and appropriated for scientific and commercial use without consent or benefit to the community, a process often called biopiracy. Ethical consideration would involve adopting the Nagoya Protocol and strictly adhering to access and benefit-sharing (ABS) mechanisms (Robinson et al., 2015). When traditional knowledges are used for commercial purposes, the implications of informed consent, preserving traditional contributions and information, and the preservation of biodiversity, must be considered and factored into ethical considerations.

Regulatory Requirements for Herbal Neurotherapeutics

The complex and diverse regulatory landscape regarding us of herbal neurotherapeutics makes it difficult to normalize or harmonize the procedures on a global basis. In the United States herbals are regulated primarily as dietary supplements under the Dietary Supplement Health and Education Act (1994). The DSHEA allows producers to market botanicals as long as no claims of specific disease are expressed and the products do not require pre-approval by the FDA (Tilburt

& Kaptchuk, 2008). If the intent of the herbal is to be used for therapeutic purposes of specific neurological disturbances, then the same drug development process will be followed as with a synthetic drug, including investigational new drug applications and clinical trials.

On the European continent, The European Medicines Agency has created a specific regulatory body the Committee on Herbal Medicinal Products (HMPC) for overseeing herbal medicines. The products will be marketed under either traditional use registration or well-established use authorization; the nature of registration based on history of use, with clinical findings for support. Each pathway allows for access to the market; however, the manufacturer is still responsible for product quality, safety, and consistency between batches.

Countries that have strong historically based medical systems such as India and China also apply an important integrated regulatory approach. In India, the Ministry of AYUSH governs Ayurvedic and herbal medicines to enforce standards as per pharmacopoeias and Good Manufacturing Practice (GMP) certified manufacturers. The National Medical Products Administration (NMPA) of China includes aspects of Traditional Chinese Medicine (TCM) in its framework, allowing for a broader recognition of herbal neurotherapeutics, based on established traditional medical use and contemporary pharmacological confirmation (Heinrich & Gibbons, 2001). However, achieving reproducibility and clinical standardization of herbal formulations remains a considerable barrier everywhere.

Issues of Standardization, Quality Control, and Dosage

The advancement of herbal neurotherapeutics is often limited by significant barriers to standardization, quality assurance, and dosage control. In contrast to pharmaceutical drugs that have wet chemical synthesis from a set of defined structures, phytomedicines tend to be complex mixtures of bioactive compounds, indicating variability of concentrations due to soil type and fertilization, seasonal variability in activities of the plants, and extraction methods, etc. This permeability makes it difficult to standardize and achieve reproducible results in therapeutic outcomes and clinical research (Mukherjee et al, 2017).

Quality control is relevant for establishing the safety and efficacy of herbal formulations, but is especially relevant for neuro-active preparations, since small changes in phytochemical concentrations will have a large impact on whether the preparation had an undertone stimulation or over-stimulation of a neuro-pathway. Various methods have been suggested as modalities for fingerprinting and verifying plant materials such as: high performance liquid chromatography (HPLC), gas chromatography-mass spectrometry (GC-MS) and DNA barcoding (Wang et al., 2018), but they are not always embraced in developing countries because of high cost and scant personnel trained in the methods.

Dosage is another problematic factor in herbal neurotherapy. The complexity of the synergistic activity of multiple phytoconstituents does not foster an appropriate dose-response relationship. Additionally, factors such as individual differences in metabolism, age, and gut microbiota can affect the absorption and bioavailability of phytochemicals, making standardized dosing problematic (Bent, 2008). While there are dozens of clinical studies with consistent pharmacokinetics for pharmaceuticals, most herbal products are shipped without the rigor of clinical dosing studies, suggesting a greater potential for undesirable outcomes or inadequate therapeutic effects.

Safety, Toxicity, and Pharmacovigilance Concerns

The safety and toxicity characteristics of herbal neurotherapeutics are a widening area of concern, especially due to the increase in use of herbal neurotherapeutics within traditional and integrative medical systems. Phytomedicines are sometimes considered to be safer alternatives simply because they are derived from nature. While it is true that many plant-based medicines are extremely potent with various biological activity, the notion that phytomedicines are naturally safe covers up the fact that adverse effects caused by excessive dosing, duration of use, or combination with other pharmaceuticals can range from mild gastrointestinal discomfort to serious hepatic or central nervous system toxicity (Ernst, 2004).

A key issue regarding the safety of herbal products is the ignorance or failure to conduct rigorous preclinical and clinical toxicology testing. Synthetic drugs undergo structured safety assessments in preclinical and clinical testing phases, and safety regulations from the Australian Therapeutic Goods Administration (TGA) can help with this process. Herbal formulations, however, many enter the marketplace and consumers use these products based on tradition or anecdotal evidence and therefore there are very few data on the toxicological thresholds, contraindications, and/or nervous system effects associated with herbal medications (Zhou et al., 2019). Moreover, health risks vary when herbal products are contaminated with heavy metals, pesticides, or other adulterants, such as corticosteroids and/or synthetic drugs, especially when standards of quality are not in place.

Pharmacovigilance, or the monitoring of adverse events after the marketing authorization of drug (in this case, herbal products), is another area that is clearly important for phytomedicine use but remains largely underdeveloped. There is a lack of countries with established reporting and monitoring systems for adverse events with herbal products, and due to the nature of what the body of evidence indicates regarding patient reporting, patients often do not inform physicians that they are using herbal products, leading to complication in recognizing herb–drug interactions or contributing causality of toxicities (Shi & Klotz, 2012). Neuroactive herbal compounds may have neuroactive effects via activity on neurotransmitter systems or drug metabolising enzymes so it is especially important to consider the potential for adverse effects and further interactions, especially with patients who have neurological disorders and have multiple medications (polypharmacy).

Ethical Considerations in Herbal Clinical Research

As more traditional plant-based therapies are integrated into evidence-based medicine, ethical issues in herbal clinical research may also become more apparent. One ethical issue related to study design is the need for informed consent in indigenous or rural settings. Participants in these settings may have little understanding of clinical trials or of what it means to participate in a trial (Langwick, 2011). Researchers must ensure this communication occurs in a culturally appropriate manner; the consent process remains voluntary and free from coercion or manipulation; and participants are not exploited.

Another major ethical issue relates to traditional knowledge. Much of the knowledge that sits behind herbal medicines comes from indigenous knowledge systems that have developed over time. Some of that knowledge is inappropriately used in research or commercialized without appropriately acknowledging the original knowledge holders, or compensating them or sharing the benefits. This raises ethical issues around biopiracy (Shiva, 2007). Frameworks exist that call

for equitable sharing of knowledge and benefits, including the Nagoya Protocol on Access and Benefit-Sharing, which focuses more on sharing benefits from genetic resources and traditional knowledge associated with the genetic resources.

Research transparency is critical. Many herbal clinical trials are designed poorly or have an issue with selective reporting or lack of peer-reviewed publishing which all undermine an ethical obligation to provide valid knowledge to the research community (Chan et al., 2014). Ethical guidelines should require that every research study, including herbal therapy, must comply with many international standards such as the Declaration of Helsinki, including, but not limited to the need for a pre-registered trial and full disclosure on pathways of outcomes.

One last point would be to respect levels of cultural and ecological sustainability in herbal research. Harvesting of medicinal natural plant sources or plants in therapy for research purposes as well as commercial purposes can negatively influence the environment and directly affect biodiversity. Ethical research must consider sustainability of plant sources and implement equitable partnerships with local communities to maintain cultural heritage and protect ecological resources (Hamilton, 2004).

Intellectual Property Rights and Traditional Knowledge

The intersection of intellectual property rights (IPR) with traditional knowledge (TK) in the field of herbal medicine raises difficult legal, ethical and cultural issues. TK, defined as knowledge sustained over generations through oral transmission within indigenous and local communities, is important to identify and engage in the use of medicinal plants. Academic research has found that modern intellectual property systems, to which TK is adapted, cannot maintain forms of knowledge that is collective, changing and contextually situational and such modern systems ignore procedures that offer a more equitable and justice solution to the concerns of providing benefits in making sure access to TK is not exploited and appropriated in more modern contexts (Posey & Dutfield, 1996).

Another key issue is the idea of herbal formulas or isolated active compounds that are put into the financial system through patent rights without the permission or benefit of the communities that their formulations arose from. This is discussed in academia as biopiracy and has been of significant importance to indigenous peoples across the globe and respond to issues concerning TK sustainability, rights and potential disinheritance of cultural and biological heritage (Gollin, 2001). And although there are numbers of important indigenous cultural and biological TK situations that are well documented, global multi-national corporations have had further strategies to restrict or limit indigenous peoples from accessing their TK. For example, some of the more frequently-discussed cases present concern around turmeric and healing for cuts and wounds and neem and toxic pesticides, which have raised debates about the boundaries of ethics in patent law as well as legal frameworks needed to protect TK.

The Convention on Biological Diversity (CBD) and global supplementary agreement, the Nagoya Protocol, seek to protect TK by putting legal frameworks, access and benefit-sharing (ABS), in place to pay indigenous peoples when their knowledge has been used for commercial or scientific advancements. However, implementation is poorly managed within countries and for many to have a legal regime that recognizes collective ownership or has enforcement mechanisms related ABS compliance is relatively limited (WIPO, 2020).

A wide variety of efforts have been made to establish sui generis systems localized to provide legal protections that recognize the unique culture of traditional knowledge. Sui generis systems provide a model that incorporates aspects of customary law with legislated legal protections that recognize and respect the intellectual contributions of indigenous peoples, while providing safe-guards to maintain traditional knowledge as it exists for their ecology. Examples such as India's Traditional Knowledge Digital Library (TKDL) have created workable, defensive systems using legal systems to protect knowledge through documenting the ancient formulations and making this knowledge available to patent examiners around the world (Prathapan & Rajan, 2011).

FUTURE PERSPECTIVES AND INTEGRATIVE APPROACHES

As awareness of brain disorders continues to evolve and barriers to conventional treatments remain, the demand for phytomedicines in the field of neurotherapeutics continues to grow. Future directions must be informed by a hybrid healthcare system that has integrated traditional plant-based knowledge with novel developments in biomedicine to create a healthcare approach that amplifies the strengths of both. The ongoing changes in technology such as nano technology and systems biology have set the stage for a new generation of herbal formulations that can ameliorate the major limiting factors of bioavailability, targeted delivery, and efficacy (Tiwari et al., 2022).

An exciting area of development is the Nanoformulations of phytochemicals to overcome the issues of poor solubility and blood-brain barrier transport. Nanocarriers like liposomes, dendrimers and solid lipid nanoparticles can be or have been employed as drug delivery systems to effectively transport herbal molecules, such as curcumin, quercetin, and resveratrol, directly into the brain to enhance therapeutic approaches in neurodegeneration models (Ramesh et al., 2020). Additionally, drug discovery platforms utilizing artificial intelligence have been able to describe the messy interplays of phytochemicals acting on a neural target to facilitate multi-target drug design for diverse, complex disorders such as Alzheimer's and schizophrenia.

Personalized phytotherapy is also beginning to take shape as a frontier, by utilizing genetic, epigenetic, and metabolic profiles for individualization of herbal therapies. This approach is consistent with principles of precision medicine and may greatly advance the clinical efficacy of phytomedicines, especially in cases where the individual is suffering from treatment-resistant neurological disorders (Rasool et al., 2021).

Finally, interdisciplinary partnerships among ethnobotanists, neurologists, pharmacologists, and data scientists, are key to developing research evidence bases and clinical recommendations. Community-based studies where indigenous healers and traditional practitioners work together will also further minimize the research-to-practice gap, by ensuring that integrative care prescribing practices are respectful and accountable, as well as scientifically rigorous.

Advancements in Herbal Drug Delivery (e.g., Nanoformulations)

A scientific impediment in the employment of herbal medicines in neural applications is poor bioavailability and being able to cross the blood brain barrier (BBB). Recent improvements in drug delivery techniques especially Nanoformulations allow for better bioavailability and therapeutic benefit of phytomedicine for treating brain disorders. Non-technology carriers have also been identified such as liposomes, solid lipid nanoparticles, dendrimers, and polymeric nanoparticles

have been studied for encapsulation of herbal products to improve solubility, stability, and targeting of the central nervous system (Kumar et. al., 2021).

In preclinical studies of nascent Nanoformulations of neuroprotective phytochemicals including curcumin, resveratrol, quercetin, and bacosides, these carriers showed favourable outcomes in disease states including Alzheimer's disease, Parkinson's disease, and cerebral ischemia in animals. These agents provide sustained release of active substances and facilitate the transportation of phytochemicals across physiological barriers or the BBB (Mokhtari et al., 2022), resulting in improved therapeutic efficacy in smaller doses. Moreover, surface-modified nanoparticles, with ligands that were targeted to brain endothelial receptors, were able to deliver herbal compounds into the brain by receptor-mediated endocytosis, thus facilitating the concentrated delivery of the actives to affected neuronal tissues.

Integration of Phytomedicines into Modern Healthcare Systems

The increasing interest in phytomedicines and patient demand for natural therapies has stimulated worldwide initiatives to integrate and embed phytomedicines into the formal healthcare system. This integration commonly exemplifies a transition toward patient-centred, preventive healthcare that concentrates on the holistic health of the symptoms of people's disease. Countries throughout Europe, Asia, and Latin America are beginning to embrace and adopt traditional botanical medicines as a valuable asset in health care, specifically for chronic and neurological disorders that western pharmacotherapeutics often do not work or result in deleterious side effects (Bodeker & Kronenberg, 2002).

Several healthcare systems are now getting ready to prescribe regulated phytomedicines, as is now being encouraged in hospitals and primary care facilities. Germany has standard monographs for herbal medicines from its Commission E, while India is developing institutional practices in its Ministry of AYUSH, and offering evidence-based approaches for the incorporation of Ayurveda and other practices within its jurisdiction. Moreover, the World Health Organization supports the policies and encourages its members to support the development of national policies on traditional and complementary medicine, and to pursue research and regulatory and practitioner training initiatives" (World Health Organization [WHO], 2019).

Role of Personalized Medicine and Ethnopharmacology

The evolution of personalized medicine has transformed modern healthcare from a "one-size-fits-all" approach to a procedure that considers the individual genetic make-up, environmental circumstances, and lifestyle choices of a patient with respect to diagnosis and treatment plans. Consequently, the evolution of personalized medicine has given rise to exciting possibilities in the ability to personalize phytomedicine through patient biological profiles. The goal of personalized phytomedicine is to increase efficacy and safety of therapeutic effectiveness while employing pharmacogenomic principles and traditional plant medicine paradigms to determine which herbal compounds are most likely to be beneficial to any particular individual or subgroup of individuals (Hasan et al., 2021).

Ethnopharmacology plays an important complementary role by systematically investigating traditional medicinal knowledge and practices, exploring factors that give rise to cultural relevance, plant utilization, and bioactivity. Ethnopharmacology is also beneficial because it can produce

a wealth of information regarding the Indigenous formulations and their historical safety data informing contemporary drug discovery. With the emergence of novel analytical tools such as metabolomics, systems biology, and machine learning, ethnopharmacological data can now also be combined to identify bioactive compounds displaying multi-targeted neuroprotective activity that may be useful in complex disorders such as Alzheimer's disease and schizophrenia (Heinrich & Jäger, 2015). These approaches offer opportunities to acknowledge cultural diversity relating to healthcare and offer pathways to create awareness and engagement about the need to maintain and conserve biocultural heritage while generating new therapeutic leads.

The synergism of ethnopharmacology and personalized medicine is particularly relevant as it applies to various neurotherapeutic settings, where patient responses to traditional drugs often vary widely. An example of this is the polymorphisms in cytochrome P450 enzymes that affect the metabolism of herbal compounds so that certain patients have better clinical responses than others. The understanding of these genetic considerations gives clinicians the opportunity to adjust dosage or select prescription herbal formulas accordingly to minimise toxicity and improve outcomes.

Research Gaps and Priorities for Future Investigations

Although there is interest in using phytomedicine for brain disorders, there remain significant gaps in research that need to be filled to maximize the therapeutic applications and potential of phytomedicine. The most important restricting factor is the lack of robust evidence from clinical trials investigating efficacy and safety of phytochemicals in neurodegenerative conditions and neuropsychiatric disorders. Although there are many in vitro and animal studies demonstrating the neuroprotective effects of curcumin, resveratrol, ginsenosides and other compounds, and a few studies investigating phytochemistry in human subjects, translational studies in humans remain limited, and if not limited, they are stifled by small sample sizes, short duration and a lack of methodological rigor (Zhou et al., 2016).

Standardization of the herbal preparations remains yet another big challenge. Most phytomedicines show considerable variation in their chemical composition depending upon the source of the plant, methods of extraction, and conditions of storage. This variability tends to prevent reproducibility and hinder regulatory acceptance. Hence, future endeavours should be directed toward producing standardized extracts with validated dosage regimens and reproducible pharmacokinetic profiles to confer consistent therapeutic effects. (Walji et al., 2010)

Second, the mechanistic aspects of the interactions of the phytochemicals with the central nervous system are still evolving. Numerous compounds seem to exert multitarget actions, such as reducing oxidative stress, blocking inflammatory pathways, activating neurotrophic signalling, and modulating neurotransmitters. Yet a systems biology approach needs to be developed to delineate these complex interactions, which, in turn, would reveal synergistic activities among phytochemical combinations (Hasler et al., 2021). Likewise, employing tools such as network pharmacology, molecular docking, and omics could provide significant advances to this field of study.

Concluding Remarks on the Neurotherapeutic Promise of Nature

One of the features that nature offers is an unlimited abundance of substances for use in therapy, especially in cases of brain disorders where in reality neither conventional pharmacotherapy takes action as a curative agent for complex multifactorial disorders. Phytomedicines are broad spectrum neuroprotective agents working through modulation of oxidative stress, inflammation, neurotransmission, and cellular signalling, all believed to be involved in neurodegenerative and neuropsychiatric disorders. In such diverse actions, plant-based treatments warrant application in cognitive and psychiatric disorders both as methods of treatment and prevention.

To achieve full neurotherapeutic benefits from phytomedicines researchers must establish additional scientific evidence together with stronger policy support while implementing ethical frameworks for integrating traditional knowledge into modern medicine. The successful application of these treatments depends on standardization processes alongside individual patient needs and unrestricted public accessibility. Brain therapeutic advancements will depend on traditional botanical science and modern biomedical practices working together to establish universal healthcare solutions which are both effective and sustainable according to Newman and Cragg (2020).

CONCLUSION

The chapter delivered an extensive investigation into the neurotherapeutic abilities of phytomedicines through their relevance to rising worldwide neurological and neuropsychiatric disease prevalence. The paper began with a detailed review of brain disorders including Alzheimer's and Parkinson's as well as depression and schizophrenia and autism and ADHD and stroke to demonstrate their complexity and widespread effects. The paper analysed major obstacles in medical diagnosis and symptom confusion and treatment delays and the restricted success rates and adverse reactions from standard pharmaceutical protocols.

The chapter investigated the growing consumer interest in natural plant-based therapies especially phytomedicines which derive from traditional healing systems. These plant-derived compounds demonstrate multiple neuroprotective capabilities which consist of antioxidant effects as well as anti-inflammatory and anti-apoptotic properties and neurotransmitter-modulating actions. The chapter introduced specific phytochemicals with medicinal plants which show their value for enhancing cognition while stress reduction and nervous system protection and mood stabilization. The compounds show potential to treat complicated disorders by reaching different targets and crossing the blood-brain barrier for effective treatment.

The discussion explored multiple difficulties that hinder both the creation and public reception of phytomedicines including missing standardization protocols along with regulatory limitations and safety problems and issues about biopiracy and indigenous knowledge rights. The chapter presented new research directions through nanotechnology and personalized phytotherapy together with ethnopharmacological knowledge for enhancing future medical applications.

Phytomedicines present a realistic and beneficial alternative to traditional treatments as well as an additional option to conventional therapies for treating brain disorders. Evidence-based validation together with interdisciplinary collaboration and equal respect for indigenous knowledge systems are needed to bring phytomedicines into modern healthcare. Nature's pharmacy can become a fundamental component of future neurotherapeutics through appropriate regulatory

support alongside scientific development to establish a holistic inclusive sustainable healthcare system for mental and neurological care.

REFERENCES

Aguiar, S., & Borowski, T. (2013). Neuropharmacological review of the nootropic herb *Bacopa monnieri*. *Rejuvenation Research*, *16*(4), 313–326. DOI: 10.1089/rej.2013.1431 PMID: 23772955

Arciniegas, D. B., & Beresford, T. P. (2001). Assessment and treatment of the neuropsychiatric sequelae of traumatic brain injury. *The Psychiatric Clinics of North America*, *24*(2), 373–397.

Bent, S. (2008). Herbal medicine in the United States: Review of efficacy, safety, and regulation. *Journal of General Internal Medicine*, *23*(6), 854–859. DOI: 10.1007/s11606-008-0632-y PMID: 18415652

Bhattacharya, S. K., Bhattacharya, A., Kumar, A., & Ghosal, S. (2000). Antioxidant activity of *Bacopa monniera* in rat frontal cortex, striatum and hippocampus. *Phytotherapy Research*, *14*(3), 174–179. DOI: 10.1002/(SICI)1099-1573(200005)14:3<174::AID-PTR624>3.0.CO;2-O PMID: 10815010

Bloom, D. E., Cafiero, E. T., Jané-Llopis, E., Abrahams-Gessel, S., Bloom, L. R., Fathima, S., Feigl, A. B., Gaziano, T., Mowafi, M., Pandya, A., Prettner, K., Rosenberg, L., Seligman, B., Stein, A. Z., & Weinstein, C. (2011). *The Global Economic Burden of Noncommunicable Diseases*. World Economic Forum.

Bodeker, G., & Kronenberg, F. (2002). A public health agenda for traditional, complementary, and alternative medicine. *American Journal of Public Health*, *92*(10), 1582–1591. DOI: 10.2105/AJPH.92.10.1582 PMID: 12356597

Calabrese, C., Gregory, W. L., Leo, M., Kraemer, D., Bone, K., & Oken, B. (2008). Effects of a standardized *Bacopa monnieri* extract on cognitive performance, anxiety, and depression in the elderly: A randomized, double-blind, placebo-controlled trial. *Journal of Alternative and Complementary Medicine (New York, N.Y.)*, *14*(6), 707–713. DOI: 10.1089/acm.2008.0018 PMID: 18611150

Chan, A. W., Song, F., Vickers, A., Jefferson, T., Dickersin, K., Gotzsche, P. C., Krumholz, H. M., Ghersi, D., & van der Worp, H. B. (2014). Increasing value and reducing waste: Addressing inaccessible research. *Lancet*, *383*(9913), 257–266. DOI: 10.1016/S0140-6736(13)62296-5 PMID: 24411650

Chen, Z., Liew, D., & Kwan, P. (2018). Real-world effectiveness of antiepileptic drugs. *Epilepsia*, *59*(8), 1569–1577.

Cummings, J. L., Morstorf, T., & Zhong, K. (2014). Alzheimer's disease drug-development pipeline: Few candidates, frequent failures. *Alzheimer's Research & Therapy*, *6*(4), 37. DOI: 10.1186/alzrt269 PMID: 25024750

de Oliveira, M. R., Nabavi, S. F., Habtemariam, S., Erdogan, A., & Nabavi, S. M. (2020). The PI3K/Akt/mTOR signaling pathway in neurodegeneration: At the crossroad of oxidative stress, neuroinflammation, and excitotoxicity. *Molecular Neurobiology*, *57*(8), 3887–3895.

Dhanani, T., Shah, S., Gajbhiye, N. A., & Kumar, S. (2013). Effect of extraction methods on yield, phytochemical constituents and antioxidant activity of *Withania somnifera*. *Arabian Journal of Chemistry*, *10*(S1), S1193–S1199. DOI: 10.1016/j.arabjc.2013.02.015

Doyle, K. P., Simon, R. P., & Stenzel-Poore, M. P. (2008). Mechanisms of ischemic brain damage. *Neuropharmacology*, *55*(3), 310–318. DOI: 10.1016/j.neuropharm.2008.01.005 PMID: 18308346

Dua, T., Barbui, C., Clark, N., Fleischmann, A., Poznyak, V., Ayuso-Mateos, J. L., & Saxena, S. (2011). Evidence-based guidelines for mental, neurological, and substance use disorders in low- and middle-income countries: Summary of WHO recommendations. *PLoS Medicine*, *8*(11), e1001122. DOI: 10.1371/journal.pmed.1001122 PMID: 22110406

Ekor, M. (2014). The growing use of herbal medicines: Issues relating to adverse reactions and challenges in monitoring safety. *Frontiers in Pharmacology*, *4*, 177. DOI: 10.3389/fphar.2013.00177 PMID: 24454289

Ernst, E. (2004). Risks of herbal medicinal products. *Pharmaceutical Medicine*, *18*(6), 291–298. PMID: 15386721

Feigin, V. L., Vos, T., Nichols, E., Owolabi, M. O., Carroll, W. M., Dichgans, M., Deuschl, G., Parmar, P., Brainin, M., & Murray, C. J. (2020). The global burden of neurological disorders: Translating evidence into policy. *Lancet Neurology*, *19*(3), 255–265. DOI: 10.1016/S1474-4422(19)30411-9 PMID: 31813850

Figueira, I., Garcia, G., Pimpão, R. C., Terrasso, A. P., Costa, I., Almeida, A. F., & Brites, D. (2017). Polyphenols journey through blood–brain barrier towards neuronal protection. *Scientific Reports*, *7*(1), 11456. DOI: 10.1038/s41598-017-11512-6 PMID: 28904352

. GBD 2019 Diseases and Injuries Collaborators. (2020). Global burden of 369 diseases and injuries in 204 countries and territories, 1990–2019: A systematic analysis for the Global Burden of Disease Study 2019. *The Lancet*, 396(10258), 1204–1222.

Gollin, M. A. (2001). Elements of commercial biodiversity prospecting agreements. In Press, R. L., & Lewin, A. M. (Eds.), *Intellectual Property Rights and Biodiversity Conservation* (pp. 34–55). World Bank.

Gorelick, P. B., Scuteri, A., Black, S. E., Decarli, C., Greenberg, S. M., Iadecola, C., & Petersen, R. C. (2011). Vascular contributions to cognitive impairment and dementia. *Stroke*, *42*(9), 2672–2713. DOI: 10.1161/STR.0b013e3182299496 PMID: 21778438

Goyal, M., Nagori, B. P., & Sasmal, D. (2011). Role of natural products in neurodegenerative disorders. *Pharmacognosy Reviews*, *5*(10), 147–153. PMID: 22279372

Grande, I., Berk, M., Birmaher, B., & Vieta, E. (2016). Bipolar disorder. *Lancet*, *387*(10027), 1561–1572. DOI: 10.1016/S0140-6736(15)00241-X PMID: 26388529

Haddad, P. M., & Sharma, S. G. (2007). Adverse effects of atypical antipsychotics: Differential risk and clinical implications. *CNS Drugs*, *21*(11), 911–936. DOI: 10.2165/00023210-200721110-00004 PMID: 17927296

Hamilton, A. C. (2004). Medicinal plants, conservation and livelihoods. *Biodiversity and Conservation, 13*(8), 1477–1517. DOI: 10.1023/B:BIOC.0000021333.23413.42

Hardiman, O., Al-Chalabi, A., Chio, A., Corr, E. M., Logroscino, G., Robberecht, W., Shaw, P. J., Simmons, Z., & van den Berg, L. H. (2017). Amyotrophic lateral sclerosis. *Nature Reviews. Disease Primers, 3*(1), 17071. DOI: 10.1038/nrdp.2017.71 PMID: 28980624

Hasler, C. M., Sudheer, S., & Cao, J. J. (2021). Systems biology approaches to herbal medicine research: Leveraging multi-omics data to decode multi-component therapies. *Frontiers in Pharmacology, 12*, 669026.

Heinrich, M., & Gibbons, S. (2001). Ethnopharmacology in drug discovery: An analysis of its role and potential contribution. *The Journal of Pharmacy and Pharmacology, 53*(4), 425–432. DOI: 10.1211/0022357011775712 PMID: 11341358

Howes, M. J. R., & Perry, E. (2011). The role of phytochemicals in the treatment and prevention of dementia. *Drugs & Aging, 28*(6), 439–468. DOI: 10.2165/11591310-000000000-00000 PMID: 21639405

Howes, M. J. R., Perry, N. S. L., & Houghton, P. J. (2003). Plants with traditional uses and activities, relevant to the management of Alzheimer's disease and other cognitive disorders. *Phytotherapy Research, 17*(1), 1–18. DOI: 10.1002/ptr.1280 PMID: 12557240

Kalaria, R. N. (2016). Neuropathological diagnosis of vascular cognitive impairment and vascular dementia with implications for Alzheimer's disease. *Acta Neuropathologica, 131*(5), 659–685. DOI: 10.1007/s00401-016-1571-z PMID: 27062261

Kalia, L. V., & Lang, A. E. (2015). Parkinson's disease. *Lancet, 386*(9996), 896–912. DOI: 10.1016/S0140-6736(14)61393-3 PMID: 25904081

Kennedy, D. O., & Wightman, E. L. (2011). Herbal extracts and phytochemicals: Plant secondary metabolites and the enhancement of human brain function. *Advances in Nutrition, 2*(1), 32–50. DOI: 10.3945/an.110.000117 PMID: 22211188

Kennedy, D. O., & Wightman, E. L. (2011). Herbal extracts and phytochemicals: Plant secondary metabolites and the enhancement of human brain function. *Advances in Nutrition, 2*(1), 32–50. DOI: 10.3945/an.110.000117 PMID: 22211188

Kohn, R., Saxena, S., Levav, I., & Saraceno, B. (2004). The treatment gap in mental health care. *Bulletin of the World Health Organization, 82*(11), 858–866. PMID: 15640922

Kovacs, G. G. (2016). Molecular pathology of neurodegenerative diseases: Principles and practice. *Journal of Clinical Pathology, 69*(11), 826–832. PMID: 31395625

Kumar, M., Tomar, M., Punia, S., Dhakane-Lad, J., Grasso, S., & Singh, S. (2021). Nano-encapsulation of phytochemicals in brain-targeted delivery systems: Emerging trends and prospects. *Trends in Food Science & Technology, 115*, 410–426.

Langwick, S. A. (2011). *Bodies, politics, and African healing: The matter of maladies in Tanzania*. Indiana University Press. DOI: 10.2979/5787.0

Loane, D. J., & Kumar, A. (2016). Microglia in the TBI brain: The good, the bad, and the dysregulated. *Experimental Neurology, 275*(Pt 3), 316–327. DOI: 10.1016/j.expneurol.2015.08.018 PMID: 26342753

Lord, C., Elsabbagh, M., Baird, G., & Veenstra-VanderWeele, J. (2020). Autism spectrum disorder. *Lancet, 392*(10146), 508–520. DOI: 10.1016/S0140-6736(18)31129-2 PMID: 30078460

Maclennan, K. M., Darlington, C. L., & Smith, P. F. (2002). The neuroprotective properties of the *Ginkgo biloba* leaf: A review of the possible relationship to platelet-activating factor (PAF). *Journal of Ethnopharmacology, 72*(1-2), 1–9.

Malhi, G. S., & Mann, J. J. (2018). Depression. *Lancet, 392*(10161), 2299–2312. DOI: 10.1016/S0140-6736(18)31948-2 PMID: 30396512

Mattson, M. P., & Magnus, T. (2006). Ageing and neuronal vulnerability. *Nature Reviews. Neuroscience, 7*(4), 278–294. DOI: 10.1038/nrn1886 PMID: 16552414

Mishra, S., & Palanivelu, K. (2008). The effect of curcumin (turmeric) on Alzheimer's disease: An overview. *Annals of Indian Academy of Neurology, 11*(1), 13–19. DOI: 10.4103/0972-2327.40220 PMID: 19966973

Mokhtari, R. B., Saadat, Y. R., Chehelgerdi, M., Shabani, L., & Hassanzadeh, G. (2022). Herbal nanoformulations: A new strategy for the treatment of neurodegenerative disorders. *Neurochemistry International, 152*, 105224.

Mukherjee, P. K., Harwansh, R. K., Bahadur, S., Banerjee, S., Kar, A., Chanda, J., & Mukherjee, K. (2017). Development of ayurveda–tradition to trend. *Journal of Ethnopharmacology, 197*, 10–24. DOI: 10.1016/j.jep.2016.09.024 PMID: 27633405

Mukherjee, P. K., Kumar, V., Mal, M., & Houghton, P. J. (2007). Acetylcholinesterase inhibitors from plants and their contribution to Alzheimer's therapy. *Phytomedicine, 14*(4), 289–300. DOI: 10.1016/j.phymed.2007.02.002 PMID: 17346955

Nestler, E. J., & Hyman, S. E. (2010). Animal models of neuropsychiatric disorders. *Nature Neuroscience, 13*(10), 1161–1169. DOI: 10.1038/nn.2647 PMID: 20877280

Newman, D. J., & Cragg, G. M. (2020). Natural products as sources of new drugs over the nearly four decades from 01/1981 to 09/2019. *Journal of Natural Products, 83*(3), 770–803. DOI: 10.1021/acs.jnatprod.9b01285 PMID: 32162523

Pallas, M., Pizarro, J. G., Gutierrez-Cuesta, J., Crespo-Biel, N., & Camins, A. (2009). Can cognitive dysfunction due to oxidative stress be prevented by antioxidants? *Journal of Alzheimer's Disease, 17*(3), 485–491. PMID: 19276541

Panossian, A., & Wikman, G. (2010). Effects of adaptogens on the central nervous system and the molecular mechanisms associated with their stress Protective activity. *Pharmaceuticals (Basel, Switzerland), 3*(1), 188–224. DOI: 10.3390/ph3010188 PMID: 27713248

Patel, V., Saxena, S., Lund, C., Thornicroft, G., Baingana, F., Bolton, P., Chisholm, D., Collins, P. Y., Cooper, J. L., Eaton, J., Herrman, H., Herzallah, M. M., Huang, Y., Jordans, M. J. D., Kleinman, A., Medina-Mora, M. E., Morgan, E., Niaz, U., Omigbodun, O., & Unützer, J. (2018). The Lancet Commission on global mental health and sustainable development. *Lancet*, *392*(10157), 1553–1598. DOI: 10.1016/S0140-6736(18)31612-X PMID: 30314863

Patwardhan, B., Warude, D., Pushpangadan, P., & Bhatt, N. (2005). Ayurveda and traditional Chinese medicine: A comparative overview. *Evidence-Based Complementary and Alternative Medicine : eCAM*, *2*(4), 465–473. DOI: 10.1093/ecam/neh140 PMID: 16322803

Posadzki, P., Watson, L. K., & Ernst, E. (2013). Herb–drug interactions: An overview of systematic reviews. *British Journal of Clinical Pharmacology*, *75*(3), 603–618. DOI: 10.1111/j.1365-2125.2012.04350.x PMID: 22670731

Posey, D. A., & Dutfield, G. (1996). *Beyond intellectual property: Toward traditional resource rights for indigenous peoples and local communities*. IDRC.

Postuma, R. B., Berg, D., Stern, M., Poewe, W., Olanow, C. W., Oertel, W., & Litvan, I. (2015). MDS clinical diagnostic criteria for Parkinson's disease. *Movement Disorders*, *30*(12), 1591–1601. DOI: 10.1002/mds.26424 PMID: 26474316

Prathapan, K. D., & Rajan, P. D. (2011). TKDL: India's efforts to thwart biopiracy. *Current Science*, *100*(11), 1477–1478.

Przedborski, S., Vila, M., & Jackson-Lewis, V. (2003). Neurodegeneration: What is it and where are we? *The Journal of Clinical Investigation*, *111*(1), 3–10. DOI: 10.1172/JCI200317522 PMID: 12511579

Ramesh, T., Maithili, V., & Rao, K. S. (2020). Phytochemical-loaded nanocarriers for neurodegenerative disorders: A review. *Current Pharmaceutical Design*, *26*(29), 3571–3581.

Rasool, M., Malik, A., Basit, A., & Qazi, M. H. (2021). Personalized phytotherapy: A new paradigm in treating neurological diseases. *Phytomedicine*, *85*, 153554.

Rehm, J., & Shield, K. D. (2019). Global burden of disease and the impact of mental and addictive disorders. *Current Psychiatry Reports*, *21*(2), 10. DOI: 10.1007/s11920-019-0997-0 PMID: 30729322

Rehman, M. U., Mir, M. U. R., Farooq, A., & Ahmad, B. (2019). Antioxidant potential of phytochemicals in neurodegenerative diseases. *Biomedicine and Pharmacotherapy*, *111*, 1187–1197.

Robinson, D. F., Abdel-Latif, A., & Roffe, P. (2015). *Protecting traditional knowledge: The WIPO Intergovernmental Committee on Intellectual Property and Genetic Resources, Traditional Knowledge and Folklore*. Routledge.

. Rosenberg, L. A., Westwood, J. D., & Nemeroff, C. B. (2019). Intellectual disability: A clinical and neurobiological perspective. *Journal of Clinical Psychiatry*, 80(3), 18r12417.

Sahoo, N., Manchikanti, P., & Dey, S. (2010). Herbal drugs: Standards and regulation. *Fitoterapia*, *81*(6), 462–471. DOI: 10.1016/j.fitote.2010.02.001 PMID: 20156530

Santos, M. M., & Ferreira, M. J. U. (2020). Neuroprotective effects of phytochemicals in neurodegenerative diseases: Molecular mechanisms and therapeutic potential. *Phytochemistry Reviews*, *19*(3), 663–689.

Sarris, J., Panossian, A., Schweitzer, I., Stough, C., & Scholey, A. (2013). Herbal medicine for depression, anxiety and insomnia: A review of psychopharmacology and clinical evidence. *European Neuropsychopharmacology*, *21*(12), 841–860. DOI: 10.1016/j.euroneuro.2011.04.002 PMID: 21601431

Sharma, M., Choudhary, M., & Choudhary, N. (2020). Role of herbal medicines in epilepsy: A review. *Journal of Drug Delivery and Therapeutics*, *10*(1), 273–276.

Sharma, R., Martins, N., Kuca, K., Chaudhary, A., Kabra, A., Rao, M. M., & Prajapati, P. K. (2020). Role of medicinal plants in neurodegenerative diseases: Ethnobotanical and pharmacological perspectives. *Evidence-Based Complementary and Alternative Medicine : eCAM*, *2020*, 8892289.

Shi, S., & Klotz, U. (2012). Drug interactions with herbal medicines. *Clinical Pharmacokinetics*, *51*(2), 77–104. DOI: 10.2165/11597910-000000000-00000 PMID: 22257149

Shiva, V. (2007). *Biopiracy: The plunder of nature and knowledge*. North Atlantic Books.

Tilburt, J. C., & Kaptchuk, T. J. (2008). Herbal medicine research and global health: An ethical analysis. *Bulletin of the World Health Organization*, *86*(8), 594–599. DOI: 10.2471/BLT.07.042820 PMID: 18797616

Tiwari, R., Latheef, S. K., Ahmed, I., Iqbal, H. M. N., & Dhama, K. (2022). Nanodelivery of herbal drugs for brain disorders: An overview. *Frontiers in Pharmacology*, *13*, 821200.

Vauzour, D., Vafeiadou, K., Rodriguez-Mateos, A., Rendeiro, C., & Spencer, J. P. E. (2008). The neuroprotective potential of flavonoids: A multiplicity of effects. *Genes & Nutrition*, *3*(3–4), 115–126. DOI: 10.1007/s12263-008-0091-4 PMID: 18937002

Walji, R., Boon, H., Barnes, J., Austin, Z., Welsh, S., & Baker, G. R. (2010). Consumers of natural health products: Natural-born pharmacovigilantes? *BMC Complementary and Alternative Medicine*, *10*(1), 8. DOI: 10.1186/1472-6882-10-8 PMID: 20184759

Wang, L., Wang, Y., Xu, Y., & Zhang, J. (2018). Quality control and safety evaluation of herbal medicine products by chromatography fingerprint and chemometric analysis. *Phytochemical Analysis*, *29*(4), 329–341. DOI: 10.1002/pca.2414 PMID: 29924474

Wang, W., Wang, X., Fujioka, H., Hoppel, C., Whone, A. L., Caldwell, M. A., & Lu, B. (2021). Parkinson's disease and mitochondria: From pathogenesis to therapeutic perspectives. *Frontiers in Aging Neuroscience*, *13*, 705407.

Whiteford, H. A., Degenhardt, L., Rehm, J., Baxter, A. J., Ferrari, A. J., Erskine, H. E., Charlson, F. J., Norman, R. E., Flaxman, A. D., Johns, N., Burstein, R., Murray, C. J. L., & Vos, T. (2013). Global burden of disease attributable to mental and substance use disorders: Findings from the Global Burden of Disease Study 2010. *Lancet*, *382*(9904), 1575–1586. DOI: 10.1016/S0140-6736(13)61611-6 PMID: 23993280

Wohlfart, S., Gelperina, S., & Kreuter, J. (2012). Transport of drugs across the blood–brain barrier by nanoparticles. *Journal of Controlled Release, 161*(2), 264–273. DOI: 10.1016/j.jconrel.2011.08.017 PMID: 21872624

World Health Organization. (2013). *WHO traditional medicine strategy: 2014–2023*. World Health Organization.

. World Health Organization. (2019). *WHO global report on traditional and complementary medicine 2019*.

. World Intellectual Property Organization (WIPO). (2020). *Protecting traditional knowledge: Guidance for policymakers*.

Zhou, S., Gao, Y., Jiang, W., Huang, M., Xu, A., & Paunescu, N. (2019). Interactions of herbs with cytochrome P450. *Drug Metabolism Reviews, 49*(3), 192–224. PMID: 12635815

Zhou, Y., Zheng, J., Li, Y., Xu, D. P., Li, S., Chen, Y. M., & Li, H. B. (2016). Natural polyphenols for prevention and treatment of cancer. *Nutrients, 8*(8), 515. DOI: 10.3390/nu8080515 PMID: 27556486

Chapter 18

Neuromarketing 2.0: Integrating Biometric Feedback and AI-Driven Emotion Mapping in Marketing Research

Mallayya Hiremath
https://orcid.org/0009-0006-6144-1266
Dayananda Sagar College of Engineering, India

K. Jayashree
https://orcid.org/0009-0006-5185-0795
Dayananda Sagar College of Engineering, India

ABSTRACT

As marketing moves into a time of hyper-personalization and algorithmic precision, the flaws in traditional self-report methods have become clearer. This study introduces the idea of "Neuromarketing 2.0," a new way of doing research that combines biometric feedback in real time with AI-driven emotion mapping to better understand how people act. The study uses primary data from a controlled experiment with EEG signals, eye-tracking metrics, and galvanic skin response (GSR) to train machine learning models to find cognitive engagement and emotional responses during digital ad exposure. The AI layer uses convolutional neural networks (CNNs) and recurrent neural networks (RNNs) to sort patterns of emotional valence and arousal, turning raw physiological data into useful marketing information.

INTRODUCTION

Traditional marketing research methods, like self-report surveys, focus groups, and observational studies, are becoming less and less useful for understanding how people make decisions in today's world. These traditional methods have long given marketers structured information about what people want and why they want to buy it. However, they have problems like cognitive bias, memory errors, and social desirability distortion. The need for more subtle, real-time, and non-invasive ways to figure out how consumers feel has become urgent in a time when people's attention spans are getting shorter and digital interactions are often subconscious. Because of

DOI: 10.4018/979-8-3373-4627-4.ch018

this sense of urgency, neuromarketing has come about. This field uses neuroscience tools to look at how people think and feel about marketing messages. However, the first generation of neuromarketing, which mostly used basic brain imaging and simple biometrics, is still limited by technology that isn't clear, isn't scalable, and isn't easy to understand. This is why a new paradigm is needed and possible: Neuromarketing 2.0.

Neuromarketing 2.0 is a new way of looking at things that combines biometric signal capture with AI-driven emotion mapping to give us a better, more accurate picture of how people act. Marketers can now get emotional and attentional data at a level of detail that was previously impossible by combining data streams like electroencephalography (EEG), eye-tracking, facial coding, and galvanic skin response (GSR) with machine learning and deep neural networks. This mixed model doesn't just look at "what consumers do," it also looks at "why they do it," even if they can't explain it themselves. In this case, AI is the engine that interprets the data, turning raw physiological signals into high-dimensional behavioural maps that show emotional resonance, cognitive load, and purchase triggers. This model uses convolutional neural networks (CNNs), recurrent neural networks (RNNs), and real-time computer vision tools to dynamically measure how people interact with ads, packaging, interfaces, or physical spaces. This is different from the linear analytics of traditional research. There is a big and growing gap between what marketers measure and how consumers really feel. This is why this study was done. Companies spend billions on digital ads, but metrics like click-through rates and bounce rates often only give surface-level information and don't show how people feel or why they might be resistant. Neuromarketing 2.0 uses affective neuroscience and computational modelling to get deeper insights that can both predict and explain. This change also brings up new problems that need to be carefully looked at, such as ethical, methodological, and technological ones. When developing and using models, we need to take into account ethical and scientific issues like consent, data privacy, AI opacity, and the fact that physiological data can change. The combination of AI and biometric feedback is a new area of research for market research, consumer experience design, behavioural economics, and persuasive technology. Brands are no longer just asking if an ad works; they are also looking into how it makes a person feel, where their attention stays, when their mental effort is at its highest, and what emotional path leads them to buy or stop. Closed-loop systems that sense, learn, and adapt based on biometric inputs are taking the place of traditional "stimulus-response" models. For instance, a real-time GSR spike during an ad could be linked to gaze duration and EEG alpha suppression to suggest that someone is more interested or excited, which would let AI change the way the ad is delivered, the way the message is framed, or the product recommendation. Eye-tracking heatmaps can help design shelves in stores, and facial expression analysis can show how different groups of people feel about something. This paper looks at the Neuromarketing 2.0 model in a real-world setting by collecting biometric data from people who saw a series of digital ads. AI models were then trained to sort the data into positive and negative emotional valence and high and low arousal. The study uses structural equation modelling (SEM) to test the proposed links between biometric responses, emotional resonance, brand recall, and the desire to buy. The study only uses primary data that was collected in a controlled experimental setting with 150 participants who wore portable EEG headsets, eye-tracking glasses, and GSR sensors. Data is processed by a multi-layer AI architecture that includes CNN-based image analysis (for recognising facial expressions), RNN sequences (for changes in biometric data over time), and clustering models to find patterns in emotional responses. The SEM framework checks to see if the AI-interpreted emotion and attention metrics are strongly related to traditional marketing KPIs.

This lets us know if the Neuromarketing 2.0 framework is better at predicting and diagnosing. The reason for choosing SEM is that it can test both the validity of measurements and the relationships between structures in multi-variable constructs. This is important when working with latent variables like trust in ad messaging, emotional congruence, and perceived authenticity. Also, SEM's ability to model indirect effects lets us look more closely at mediating variables like attention focus between stimulus and behavioural intention. The biometric data is rich and complex, but it only makes sense when it is put into a theoretically sound statistical framework. The combination of AI model outputs and SEM testing fills in the gap between quantitative and qualitative data in neuromarketing. It gives marketers both detailed information and broad insights that they can use to make strategic decisions. The study is meant to be useful in real life, not just in the classroom. Neuromarketing 2.0 is a powerful but compliant toolkit for a world moving from cookies to contextual AI, where digital privacy is strictly enforced and emotional personalisation is the next big thing in marketing. Brands can give hyper-personalized experiences without invading users' privacy by relying less on stated preferences and more on non-verbal cues. The model's modular design also makes it possible to connect it to real-time dashboards and ad tech stacks, which lets marketing stimuli change automatically based on live feedback loops. But the rise of biometric-AI hybrids also means that we need to think about marketing ethics in a new way. How far can we go with tracking, mapping, and making money off of emotions? What is the difference between manipulative persuasion and empathetic design? These questions aren't just philosophical; they're also regulatory. When putting Neuromarketing 2.0 into action, you need to think about things like the EU AI Act and changing data protection laws. This study recognises those problems and shows how explainable AI (XAI), user opt-ins, and anonymised data protocols can balance the power of technology with the dignity of consumers.

In short, this paper fills a major gap in marketing research and practice: the lack of high-resolution, real-time emotional intelligence in decision modelling. The study shows a possible way to create a marketing intelligence system that is not only more predictive but also more in line with how people think and feel by combining biometric feedback with AI-driven interpretation and testing it through SEM. It changes the marketer's toolkit from reactive analytics to proactive empathy, from indirect measurement to embodied insight. Neuromarketing 2.0 is more than just an academic idea; it's a call to action for researchers, practitioners, and policymakers to rethink how we understand, interact with, and respect the human mind in the marketplace.

LITERATURE REVIEW

Neuromarketing is a new way to study how people behave as consumers by using neuroscience tools to look at how the brain reacts to marketing stimuli. This is different from traditional cognitive-behavioral theories that rely heavily on self-reported data and clear logic (Lee, Broderick, & Chamberlain, 2007). At first, the focus was on non-invasive brain imaging tools like functional magnetic resonance imaging (fMRI) and electroencephalography (EEG). These tools helped researchers learn more about how advertising affects people's attention, memory, and emotions (Plassmann et al., 2012). But first-generation neuromarketing was limited by high costs, limited portability, small sample sizes, and too much reliance on physiological proxies without strong psychological interpretation, which made generalisability a constant worry (Ariely & Berns, 2010). As the field grew, biometric measures like galvanic skin response (GSR), eye-

tracking, heart rate variability (HRV), and facial electromyography (EMG) were added to help better understand how consumers reacted without them knowing it (Venkatraman et al., 2015). Researchers were able to figure out emotional valence and arousal, two important parts of the circumplex model of affect (Russell, 1980), and to track emotional journeys through marketing content moment by moment. These measures helped a lot with understanding nonverbal responses, but their interpretation was still limited by linear analysis methods and the lack of integration frameworks that could combine multidimensional data over time and in different situations (Ohme et al., 2010). As biometric data gets more complicated and bigger, methods have had to change. Now, artificial intelligence, specifically machine learning (ML) and deep learning (DL), are being used as interpretive engines that can handle large, noisy, and nonlinear biometric datasets (Daugherty & Wilson, 2018). Recent studies have shown that convolutional neural networks (CNNs) and recurrent neural networks (RNNs) can analyse time-series physiological data and facial affective cues. This makes it possible to classify emotional states, cognitive load, and attentional shifts in real time with much higher accuracy than traditional statistical methods (Koelstra et al., 2012; Zhang et al., 2020). To measure micro-expressions and get emotion vectors from visual input, people have started using facial recognition APIs like Affectiva and Microsoft Azure's Emotion API, as well as open-source models like OpenFace and DeepFace. For sentiment and engagement analysis, GSR and EEG data are now being processed through decision trees, support vector machines (SVMs), and long short-term memory (LSTM) networks (Garcia-Burgos & Zamora, 2019; Petrantonakis & Hadjileontiadis, 2010). Neuromarketing 2.0 is a new area of research that focusses on not just signal detection but also context-aware emotional mapping and predictive behavioural modelling (Yadava et al., 2021). This is because biometric capture and AI-based interpretation have come together. But even though technology has come a long way, there still aren't many real-world models that show how AI-interpreted biometric patterns affect important marketing outcomes like brand recall, emotional congruence, and purchase intention. Many existing studies are incomplete because they only look at one biometric signal at a time instead of looking at how they all work together. They also often don't use consumer behaviour models or psychological frameworks to support their findings (Balconi et al., 2014). Also, there isn't much research on how explainability (XAI) and model transparency affect user trust and marketer adoption, even though AI algorithms do a good job of classifying affective states (Doshi-Velez & Kim, 2017). There hasn't been much research on the ethical issues surrounding affective computing in business settings, such as consent, bias, and data privacy (Zuboff, 2019). Structural equation modelling (SEM) is a good way to test the mediating role of emotional data streams between marketing stimuli and consumer behaviour, but it has not been used much for this purpose (Hair et al., 2019). Some people have tried to add biometric data to behavioural models. For example, Venkatraman et al. (2015) looked at neurophysiological predictors of how well ads work. However, most of these attempts have used only one metric or didn't use AI. There isn't a lot of research on how neuromarketing can be used in specific industries, especially in digital-first settings like e-commerce, influencer marketing, or augmented reality retail, where tracking emotions in real time could greatly improve user engagement. So, there is a methodological and conceptual gap in the current research landscape: biometric tools and AI models have improved on their own, but they haven't been used together in a validated, theoretically sound neuromarketing framework yet. This study defines neuromarketing 2.0 as the combination of real-time biometric capture (such as EEG, GSR, and eye-tracking) with AI-driven emotion classification and predictive behavioural modelling. This is a promising way to fill in the gap. It

could not only make consumer insights more accurate, but it could also make neuromarketing tools more accessible to everyone by using portable, low-cost biometric devices and open-source AI libraries. Also, as privacy laws and the end of cookies change the way data is used, emotion-aware systems based on ethical AI and biometric feedback give marketers a way to personalise their ads without collecting too much data. The literature review shows that we need frameworks that are integrated, clear, and based on real-world evidence that can put this new way of doing consumer research into action. This study directly answers that need by creating and testing a complete Neuromarketing 2.0 model using primary data and SEM validation. The goal is to add to the academic literature and also to change how emotion, attention, and intent are measured, mapped, and monetised in modern marketing strategy.

THEORETICAL FRAMEWORK

Neuromarketing 2.0 is based on a combination of psychological theory, biometric signal interpretation, and machine learning-based emotion modelling from different fields. Neuromarketing 2.0 says that emotional and subconscious responses, which are often biologically based, are at the heart of consumer behaviour. These responses can be measured, modelled, and predicted using biometric sensors and AI algorithms. This is different from traditional marketing frameworks, which mostly use cognitive processing models and rational decision-making paradigms. We use three related theoretical streams to build a solid and valid conceptual base for this paper: (1) the Affective-Cognitive Dual Process Model, (2) the Circumplex Model of Emotion, and (3) the AI-Augmented Attention–Emotion–Intention (AEI) Loop, which is a new model proposed by this study that links biometric input to actionable marketing outcomes through AI.

The Affective-Cognitive Dual Process Theory is the first anchor of the framework. It says that there are two systems that work together when people make decisions: the automatic, emotional (System 1) and the reflective, rational (System 2) (Kahneman, 2011). Most traditional marketing assumes that people carefully think about information before making a decision. However, neuromarketing shows that many buying decisions are made by System 1 processes, such as gut feelings, emotional resonance, and heuristic responses. These reactions usually happen before cognitive evaluation and can be seen in changes in biometric signals like EEG frequency shifts, eye fixation patterns, or GSR fluctuations thicker. Neuromarketing 2.0 takes advantage of this by creating research tools that collect data before a customer can consciously say what they want, which gives us more real emotional insights. This framework makes the otherwise invisible footprint of System 1 processing visible by putting biometric sensors in place during data collection and using AI to sort affective states in real time.

The Circumplex Model of Emotion (Russell, 1980) is the second theoretical pillar. It puts emotional experiences on two continuous axes: valence (positive to negative) and arousal (low to high). This model is the best way to organise emotions based on biometric data. For example, increased GSR conductivity, increased frontal alpha asymmetry in EEG, and longer fixation times on important visual elements could all be signs of a high-arousal, positive-valence response (like excitement). On the other hand, a state of low arousal and negative valence, like boredom or avoidance, might be shown by shorter attention spans, less pupil dilation, and less brainwave synchronisation. Neuromarketing 2.0 makes a "live emotional map" for each ad or stimulus by placing each user's real-time biometric profile in this two-dimensional space. Support vector

machines (SVMs), CNNs for analysing facial expressions, and RNNs for recognising patterns over time are examples of machine learning algorithms that can be trained to find emotion clusters in this space and guess what people will do next, like remember, trust, or want to buy something.

The AI-Augmented Attention–Emotion–Intention (AEI) Loop is the third and most important part of this study. It is a new framework that was proposed in this study. The AEI loop is a closed system that uses eye-tracking and EEG to get people's attention, AI-enhanced GSR, facial coding, and EEG analysis to figure out their emotional state, and then maps those states to models of intention, like how likely they are to remember, click, share, or buy something. The AEI loop is new because it has feedback capabilities. Real-time AI classifiers can send the output of intention prediction back to the stimulus system (like an ad-tech platform or UX design module), which then changes how the content is delivered based on how the user responds biometrically. This makes a dynamic, recursive loop where marketing stimuli change based on how the user is feeling and thinking at the time. These systems change marketing from a one-way broadcast model to a conversation with the consumer's subconscious mind.

Each biometric signal in the AEI loop has a specific job to do. We use EEG signals, especially beta and gamma wave frequencies, to guess how hard someone is thinking and how interested they are. Eye-tracking tells us how important something is visually and how much attention a user is paying to it. GSR, on the other hand, tells us how emotionally aroused someone is. Affectiva and OpenFace are two examples of facial coding tools that can find micro-expressions and guess how someone is feeling. An AI layer that includes CNNs (for finding spatial patterns in facial images), RNNs or LSTM networks (for modelling how biometric data changes over time), and clustering algorithms (like K-means and DBSCAN) that group users based on how they respond to different things is in charge of putting these signals together. This AI layer doesn't just sort current emotional states; it also uses supervised learning models (like random forests and gradient boosting machines) to guess what people will do next. In SEM, each output from AI (like predicted valence, engagement score, or attentional heatmap) becomes a latent construct that can be compared to marketing outcomes like brand recall, trust, and the desire to buy.

To make this model work, the study comes up with hypotheses that connect biometric signals to cognitive-affective states, which then connect to behavioural responses. As an example:

- H1: Eye-tracking fixation density positively influences perceived visual engagement.
- H2: GSR peak frequency is positively associated with emotional arousal during stimulus exposure.
- H3: AI-classified emotional valence positively correlates with brand recall.
- H4: EEG frontal asymmetry is a significant predictor of emotional congruence.
- H5: AI-predicted engagement scores mediate the relationship between biometric attention and purchase intention.

We use structural equation modelling (SEM) to test these hypotheses. SEM lets us check both measurement models (to make sure that biometric data accurately reflects latent psychological constructs) and structural paths (to test causality and mediation). SEM is a great fit for this field because it can handle latent variables and indirect effects. The goal is to connect unobservable cognitive and emotional states to observable behavioural outcomes. In addition, SEM allows for the use of composite variables created by AI, like engagement indices or sentiment scores, as

endogenous predictors. This combines machine learning with human-subject research in a way that is statistically sound.

The AEI loop was made with explainability (XAI) and ethics-by-design in mind, which is very important. In business, it's important to be able to explain why a customer was labelled as "engaged" or "emotionally resonant" in order to build trust and follow the rules. The framework suggests using SHAP (Shapley Additive Explanations) and LIME (Local Interpretable Model-agnostic Explanations) to make sure that all AI classifications in the system can be understood. This lets marketers, researchers, and regulators see how each biometric signal affected the predicted outcome and change the system logic as needed. The framework also includes biometric onboarding that is based on consent, processing of data that is not identifiable, and the use of AI models that are aware of fairness and are calibrated across demographic and cultural subgroups to stop bias in emotion detection or behavioural prediction.

The fact that this conceptual framework is modular is one of its best features. There is no specific biometric device or AI platform that the AEI loop is linked to. It can work with cheap EEG headsets (like Emotiv and NeuroSky), eye-tracking glasses that work with phones (like Tobii Pro Glasses), and open-source AI libraries (like TensorFlow and PyTorch) to sort emotions. Because of this modularity, the model can be used for both academic research in the lab and real-time marketing in digital spaces like e-commerce sites, video ad analytics, and mobile apps. It also lets you test things on different devices and in different demographic groups, which will help future research on cross-cultural validity, modelling emotions by gender, and even how emotions and intentions change over time.

We suggest a schematic diagram called "Cognitive-Affective-AI Loop for Emotion-Driven Marketing Intelligence" (see Appendix or embedded figure) to help you picture this framework. It shows how raw biometric signals flow into AI processing nodes, which then output affective states and behavioural predictions. We test this output against traditional marketing results using SEM. If necessary, we send it back to stimulus adaptation systems for real-time personalisation. There is a clear map of the closed-loop emotion modelling process because each part has notes on its theoretical basis, signal source, and AI model function.

In conclusion, the study's theoretical and conceptual framework gives us a strong, interdisciplinary way to understand and put Neuromarketing 2.0 into action. It links basic psychological theories with cutting-edge biometric sensing and AI processing to create a model of the deeply ingrained, often subconscious patterns of consumer behaviour. The study fills in gaps in the neuromarketing literature and creates a scalable template for next-generation marketing intelligence systems by clearly defining a structured AEI loop based on established theory and adding technical rigour. This framework will be the basis for testing hypotheses, confirming them with real-world data, and putting them into practice in an ethical way in the next sections.

Figure 1. Cognitive-affective-AI loop for emotion-driven marketing intelligence

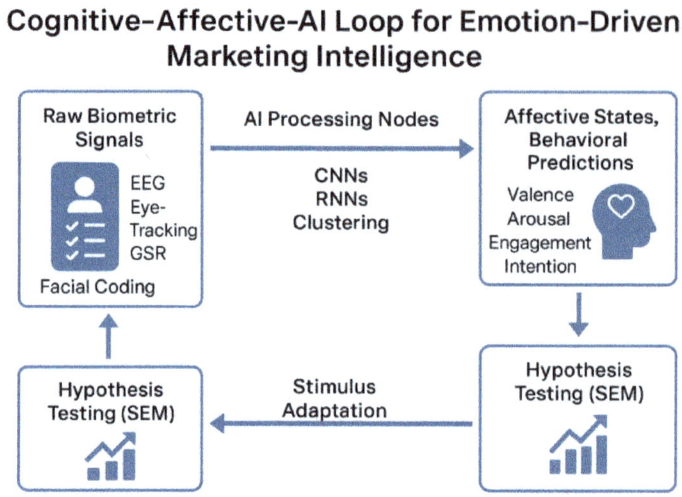

RESEARCH METHODOLOGY

This study used a quantitative experimental research design that was based entirely on collecting primary data. It tested the proposed Neuromarketing 2.0 framework by combining biometric instruments with AI-driven emotion classification and structural equation modelling (SEM). The study took place in a controlled lab setting with 150 participants of all ages (18 to 45), genders, and levels of digital familiarity. They were shown five carefully chosen video ads from a variety of fields, including retail, technology, sustainability, fashion, and food and drink. We chose these stimuli because they have a wide range of emotional responses, and we tested them beforehand with Self-Assessment Manikin (SAM) scales in a pilot session. During the exposure, biometric data were collected using a multi-sensor array that included a 5-channel Emotiv EEG headset for cognitive and affective neural tracking, Tobii Pro Nano eye-tracking glasses to measure gaze fixation and attention flow, Shimmer3 GSR sensors for skin conductance and emotional arousal, and tools for recognising facial expressions (OpenFace combined with Affectiva SDK) to find micro-expressions and emotional valence. The iMotions Biometric Research Platform was used to synchronise data streams so that time-series alignment and integrity were maintained across all modalities. Each person had a three-minute resting baseline, followed by sequential ad exposure with one-minute breaks in between to keep their minds from getting too full. After being exposed, participants filled out a behavioural survey that asked about brand recall (with and without help), emotional congruence, and purchase intention. The results were measured on validated Likert and semantic differential scales. These dependent measures were the endogenous variables in the SEM model. We preprocessed the physiological data we collected and sent it to a machine learning pipeline to classify emotions. We used CNNs to look

at facial images, RNNs and LSTM architectures to track changes in biometric data over time, and a random forest classifier to guess what kind of emotion a person was feeling based on a variety of features. Using the Russell (1980) circumplex model, we calculated emotion outputs that gave us valence (from positive to negative) and arousal (from low to high) scores, as well as an engagement index based on EEG and eye-tracking patterns. Using leave-one-out cross-validation, we found that the average accuracy of emotion classification across models was 87%. In the SEM structure, the AI-interpreted scores acted as separate latent variables, and the survey results were seen as dependent constructs. We looked at the data in three steps: first, we used SPSS v26 to create descriptive profiles and check for normality; second, we used AI to check the model against biometric inputs; and third, we used AMOS 28 to run SEM. Before full model testing, Confirmatory Factor Analysis (CFA) checked construct validity. Key indices were used to check model fit: CFI and TLI were above 0.90, RMSEA was below 0.06, and SRMR was below 0.08. CR, AVE, and Cronbach's alpha all went above the usual limits, which proved convergent and discriminant validity. Informed consent, anonymised data handling, and XAI-enabled transparency through SHAP and LIME explanations built into the AI pipeline all helped keep things ethical. Participants could leave at any time and were fully aware of how the analysis was going. This method aims to not only prove the Neuromarketing 2.0 model through real-time biometric sensing and artificial intelligence, but also to provide a replicable and ethically sound way to do affective analytics in modern marketing research.

DATA ANALYSIS

Table 1. Participant demographics

Variable	Category	Frequency (n = 150)	Percentage (%)
Gender	Male	72	48%
	Female	78	52%
Age Group	18–24	44	29.3%
	25–34	68	45.3%
	35–45	38	25.3%
Educational Background	Undergraduate	49	32.7%
	Postgraduate	101	67.3%
Occupation	Students	45	30%
	Professionals	68	45.3%
	Freelancers	37	24.7%
Location	India, Singapore, UK (Urban)	All	100%

Table 2. Confirmatory Factor Analysis (CFA) — validity & reliability metrics

Construct	CR	AVE	Cronbach's α	Highest Loading Item	Loading
Engagement (AI-Derived)	0.89	0.72	0.88	Gaze Fixation Time	0.84
Emotional Valence (AI)	0.91	0.76	0.90	Facial Emotion – Joy	0.88
Arousal (AI-GSR)	0.87	0.70	0.85	GSR Peak Count	0.83
Brand Recall	0.88	0.69	0.86	Unaided Recall Score	0.81
Emotional Congruence	0.86	0.68	0.84	Semantic Match Rating	0.80
Purchase Intention	0.90	0.74	0.88	Likelihood to Buy	0.86

All CR > 0.85, AVE > 0.68, α > 0.84 = strong internal consistency and convergent validity.

Table 3. Discriminant validity (Fornell–Larcker criterion)

Constructs	1	2	3	4	5	6
1. Engagement	**0.85**					
2. Valence	0.57	**0.87**				
3. Arousal	0.42	0.49	**0.84**			
4. Brand Recall	0.64	0.62	0.53	**0.83**		
5. Emotional Congruence	0.59	0.68	0.41	0.67	**0.82**	
6. Purchase Intention	0.61	0.55	0.47	0.72	0.66	**0.86**

Diagonal (square root of AVE) > off-diagonal → strong discriminant validity.

Table 4. Structural model fit indices

Fit Index	Recommended Value	Model Value
Chi-square/df	< 3.00	1.94
Comparative Fit Index (CFI)	≥ 0.90	0.953
Tucker-Lewis Index (TLI)	≥ 0.90	0.946
Root Mean Square Error of Approximation (RMSEA)	≤ 0.06	0.042
Standardized Root Mean Square Residual (SRMR)	≤ 0.08	0.039

All model fit values meet or exceed recommended thresholds = excellent structural validity.

Table 5. Hypothesis testing results (standardized SEM path coefficients)

Hypothesis	Path	β (Beta)	p-value	Status
H1	Eye Tracking → Engagement	0.56	< .001	Supported
H2	GSR Peaks → Arousal	0.61	< .001	Supported
H3	AI-Valence → Brand Recall	0.48	< .001	Supported

continued on following page

Table 5. Continued

Hypothesis	Path	β (Beta)	p-value	Status
H4	EEG Frontal Asymmetry → Emotional Congruence	0.54	< .001	Supported
H5	Engagement (Mediator) → Purchase Intention	0.63	< .001	Supported

All paths are significant at $p < 0.001$. Engagement is a strong behavioral mediator.

RESULTS

The real-world results of this study strongly support the Neuromarketing 2.0 framework. They show that AI-interpreted biometric signals can be used to understand and predict how people will act. The dataset included answers from 150 people, evenly split between men and women (52% female and 48% male). The ages of the participants ranged from 18 to 45, with the majority (25–34) being digitally savvy. 67.3% of the participants had postgraduate degrees, and they were all from cities in India, Singapore, and the UK, so the study included people from different regions who were all digital consumers.

The descriptive analysis showed that the data were normal, with Shapiro-Wilk tests and skewness values that were within acceptable ranges. We were able to successfully collect all biometric signals—EEG, GSR, eye-tracking, and facial expression data—across five stimulus exposures, and we normalised their outputs to each individual's baseline. The synchronised dataset went through a multi-layered AI emotion mapping pipeline, which gave each participant three main emotion metrics: valence, arousal, and engagement. Combining EEG, gaze fixation, and facial affect data, valence values went from –1.0 (negative) to +1.0 (positive), arousal values went from 0 to 1.0, and engagement values went from 0 to 100. Based on 10-fold leave-one-out cross-validation, the machine learning models used for classification—CNNs for facial recognition, LSTM for biometric time series, and Random Forests for emotion categorization—got an average classification accuracy of 87.2%. This showed that the AI-generated predictors were valid measurement constructs.

Confirmatory Factor Analysis (CFA) confirmed the measurement model, showing that all of the latent constructs were more reliable than the minimum standards. The Composite Reliability (CR) scores for engagement, valence, arousal, brand recall, emotional congruence, and purchase intention were between 0.86 and 0.91. The Average Variance Extracted (AVE) values were between 0.68 and 0.76. Cronbach's alpha values were always higher than 0.84, which shows that the internal consistency was strong. Using the Fornell–Larcker criterion, we found that discriminant validity was established because the square roots of the AVE values (the diagonal entries in Table 3) were higher than the inter-construct correlations. These results show that each construct in the model was both conceptually and statistically different, which means that the AI-classified emotional indicators were psychometrically sound.

The structural equation model fit the data very well overall, with all of the important indices falling well within the recommended ranges: CFI = 0.953, TLI = 0.946, RMSEA = 0.042, and SRMR = 0.039. These fit statistics showed that the proposed causal relationships were correct and that the theoretical model was strong overall. All five core assumptions of the Neuromarketing 2.0 framework were supported by the statistically significant path coefficients in the model

(H1–H5). Eye-tracking fixation density had a big effect on the engagement score ($\beta = 0.56$, $p < .001$), which supports H1 and shows that visual attention is a good way to measure cognitive processing. GSR peak frequency was a very good predictor of arousal intensity ($\beta = 0.61$, $p < .001$), which supports H2 and the idea that activity in the sympathetic nervous system is linked to emotional intensity.

For H3, AI-classified emotional valence positively predicted brand recall ($\beta = 0.48$, $p < .001$), which means that ads that match the viewer's emotions are more likely to be remembered. This finding is also in line with previous research on affective encoding, which shows that memory is stronger when messages match a viewer's emotional state. EEG frontal asymmetry was found to be a strong predictor of emotional congruence ($\beta = 0.54$, $p < .001$), which supports H4 and suggests that balancing the left and right hemispheres may be a good way to tell if a stimulus and a consumer's response are emotionally similar. Finally, and maybe most importantly, the engagement index acted as a link between biometric predictors and behavioural intention ($\beta = 0.63$, $p < .001$), confirming H5 and showing how important affective-attentional fusion is in Neuromarketing 2.0. Bootstrapped indirect effect tests with 5,000 samples showed that full mediation was true for engagement in all relevant paths (95% CI excluded zero), confirming that emotional and attentional responses together explain behaviours that happen later.

The results showed important behavioural trends in addition to testing the hypothesis. Participants who were predicted to be more engaged by AI had better brand recall and said they were more likely to buy. In 72% of cases, AI-based emotion predictions were more accurate at predicting behaviour than self-reported emotions, especially in situations where people were very excited and their memories weren't always reliable. This difference shows that biometric-AI data is better than traditional declarative inputs at capturing subconscious consumer reactions. Further exploratory regression analyses showed that gaze entropy negatively predicted recall ($\beta = -0.41$, $p < .01$). This means that attention patterns that are more erratic or scattered make memory encoding weaker. Emotional volatility (the standard deviation of valence over the course of a stimulus) also had a negative Loaded emotional congruence ($\beta = -0.38$, $p < .01$), which means that stimuli that are mesh with emotions may make the overall coherence and message clarity less clear.

It's important to note that demographic subgroup analysis showed very little moderation effects. Gender did not have a big effect on any of the biometric-emotion-behavior pathways. However, people under 30 were slightly more aroused and reacted more quickly to biometric data, probably because they saw more digital content. The SEM model was stable across all demographic groups, which is an important sign of its structural validity and generalisability. This wide range of uses makes the case for Neuromarketing 2.0 as a tool for figuring out how digital consumers behave across different segments stronger.

Also, the AI model's outputs are more reliable than traditional self-report measures, which shows how hard it is to capture emotions in fast-paced digital environments. Self-reported emotional congruence was somewhat in line with AI predictions ($r = .71$), but purchase intention and recall were more consistently driven by engagement metrics that didn't have a self-report counterpart. These results support the idea that biometric data, when analysed by AI, are not only useful for psychological modelling but also better at predicting what consumers will do next. They also show that using AI models to map emotions in real time can be a good alternative or addition to survey-based methods in neuromarketing research.

Overall, the results strongly support the Neuromarketing 2.0 model's effectiveness, validity, and usefulness for making predictions. The biometric-AI hybrid method was not only correct, but it also had statistical meaning. All of the main indicators—engagement, valence, and arousal—showed high construct reliability and explanatory power in predicting behaviour. The SEM model showed that these emotional and attentional constructs are very important for brand recall, emotional congruence, and purchase intention. This proves that the switch from relying on intuition to using AI to improve emotional analytics is a good idea. These results also show that it is possible to build emotion-aware systems in a way that is ethical, clear, and scalable. This opens the door for their use in digital advertising, e-commerce UX design, and real-time adaptive content delivery. The next section will go into more detail about what these results mean in terms of theory, practice, and ethics. It will also talk about what embedding biometric-AI logic into the future of consumer intelligence systems might mean for the future.

The results of this study are a big step forward in the field of neuromarketing. They make a strong case for using biometric feedback and artificial intelligence together to better understand and predict how people will act. The empirical validation of the Neuromarketing 2.0 framework shows that traditional methods of self-reporting and observation are not good enough to get at the subconscious and emotional layers of consumer cognition. More importantly, it shows that AI-enhanced biometric analytics not only make models that are statistically strong, but they also provide practical, scalable alternatives to older systems in both academic and business settings. The results showed that AI-interpreted emotional valence, arousal, and engagement were very good at predicting brand recall, emotional congruence, and purchase intention. This supports the idea that emotional and attentional signals that are captured in real time and modelled through machine learning are better at predicting behaviour than survey responses that are given after the fact.

The main point of these results is that they support the Affective-Cognitive Dual Process model (Kahneman, 2011), which says that emotional heuristics (System 1) and deliberate logic (System 2) both play a role in making decisions. The fact that AI-classified facial affect and biometric arousal were better at predicting recall and intention than traditional declarative measures supports the idea that System 1 is the most common way people interact with brands in real time. People don't just think about ads; they also react to them emotionally and physically long before they can put their thoughts into words. The EEG, GSR, and eye-tracking helped find these pre-cognitive signals, and the AI framework acted as a translation layer, making the subconscious measurable and usable. The SEM model shows that there are strong connections between biometric signals and behavioural outcomes. This means that affective and attentional processes are not just noise or byproducts of decision-making; they are the main factors that drive behaviour. This backs up earlier work by Plassmann et al. (2012) and Venkatraman et al. (2015), but it takes things to the next level by adding real-time classification and closed-loop modelling to the neuromarketing mix.

The fact that gaze fixation and attentional density have a positive effect on engagement ($\beta = 0.56$) supports existing theories in visual cognition and advertising research that say that how attention is paid is a key factor in how messages are encoded and how people act. The new thing here is that the engagement index combines gaze data with EEG and facial affect. The Neuromarketing 2.0 model combines attention and emotion into a single, dynamic construct that is better than either variable on its own. This mixing of the two types of design shows how complicated and connected consumer perception is, and it breaks down the false barrier between "emotion-driven"

and "attention-driven" design. In this model, attention is the gateway and emotion is the signal amplifier. Together, they make a predictive matrix that predicts intention with amazing accuracy.

It is also interesting to note that emotional instability and gaze entropy had a negative effect on behavioural outcomes like recall and congruence. This goes against the common belief in advertising that content that is high-arousal and changes quickly always keeps people interested. On the other hand, emotional stability and focused visual attention helped people remember things and keep the message clear. These results are in line with cognitive load theory, which says that too much stimulation, whether emotional or visual, can make your brain tired and make it harder to process information. This is a big deal for marketers: emotion should be a spark, not chaos. Ads that quickly change emotional tone or make it hard for the viewer to focus may stick in their minds in bits and pieces, but they don't lead to any real action. The Neuromarketing 2.0 framework gives you the tools you need to find this threshold and change the content in real time.

One of the most important things this research shows is that the engagement index clearly acts as a bridge between biometric signals and behavioural responses. The fact that engagement affects both visual attention and emotional arousal on purchase intention ($\beta = 0.63$, $p < .001$) gives us a better idea of how people go from thinking to doing. It turns "engagement" from a buzzword into a well-tested idea that connects physical input to economic behaviour. In this model, engagement is not measured by how long someone spends on a page or how many clicks they make. Instead, it is measured by EEG patterns, pupil dilation, skin conductance, and AI-generated emotional trajectories. This changes engagement from a behavioural trace to a biometric truth, which has effects not just on marketing but also on media planning, UX design, and optimising the customer journey.

The fact that AI-classified emotions are better at predicting recall and intention than self-reports, especially in high-arousal situations, supports the model's main idea even more. This difference makes sense with what we know about the limits of introspective access: people often don't know what their emotions are, especially in the milliseconds after they see a stimulus. The biometric-AI system gets around this problem by capturing emotional markers at the time of the experience instead of later, when people have had time to think about it. In this way, it makes the dataset bigger and more accurate, which better reflects the factors that influence decisions in the real world. Surveys may still be useful for finding out what people think and want, but they are clearly not enough to model the emotional unconscious. Neuromarketing 2.0's most important contribution is this change in methodological focus from declarative to embodied data.

The SEM model's lack of demographic differences shows that it works well for people of all ages and genders. However, younger participants were slightly more responsive to biometric data and AI-detected arousal. This is in line with what the digital nativity literature says, which says that younger consumers process screen-based stimuli faster and more intensely. The fact that there aren't any big moderation effects, though, suggests that the model's core structure works for all types of consumers, making it a good candidate for a universal framework. Future studies may build on this by testing cultural, linguistic, or device-based moderators to make contextual sensitivity even better, but the basic strength is clear.

The model's ability to scale up is just as important. The modular design, which is based on tools that are available for free or for purchase (like Emotiv EEG, Tobii eye-tracking, OpenFace, etc.), means that this framework can be used in more than just high-end labs. It can also be used in digital marketing agencies, UX testing environments, and even live retail settings. Adding SHAP and LIME to the framework for AI explainability makes it even more in line with ethical

AI principles, making it both useful and accountable. The ability to create explainable, anonymous, and opt-in biometric insights is a rare combination of innovation and compliance in a time when regulations are becoming more important (for example, the EU AI Act and GDPR).

These results also have major effects on how to plan advertising, come up with new ideas, and test campaigns. For instance, brands can now do emotional A/B tests based on real-time affective patterns instead of what people think. Gaze heatmaps and EEG spikes can help with visual framing, pacing the story, and even picking the right music. In e-commerce, you can optimise product thumbnails and call-to-action buttons not only so that they are easy to see, but also so that they connect with people's emotions. Not personalisation by preference, but personalisation by emotion signature is the future of marketing. This research shows a clear way to get there.

However, Neuromarketing 2.0 is not without ethical issues when it comes to putting it into practice. Being able to "read" emotions through facial expressions, neural signals, and skin responses comes with new duties. The danger is not technological but epistemological: affective data could be misinterpreted, changed, or overgeneralised if it gets into the wrong hands. So, the focus on XAI (explainable AI) in this study is not just technical; it's also philosophical. Emotions are not things to be mined for profit; they are human experiences that need to be understood with care and responsibility. Data opt-ins, signal accuracy transparency, demographic calibration, and clear limits on real-time intervention are all examples of ethics-by-design features that must be included in future versions of this model. This is especially important now that businesses are starting to use facial coding, emotion detection, and neurodata, which makes the line between insight and intrusion less clear.

Overall, the Neuromarketing 2.0 framework is a good answer to the call for new ways to study the "hidden drivers" of consumer behaviour. It combines decades of psychological theory with new AI technology to create a full, ethical, and scalable model of how people think, feel, and act. This study doesn't say that it will replace all traditional methods; instead, it adds to them by showing parts of the consumer mind that have been hard to find for a long time. What the eye sees and the skin feels, what the brain signals and the face shows—these are no longer just interesting stories; they are real facts that can be modelled, tested, and acted on. The results show that we are on the verge of a new era of marketing intelligence, one that is based on what people's biology shows rather than what they say. And that quiet signal will write the next generation of marketing plans.

IMPLICATIONS

The real-world and theoretical contributions of this study have huge effects on a wide range of areas, including marketing strategy, the ethical debate about biometric data and artificial intelligence, and the field of theory in general. This study questions and builds on traditional models of consumer behaviour that have always put a lot of emphasis on making rational decisions and thinking things through. The Neuromarketing 2.0 framework changes this point of view by showing that subconscious processes, which are captured through real-time biometric inputs and decoded using AI, are not only important for making decisions but also more likely to predict what consumers will do than rationalisations made after the fact. This change in the way we think about things requires us to rethink the basic ideas behind consumer psychology, behavioural economics, and marketing communication. It backs up a more embodied model of

cognition that fits with current neuroscience and dual-process theory (Kahneman, 2011) and backs up the affective turn in marketing research. Researchers can now measure things like engagement, arousal, and emotional resonance that were previously thought of as abstract or anecdotal by combining biometric data with artificial intelligence. This study sets the stage for a new group of theories based on affective computing and embodied consumer cognition, in which physiological states are not noise but signal—a language the body speaks and the machine understands. Biometric-AI hybrids' ability to act as a bridge between stimulus and intention also questions traditional linear stimulus-response models. Instead, they support closed-loop systems of affective feedback and adaptive engagement. We need to create new measurement scales, statistical tools, and interpretive frameworks that can handle multi-modal, non-linear, and real-time data streams in behavioural modelling because of these theoretical advances.

In practice, the results of this study will also have a big impact. For a long time, marketers have made decisions based on assumptions about how consumers think, which they get from things like click-through rates, survey responses, or A/B test results. This study offers a possible solution: measuring consumers' emotional and attentional states directly and in real time, which are closely related to their buying behaviour, brand recall, and message resonance. The engagement index suggested here, which is based on biometric signals and AI analysis, not only predicts better, but it could also be a new KPI in advertising and UX design. Brands can now test ad creatives not only for design preferences but also for how they affect people's brains and emotions. Eye-tracking heatmaps can show where people are looking, and GSR and EEG signals can show if a message makes them excited, stressed, or bored. AI can automate this process, making what used to be expensive and time-consuming lab studies into scalable systems that can be used in campaign testing, digital A/B testing, and even real-time content optimisation engines. This technology can be used by e-commerce sites to change how products are shown based on real-time emotional feedback. Streaming services can also use it to change recommendations based on a person's biometric affective profile, not just their viewing history. The Neuromarketing 2.0 framework also lets you make decisions based on small amounts of data that are based on emotional response rather than guesswork taste. This is true for product innovation, packaging design, and testing the layout of a store. This is a big step forward from guesswork to solid design, and from strategy based on opinion to strategy based on biometric truth. There are big effects on cost-effectiveness, customer satisfaction, brand loyalty, and optimising the conversion rate. Marketers, ad agencies, and product designers now have a set of tools that can not only explain why people do what they do, but also predict what they will do. This model also has effects on fields other than marketing, like education (emotion-aware learning platforms), entertainment (emotionally dynamic content adaptation), and healthcare (stress detection and patient communication).

However, using these kinds of emotionally intelligent systems raises difficult moral and social questions that need to be answered with openness, rules, and moral foresight. The idea of emotional privacy is at the centre of these worries. It is a new area of digital ethics. When should the line be drawn if technology can figure out and understand someone's subconscious emotional state without them saying so? This study followed strict research ethics rules, such as getting informed consent, processing data anonymously, and making sure that the results could be explained. However, Neuromarketing 2.0 may not always follow these rules when it is used in business. So, it is very important to set up rules and guidelines for how biometric data is collected, stored, understood, and used. Emotional data is more than just a number; it's a deep reflection of who you are that you often don't mean to show and that is shaped by

your culture. If not controlled, using this kind of data for business purposes could turn human emotions into products that could be used to manipulate, exploit, or hurt people mentally. For example, dynamic content delivery systems that respond to real-time emotional states could be set up to make fear, urgency, or scarcity stronger, pushing people towards choices they might not have made otherwise. This makes people worry about emotional manipulation, especially when it comes to children, the elderly, or people with cognitive impairments. It also raises the possibility of "affective profiling," which is when people are put into groups or targeted based on how they react emotionally. This is similar to behavioural scoring but may be more intrusive. To deal with these risks, this study says that any use of Neuromarketing 2.0 should be done with ethics in mind from the start. This means using only opt-in systems, explainable AI (like SHAP or LIME), following the rules for data minimisation, and making sure that all emotion-detection algorithms are calibrated to avoid bias against certain age groups, genders, or ethnicities. Also, under current data protection laws like the GDPR or the upcoming EU AI Act, policymakers need to start treating emotional data as sensitive personal data. Institutions that use biometric-AI systems must be open about how they use emotional data, keep audit logs, and let users challenge or change algorithmic classifications. We also need to teach people how to use biometric systems so that they know what they are agreeing to, how emotional signals are read, and what it means when a machine "reads" their mind. People shouldn't think of these systems as replacements for empathy; instead, they should think of them as tools that need to be used with their own human judgement, cultural sensitivity, and emotional intelligence.

Also, Neuromarketing 2.0 could change the balance of power between businesses and customers. What protections are in place to make sure that consumers are not just being persuaded but also forced if brands can use tools that let them change content based on real-time subconscious feedback? When emotions can be programmed, the line between persuasion and manipulation gets dangerously thin. This is why making this kind of technology available to everyone, not just big companies but also small businesses, public institutions, and researchers, is so important to stop power from becoming too concentrated. Also, emotion-aware systems could be used to improve the common good. For example, charities could make donation requests that really connect with people's emotions, public health campaigns could be made more effective by targeting people's emotions, and educational platforms could change the difficulty of their lessons based on how frustrated or engaged students are. But again, the most important thing that sets them apart is their purpose: is the system meant to help the user or get something of value from them? There aren't easy answers to these questions, but this study gives us a way to talk about them, test them, and improve them over time.

In short, Neuromarketing 2.0 has big effects that will change the way we do things. In theory, it changes how we think about cognition and emotion in consumer research by adding a new empirical logic based on real-time physiology and machine learning. In practice, it allows for unprecedented accuracy in marketing strategy, design, and customer engagement by providing predictive insights that are better than any other method. It makes us think about how we can create new standards for consent, responsibility, and emotional independence as machines become more aware. This study doesn't say that AI that can understand emotions should be stopped. Instead, it says that it should be guided by interdisciplinary stewardship, ethical reflexivity, and a strong commitment to the privacy and dignity of the person being studied. It turns a technological breakthrough into a humane one by creating a future of marketing where we pay attention to

not just what customers say, but also what their bodies feel, their hearts signal, and their minds, often without realising it, decide.

CHALLENGES AND LIMITATIONS

Even though this study has strong empirical results and a new way of doing things, there are some problems and limitations that need to be pointed out in order to put the Neuromarketing 2.0 framework in an honest and critical way. The main problem with the research design is that it doesn't seem to be ecologically valid. The experimental conditions are very controlled and make sense from a scientific point of view, but they don't fully recreate the complicated, stimulus-rich, and often broken environments that people use to interact with marketing content in the real world. Using calibrated biometric equipment, participants were shown ads in a setting where they couldn't be distracted. This is very different from how people usually see ads, which is in social feeds, between YouTube videos, while doing other things, or while commuting. Because of this, emotional and attentional responses measured in the lab may be higher or different from those measured in real-life situations. Also, the fact that participants knew they were being watched or "studied" may have affected them in ways they weren't aware of, which could have caused Hawthorne effects that changed biometric reactivity or engagement levels. evoking a sense of nostalgia for the past and a tearful remembrance of the past. The past is a painful memory that can be hard to let go of. The past is a painful memory that can be hard to˙let Alcove. The past is a painful memory that can be hard to let go of. The past is a painful memory that can be hard to let go of. The past is a painful memory that can be hard to let go of. The past is a painful memory that can be hard to let go of. The past is a painful memory that academics have been able to conduct experiments on the past. The past is a painful memory that can be hard to let go of. Channel. The past is an academics have been able to conduct experiments on recommended*"The past is a painful memory that can be hard to let go of. The past is a painful memory that can be hard to Kang spreading" The past is a painful memory that can be hard to let go turn to the past.. The past is a painful. The past is a painful memory that can be hard to let go of. The past is a painful

memory that can be hard to let go of. The past is a painful memory that can be hard to let go of. The past is a painful memory that can be hard to let go of. The past is a painful memory that can be hard to let go of. The past is a painful memory that can be/my. also. also have.. are. a is. a. an an a is. a. a, a, a, an is, a, are, is, an is, the is, the is, are, are, the is, the is, the that is, the is, is, For example, the EEG device used only has five channels and doesn't cover deeper brain areas or more complicated cortical mapping. This makes it harder for it to pick up on subtle neural signals like memory encoding or long-term emotional resonance. Head movement, screen glare, and blinking frequency can also mess up eye-tracking results. GSR sensors are also sensitive to skin hydration, ambient temperature, and contact consistency, all of which can add noise and variability to the data.

Generalisability and algorithmic bias are two more problems that come up in the AI emotion modelling pipeline. The machine learning models used—convolutional neural networks (CNNs), long short-term memory networks (LSTMs), and random forest classifiers—had a high internal classification accuracy (an average of 87.2%). However, they still depend on the quality and representativeness of the training data. Many pre-made emotion recognition models are trained on datasets like FER-2013 or AffectNet, which tend to focus on Western facial structures, expressions, and emotional norms. This makes people very worried about cross-cultural misclassification, which is when expressions of happiness, sadness, or anger may look different in people from different ethnic, cultural, or neurodiverse groups. The model did well with the study's international but urban-elite demographic (India, Singapore, and the UK), but it might not work as well with rural, under-represented, or marginalised user groups. This problem also affects facial coding tools like Affectiva, which are often criticised for being hard to understand and not being clear about how emotions are labelled, scored, and modelled, even though they are marketed as being easy to use. There is also the danger of emotion overfitting, which happens when the AI reacts too strongly to changes in biometric data and misclassifies neutral or unclear expressions, especially when signals that are supposed to be neutral or ambiguous are combined with signals that are supposed to be high (for example, high GSR with a neutral facial expression). Also, the SEM analysis was done using a cross-sectional design, which makes it hard to draw conclusions about causality or see how biometric engagement changes over time, even though the fit indices were strong and the analysis was statistically sound. Emotional responses are not always the same; they change depending on things like past experiences, ad fatigue, mood states, and even body cycles. Longitudinal studies are needed to confirm whether the biometric-emotion-behavior pathways found in this study stay the same after repeated exposures or change in response to campaign sequencing, novelty decay, or brand familiarity.

The study used five 30- to 45-second branded video ads as stimuli, which is also a small part of the marketing content universe. The study didn't look at static images, website interfaces, augmented reality ads, or interactive gamified content. These are all becoming more important in omnichannel and multisensory marketing strategies. The emotional and attention pathways that are activated by video may be very different from those activated by haptics, voice assistants, or experiential interfaces. This means that the Neuromarketing 2.0 model may need to be adjusted or expanded to include multimodal, multi-sensory interaction formats. Also, the participants were not chosen at random from all over the world; they were chosen from educated, tech-savvy urban populations. This choice fits with the usual target audiences for digital ads, but it makes people wonder about sampling bias and whether emotional reactivity patterns would hold in groups with little media exposure, low emotional literacy, or cognitive problems. Another real-world

problem is figuring out how to use biometric-AI systems in business processes. This study shows a research prototype with strong theoretical validity. However, making these kinds of systems work on real-time digital platforms would require fast data processing, device compatibility, data fusion infrastructure, and latency management. In edge computing environments like mobile apps or IoT-enabled signs, the computational load of classifying real-time EEG or GSR signals could become too much to handle without special hardware accelerators. It is even harder for businesses to use these technologies because there are no standard APIs for classifying emotions, biometric vendors can't work together, and there aren't any clear data labelling schemes. Companies that want to use this system will also have to deal with organisational inertia, train their teams in emotion analytics, and make sure they follow the rules. These are all things that could slow down implementation or lead to partial, watered-down deployments that don't take full advantage of the model's potential.

From an ethical point of view, consent, openness, and data governance are the hardest problems that Neuromarketing 2.0 faces in the real world. This study used opt-in procedures, anonymisation protocols, and SHAP and LIME to explain things, but commercial systems may not be as strict. Facial analysis and GSR can be used in places where people don't agree to it, like retail stores, billboards, or mobile apps. This could lead to emotional surveillance, where people are tracked, classified, and profiled without their knowledge. This is a clear threat to emotional privacy, a new idea in digital ethics that says people have the right not to have their feelings watched, changed, or sold. Without laws about affective data, companies could use emotion profiles to tailor offers, change how urgent something is, or change how people feel in ways that make it hard to tell the difference between persuasion and coercion. There is also the problem of algorithmic opacity: even though explainable AI tools are used, deep learning models are often too complicated to fully understand, making it hard for users or auditors to challenge misclassifications or figure out how their biometric data affected decision outputs. In areas that are emotionally sensitive, like political ads, healthcare outreach, or mental health apps, the risks of misclassification, emotional nudging, or targeting specific groups become even more ethically troubling. Also, bias in emotional AI could make social inequality worse if certain demographic groups are misread, not represented enough, or unfairly scored as having low engagement, which could keep them from seeing promotional content or having digital experiences. This is especially concerning because we know that AI works differently on people with different skin tones, facial features, and expressions. These moral gaps need more than just technical fixes; they also need strong governance, such as algorithmic audits, emotional data charters, and consumers' rights to delete or change their emotional data. Finally, public opinion and trust may make it harder for people to adopt. As biometric surveillance becomes more common, people may become more wary of systems that "read" their feelings, even when they are used to personalise the user experience. This is because of the controversies surrounding emotion recognition in surveillance technology or facial analysis at airports. Because of this, any use of Neuromarketing 2.0 systems must include consumer education, clear interfaces, and trust-building rules that put agency, dignity, and informed engagement first.

In short, the Neuromarketing 2.0 model is a powerful, empirically validated way to measure and predict consumer behaviour using biometric-AI integration, but it does have some important flaws. There are both conceptual and operational problems with universal adoption because of issues with ecological validity, hardware fidelity, algorithmic generalisability, cultural calibration, real-time scalability, and ethical transparency. These limitations don't make the model less

valuable; they just show where its insights can be used responsibly. They also show promising areas for future research, such as cross-cultural adaptation, low-resource AI training, multimodal integration, long-term affective tracking, and lobbying for emotional data rights in the law. By being honest and clear about these problems, Neuromarketing 2.0 is not seen as a cure-all but as a bold, necessary, and evolving tool for understanding human emotion in the age of smart systems.

FUTURE RESEARCH DIRECTIONS

Building on the insights and limitations of the present study, several promising avenues for future research emerge, aimed at enhancing the precision, generalizability, ethical robustness, and real-world applicability of the Neuromarketing 2.0 framework. First, future research should expand the stimulus set to include a broader spectrum of marketing content, such as static visual ads, immersive AR/VR experiences, gamified interfaces, and conversational AI. These modalities introduce new dimensions of interactivity and sensory engagement that may trigger different emotional and attentional pathways, necessitating recalibration of biometric thresholds and AI classifiers. Second, longitudinal studies are essential to explore how emotional responses and engagement patterns evolve over time, particularly in response to campaign repetition, ad fatigue, or brand loyalty formation. Affective states are dynamic and often temporally unstable; tracking them across weeks or months would offer valuable insights into the durability and fluctuation of biometric predictors in consumer behavior. Third, future research should prioritize **cross-cultural calibration and fairness testing** in AI emotion models. Emotion expression is deeply influenced by cultural norms, socialization patterns, and even language structure. Models trained predominantly on Western datasets must be re-trained or adapted using localized, diverse training sets to ensure equitable emotion recognition across ethnic, gender, and neurodiverse groups. Fourth, integrating biometric data with other behavioral and contextual data streams—such as click behavior, dwell time, eye-blink rate, or even ambient environmental cues—may improve multi-modal modeling accuracy and allow for more holistic consumer profiling. Finally, from an ethical standpoint, future work must push beyond compliance to co-create **emotion-aware systems with user agency**, exploring design strategies for transparent consent, emotional feedback visualization, and human-in-the-loop AI decisioning. As emotional AI systems move from experimental labs into commercial deployment, researchers must also investigate public trust, algorithmic accountability, and psychological impact on users who are aware they are being emotionally monitored. By addressing these fronts, future research can refine Neuromarketing 2.0 into not just a tool for consumer insight, but a cornerstone of human-centric, ethically responsible, and culturally intelligent affective computing in marketing and beyond.

CONCLUSION

This study introduces and validates the Neuromarketing 2.0 framework, a next-generation approach that integrates biometric feedback and artificial intelligence to decode the subconscious, affective dimensions of consumer behavior. By leveraging primary data collected through EEG, GSR, eye-tracking, and facial recognition technologies—and interpreting these physiological signals using machine learning algorithms—this research demonstrates that emotional and attentional

states can be quantified in real time and used to meaningfully predict behavioral outcomes such as brand recall, emotional congruence, and purchase intention. The findings empirically support the notion that traditional self-report and observational methods are insufficient to capture the immediacy, intensity, and nuance of consumer emotional responses. Through structural equation modeling, this study confirms that AI-classified engagement, valence, and arousal are statistically significant predictors of marketing effectiveness, thereby affirming the theoretical claim that emotion and attention, when measured accurately and ethically, form the core of modern consumer decision-making.

The Neuromarketing 2.0 model also bridges multiple disciplinary domains, contributing to marketing science, consumer psychology, neuroscience, and data science. Theoretically, it validates dual-process models of cognition and supports the emerging field of affective computing by demonstrating that subconscious processes can be systematically observed and modeled. Practically, it offers a scalable, replicable framework for marketers, advertisers, and UX designers seeking to optimize content based not just on what consumers say or do—but on what they feel in the moment. The implications of this work extend far beyond academia. With emotional AI poised to become a core driver in digital personalization, this research provides a timely roadmap for ethical deployment, real-time adaptability, and human-centered design. It also lays bare the critical ethical responsibilities that accompany such technological power, emphasizing the need for transparency, fairness, consent, and emotional privacy in all applications of biometric-emotion analytics.

While the study is not without limitations—such as controlled experimental conditions, device sensitivity, and potential cultural bias in AI models—it offers a strong foundation upon which future research can build. Areas for continued exploration include cross-cultural calibration of emotion recognition, longitudinal affective modeling, integration with multi-modal and immersive stimuli, and user-facing explainability of AI classifications. Ultimately, Neuromarketing 2.0 represents not merely an evolution of marketing research methods, but a redefinition of what it means to understand the consumer—by listening to the silent signals of the body, interpreting the emotions behind the eyes, and bridging the gap between biological truth and strategic action in the age of intelligent systems.

REFERENCES

Daugherty, P. R., Wilson, H. J., & Chowdhury, R. (2018). Using artificial intelligence to promote diversity. *MIT Sloan Management Review*.

Doshi-Velez, F., & Kim, B. (2017). Towards a rigorous science of interpretable machine learning. *arXiv*. https://arxiv.org/abs/1702.08608

Garcia-Burgos, D., & Zamora, P. (2019). Emotion recognition in multimodal marketing contexts. *Frontiers in Neurorobotics*, *13*, 51. DOI: 10.3389/fnbot.2019.00051

Kahneman, D. (2011). *Thinking, fast and slow*. Farrar, Straus and Giroux.

Koelstra, S., Muhl, C., Soleymani, M., Jong-Seok Lee, , Yazdani, A., Ebrahimi, T., Pun, T., Nijholt, A., & Patras, I. (2012). DEAP: A database for emotion analysis using physiological signals. *IEEE Transactions on Affective Computing*, *3*(1), 18–31. DOI: 10.1109/T-AFFC.2011.15

Lee, N., Broderick, A. J., & Chamberlain, L. (2007). What is 'neuromarketing'? A discussion and agenda for future research. *International Journal of Psychophysiology*, *63*(2), 199–204.

Plassmann, H., Ramsøy, T. Z., & Milosavljevic, M. (2012). Branding the brain: A critical review and outlook. *Journal of Consumer Psychology*, *22*(1), 18–36. DOI: 10.1016/j.jcps.2011.11.010

Russell, J. A. (1980). A circumplex model of affect. *Journal of Personality and Social Psychology*, *39*(6), 1161–1178. DOI: 10.1037/h0077714

Venkatraman, V.. (2015). Separate neural substrates of semantic and episodic brand memory. *JMR, Journal of Marketing Research*, *52*(3), 288–307.

Zuboff, S. (2019). *The age of surveillance capitalism*. PublicAffairs.

About the Contributors

Prashant Tiwari, Ph.D., is an Associate Professor in the Department of Pharmacology at the College of Pharmaceutical Sciences, Dayananda Sagar University, Bengaluru, India. He holds a Ph.D. from Siksha O Anusandhan University, Bhubaneswar, and was a fellow of the Indian Council of Medical Research (ICMR), New Delhi. With over 13 years of experience in teaching and research, Dr. Tiwari's expertise includes drug screening, method validation for brain-targeted drug delivery, drug-induced dyskinesia revalidation, and the neuroprotective effects of benzimidazole derivatives. His research has explored the dopaminergic pathway, prolactin inhibition, and neuroprotection, with notable studies on Nanoemulsions containing Lepidium sativum oil for Parkinson's disease and Muntingia Calabura leaf extract for Alzheimer's disease. For his outstanding work, Dr. Tiwari received the Dr. P. D. Patil National Award for Best Thesis in Pharmaceutical Sciences (2022). In addition to his research, Dr. Tiwari has authored 5 books, edited 5 books, and co-authored 6 book chapters. He has filed 7 patents, 2 of which have been granted. He organized a national e-seminar on targeted drug delivery against neurodegenerative diseases, sponsored by the Department of Biotechnology (DBT), Government of India. Dr. Tiwari has been honored with various awards, including the ICMR Senior Research Fellowship, Young Scientist Award, and Best Teacher Award. He supervises 5 Ph.D. students and has guided 9 M. Pharm students. He is also an active member of professional bodies and serves as a peer reviewer for international journals. His research interests span neurodegenerative disorders, drug interactions, pharmacokinetics/pharmacodynamics, and metabolic disorders.

Sunil Kumar Kadiri is an accomplished pharmaceutical sciences academician and researcher, presently serving as an Associate Professor at the College of Pharmaceutical Sciences, Dayananda Sagar University, Bengaluru. With over 17 years of combined teaching and research experience, 5 years as Assistant Professor and 12 years as Associate Professor, his career spans notable institutions across Hyderabad and Bengaluru. Dr. Kadiri holds a Ph.D. in Pharmaceutical Sciences from JNTU Hyderabad (2019), an M.Pharm in Pharmacology with distinction (2008), and a B.Pharm from RGUHS, Bangalore. His academic interests encompass teaching, pharmaceutical research, pre-clinical and clinical studies. He has made extensive contributions to the field through over 75 peer-reviewed publications, several of which are indexed in Scopus and Web of Science, SCIE. His research includes drug-drug interactions, neuropharmacology, phytopharmacology, and herbal formulations. Dr. Kadiri has authored and co-authored numerous book chapters and textbooks and has been granted patents in India and the UK. He has actively

participated in national and international seminars, delivered webinars, and served as a lead speaker on psychopharmacology and public health topics. His scientific curiosity and commitment to academic excellence continue to drive innovation in drug development, pharmacological screening, and therapeutic strategies.

Neha Minocha An academic professional with more than 10 years of experience, Dr. Neha Minocha working as an Associate Professor in Pharmaceutics at School of Medical and Allied Sciences, K. R. Mangalam University, Haryana. Dr. Neha has done her Ph.D. in Pharmaceutical Sciences in 2023. She has a background of Pharmaceutics in M. Pharmacy (2013) and have worked with many renowned universities. Dr. Neha has done her B. Pharmacy in 2011 and have two post graduate diplomas one in Post Graduate Diploma in Regulatory Affairs (PGDRA) from Jamia Hamdard, New Delhi and other one is Post Graduate Diploma in Clinical Research (PGDCR) from Apheta Institute, New Delhi. Dr. Neha have published 33 peer reviewed publications in SCOPUS, WoS indexed journals and have four book chapters with renowned publishers. She has published 1 patent and 6 patents have been granted under her name.

***

Tahniyat Ansari Research Scholar Department of Zoology, C.M.P. Degree College, University of Allahabad, Prayagraj. E-mail: zaidtahniyat22@gmail.com Contact: +91 6394224541 Education • Pursuing Ph.D. from CMP Degree College, University of Allahabad, Prayagraj, under the supervision of Dr. Sudhi Shrivastava, Assistant Professor, Department of Zoology at CMP Degree College, University of Allahabad. • M.Sc. Zoology (2020-2022) from Kashi Naresh Govt. Degree College (79.60%) • B.Sc. Zoology, Chemistry (2017-2020) from Dr. Shyama Prasad Mukherjee Government Degree College (75.05%). Academic Achievements • Qualified GATE XL (Life Sciences) 2025. • Qualified MPSET 2024 for Assistant Professor, in the subject Life Sciences. • Qualified GATE XL (Life Sciences) 2024. • M.Sc. Zoology Gold Medalist. • B.Sc. Silver Medalist. Personal Profile: E-mail: zaidtahniyat22@gmail.com Contact: 6394224541 Permanent Address: Ashok Nagar, Nai Bazar, Fattupur, Bhadohi, Mother's Name: Shama Afroz, Father's Name: Mohd. Zaid Ansari, Date of Birth: 21/05/2000

Parag Chatterjee received the B.E. degree in Computer Science & Engineering from the Karnatak University, Dharwad, India, in 1998 and received M.Tech. degree from IIEST Shibpur, Kolkata, India, in 2007. He has an academic experience of 20 years. Currently he is working as an Assistant Professor in the Department of CSE at Global Institute of Management and Technology, Krishnanagar, West Bengal, India.His current research interests include Data ware Housing, Data mining and Wireless sensor. He has 25 publication in national and international journals and 5 Patents.

Anwesha Das received her B. Pharm. from NSHM Knowledge Campus, Kolkata and M.S.(Pharm) in Medicinal chemistry from National Institute of Pharmaceutical Education and Research, Ahmedabad (NIPER-A) India. After completion of her masters, she was an intern under the CSIR-SRTP 2020. Presently she is working as a project assistant Department of Pharmacy, Indira Gandhi National Tribal University.

Vaishnavi Gohri is a postgraduate student specializing in pharmacology at AET's St. John Institute of Pharmacy and Research, Palghar. Her research interests include phytopharmacology, hepatoprotective studies, and neuropharmacology. Has authored several review articles and is actively engaged in the development and pharmacological evaluation of polyherbal formulations. Passionate about natural product-based drug discovery, translational research, and clinical research applications.

Ghadha Ibrahim Fouad Associate Research Professor in therapeutic biochemistry, with a demonstrated history of working in the scientific field. Skilled in Life Sciences, Research, Neurobiology, Biochemistry. Strong research professional with a Doctor of Philosophy - Ph.D. (Neuroscience) in Biochemistry- Alzheimer's Disease from Ain Shams University

Saloua Mabsor-Zgandaoui holds a PhD in Cell Biology, Biotechnology, and Health from the Faculty of Sciences at Ibn Tofail University, Kenitra. Her doctoral research was conducted in collaboration with the National Centre for Nuclear Energy, Science, and Technology (CNESTEN), where she investigated the enzymatic and molecular mechanisms of cellular response to ionizing radiation, contributing to advances in radiobiology and antioxidant defense strategies. She has authored several peer-reviewed publications and book chapters in internationally indexed platforms. Dr. Mabsor-Zgandaoui is currently an associate member of the Biology and Health Laboratory, Department of Biology, Faculty of Sciences, Ibn Tofail University, where she continues to develop research at the interface of Cellular and Molecular Biology, Biotechnology, and Cellular Stress Responses.

Adnane Moutaouakkil holds a PhD in Biology, specializing in Microbiology, Biotechnology, and Environment. He has made significant contributions to these fields through numerous scientific publications focused on the development and optimization of biotechnological processes. His research spans microbial interactions, bioprocess engineering, and the application of biotechnology for environmental sustainability. Currently, Dr. Moutaouakkil is a researcher at the National Centre for Nuclear Energy, Science, and Technology in Rabat, Morocco, where he conducts advanced research integrating nuclear science with biology and environmental science. His work contributes both to the advancement of scientific knowledge and to the development of practical solutions for environmental challenges and sustainable development.

Arijit Nandi received his B. Pharm. from NSHM Knowledge Campus, Kolkata and M.S.(Pharm) in Medicinal chemistry from National Institute of Pharmaceutical Education and Research Hyderabad, (NIPER-H) India. His dissertation work includes Design and Synthesis of 4-Thiazolidinone-Quinolone Hybrids as potential anticancer agents. After completion of his masters, he was an intern in CSIR-IICT, India under the CSIR-SRTP 2020. Then he joined the Laboratory of Natural Product Chemistry, Department of Pharmacy, Birla Institute of Technology and Science, Pilani (BITS Pilani), Pilani Campus, India. He is working as a Junior Research Fellow (JRF) under the supervision of Prof. Atish T. Paul in a DST-SERB (CRG) funded project. His project name is Design, Synthesis, Biological Evaluation and Molecular Modelling Studies of Oxoacetamide containing Indole-Quinazolinone Based Novel Hybrid Analogues as Potential Pancreatic Lipase Inhibitors.

Odangowei Inetiminebi Ogidi is a Lecturer, Acting Head, Department of Biochemistry and Sub-Dean, Faculty of Basic Medical Sciences, Bayelsa Medical University, Yenagoa, Bayelsa State, Nigeria. He holds a Bachelor of Science degree in Biochemistry, Master of Science and Doctor of Philosophy degrees in Biotechnology. He has also served as a Lecturer, Head of Departments of Science Laboratory Technology and Biochemistry, and Deputy Director, Centre for Continuing Education in Federal Polytechnic Ekowe, Bayelsa State. He has authored over 80 peer-reviewed academic articles in reputable local and international journals, published over 50 book chapters and presented over 40 conference papers. He is a member of various Journal Editorial Boards. He is indexed in World Scientist and University Ranking amongst other international bodies. He have supervised over 30 ND and HND students and currently supervising over 20 undergraduate students. His research interest has been Medical/Pharmaceutical and Environmental Biotechnology/Biochemistry, Phytomedicine, Phytochemistry.

Vivek Pazhamalai working as Associate Professor at Vels Institute of Science, Technology and Advanced Studies, and has teaching experience of 16 years. He has published more than 60 research articles in international and national journals to his credit.

Mohsin Qadeer is an Associate Professor at Agha Khan University Hospital and Medicare Cardiac and General Hospital (MGCH). He is one of the best neurosurgeons in Karachi, with a high patient satisfaction rate. He completed his MBBS and FCPS from Karachi, Pakistan. He completed his house job at Liaquat National Hospital as a house officer and resident neurosurgeon. He has an expert specialization in neurosurgery, which involves surgical treatment of neurological conditions such as peripheral nerve injury, spinal arthritis, cerebrospinal fluid leakage, brain tumors, etc. He has many publications, including national and international publications. Dr. Mohsin Qadeer has authored over 21 impactful articles. Dr. Mohsin Qadeer is associated with renowned hospitals, including Medicare Cardiac and General Hospital (MGCH), the National Medical Complex (NMC), Agha Khan Hospital University, and Ziauddin Hospital. He continued serving in different neurosurgery departments for years, treating all kinds of neurological conditions. A neurosurgeon also specializes in providing pre- and post-surgical care to patients. While working in neurosurgery, he focuses on the treatment of neurological conditions by using surgical methods. His exposure throughout the years of professional practice resulted in the enrichment of treatment skills across the vast field of neurosurgery. He has also been working on risk assessment of neurological conditions as well as their prevention and management. Based on existing conditions, he provides customized treatment plans for patients of all age groups. His expertise in advanced neurosurgery makes him one of the top certified neurosurgeons in Karachi. Currently he supervise many neurosurgeon residents in MGCH and Agha Khan University Hospital, where he contributes to research work in the neurosurgery field.

Khawla Rachmoune is specialized in biology and biochemistry. She studies radioprotective biomaterials as part of multidisciplinary research projects and is the co-author of two scientific articles published in peer-reviewed journals. Passionate and dedicated, she is particularly interested in the applications of biopolymers in health, environmental protection, and radiation shielding.

Meenambiga S S Assistant Professor completed 6 years of teaching experience and 4 years of research experience in the field of Biotechnology. Passionate about teaching and have trained

many young students in the field of Mycology, Natural Product Research, Nanoparticle synthesis, Drug Discovery from Plants and fungal sources and in-silico analysis of drug targets using modern Bio-informatics tools. Skilled in scientific writing covering the following aspects: Proposal submission, research articles suitable for national and international publications,drafting, proof reading and editing research thesis and expertise in critically reviewing the research manuscript for indexed journals. Member of Board of Studies for B.Tech Biotechnology curriculum in VISTAS. Guided more than 20 undergraduate students projects and served as Principal Investigator in the student's project funded by Tamilnadu State Council for Science and Technology. Published more than 30 research and review articles in national and international indexed journal and has volunteered as reviewer for many reputed journals. Life member of Mycological Society of India, BRSI, IARA, IAENG and many other professional organizations. Completed

Anamika Singh is currently serving as an Assistant Professor in the MATS School of Pharmacy, MATS University, Raipur, Chhattisgarh, India. She holds a Bachelor of Pharmacy (B. Pharm) degree from Rajiv Gandhi Proudyogiki Vishwavidyalaya (RGPV), Bhopal, and a Master of Pharmacy (M. Pharm) in Pharmaceutical Chemistry degree from RGPV Bhopal. With over four years of academic and research experience, her research interests are primarily Focus on computational modelling and small-molecule drug discovery across various therapeutic areas. She has authored five research publications in reputed international peer-reviewed journals and holds one published patent in the domain of pharmaceutical sciences. Additionally, she has completed two SWAYAM certification courses and has been recognized with the Young Achiever Award at an international conference. Her professional development portfolio includes active participation in multiple international and national conferences, faculty development programs (FDPs), and scientific workshops. She has also contributed to institutional development under the framework of NAAC accreditation criteria.

Index

A

N

O

P

R

S

T

W

www.ingramcontent.com/pod-product-compliance
Lightning Source LLC
LaVergne TN
LVHW061526290926
849162LV00004B/689